MW01042349

ASSESSMENT AND TREATMENT OF SPEECH SOUND DISORDERS IN CHILDREN

THIRD EDITION

Assessment and Treatment of Speech Sound Disorders in Children
A Dual-Level Text

THIRD EDITION

Adriana Peña-Brooks

M. N. Hegde

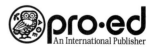
pro·ed
An International Publisher

8700 Shoal Creek Boulevard
Austin, TX 78757-6897
800/897-3202   800/397-7633
www.proedinc.com

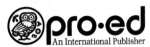
An International Publisher

© 2015, 2007, 2000 by PRO-ED, Inc.
8700 Shoal Creek Boulevard
Austin, Texas 78757-6897
800/897-3202   Fax 800/397-7633
www.proedinc.com

All rights reserved. **Except as indicated below**, no part of the material protected by this copyright notice may be reproduced or used in any form or by any means, electronic or mechanical, including photocopying, recording, or by any information storage and retrieval system, without prior written permission of the copyright owner.

This product includes a CD with reproducible pages.

Limited Photocopy License
PRO-ED, Inc. grants to individual purchasers of this material nonassignable permission to reproduce the reproducible forms on the CD. This license is limited to you, the individual purchaser, for use with your clients. This license does not grant the right to reproduce these materials for resale, redistribution, or any other purposes (including but not limited to books, pamphlets, articles, video- or audio- recordings, Web sites, and handouts or slides for lectures or workshops).
Permission to reproduce these materials for these and other purposes must be obtained in writing from the Permissions Department of PRO-ED, Inc.

Library of Congress Cataloging-in-Publication Data

Peña-Brooks, Adriana, author.
  [Assessment and treatment of articulation and phonological disorders in children]
  Assessment and treatment of speech sound disorders in children : a dual-level text / Adriana Peña-Brooks, M.N. Hegde. — Third edition.
      p. cm.
  Preceded by Assessment and treatment of articulation and phonological disorders in children : a dual-level text / Adriana Peña-Brooks, M.N. Hegde. 2nd ed. c2007.
  Includes bibliographical references and index.
  ISBN 978-1-4164-0580-1
  I. Hegde, M. N. (Mahabalagiri N.), 1941- author. II. Title.
  [DNLM: 1. Speech Disorders—therapy. 2. Child. 3. Speech—physiology. 4. Speech Disorders—diagnosis. 5. Speech Therapy—methods. WL 340.2]
  RJ496.S7
  618.92'855—dc23
                                                                      2013032626

Art Director: Jason Crosier
Designer: Tina Brackins
This book is designed in Janson Text and Trade Gothic.

Printed in the United States of America

2 3 4 5 6 7 8 9 10   23 22 21 20 19 18 17 16 15

I dedicate this book to God, my fortress. To my husband, Ryan Brooks, for his love and support. To my beautiful nine-year-old triplets Jordan, Jacob, and Nolan, for bringing me more joy than any one person deserves. And to my mother, Maria Peña, who from an early age taught me the importance of strength and character. I love you all!

—APB

CONTENTS

All speech, written or spoken, is a dead language, until it finds a willing and prepared hearer.

—*Robert Louis Stevenson*

Thank you for listening to what we have to say. We hope that this text finds many who are willing and prepared to hear. We are excited to offer you a text that reviews the basic and advanced information on speech sound disorders. A unique feature of this book is its modular organization. It is organized to serve as both an introduction text and an advanced text for graduate seminars.

In most university programs in speech–language pathology, students take an introductory undergraduate course and an advanced graduate course on speech sound disorders. When vastly different books are used at the undergraduate and graduate levels of instruction, some students may fail to see continuity from their undergraduate knowledge base to the more advanced graduate information. Also, for most students, several years will have elapsed since their undergraduate study before they take the graduate seminar on speech sound disorders. Almost all students need to review the undergraduate material before they can effectively participate in a graduate seminar and understand and integrate the material presented at the two levels of instruction. Unfortunately, not all graduate texts summarize the basic information for a review at the graduate level. Also, sometimes opinions differ as to what is basic and what is advanced. Simply omitting certain materials from a text because it is judged basic or advanced makes it harder for the instructors to use a text, especially if they disagree about the distinction the author or authors have made.

The modular organization of this text helps resolve this problem to some extent. To supplement a text, graduate seminar instructors typically use multiple sources, including other books and journal articles. We do not pretend that our distinction between basic and advanced information will be acceptable to all instructors. However, we do hope that the organization of the book will make it easier for students and instructors to use material as they see fit at the two levels of instruction. For example, those who wish to avoid theoretical or more complicated information in their undergraduate classes can easily skip the advanced units or use that information selectively. All graduate students can find the basic information in the text so they can review the assigned chapters before their participation in graduate seminars. We are grateful to the students, instructors, and reviewers who have affirmed our organization of the text as a unique and useful feature.

Besides giving the book a two-tier organization, we have tried to use a student-friendly writing style. We have minimized the use of jargon, and all relevant technical terms are introduced and defined. Our goal was to write the book in a way that makes it easier for students to understand phonology's basic vocabulary, approaches, perspectives, theories, and assessment and treatment techniques for speech sound disorders. Some students and our reviewers have repeatedly confirmed that we have succeeded in writing a user-friendly text.

Those who are familiar with the second edition of the text will notice the change in the title of the book. We have changed the title from *Assessment and Treatment of Articulation and Phonological Disorders in Children* to *Assessment and Treatment of Speech Sound Disorders in Children*. This change reflects the current trend in the profession to use the term *speech sound disorders* to include both articulation disorders and phonological disorders. It is also a change recommended by our reviewers and instructors in universities.

This third edition includes substantial and significant revisions and additions to reflect advances in the study and treatment of speech sound disorders. In addition to updating research in each chapter, we have added two new chapters to this edition.

We have written a new introductory chapter (Chapter 1) to define and describe speech sound disorders and to distinguish articulation disorders from phonological disorders. We give a brief historical account to help students understand what theoretical trends have forced the distinction. In this new chapter, we also provide a brief overview of the different types of speech sound disorders discussed in the clinical and research literature.

The second new chapter, Chapter 9, addresses the issue of phonological awareness as it relates to speech sound disorders. Our second edition included basic perspectives on this popular topic, but the growing body of information justified an entire chapter. We discuss the relevant issues related to the definition, description, and development of phonological awareness skills in children learning their speech sounds. We give an overview of phonological intervention and offer a critical review of the research literature on the necessity of teaching phonological awareness skills to children with speech sound disorders.

The remaining chapters have all been revised to reflect recent trends, research, and theories. We have reorganized several chapters to facilitate a better flow of information. Chapters that provide background information that may not be covered in detail by most instructors have been summarized more succinctly. As recommended by several of our reviewers, we have placed our comprehensive treatment approach chapter ahead of the chapter on specific treatment programs.

Chapter 2 gives an overview of the anatomy and neuroanatomy of speech production. The chapter in this new edition provides information in a more succinct form than the chapter in the earlier edition. We have retained all the illustrations that are helpful to students in visualizing anatomic structures and their relationships.

Chapter 3 offers the basic perspectives on phonetics and phonology of speech sound disorders. We explore the interrelatedness and interaction of these two disciplines that contribute to an understanding of speech sound disorders. We have added new sections to clearly highlight the differences in how linear and nonlinear phonological theories handle speech sound production, learning, disorders, and assessment and treatment of those disorders. The advanced unit of Chapter 3 includes phonetic, linear phonological, and nonlinear phonological theories and their critical evaluation.

Chapter 4 describes the typical learning of speech sounds as reported in normative research. It includes research on infant speech perception, as well as the extensive normative information on phonological patterns during the early years of speech sound learning and their eventual disappearance. The early speech learning stages have been revised to be consistent with current research and thinking. A discussion of variables related to typical learning of speech sounds, previously offered in a separate chapter, is now included in this chapter to better integrate the normative information. The advanced unit of this chapter is devoted to an examination of methodological and theoretical issues in studying speech sound learning, including infant speech perception.

Chapter 5 includes an examination of the relation between culture and communication. The chapter addresses bidialectal and bilingual issues associated with the typical learning of speech sounds and clinical issues related to assessment and treatment of speech disorders in ethnoculturally diverse children. In the advanced unit of this chapter, we discuss theories and hypotheses that have been advanced to explain speech and language learning in bilingual children.

Chapter 6 examines assessment approaches and methods, providing a comprehensive framework for assessing speech sound disorders in children. We have added current methods of analyzing assessment data including whole-word measures, error frequency and distribution approaches, and nonlinear methods. We have omitted the summaries of many articulation and phonological assessments and instead referred the reader to ASHA's online directory of assessment instruments for the latest and most current information. We incorporate preferred terms in the diagnosis of speech sound disorders. The advanced unit of this chapter continues to include an overview of speech sound disorders associated with organic and neurogenic problems; however, in this edition we have focused exclusively on those found in childhood.

As previously indicated, we have reorganized the order of Chapters 7 and 8 at the recommendation of our reviewers, who suggested going back to the way we sequenced them in the first edition. Chapter 7 now includes our comprehensive, step-by-step program that takes advantage of research evidence in the treatment of speech sound disorders in children of varied backgrounds. We continue to emphasize that the program, although detailed and specific, is adaptable to include such specific strategies as treating individual sound production, concurrent and variable treatment, phonological process elimination, minimal pairs approach, maximal oppositions or multiple oppositions, sound and word complexities, phonological constraints, and so forth.

In Chapter 8, we have made extensive changes and provide the reader with an overview of some now classic and some newer treatment approaches. We have eliminated various programs that have fallen out of favor in clinical practice or include published components that are no longer readily available. To help clinicians make informed decisions on treatment selection, this chapter also offers a brief evaluation of the research evidence supporting each approach.

We have added text boxes and various activities in each chapter to help the student integrate newly learned information. The text also now includes a companion CD that includes a modifiable PowerPoint outline of each chapter. Instructors may find this a useful feature for their lecture preparation. The CD also includes a variety of resources previously found in the resource manual, *Articulation and Phonological Disorders: Assessment and Treatment Resource Manual,* that accompanied the second edition. Clinically friendly materials such as diagnostic reports; sound evoking techniques; baseline, treatment, and probe documentation forms; sound stimulability recording forms; informal screening measures; and the like are now located in the CD that accompanies the third edition.

We would like to extend our deepest gratitude to the book reviewers, who provided us with valuable feedback; their suggestions helped guide many of the changes found in this third edition. We have made rigorous efforts to incorporate all of the proposed changes. We would also like to thank the many children in our professional lives, who have taught us more about speech sound disorders than any research study ever could. Their uniqueness affirms that all children are individuals and cannot be put into a universal framework. Their uniqueness makes assessment and treatment of speech sound disorders stimulating, exciting, and extremely rewarding. The delight that comes in helping children achieve better communication with the important people in their lives is immeasurable. We hope that our presentation of speech sound disorders excites and prepares the clinician to take on this gratifying and worthwhile endeavor.

SPEECH SOUND DISORDERS IN ALL OF THEIR NAMES: AN INTRODUCTION

Speech is the mother, not the handmaid, of thought.

—Karl Kraus

Importance of Speech Sound Disorders

Speech sound disorders (SSDs) are among the more common disorders of communication. As speech disorders, SSDs are typically distinguished from language disorders, in which the affected aspects are morphologic, syntactic, semantic, and pragmatic. Speech disorders include stuttering and cluttering, apraxia of speech, and dysarthria. Speech sounds are the building blocks of the larger language skill. Therefore, a discussion of speech sound mastery and disorders takes place in the context of language learning and impairments in that learning.

A distinction between speech disorders and language disorders is practical and clinically useful. While some speech sound disorders may coexist with a language disorder, other speech disorders, such as stuttering, may or may not be associated with a language impairment. In assessment and treatment, clinicians tend to separate speech production difficulties from language production problems for practical considerations. Speech sound treatment targets are obviously different from language treatment targets, which may include multiple skills (e.g., morphologic, syntactic, semantic, and pragmatic skills).

Speech–language pathologists (SLPs) working in public schools spend a significant amount of time with children who have SSDs. A survey reports that 56% of a typical school-based SLP's caseload may involve children with SSDs (Mullen & Schooling, 2010). A recent survey found that 91% of clinicians working in the public schools served children with speech sound disorders (American Speech-Language-Hearing Association, 2006), some of whom may receive treatment for coexisting language or other communication disorders and may experience academic difficulties, especially problems of literacy in later years (see Chapter 9 for details). It is evident that SSDs are a significant communication problem in school-age children. Considerable amounts of professional resources are spent on assessing and treating children with SSDs, which indicates its importance to the profession.

Prevalence and Risk Factors for Speech Sound Disorders

The prevalence of SSDs among children is quite high. It is estimated that nearly 10% of the population has a disorder of communication. Of this percentage, 50% to 80% may have an SSD. In certain professional settings, especially in public schools, clinicians serve a large number of children with SSDs. In spite of many studies, the precise prevalence rate of SSDs in children has been difficult to estimate (see Shriberg et al., 2005, and Shriberg, Tomblin, & McSweeny, 1999, for summative reviews). Available evidence suggests that the prevalence rate of SSDs in 6-year-old children is about 3.8%. Speech disorders may be found in roughly 15% to 16% of 3-year-olds (Campbell et al., 2003). Some 75% of them achieve normal articulation by age 6, however—hence, the lower prevalence rate at age 6 (Shriberg et al., 2005; Shriberg, Tomblin, & McSweeny, 1999). A differential prevalence rate of SSDs is typically reported for boys (4.5%) versus girls (3.1%).

A few risk factors have been noted for SSDs. Campbell et al. (2003) investigated potential risk factors for speech delay of unknown origin in 100 3-year-old children diagnosed with speech delay and 539 who did not meet the criterion for the diagnosis. Based on prior research findings, the authors considered six potential risk factors: male gender, family history of SSDs, low maternal education, low socioeconomic status, African American race, and prolonged otitis media with effusion (OME). Their odds ratio analysis found only three were risk factors for speech delay of unknown origin: male gender, low maternal education, and family history of SSDs. Several large-scale studies on the effects of OME have not consistently linked it with significant difficulty in learning to produce speech sounds (see Roberts, Rosenfeld, & Zeisel, 2004, for a review and meta-analysis of studies). Nonetheless, some researchers consider it a risk factor. Based on the results of other studies, Shriberg (2010) has concluded that early mild-to-moderate hearing loss of 35 to 45 dB HL associated with OME is a risk factor for SSD, affecting especially the production of sibilants /s/ and /z/. It is possible, however, that lower socioeconomic status of the families is the real variable, as OME is significantly higher in that group; independent studies have shown that lower socioeconomic status, possibly confounded with low maternal education, is associated with SSDs (Paradis et al., 2000). The same logic may apply to suggested risk of African American race; it may be a lower socioeconomic condition, rather than race, that poses risks. Again, lower socioeconomic condition may be confounded with low maternal education, low literacy resources at home, and other possible negative effects of an extremely limited home environment.

Several other variables may be risk factors if they are outside the normal range. For instance, intelligence within the normal range is not significantly associated with SSDs, but intelligence below the normal range is; mild hearing loss may not be, but significant hearing loss is; speech motor skills within the normal range may not be, but motor impairments are; and so forth. See Chapter 4 for details on variables that may affect speech sound learning in children.

Historical Perspectives on Changing Nomenclature

We will shortly define and distinguish the different names used to describe speech sound errors children make, but first we will provide a brief historical introduction to changing times. The diagnostic name for the difficulty children experience in learning to produce their speech sounds has been in flux, with a certain degree of disagreement among clinicians and researchers. This is partly because speech–language pathology, though a clinical discipline, rides on the linguistic tides, riding high or low and often radically changing direction. In the past, and at the beginning of study in this area (the 1940s through the mid-1970s or early 1980s), children's speech sound errors were simply called *articulation disorders*. Each sound a child produced in different word positions, as found in a speech sample, was evaluated as being correctly or incorrectly articulated. Incorrect individual speech sound articulations indexed an articulation *disorder*. There were no perspectives or analytical methods available in the 1950s and 1960s for grouping the errors into patterns beyond the classic phonetic classification of speech sounds (e.g., manner, place, and voicing features, which were not then thought of as *sound patterns*). Articulation disorders were described mostly from a descriptive linguistic viewpoint (Winitz, 1969) and were considered mostly a speech sound *production* problem.

Linguistics began to change radically in the late 1950s, and change continued throughout the 1960s and beyond. Chomsky's publication of *Syntactic Structures* in 1957 affected how language was viewed and studied. His theory rejected the previous descriptive linguistics as inadequate; it also claimed that language production and the social conditions under which adults and children talked were irrelevant to a deeper understanding of language. The central element of Chomsky's rational (nonempirical) analysis of language was his belief in an innate and universal knowledge of grammar. SLPs soon adopted this widely hailed "revolutionary" view of language. Eleven years later, Chomsky and Halle (1968) presented another revolutionary view of speech sounds. Known as the *distinctive feature theory*, it claimed that speech sounds are a bundle of unique (as well as shared) features that help distinguish one sound from the other; because there were no assumptions of a hierarchical arrangement among the features, Chomsky's is the classic "linear" phonological theory. This newer Chomskyan approach emphasized an *innate knowledge* of a universal grammar and of the sound systems of languages in general. SLPs soon began to analyze speech sound disorders in terms of distinctive features, with the assumption that typical learners of speech sounds have an innate knowledge of the universal sound system and fine-tune this knowledge from what they hear in their environment (i.e., their home language). Consistent with this assumption, it was further assumed that children who experience difficulty learning their speech sounds in fact had difficulty acquiring knowledge of the sound system. Note that the emphasis shifted from learning or failing to learn speech sound productions to acquiring abstract knowledge of distinctive features.

Procedures to assess and treat distinctive features began to appear in clinical literature (Costello & Onstine, 1976; McReynolds & Engmann, 1975; Weiner & Bankson, 1978). This approach, however, did not survive. Around the same time that the new distinctive feature approach was being advocated, a newer *phonological* approach quickly overshadowed it (Ingram, 1976). Soon several publications began to promote a *phonological process analysis* of speech sound errors (Grunwell, 1982; Stoel-Gammon & Dunn, 1985). Publication of phonological assessment instruments encouraged clinicians to adopt this new approach to diagnose speech sound disorders in children (Hodson, 1986; Khan & Lewis, 1986). Consequently, the term *phonological disorders* began to be used commonly, along with the term *articulation disorders*.

Phonological process analysis of speech sound errors, though a shift from the distinctive feature analysis, also was based on the assumption that not all speech sound errors may be understood as production problems. Linguists assume that in some children, speech sound errors may be due to a failure to acquire *phonological knowledge* of their language. In a theoretical sense, phonological process analysis was not (and still is not) too different from the distinctive feature approach, though the error patterns analyzed are different. Although many currently popular phonological theories (e.g., Goldsmith, 1979, 1990; Prince & Smolensky, 1993) are nonlinear in their assumptions (hence unlike the linear Chomskyan theory), they do assume, as the Chomskyan generative grammar theory does, that the main task in acquiring the speech sounds of a language is essentially a matter of acquiring an abstract phonological knowledge system. Most if not all phonological theories assume that there is an unobservable underlying representation (UR) of a sound system in the minds of speakers, which is not the same as their sound production patterns, called the surface representation (SR). These concepts are similar to Chomsky's underlying mental language competence or universal grammar (UG) and imperfect surface forms. When a phonological analysis is found appropriate for a child, phonological theories downplay the problems of "motoric" production of speech sounds, in spite of the clinical necessity of teaching the production of sounds that are in error. (Because there are no nonmotoric sound productions, the term *motoric production* is redundant.)

From the early 1980s to the recent past, clinicians used the term *articulation and phonological disorders*, making a distinction when called for. During the past few years, however, still another shift in terms has taken place. Former articulation and phonological disorders are now subsumed under a single umbrella term, *speech sound disorders*. While the previous terminological shifts were theoretically based, it is difficult to identify a new linguistic theory for this latest shift. Regardless of the reason, this is a welcome change, and we have adopted it for the title of the current edition of this book. Minimally, *speech sound disorders* avoids the lengthy and awkward term articulation and phonological disorders. More important, the term is inclusive and possibly less theoretical (Shriberg, 2010). It should be noted, however, that not everyone considers speech sound disorders an umbrella term for articulation disorders and phonological disorders. Shriberg (1993, 1994), whose classification of speech sound disorders is described in a later section, is a case in point.

Two more terminological variations, if not shifts, and we may be done for the time being. One variation refers to *phonological process* versus *patterns* versus *error patterns*. Phonological process was the preferred term for many years and is still the term to use when referring specifically to the linear theory of natural phonology (Stampe, 1969, 1979), which describes phonological processes as a child's way of simplifying adult productions. Also, according to the linear theories, phonological processes may be correctly described as error patterns. On the other hand, in nonlinear theories, a child's problematic productions may be *errors* or *mismatches*, as described later. The other variation is in *phonological rules* versus *phonological constraints*. Linear phonological theories describe phonological rules that force phonological processes. Nonlinear theories describe constraints instead of rules that cause specific patterns of speech sound productions. See Chapters 3 and 4 for phonological theories.

If all these shifts and variations make you feel like you are walking on a beach with waves stealing sand from under your feet, please take a look at Text Box 1.1. Shifting terms are not the only problems.

Text Box 1.1. Disordered phonology?

It is common to define *phonology* as the study of speech sounds and their patterns in language. As such, it is an academic discipline. Unfortunately, it currently is also the most misused term in speech–language pathology, and maybe in linguistics, as well. After defining the term as a field of study, most writers then use it in many imprecise ways. We need not give references to such uses, because the reader who picks up any article or book on the subject may encounter some of the following examples:

- *Disordered phonology:* This could only mean that phonology as an academic discipline is disordered. A sarcastic linguistic colleague of ours—a fierce critic of phonological theories—said, "Indeed! The discipline is in disarray!" Surely, no one would use the term *disordered biology* or *disordered linguistics.*

- *Phonology disorder:* A cousin is *phonology impairment.* Should we call clinical anxiety a *psychology disorder* or apraxia a *neurology impairment*?

- *Children with disordered phonology:* If this were correct, then the term *disordered cardiology* should apply to people who have had a heart attack. A person with a genetic disorder might have *disordered genetics.* The phrase "children with phonological disorders" has almost the same four words, but its meaning is accurate.

- *Two-year-old phonology:* No, it does not refer to the age of phonology; it refers to the phonological skills of *two-year-old children.*

- *Age-appropriate phonology* (following treatment): If this were correct, children who have been successfully treated for a seizure disorder would have *age-appropriate neurology*, and children who are successfully treated for a language disorder would have *age-appropriate linguistics.*

- *Spoken phonology:* It is not the speech or language that is spoken, it is phonology (and may be even *morphology*, another field of study) that is spoken. Children don't just speak, they speak linguistics.

- *Development of phonology:* It does not mean the progress phonology as a discipline makes; it is intended to refer to the development of phonological skills in children.

We make heroic efforts to avoid indiscriminate use of the pronoun "he" to refer to all children or adults; we make even more elaborate efforts to put the person first and the disability or the disorder next—so why not simply write "phonological disorders" when we mean disorders rather than the discipline that studies them?

What Are Speech Sound Disorders?

For the sake of convenience and simplicity, not necessarily because we agree with some of the linguistic theoretical underpinnings, we use the term *speech sound disorders* to include articulation disorders and phonological disorders. Articulation disorders have a longer history than phonological disorders and were reconceptualized after the acceptance of linguistic theories. Purely from a clinical (and nontheoretical) perspective, **speech sound disorders** are errors in producing speech sounds. Additional and often theoretical considerations dictate further distinctions, elaborations, and qualifications.

The term *articulation* in the context of speech production means the movement of speech structures to vary the vocal tract configurations and make specific contacts between some of the structures to produce speech sounds. Imprecise or otherwise impaired movements of the articulators were formerly thought to result in a disorder of articulation. Therefore, **articulation disorders** were traditionally defined as difficulties in correctly producing individual speech sounds. In simple terms, articulation disorders are speech sound errors; anything added to that description is often analytical and theoretical. Some classic writers considered articulation disorders as a *faulty habit* of articulation (Morley, 1957).

The *unqualified* definition of the term *articulation disorder* included all kinds of speech sound production errors (omissions, substitutions, and distortions) until phonological process analysis came to influence the study of speech sound disorders. Phonological theories began to qualify that traditional definition so that a distinction between articulation and phonological disorders could be sustained. Phonological theories also began to limit articulation disorders to speech sound *distortions*. Omissions and substitutions became the province of phonological theories, and distortion errors that those theories could not explain were relegated to articulation disorders. Accordingly, *articulation disorder* was redefined as an SSD involving a difficulty in "motoric" or phonetic production of only a few speech sounds, mostly speech sound distortions that could not be organized into a phonological pattern without losing phonemic contrasts (i.e., without affecting intelligibility), and not due to problems in underlying cognitive or linguistic representations. The basic phonological-theoretical assumption was that the multiple and nonmotoric difficulties producing speech sounds were due to a problem acquiring knowledge of the sound system. This assumption, however, could not be applied to children whose relatively few errors did not seem to follow phonological rules or patterns. Therefore, the scope of the more generally used diagnostic category of *articulation disorder* began to be restricted in order to justify phonological disorders that are attributed to more central, mental, cognitive, innate, and underlying difficulties.

Articulation disorders as understood in the post-phonological pattern era are said *not* to affect speech intelligibility to any significant extent. They include errors of speech sound production that are few, mild, and typically distorted with maintained phonemic contrasts (i.e., acceptable intelligibility and distinction between sounds and words). For example, the speech of a child whose /s/ is distorted because of a lateral lisp in the production of the word *soup* is still intelligible because the distorted /s/ retains contrast with other sounds (Lowe, 1994). In social interactions, listeners do not confuse the lateralized /s/ with another sound; they react to the child's speech as though the child said the word correctly. Similarly, a mild distortion of /r/ is an articulation error that results in nonstandard English productions but does not typically affect the understanding of words, although severe distortions can. When a student of ours enthusiastically shared with her third-grade teacher that her father was a farrier (an equine blacksmith), her bewildered teacher understood the word as "failure" due to the severe nature of the child's /r/ distortion.

If one adheres to this fine distinction between articulation and phonological errors, the term *articulation disorder* could be used to diagnose only a limited number of speech sound errors (mostly distortions) that do not affect the understood meaning of words or neutralize the phonemic contrast in the language. It is likely that most clinicians do not make such a fine discrimination. Being more practical, clinicians typically diagnose an articulation disorder when a child's sound production errors are among the following descriptions:

- not typical of the speech of other children of the same age
- limited to only a few sounds and not necessarily restricted to distortions
- without an identifiable pattern
- do not compromise intelligibility to any significant extent, though there may be an occasional misunderstanding
- (optionally) associated with an organic, structural, or neurological origin (whether they are phonetic, phonological, or both)

In most cases, articulation disorders are not associated with obvious structural (organic) or neurological impairments. Therefore, they are often described as "functional articulation disorders," implying that faulty learning may have caused the disorder. Speech sound errors associated with organic, structural, or neurological origin may also be described as articulation disorders. These disorders are found in a heterogeneous group. Some may be purely organic, as in children with clefts of the lip or palate. However, when there are neurological or neuromuscular impairments, clinicians may use such special diagnostic categories as *childhood apraxia of speech* or *developmental dysarthria*, as described in Chapter 6, Advanced Unit. Especially in the case of developmental dysarthria, more than just speech sound disorders will be evident.

It is well known that clinicians generally compare a child's speech sound productions to those of his or her peers in the normative sample to make a clinical decision as to whether the child has a speech sound disorder. The bulleted list above suggests that in addition to norms, the presence of an organic condition, the number of sounds in error, the extent to which intelligibility is affected, and the question of whether the errors form a pattern are considerations in diagnosing an articulation disorder, as opposed to a phonological disorder. Some of these considerations are not easy to quantify and are open to interpretation. For instance, how many sound errors are few, and how many are too many? What threshold should speech intelligibility not cross to make a valid diagnosis of articulation disorder? Most likely, clinicians make their own judgments about these variables, following some rough guidelines offered by normative research.

A traditional error analysis in diagnosing an articulation disorder includes omissions, substitutions, and distortions. A child's production of each sound may be evaluated for such errors in word initial, medial, and final positions. The child productions are evaluated against the adult models.

Phonological disorders (PDs) are multiple speech sound error *patterns* or adult–child production mismatches that persist beyond certain age levels, often losing phonemic contrasts, significantly impairing speech intelligibility, and are presumably due to an underlying problem in phonological representation or knowledge. Therefore, PDs are not due to a pure production problem. Shorter versions of this comprehensive definition are available. For example, PDs have also been defined simply as multiple errors of speech sounds that may be organized into patterns. Operation of phonological rules or constraints that underlie those errors is always implied. Decreased intelligibility would then be implied by multiple errors exhibited. The loss of phonemic contrasts is the main problem of reduced intelligibility. A child who says *gun* instead of *fun* is said not only to lose the phonemic contrast, but also to severely compromise his or her intelligibility. Note that the child in this example did not articulate any sound badly; substitution is the error in this case.

A brief definition of questionable validity is that of the American Speech-Language-Hearing Association (2008), which states that "a phonological disorder is an impaired comprehension of the sound system of a language, and the rules that govern the sound combinations." This surprising definition makes no reference to speech sound production. Impaired *comprehension* of the sound system and the rules that govern the sound combinations may be a part of the disorder, but not mentioning any speech sound production problems is a serious omission. Most clinicians assess speech sound production to diagnose (or rule out) a speech sound disorder, including a phonological disorder.

Phonological disorders, more than articulation disorders, may be associated with language problems. Several researchers believe that phonological disorders are a part of a language disorder. Phonological and language disorders tend to coexist; word learning and learning of other elements of language may be impaired to varying degrees in children with phonological disorders. Shriberg and Austin's (1998) review of studies linking speech sound disorders and language disorders shows wide discrepancy among those studies: from a low comorbidity rate of 21% in one study (Ruscello, St. Louis, & Mason, 1991) to a high of 66% in another (Shriberg & Kwiatkowski, 1994), although a majority of studies show a rate between 45% and 66%. Literacy problems (reading and writing difficulties) may also coexist with phonological disorders (see Chapter 9 for details). These observations may provide yet another contrast between *articulation* disorders, which may be restricted in their scope and cause fewer negative effects, and *phonological* disorders, which may have a broader basis and produce wider effects.

In contrast to articulation disorders, phonological disorders are thought to be caused by processes, rules, and constraints specified in phonological theories. In linear phonological theories (LPTs), a process is thought to force an error: A child deletes the final consonants in words because of the operation of a simplifying final consonant deletion process (Stampe, 1969, 1979). In nonlinear phonological theories (NPTs), some speech sound production difficulties are **errors**, whereas others are **mismatches** (Bernhardt & Stoel-Gammon, 1994). Such difficulties found through a phonological process analysis done according to LPTs (e.g., the natural phonological theory) are errors. In this case, the child's misarticulations (errors) are evaluated against an adult's correct productions. (In NPTs, the main concern is to analyze the child's productions, with only a secondary goal of comparing them with the adult models.) When the form (topographic feature) of the child's productions is the same as that of the adult, the term used is *match*; when the child's productions are different from the adult's, the term used is *mismatch* (Bernhardt & Stoel-Gammon, 1994). From a clinical standpoint, however, phonological disorders include only omissions and substitutions.

Specifying presumed causes of phonological disorders with such underlying entities as mental representations of speech sounds, phonological processes, or phonological rules and constraints poses risks to the clinician because of the changing phonological theories that switch their underlying assumptions. If the presumed causal part of the definition is omitted, the only difference between articulation and phonological disorders is that the latter are more severe than the former. It is not necessary to use phonological theories to see patterns in a child's speech sound errors. Such errors may be grouped to see patterns based on the traditional phonetic principles (e.g., place, manner, voice). From a treatment standpoint, patterns that are more valid than any based on phonological theories can be described by documenting which treated individual sounds result in generalized production of which other sounds. Most likely, phonetic (physiological) variables affect sound grouping and generalization from one or more sounds taught in the clinic to the generalized production of other sounds. See Chapter 7 on generalized production of treated phonemes to untreated phonemes, words, and speaking situations. Furthermore, as pointed out by Rvachew and Brosseau-Lapré (2010), there is no evidence to justify the distinction between speech sound distortions being articulatory (motoric) and substitutions and omissions being cognitive and linguistic (phonological). They further point out that because distortions, substitutions, and omissions often coexist in the same child, the possibility that all types of errors have a common origin cannot be ruled out. In treatment, targeted correct production of any kind of an error is taught only as a motoric response, through such behavioral procedures as modeling and positive reinforcement. There are no cognitive-linguistic treatment procedures.

In diagnosing a phonological disorder, few clinicians are likely to follow the strict guidelines offered by phonological theories. It is possible, indeed probable, that most clinicians use error patterns or the patterns of LPTs as against the various guidelines given in NPTs. Even though nonlinear approaches to assessment and treatment have been advocated and recommended to clinicians for several years (Bernhardt & Stoel-Gammon, 1994; Gierut & Morrisette, 2005), the phonological patterns (processes) of LPTs seem to be better known to, and used by, most practitioners. The available standardized phonological process assessment tools (Hodson, 2004) and a lack of similar tools for nonlinear analysis may be a reason process analysis continues. Rvachew and Brosseau-Lapré (2012) have written that in spite of their application since the early 1990s (Bernhardt, 1992), nonlinear approaches in speech–language pathology have not been widely applied by clinicians because the method is excessively time consuming. Another reason might be that most clinicians do not receive the necessary training in nonlinear analysis of speech sound errors.

Therefore, most clinicians are likely to make a diagnosis of a phonological disorder when one or more of the following is true:

- Phonological processes (error patterns) that should have disappeared persist beyond the expected age for those processes.

- The patterned sound production errors may be analyzed for some underlying rules or constraints.

- The speech intelligibility is very poor, regardless of other variables (e.g., the number of phonemes involved).

Whether a phonological pattern analysis will be replaced by nonlinear analysis of speech sound errors, and if so how soon, is a question that awaits an answer. If history offers any lessons, there is a potential problem here: Even before many clinicians gain expertise in using nonlinear approaches, a new theory may emerge, creating even more ambivalence among clinicians.

Are There Subtypes of Speech Sound Disorders?

Whether the concept of speech sound disorders is unitary or includes heterogeneous groups with possibly different etiologies, topographic features (symptoms or error patterns), prognoses, and treatment implications has been a concern for several researchers and clinicians. Obviously, answers to these questions obtained through empirical research will affect clinical practice. The distinction made between **articulation** and **phonological** disorders constitutes a well-established classification of SSDs. We noted earlier that a distinction between **phonetic** and **phonological** disorders (Lowe, 1994) corresponds roughly to the distinction between articulation and phonological disorders. Traditionally, SSDs are grouped according to their rated **severity levels** (e.g., mild, moderate, and severe); such levels also suggest classification of subtypes. The severity levels, however, may be applied to both articulation (phonetic) and phonological disorders. We will now summarize a few other ways of classifying SSDs.

Some classifications of SSDs are **typological**—they are based on the behavioral characteristics (symptoms) of SSDs (Dodd, 2005; Shriberg et al., 2010). Errors in speech sound productions are the main basis for this type of classification. Typological classifications are not entirely new, because they are similar to traditional classifications of articulation and phonological disorders. Other classifications are **etiological**; these are based on presumed causation of the disorder (Shriberg et al., 2010). Still other classifications are **endophenotypic** (Gottesman & Gould, 2003); as used in classifying SSDs, *endophenotypes* are related or underlying skills or processes that affect a phenotype (an observable speech disorder). Underlying variables that affect speech sound learning include oral–motor skills, phonological memory, phonological awareness, speed of processing, vocabulary, and such other variables (Lewis et al., 2011). Endophenotypes are supposed to have significant genetic influence. Endophenotypic classifications are similar to those based on **underlying deficits**, such as impaired cognitive processing (Stackhouse & Wells, 1997). Different underlying deficits (endophenotypes) found in children with SSDs would suggest different subtypes; these are emerging subtypes in the research literature. **Comorbidity** may be yet another basis on which to classify SSDs (Lewis et al., 2011). For instance, SSDs with no other associated disorders may be different from those associated with language disorders, reading problems, intellectual impairments, hearing disorders, and so forth. Some researchers have suggested a distinction between **speech sound delay** versus **speech sound disorder** (Dodd, 2011). Others have suggested a distinction between **typical errors** versus **atypical errors** (Preston & Edwards, 2010). Classifications do not always agree fully, because different investigators have different theoretical biases, leading to divergent classifications. To accommodate new data or perspectives, the same experts change their classifications or terms within classifications.

A detailed description of all the classifications is beyond the scope of this chapter. To introduce the general approach researchers take in classifying speech sounds, we have summarized in Table 1.1 three classifications: two that are typological and one that is etiological. Dodd (2005), on the other hand, proposed only a typological classification. That classification, too, may be subject to revision. We urge readers to keep abreast of research on this topic.

Table 1.1

MAJOR SPEECH SOUND DISORDER CLASSIFICATIONS

Typological		Etiological
Shriberg et al., 2010	*Dodd, 2005*	*Shriberg et al., 2010*
Normal (0–3 years) or normalized speech acquisition (9+ years)		Speech delay—genetic
Speech delay (3–9 years)	Articulation disorder	Speech delay—otitis media with effusion
Motor speech disorders (3–9 years)	Phonological delay	Speech delay—developmental psychosocial involvement
Speech errors (6–9 years)	Consistent deviant phonological disorder	Motor speech disorders—apraxia of speech
	Inconsistent deviant phonological disorder	Motor speech disorders—dysarthria

Note. Shriberg et al. (2010) make both a typological and etiological classification. Dodd's is only typological.

Classification Based on Speech Sound Error Characteristics

Shriberg and colleagues (Shriberg, 1994, 2010; Shriberg et al., 2010) have proposed a typological classification of SSDs based on a combination of variables that include typical age-based developmental considerations, speech errors, normalization of those errors, and residual errors. This classification system is still evolving and is being revised as new data become available. What final shape the system will take is not clear. See the sources by Shriberg and his associates cited in this paragraph for details on, and the research base for, their classification. Here we offer only a brief description of each subtype (Shriberg, 2010; Shriberg et al., 2010):

1. **Normal speech or normalized speech acquisition (NSA).** The first subtype in Shriberg et al.'s (2010) classification is normal or normalized speech. *Normalized* speech is currently typical but may have been problematic in the past. It is not clear why normal speech should be the first subtype of a *disorder*.

2. **Speech delay (SD; 3–9 years).** The rationale for calling this subtype of SSD *speech delay* is that children in this category tend to achieve normal speech sound production with treatment. Speech delay is characterized by phonological patterns of deletions, substitutions, or both that persist beyond age 4 (Shriberg, 2010). As such, speech delay refers to a phonological disorder that responds well to treatment, resulting eventually in typical speech. One would expect that most children with speech sound disorders, not just the one in this category, would achieve typical speech sound production with effective treatment. Regardless, naming speech disorders that may be effectively treated as speech delay raises questions about the distinction between delay and disorders,

a distinction that reminds the clinician of the equally questionable distinction between language delay and disorders. Most clinicians would probably consider a clinical condition that requires treatment a *disorder*, not a delay.

3. **Motor speech disorders (MSDs; 3–9 years).** This subtype includes SSDs typically associated with the motor speech disorders of *childhood apraxia of speech* (CAS) and *developmental dysarthria* (DD). Significant speech production problems including distortions, omissions, and substitutions are the main features. Treatment may leave residual errors. See Chapter 6, Advanced Unit, for a description of CAS and DD.

4. **Speech errors (SEs; 6–9 years).** Found in this older age group, speech errors are of English sibilants and rhotics—usually distortions. These children do not experience literacy deficits; their speech intelligibility may be acceptable. About 5% of children below age 9 and approximately 1% to 2% of adolescents and adults may exhibit residual distortion errors. Whenever a disorder persists, the question is whether the individuals were not treated or received ineffective treatment. Until these treatment-related issues are resolved, one cannot vouch for the validity of residual problems being distinct from those problems that respond more readily to treatment.

Both speech errors and motor speech disorders may persist beyond the specified age ranges, creating additional subclassifications not summarized here. Readers are urged to check the latest publications from Shriberg and colleagues, as some inconsistencies exist among their published sources.

Dodd's typological classification of SSD (see Table 1.1) is based on the types of errors a child produces, along with consistency of errors, measured over repeated productions of the same assessment target words (Dodd, 2005, 2011). Although the classification is primarily based on speech production problems, Dodd does offer theoretical speculations about underlying linguistic processing difficulties (such as phonological awareness problems). Unlike Shriberg's (2010) classification, Dodd's is not age specific (Broomfield & Dodd, 2004). Children who begin with a specific type do not exhibit another type as they grow older. Any subtype can occur at any age. Her classification includes the following types of SSD:

1. **Articulation disorder.** Found in 11% of children with SSDs, this subtype is characterized by a few speech sounds, mostly distortions. The same type of error (distortion or substitution) must occur upon repeated production of the same sound, however, and such error consistency may be a rare finding (Rvachew & Brosseau-Lapré, 2012). Essentially, this subtype is similar to a phonetic disorder distinguished from a phonological disorder, as described previously. Deficient learning of motor movements or problems in phonetic planning may cause articulation disorders.

2. **Phonological delay.** Found in 47% of children with SSDs, this subtype may also be called *delayed phonological development*. The major observable characteristics of this subtype include the following phonological error patterns (see Chapter 4) beyond their typical age of disappearance: final consonant

deletion, cluster reduction (only two-member clusters), fronting of velars and fricatives, weak syllable deletion, stopping of fricatives and affricates, and voicing errors (Dodd, 2011). Consistency of errors across words, spontaneous speech, and imitative productions are essential to diagnose this type. No specific hypothesis is offered; delay may be due to slower neurolinguistic maturation. Most clinicians and researchers would consider this a phonological disorder, not a delay.

3. **Consistent deviant phonological disorder.** Found in 30% of children with SSDs. The following unusual (atypical) phonological error patterns justify the diagnosis of this subtype; the following examples are from Dodd (2011): backing of bilabial and palatal stops (e.g., [gɛd] for /brɛd/); initial consonant deletion (e.g., [if] for /tif/); stops substituted by fricatives (e.g., [vuk] for /buk/); clusters marked by bilabial fricatives (e.g., [θi] for /θri/); substitution of /s/ for all fricatives; intrusive vowels (e.g., [aːɛg] for /ɛg/); and extensive assimilation (e.g., [bɪb] for /pig/). This subtype is presumed to be due to a cognitive difficulty in abstracting phonological rules. Typical error patterns included under phonological delay may coexist with these atypical errors. Generally, atypical errors are uncommon (Rvachew & Brosseau-Lapré, 2012).

4. **Inconsistent deviant phonological disorder.** Found in 12% of children with SSDs, this subtype is characterized by the same atypical phonological error patterns as the consistent deviant phonological disorder above, but their productions may be inconsistent across three repeated attempts at producing at least 40% of target words. Each repeated production of the same target word may involve a different error, whereas in phonological delay, repeated attempts may involve the same kind of error. A *phonological planning deficit* (not a motor planning deficit) is thought to be the underlying problem.

Classification Based on Etiology

Shriberg and colleagues (Shriberg, 1994, 2010; Shriberg et al., 2010) have proposed an additional classification of SSD into subtypes based on etiology (causation). Etiology in most cases is hypothesized on the basis of correlation; it is difficult to confirm such hypotheses. Shriberg (2010) admits that genetic and environmental causations are speculative. This classification, too, is evolving and may change over time. Two sources published in the same year have some differences (Shriberg, 2010; Shriberg et al., 2010); the etiologic classification, according to the latter source, includes the following eight subtypes:

1. **Speech delay—genetic (SD-GEN).** Based on referral information available at a university clinic, it is estimated that this subtype of SSD may be responsible for up to 56% of children referred (Hauner, Shriberg, Kwiatkowski, & Allen, 2005; Shriberg & Kwiatkowski, 1994). Genetic studies of SSDs include those on familial prevalence, twin studies, and molecular genetic analysis. A high frequency of substitutions and deletions is found in this group, although the latter are thought to be especially indicative of genetic influence on cognitive processes that affect speech sound learning and production (Shriberg, 2010).

Language and literacy problems also may coexist with this subtype, though not in all children. See Chapter 4 for a review of research on genetic variables related to SSDs.

2. **Speech delay—otitis media with effusion (SD-OME).** Mild to moderate hearing loss that may be associated with otitis media with effusion (OME). OME is considered a risk factor for SSDs, although data on this issue are somewhat contradictory. Shriberg (2010) summarizes the results of several studies in which children with OME and fluctuating mild to moderate hearing loss had lower than typical consonant-correct scores. See Chapter 4 for more on hearing impairment and SSDs.

3. **Speech delay—developmental psychosocial involvement (SD-DPI).** This category does not suggest any psychopathology or emotional disorder. Rather, such variables as approach-related negative affect (e.g., aggressive or angry) or withdrawal-related negative affect (e.g., shy or fearful), negative emotionality or mood (e.g., easily upset or frustrated), lack of task persistence (e.g., unmotivated to work on general speech tasks or unwilling to try difficult speech tasks), and short attention span may be associated with SSDs in some children. About 12% of children assessed for SSDs may exhibit these associated conditions (Hauner et al., 2005). It is not clear how such behavioral problems could affect speech sound learning; the cause-effect direction may be just the opposite: Significant speech problems may affect patterns of behavior in some children.

4. **Motor speech disorders—apraxia of speech (MSD-AOS).** These are speech disorders presumably due to motor planning or programming problems. This subtype in the research studies of Shriberg and associates (Shriberg, 2010; Shriberg & Kwiatkowski, 1994) includes adults with known neurological problems, as well as children and adults with "acquired apraxia of speech." In the context of children, it may be appropriate to use the current term *childhood apraxia of speech* (CAS), described in the Advanced Unit of Chapter 6.

5. **Motor speech disorders—dysarthria (MSD-DYS).** In some children, dysarthria (or developmental dysarthria) may be subclinical, which means that the observed symptoms may not fully support the diagnosis. MSD in children, including both varieties (AOS and DYS), may account for only about 5% of children with SSD. See Chapter 6 for more on developmental dysarthria in children.

6. **Motor speech disorders—not specified (MSD-NOS).** This classification may be used to describe children's SSDs that suggest motor speech components, but neither CAS nor developmental dysarthria seems to fit the total clinical picture.

7. **Speech errors—sibilants (SE-S).** This subtype in characterized by transient or persistent errors in producing the sibilant /s/. Distortions are the typical errors.

8. **Speech errors—rhotics (SE-R).** This subtype is characterized by transient or persistent errors in producing the rhotic /r/. Distortions are the typical errors. Limited data suggest that mild articulation problems, including a /w/ for /r/

substitution, evoke negative reactions from peers (Crowe Hall, 1991; Silverman & Paulus, 1989).

Evaluation of Subtypes

Researchers have spent a considerable amount of time and effort investigating subtypes of SSD in the hope of finding different causal factors for different subgroups. Shriberg and his associates, among those researchers who are most dedicated to investigating this important issue, have done so since the early 1980s. Their classification is still undergoing refinements after some three decades, implying the complexity of SSDs and their classification. Frequent refinements are inevitable when the system is based on empirical findings. As empirical findings change, classification has to change.

As we noted, subgroups or types may be formed based on speech sound errors (symptoms) or on hypothesized etiology (causation). One would think that it would be less controversial to form subgroups on the basis of speech characteristics than on the basis of hypothesized causes. Unfortunately, all classifications—typological as well as etiological—have been controversial; there is no agreement on any of the classifications. As we will see throughout this book, experts disagree on precise definitions of articulation disorders, phonological disorders, phonological delay, phonological processes, childhood apraxia of speech, developmental dysarthria, typical and atypical errors, and any classification of some or all of these into categories of any kind.

All classifications have their shortcomings. A few are sampled in the following list:

• A major difficulty lies with the distinction between *phonological delay* and *disorder* (Shriberg, 2010). If both varieties have to be treated, the clinical relevance of the distinction is not clear. It would be unethical to deny treatment when the diagnosis is delay. If production of a few or several speech sounds are in error in a child who would be expected to have mastered them, the clinician has to offer treatment regardless of whether the condition is called a delay or a disorder. It is not clear why SSDs that are demonstrated to have a genetic basis should be called *speech delay*.

• A similar problem exists with *delay* versus *deviant* disorder (Dodd, 2005). Although the term *delay* may suggest a less serious problem than the term *deviant*, children who are classified as delayed need treatment just the same.

• The distinction between *consistent* and *inconsistent* speech errors is based on a weak criterion: variable production on at least 40% of words. This is below chance. A study of children with residual speech errors has reported that phonetic variability does not support a subtype of SSDs, at least in older children (Preston & Koenig, 2011), although Dodd (2005) has stated that the subtypes can occur at any age. Error variability (as a measure of consistency or lack thereof) may be high in children who have multiple substitutions for the same sound. These children may be found to show considerable variability upon repeated production of the same word, by substituting different sounds for the target sound. Children who make errors on multiple sound classes also may show variability (Tyler, Williams, & Lewis, 2006). If these observations are replicated, variability (the degree of consistency) may simply reflect severity.

• The *typical* versus *atypical* distinction is similarly problematic. We may not fully understand the atypical errors, but the clinician may still have to treat them—and treat them with the same effective treatment procedures. Types of errors change over time in the same children. Rvachew, Chiang, and Evans (2007) report that compared to older children with less severe SSDs, younger children with more severe disorders tend to produce atypical errors.

• Some classifications may simply reflect the *traditional concept of severity*, which is a valid concept in itself. For instance, Dodd (2005) has reported that children diagnosed with phonological delay produce 77% of consonants correctly; the same score for the consistent deviant is 60%, and inconsistent deviant is only 40%. If the difference is only quantitative, a categorical (qualitative) distinction between the groups is difficult to justify. As noted, variability as a measure of consistency also may reflect severity.

Two methodological problems may account for this complicated situation. First, if new data constantly force changes in definitions and classifications of SSDs, then not enough data have been gathered yet, and speculations about behavioral error patterns or causation of subtypes are premature. We will have to wait until more valid and relatively stable classifications are supported by evidence. Second, causation is difficult to establish through the kinds of research that can be done on SSDs. Almost all "etiological" research is correlational. Only experimental research can reliably isolate causes of natural phenomena. It is neither possible nor ethical to conduct experimental research on hypothesized causes to see if their manipulation causes SSDs. Higher familial prevalence does not necessarily mean a disorder is genetic; family members may share common environmental factors. Even the identification of a gene through molecular genetic research does not rule out an interaction with environmental triggers. Coexistence of behavioral or psychiatric problems determined though correlation does not support a hypothesis of causation. As noted earlier, it is difficult to determine which is the cause, which is the effect, and whether both are due to something else. Correlated events are often confounded. For example, lower socioeconomic status may be confounded with lower education of parents. Different behavioral error patterns, even if reliable across children, would not reveal causation. It is difficult to suggest causes for error patterns simply because they are atypical; we do not know the cause for typical patterns, either. When causes are hypothesized to be unobservable internal, mental, cognitive, and innate structures or processes, the causes remain hypothesized, not confirmed, because they are unverifiable.

Clinical Implications of Subtypes

Ultimately, subtype classifications of SSDs are useful if each subtype requires a different treatment procedure. There is no reason to assume automatically that different subtypes, even when they are shown to have different causes, necessarily need different treatments. Only systematic treatment research can tell. There is a tendency among researchers and clinicians to assume that when different variables are hypothesized to be causally linked to different subtypes, the treatment *has* to be different. This assumption is reasonable but not self-evident; it can be confirmed only by treatment research. Researchers should demonstrate whether the same treatment procedures would work with different subtypes; the research should further show whether only certain kinds of treatments are effective with certain subtypes.

There is reason to believe that different subtypes can be treated by the same behavioral treatment methods known to be effective in teaching correct speech sound productions. Before the onset of natural phonological theories, it was hypothesized that phonetic or articulatory disorders are caused by a failure to learn the motor movements of correct articulation. These disorders were (and still are) remediated by teaching the production of specific sounds in error. Such behavioral procedures as modeling, imitation, positive reinforcement, and discrimination and generalization procedures are necessary and effective in teaching the correct production of speech sounds. This is true regardless of whether speech errors are distortions (presumed motoric) or multiple deletions or omissions (presumed phonologic); all may be taught the same way. When phonological processes (error patterns that persist) have been identified, lack of knowledge of the sound system has been hypothesized to be the cause. But how does one eliminate such a phonological error pattern as final consonant deletion? Only by teaching the correct production of some of the final consonants deleted; there is no other procedure to impart missing knowledge. And such a teaching is accomplished by the same behavioral procedures that help eliminate phonetic disorders. Presence or absence of phonological knowledge is simply inferred from patterns of correct or incorrect speech sound productions. Such inferences lose their relevance when the same treatment procedures are effective in teaching presumably different types of a disorder. It is often claimed that a phonological error pattern analysis is economical because the clinician can teach a few sounds within an error pattern and then assess generalized production of other erred sounds; when the other untreated sounds are produced with no additional treatment, the clinician saves treatment time. This is a superfluous claim because no clinician wastes time teaching a sound that is correctly produced because of prior treatment; a nonphonological measure of generalized production of untreated speech sounds taken during treatment would accomplish the same purpose. It is further claimed that teaching a few final consonants may be sufficient to generate the remaining untreated final consonants, and that this supports the phonological *knowledge* construct. What it actually supports is the generalization principle of operant learning, because the teaching is done through the same principle.

Much research has shown that SSDs may have a genetic basis in a certain number of children. Does that mean then that children with a family history of SSDs or a genetic mutation require a new and unique kind of treatment? Maybe they do, but we do not know; if they do, we need to find out what kind of new treatments may be needed for them. So far, there is no evidence to conclude that SSDs in children with a family history of the same disorder are not as easily treated as those in children without a family history.

Unfortunately, typologies and etiological classifications flourish through correlational research, while experimental evaluation of treatment for subtypes of SSDs lags. Clinicians need more treatment research on existing types, not more subtype classifications to be verified in the future. It is important to take note of cautionary comments some researchers have made regarding clinical application of subtypes. For instance, Shriberg et al. (2010) have written that their etiological classifications of SSDs "are not intended to be used in clinical practice until validated by empirical findings" (p. 799). We would add that the empirical findings should come from controlled treatment research, not from more studies of the same kind. SSD classification systems currently provide research frameworks, not diagnostic tools or treatment procedures. Clinical applications will have to be deferred until differential treatment procedures justify different types or subtypes of SSDs.

Chapter Summary

- Speech is a part of the larger language skill; SSDs are a particular group of communication disorders commonly found in children and frequently assessed and treated by SLPs.

- Speech disorders may occur in 15% to 16% of 3-year-olds and 3.8% of 6-year-olds.

- Male gender, a family history of SSDs, low maternal education, low socioeconomic condition, and otitis media with effusion are the risk factors for SSDs.

- The currently favored term *speech sound disorders* has had different names, and some of them may still be prevalent to varying extents: phonetic disorders, articulation disorders, delayed speech, deviant speech, phonological delay, phonological disorders, disordered phonology, and so forth.

- **Speech sound disorders** are problems in correctly producing speech sounds. As an umbrella term, it includes *articulation disorders* and *phonological disorders*. **Articulation disorders** are speech sound production problems—often distortions—that are limited to a few sounds, with relatively intact speech intelligibility, with no patterns that suggest the working of phonological rules, that are not characteristic of peers who are typical learners, and that may be associated with organic problems. **Phonological disorders** are speech sound error patterns that persist beyond certain age levels, generally involving multiple sound errors, often losing phonemic contrasts, significantly impairing intelligibility, and allowing an analysis of either error patterns or child–adult production mismatches, presumably due to an underlying problem in phonological representation or knowledge and hence not due to a pure production problem.

- Several subtypes of SSDs have been described; some are typological while others are etiological. Typological classifications are based on the symptom (speech sound) complexes, and etiological are based on hypothesized causes.

- No classification is generally agreed upon; all have significant limitations. Most classifications are appropriate for research and not clinical application.

- Ultimately, subtypes should be justified by treatment research showing that different subtypes need unique treatment procedures. That kind of research has not been done to any significant extent.

ANATOMY AND PHYSIOLOGY OF SPEECH PRODUCTION

If the tongue had not been formed for articulation, man would still be a beast.

—Ralph Waldo Emerson

Basic Unit: The Structural Mechanisms and Processes of Speech Production

Knowledge of the anatomical and physiological aspects of speech production is critical in understanding both normal speech and speech sound disorders. Anatomic, neurologic, physiologic, and sensory variables associated with articulatory-phonological development will be reviewed with great detail in the Advanced Units of Chapters 4 and 6. It may be noted here that the integrity of at least some anatomical structures and the neuromuscular mechanism is essential for the typical acquisition and production of speech sounds.

In this Basic Unit we will review the structures and processes of speech production and the related auditory mechanism. Most students taking a course on speech sound disorders will have completed a course on speech and hearing anatomy and speech science. Therefore, we will offer only a brief outline of the anatomy and physiology of speech production. Students are encouraged to read current texts on the subject (Bhatnagar, 2012; Fuller, Pimentel, & Peregoy, 2011; Hixon, Weismer, & Hoit, 2013; Kent, 1997; Raphael, Borden, & Harris, 2011; Seikel, Drumright, & Seikel, 2014; Seikel, King, & Drumright, 2010) for more in-depth discussion.

Production of speech requires the complex interaction of four basic systems of speech: (1) respiration, (2) phonation, (3) resonation, and (4) articulation. In addition, adequate hearing sensitivity is necessary for the natural development of speech and language and the continuous monitoring of one's own verbal output. A normally functioning central nervous system is essential for neurological control and integration of the basic systems and their functions. Each system works both individually and in harmony with the other systems.

In this Basic Unit we will outline the four structural processes of speech and the auditory mechanism. We review the neuromotor control of speech in the Advanced Unit of this chapter.

Respiratory Mechanism

The **respiratory mechanism** provides the driving force for speech production. We speak as we exhale, and the exhaled air helps set the vocal folds into a vibration needed for vocalization that is shaped into speech. The **structures of the respiratory mechanism** include (Hixon et al., 2013):

The lungs. A paired, soft and spongy structure within which are ever-branching tubular structures called bronchi, which subdivide into bronchioles, which terminate in small elastic sacks. Figure 2.1 shows the paired lungs and related structures.

The **diaphragm,** also shown in Figure 2.1, is the chief muscle of inhalation, lying just below the lungs. It is a thick, dome-shaped muscle that separates the abdomen from the thoracic cavity. The **abdomen** below contains muscles that are active during exhalation.

The **thoracic cavity** houses the lungs. It contains the respiratory passages: the **trachea, bronchial tubes,** and lungs. The trachea is a tube formed by about 20 rings of **cartilage;** it lies just beneath the larynx and serves as the main conductor chamber for air.

The **rib cage,** shown in Figure 2.2, has 12 **thoracic vertebrae** in its posterior surface, the **sternum** in its anterior surface, and 12 pairs of bony **ribs.** The ribs run in a curved, lateral fashion from the spinal column vertebrae in the back to their own **costal cartilage** in the front. For each of the first seven ribs, the cor-

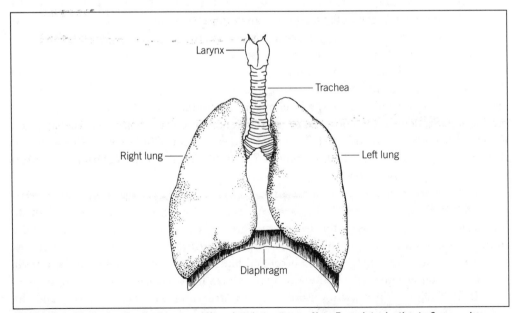

Figure 2.1. The lungs, the diaphram, and the related structures. *Note.* From *Introduction to Communicative Disorders,* 4th ed. (p. 99), by M. N. Hegde, 2010, Austin, TX: PRO-ED. Copyright 2010 by PRO-ED, Inc. Reprinted with permission.

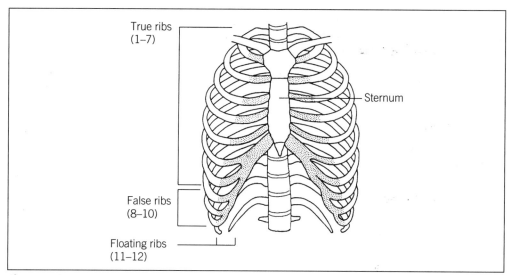

True ribs
(1–7)

Sternum

False ribs
(8–10)

Floating ribs
(11–12)

Figure 2.2. The rib cage. *Note.* From *Introduction to Communicative Disorders,* 4th ed. (p. 98), by M. N. Hegde, 2010, Austin, TX: PRO-ED. Copyright 2010 by PRO-ED, Inc. Reprinted with permission.

responding costal cartilage articulates directly with the sternum. The costal ribs 8 through 10, called the **false ribs,** do not have a direct and medial attachment to the sternum. Instead, their cartilages run superiorly to attach to the sternum. The lowest two ribs (11 and 12) remain unattached and hence are called **floating ribs.**

The muscular portion of the thoracic cavity includes the external and internal intercostal muscles and the subcostal muscles. The 11 paired **external intercostals** lift the ribs up and out to increase the diameter of the cavity for inhalation. The 11 paired **internal intercostals** are responsible for pulling the ribs down to decrease the diameter of the cavity for exhalation. The **subcostals** also pull the lower ribs down and apart to depress the thorax. The thoracic nerves 1–11 supply the internal and external intercostals for neuromotor control.

The **muscles of the respiratory mechanism** help achieve the necessary movements involved in breathing. They include both major and minor muscles (Seikel et al., 2010). The major muscles include the diaphragm, the external intercostals, and the internal intercostals. Minor muscle groups include the scalene, transverse thoracic, quadratus lumborum, pectoralis major, and pectoralis minor muscles. The diaphragm helps elevate the ribs, increasing the vertical dimension of the thoracic cage during inhalation. The external intercostals also assist in elevating the ribs in inhalation, while the internal intercostals help in depressing the ribs in exhalation. The minor muscles assist the major muscles in the inhalation and exhalation processes. The **scalene muscles** help elevate and fixate the ribs for inhalation. Two other minor muscles, **pectoralis major** and **pectoralis minor**, also help raise the ribs. The **transverse thoracic** and **quadratus lumborum muscles** assist in depressing the ribs for exhalation. See Table 2.1 for the point of origin and insertion of these muscles, their major action or function, and the nerves that supply them for neuromotor control.

Table 2.1

MAJOR AND MINOR MUSCLES OF RESPIRATION

Muscle	Origin	Insertion	Function	Nerve Supply
Diaphragm	Xiphoid process of sternum, inferior margin of rib cage, corpus of L1, transverse processes of L1–L5	Central tendon of diaphragm	Primary muscle of inspiration; depresses central tendon of diaphragm, enlarges thorax vertically, distends abdomen	Phrenic nerves arising from cervical plexus of spinal nerves C3–C5
Scalenes (anterior, medial, and posterior portions)	Mastoid process of temporal bone (anterior), transverse processes of vertebrae C3–C6 (medial), transverse processes of C5–C7	Upper surface of ribs 1 and 2	Assist with inspiration; elevate ribs 1 and 2	Cervical nerves C3–C8
Pectoralis minor	Coracoid process of the scapula	Bony ends of ribs 2–5	Assists with forced inspiration; increases transverse dimension of rib cage	Superior branch of the brachial plexus (spinal nerves C4–C7 and T1)
Pectoralis major	Head of the humerus bone	Clavicle, sternum, costal cartilages 2–6	Assists with forced inspiration; elevates sternum, increases transverse dimension of rib cage	Superior branch of the brachial plexus (spinal nerves C4–C7 and T1)
Quadratus lumborum	Posterior portion of iliac crest, iliolumbar ligament, and transverse processes of L3–L5	Lower border of rib 12 and the tendons of the abdominal muscles	Assists with exhalation; helps depress rib 12 and aids in fixing the origin of the diaphragm	Thoracic nerve T12 and L1–L4 lumbar nerves
Transverse	Inner thoracic lateral margin of sternum	Inner chondral surface of ribs 2–6	Assists with expiration, depresses rib cage	Intercostal nerves T9–T11 and subcosthoracic

During speech production, breathing patterns include a rhythmic cycle of inhalation and exhalation. To produce speech, the pressure inside the thoracic cavity must be greater than the pressure outside it, to allow air to rush into the lungs. For this to happen, the thoracic cavity must expand. To expand the thoracic cavity, the diaphragm contracts, or flattens, creating negative air pressure inside the lungs; the positive air pressure outside the lungs causes air to be inhaled through the mouth and the nose as pressure equalization is sought. As air rushes through the trachea and into the lungs (inhalation), the thoracic cavity expands even more through the actions of other respiratory muscles. This causes the air pressure inside the lungs to become greater (positive) than the air pressure outside the cavity (negative). As the diaphragm relaxes and returns to its dome-shaped position and the ribs lower, the size of the thoracic cavity decreases and air is expelled from the lungs (exhalation), creating sufficient air pressure to vibrate the vocal folds. When an unusually strong burst of air is needed to increase vocal loudness or provide emphasis, the respiratory muscles act to provide this additional pulse of energy by forceful squeezing of the thoracic cavity.

Speech production requires modification of airflow and air pressure within the oral cavity. The flow and pressure characteristics vary, depending on the type of speech sound to be produced:

- Production of vowels requires an open vocal tract (described later), a low flow of air through the oral cavity (the mouth), and minimal intraoral air pressure.

- Production of stop consonants requires a closed vocal tract, cessation of airflow during closure, and increased intraoral air pressure during closure.

- Production of nasal sounds requires an open nasal cavity, low airflow through the nasal cavity, and minimal air pressure within that cavity.

- Production of fricatives requires a constricted oral cavity, increased oral airflow, and increased intraoral air pressure.

- Production of affricates requires an initially closed and then narrowed oral cavity, initially stopped and subsequently increased oral airflow, and increased intraoral air pressure.

- Production of glides requires an open oral cavity, low airflow, and minimal air pressure.

Phonatory Mechanism

The phonatory system, particularly the **larynx**, produces sound or voice, using the air supply from the lungs. Resting just above the trachea in the anterior portion of the neck, the larynx is a cartilaginous structure suspended by muscles and ligaments attached to the U-shaped **hyoid** bone. To understand phonation, it is necessary to know how the cartilaginous framework and the muscles of the larynx are put together and function as a system.

The **cartilaginous framework** of the larynx consists of nine cartilages and their connecting membranes and ligaments. The major laryngeal structures (without the connecting membranes and ligaments) are illustrated in Figure 2.3. The three larger and unpaired cartilages are the **thyroid, cricoid,** and **epiglottis**; the smaller, paired cartilages are

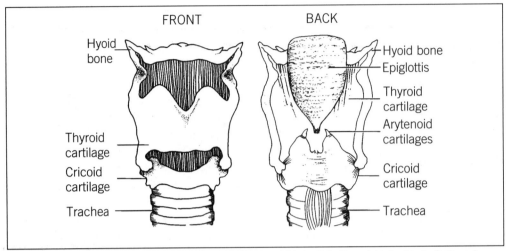

Figure 2.3. The laryngeal structures as seen from front and back. *Note.* From *Introduction to Communicative Disorders*, 3rd ed. (p. 233), by M. N. Hegde, 2001, Austin, TX: PRO-ED. Copyright 2001 by PRO-ED, Inc. Reprinted with permission.

the **arytenoids, corniculates, and cuneiforms** (the last two are not shown in Figure 2.3, as they reside within the aryepiglottic folds). Of these, the unpaired thyroid and cricoid and the paired arytenoids play the most significant role in voice production.

The **thyroid,** a large, butterfly-shaped cartilage, forms the frontal and lateral (side) walls of the larynx. It consists of two quadrilateral plates fused in front in a V-shape. The open portion faces toward the back, and the fused portion, named the **thyroid prominence (Adam's apple),** projects toward the front. The unfused portion of the plates is the V-shaped **thyroid notch,** placed just above the thyroid prominence, marking the approximate anterior attachment of the vocal folds.

Below the thyroid cartilage and above the uppermost tracheal ring sits the ring-shaped **cricoid** cartilage with a plate on the posterior side **(posterior quadrate laminae)** and a narrower band forming the front and lateral sides **(anterior arch).** The anterior arch of the cricoid contains small, oval **articular facets** on each side, which connect with the **inferior horns** of the thyroid. The articulation between the thyroid and the cricoid results in a pivot joint that permits the thyroid or the cricoid to rotate, causing the vocal folds to shorten or elongate. The paired, pyramidal arytenoid cartilages are connected to the top portion of the posterior plate of the cricoid through the **cricoarytenoid joint.** The cricoid, arytenoids, and the cricoarytenoid joint are illustrated in Figure 2.4.

Each arytenoid contains a **vocal process** and a **lateral** or **muscular process.** The vocal processes extend anteriorly, and the vocal folds are attached to them. The lateral processes have several muscles attached to them that help the vocal folds open and close.

The muscles of the larynx are either extrinsic (with one attachment outside of the larynx) or intrinsic (both attachments within the larynx). Extrinsic muscles indirectly influence sound production by both fixing the larynx in place and helping to lower or raise it. The intrinsic muscles are directly responsible for sound production.

Although several muscles are part of the laryngeal mechanism, intrinsic muscles have a leading role in phonation (the production of voice). We will describe the muscles that

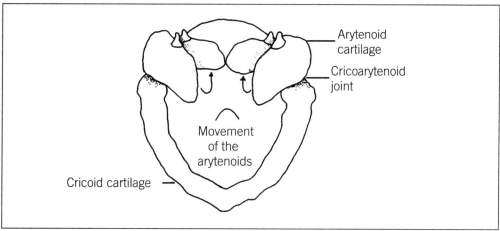

Figure 2.4. The cricoid, arytenoid, and cricoarytenoid joint. *Note.* From *Introduction to Communicative Disorders*, 4th ed. (p. 102), by M. N. Hegde, 2010, Austin, TX: PRO-ED. Copyright 2010 by PRO-ED, Inc. Reprinted with permission.

form the vocal folds, **adduct** the vocal folds (adductors), **abduct** the vocal folds (abductors), and tense and elongate the vocal folds.

The **thyroarytenoid muscle** consists of the **thyrovocalis** (or, simply, vocalis), the medial part, and the **thyromuscularis,** the lateral part. The vocalis muscle mass forms the vibrating (sound-producing) portion of the vocal folds. The anterior portion of the vocal folds attaches to the inside angle of the thyroid notch; the posterior portion attaches to the vocal process of the arytenoid cartilages. The space between the vocal folds is the **glottis,** which is open when the vocal folds are apart (as in quiet breathing) and is closed or nearly so when they are approximated. Figure 2.5 shows the vocal folds.

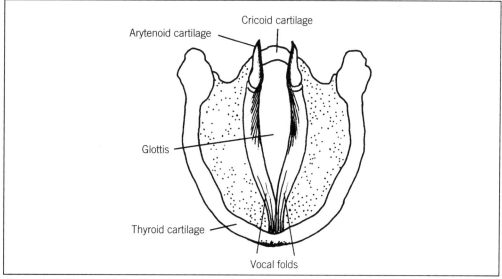

Figure 2.5. The vocal folds. *Note.* From *Introduction to Communicative Disorders*, 4th ed. (p. 103), by M. N. Hegde, 2010, Austin, TX: PRO-ED. Copyright 2010 by PRO-ED, Inc. Reprinted with permission.

The **lateral cricoarytenoid muscles,** the **transverse arytenoid muscles,** and the **oblique arytenoid muscles** help adduct (approximate) the vocal folds. These muscles are illustrated in Figure 2.6. The lateral cricoarytenoid muscles, by swiveling the arytenoid cartilages toward the middle (medially) of the larynx, help achieve partial adduction of vocal folds. Actions of the transverse and oblique arytenoid muscles help achieve complete adduction. Adduction of the vocal folds is essential for vibration of the air supplied by the respiratory mechanism in the production of voiced consonants and vowels.

To abduct, or separate, the vocal folds after their adduction, the **posterior cricoarytenoid muscles,** acting in opposition to the major vocal fold adductors, pull the vocal folds apart. These muscles originate on both sides of the posterior plate of the cricoid cartilage and attach to the lateral processes of the arytenoid cartilages. As they contract, they pull the arytenoids in a rotating fashion, making them swivel laterally, and thus pull apart (abduct) the vocal folds attached to the vocal processes of the arytenoids. Air from the lungs then travels past the vocal folds, which are open and do not vibrate, thus helping to produce unvoiced consonants.

The fan-shaped **cricothyroid muscle,** originating at the cricoid cartilage and inserting into the thyroid cartilage, consists of two parts: *pars oblique* and *pars recta*. The thyroid cartilage tilts downward when the pars recta contracts and slides forward when the pars oblique contracts, causing the vocal folds to elongate and become tense. Figure 2.7 illustrates the two parts of the cricothyroid muscle.

Phonation—the production of sound—is an aerodynamic and myoelastic phenomenon, consisting of a series of rapidly occurring events. The adducted vocal folds stop the flow of air from the lungs, building up a higher **subglottic** air pressure than the **supraglottic** pressure. Increased subglottic air pressure blows the folds apart in a vibrated manner. Opening of the vocal folds begins posteriorly, with the open space **(glottal chink)** moving

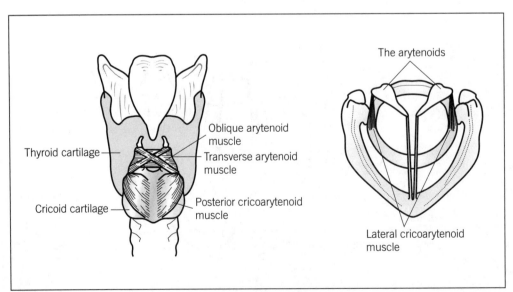

Figure 2.6. The oblique and transverse artynoid muscles, the posterior cricoarytenoid muscle, and the lateral cricoarytenoid muscle.

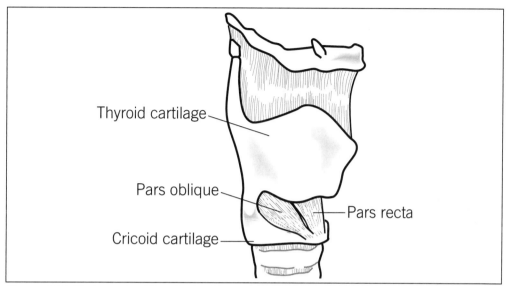

Figure 2.7. The two parts of the cricothyroid muscle.

anteriorly. This is the opening phase. Closing of the vocal folds begins when the opening phase reaches the most anterior portion of the vocal folds. Vocal folds also close from their posterior to anterior portion. Closure of the vocal folds increases the subglottic air pressure and restarts the cycle.

Increased subglottic pressure explains the opening of the vocal folds. The **Bernoulli effect** explains their closing action. According to the Bernoulli effect, as gases or liquids move through a constricted passage, velocity increases and pressure decreases. During phonation, the air (gas) traveling from the lungs passes through the slightly abducted vocal folds (a constricted passage). As the vocal folds are momentarily abducted, a puff of air is quickly released, causing a drop of air pressure directly between the vocal folds. This drop of air pressure causes a suction action to draw the vocal folds together.

The elasticity of the vocal folds is another factor that contributes to their opening and closing. Their elasticity returns them to their original position, to close again, after they have been blown apart. The **myoelastic-aerodynamic theory** of phonation states that vocal folds open and close in a cyclic manner because of the buildup of air pressure, the supra- and subglottic pressure differences (positive and negative), and the elasticity of the muscles.

Resonatory Mechanism

What we hear when someone speaks is not the sound the vocal fold vibrations produce, but the sound or voice that is *resonated* or modified to enhance or dampen certain frequency components. Various supralaryngeal structures resonate the laryngeal tone.

The vocal sound resonators that modify the laryngeal tone include: the **pharyngeal cavity (the pharynx), the oral cavity,** and the **nasal cavity.** See Figure 2.8 in the next section for an illustration of the oral, nasal, and pharyngeal cavities.

The pharynx (throat) is located superiorly and posteriorly to the larynx. Not a dynamic structure, its size and shape are modified by the vertical positioning of the larynx

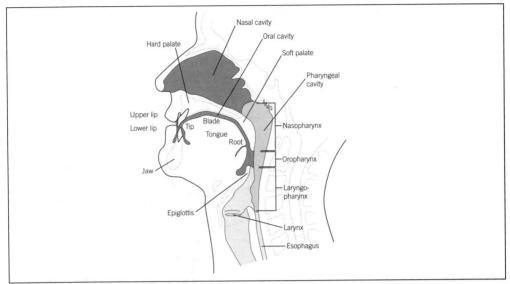

Figure 2.8. Articulators and the resonating cavities of speech. *Note.* From *Introduction to Communicative Disorders*, 3rd ed. (p. 66), by M. N. Hegde, 2001, Austin, TX: PRO-ED. Copyright 2001 by PRO-ED, Inc. Reprinted with permission.

in the neck (high or low) and by the position of the tongue in the mouth (forward or back). Because the base of the tongue is attached to the pharynx, a retracted tongue position will dampen the vocal sound at the pharyngeal level and decrease the effectiveness of oral voice projection. A forward tongue position allows a frontal resonation of sound.

The **nasal cavity** is important in the resonation of sound. Although many sounds can be produced with a nasal quality, only three English sounds should be fully nasalized: /m/, /n/, and /ŋ/. This is possible through *coupling* (the coming together) of the oral and nasal cavities. The soft palate, or **velum**, uncouples the two cavities by lifting to make contact with the posterior pharynx; it uncouples them by lowering.

The oral cavity is the resonating structure for oral sounds. Variables that affect resonance include the movement, excursion, and mass of the mandible; the size, shape, and positioning of the tongue; and the height, length, and width of the hard palate. The teeth, the cheekbones, and the contact of the velum with the posterior pharynx also play a part in oral resonance.

Besides the coupling and uncoupling of the oral and nasal cavities, articulatory movements that change the shape of the oral cavity affect resonation the most.

Articulatory Mechanism

Articulation refers to the molding of the airstream into speech sounds by the **articulators**, which are often classified into two major categories: *movable* and *immovable.* The movable articulators move toward and away from the immovable articulators. The contact between the mobile and fixed articulators may be either complete or approximate. See Figure 2.8 for the articulators and the resonating cavities.

Movable Articulators

Movable articulators include the tongue, the lips, the soft palate, and the jaw. Divided into the **tip, blade, dorsum, and root,** the tongue is the most important movable articulator because it helps shape the majority of speech sounds. The tip is the thinnest part of the tongue and rests behind the lower front teeth. The blade is next to the tongue tip and lies just below the alveolar ridge. The dorsum is the largest area of the tongue, making contact with both the hard and soft palates. The root of the tongue is its very back portion. The four **intrinsic** muscles (**superior** and **inferior longitudinals, transverse,** and **vertical**) shape the tongue into various contours. Four **extrinsic** muscles (**genioglossus, hyoglossus, palatoglossus,** and **styloglossus**) help move the tongue into various positions within the oral cavity. All are richly supplied by nerves that allow them to make rapid and precise movements (e.g., lengthening, shortening, curling up, pulling down, and flattening).

The lips are made up primarily of the **orbicularis oris** muscle. The lips are important in producing the **bilabials** /p/, /b/, and /m/, the **labiodentals** /f/ and /v/, and other consonants and vowels requiring varying degrees of lip movement.

The jaw, or **mandible,** is a large bone of the face that facilitates articulation and resonance. It is the floor of the mouth; it houses the lower set of teeth and provides a bony framework for many tongue and lip muscles. Its movements increase or decrease the size of the oral cavity.

The **velum,** or **soft palate,** begins at the end of the **hard palate** (the roof of the mouth) and extends back toward the pharynx. A small cone-shaped structure hanging from the velum is called the **uvula.** The muscles of the velum include the **levator veli palatini, tensor veli palatini, palatoglossus, palatopharyngeus,** and **uvulae,** which, acting in synchrony, allow it to move superiorly and posteriorly to make firm contact against the pharyngeal wall and achieve **velopharyngeal closure** to produce all sounds except /m/, /n/, and /ŋ/. The velum is the site of articulatory contact for the back sounds /k/, /g/, and /ŋ/.

Immovable Articulators

Immovable articulators include the hard palate, the **alveolar ridge,** and the teeth. Figure 2.8 shows the various movable and immovable articulators (plus the resonating cavities). The floor of the nose and the roof of the mouth, the **hard palate,** is a bony structure separating the oral cavity from the nasal cavity; it is made up of two paired bones called the **maxilla** and **palatine bones.** The maxilla is subdivided into the **palatine process,** the **alveolar process,** and the **premaxilla.** The palatine process is made up of two pieces of bone that grow and fuse together during the fetal stage. They make up most of the hard palate.

The **alveolar process (alveolar ridge)** contains the sockets that house the upper molar, bicuspid, and cuspid teeth. The most anterior portion of the maxillary bone that houses the four upper front teeth is called the premaxilla. In the fetal stage, the premaxilla begins as a separate structure that eventually fuses with the maxillary bone. The alveolar ridge is the place of lingual contact for several front sounds, including /t/, /d/, /s/, /z/, /n/, and /l/. The palatine process (the hard palate) is the place of lingual contact for the palatal sounds /ʃ/, /ʒ/, /tʃ/, /dʒ/, /r/, and /j/. See Figure 2.9 for a schematic representation of the hard palate.

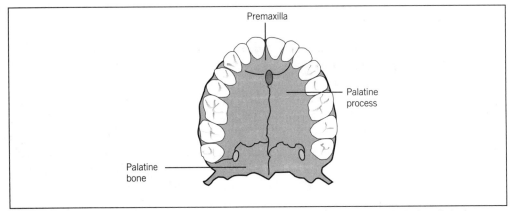

Figure 2.9. The hard palate. *Note.* From *An Advanced Review of Speech–Language Pathology*, 3rd ed. (p. 21), by C. Roseberry-McKibbin and M. N. Hegde, 2011, Austin, TX: PRO-ED. Copyright 2011 by PRO-ED, Inc. Reprinted with permission.

The teeth, along with the tongue, help produce the /f/, /v/, /θ/, and /ð/ sounds. They also help create the friction quality in the fricative sounds.

Auditory Mechanism

Children learn verbal language through hearing what is spoken to and around them. Hearing is also important in monitoring speech and modifying the rate, loudness, and clarity of what is produced.

The anatomy of the auditory mechanism includes mucous and fibrous membranes, bones, ligaments, muscles, fluid-filled canals, nerve fibers, and other supporting tissues that together make up a complex system. The gross anatomy of the human ear is typically divided into three parts: the outer ear, the middle ear, and the inner ear, as shown in Figure 2.10.

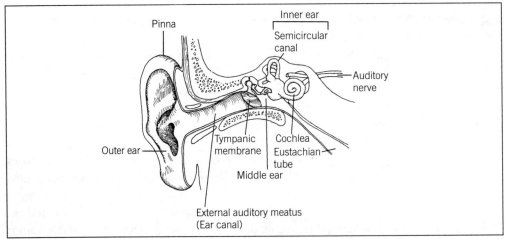

Figure 2.10. The major structures of the ear. *Note.* From *Introduction to Communicative Disorders*, 3rd ed. (p. 72), by M. N. Hegde, 2001, Austin, TX: PRO-ED. Copyright 2001 by PRO-ED, Inc. Reprinted with permission.

Outer Ear

The most visible part of the outer ear is the **auricle**, or **pinna**. The pinna collects the sound waves from the environment and directs them into the **external auditory meatus (ear canal).** The pinna also helps humans localize the sources of sound.

The **external auditory meatus** is a tubelike structure approximately 2.5 cm (1 inch) long that runs in a curved fashion and ends at the tympanic membrane (eardrum). This meatus resonates sound frequencies above 3,440 Hz, so it is important in perceiving fricative speech sounds that exceed 2,000 Hz (Raphael et al., 2011).

Middle Ear

An air-filled space lined with mucous membrane, the **middle ear** includes the tympanic membrane, the ossicular chain (three small bones), and the eustachian tube. A semitransparent, cone-shaped, luminescent structure, the **tympanic membrane** is pearl gray in its healthy appearance. Illustrated in Figure 2.11(A), this membrane is attached to the first bone of the ossicular chain. This tri-layered membrane absorbs the acoustic energy traveling through the ear canal and transforms it into mechanical energy. Sensitive to different sound frequencies, it transmits sound energy to the auditory ossicles.

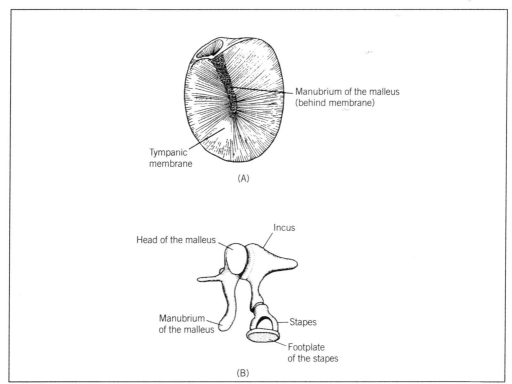

Figure 2.11. The tympanic membrane and the ossicular chain of the middle ear. *Note.* From *Introduction to Communicative Disorders,* 4th ed. (p. 496), by M. N. Hegde, 2010, Austin, TX: PRO-ED. Copyright 2010 by PRO-ED, Inc. Reprinted with permission.

The **ossicular chain** is made up of three interconnected tiny bones, illustrated in Figure 2.11(B). The first and largest bone, the **malleus,** is attached to the tympanic membrane. The second (middle) bone is the **incus,** which is connected to the malleus in a tight joint and permits very little movement. The third and last bone is the **stapes,** which articulates with the incus. The malleus and the incus receive sound energy from the vibrating tympanic membrane and transmit it to the stapes, which in turn conducts the sound to an opening called the **oval window** of the inner ear.

The **tensor tympani,** one of two small muscles in the middle ear, increases the eardrum tension to reduce its vibrations. The **stapedius,** the other muscle in the middle ear, stiffens the ossicular chain to achieve the same effect. These reactions are called the **acoustic reflex,** which protects the ear from very loud sounds and noises (Raphael et al., 2011).

Inner Ear

The beginning of the inner ear is the **oval window,** which is a small opening in the bone of the inner ear. It accommodates the foot of the stapes to receive sound vibrations. Another opening, called the **round window,** helps communicate with the middle ear. A complex system of interconnecting canals and passages called the **labyrinth** is located within the temporal bone in the inner ear. These structures are filled with a special fluid called **perilymph,** and they house the sensitive organs of the inner ear, as well as the **semicircular canals** that help maintain balance, or equilibrium.

The **cochlea** is the main inner ear structure of hearing; when fully stretched, it measures approximately 3.8 cm (1.5 inches). Shaped like a coiled hose, it is filled with a special fluid called **endolymph,** which gets moved around as the stapes pushes into the inner ear. The floor of the cochlea is the **basilar membrane.** The cochlea and the semicircular canals are illustrated in Figure 2.12.

The **organ of Corti,** the inner ear's most important structure of hearing, is located within the basilar membrane; it is bathed in the endolymph. It contains thousands of hair-like structures called **cilia,** which respond to sound.

The vibrations of the foot plate of the stapes reach the inner ear's oval window and create wavelike movements in the perilymph. These movements get transmitted to the

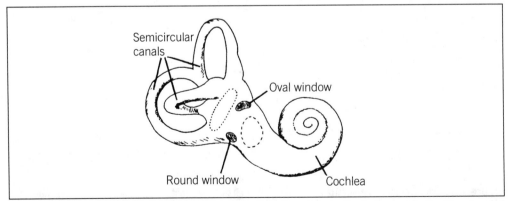

Figure 2.12. The cochlea and the semicircular canals. *Note.* From *Introduction to Communicative Disorders*, 3rd ed. (p. 74), by M. N. Hegde, 2001, Austin, TX: PRO-ED. Copyright 2001 by PRO-ED, Inc. Reprinted with permission.

endolymph through **Reissner's membrane,** which in turn transmits them to the basilar membrane.

The mechanical forces (wavelike movements of the fluids and membranes) are transformed into electrical energy within the organ of Corti so that the nerve fibers that carry the sound to the central nervous system can respond to those electrical impulses.

The electrical or neural impulses created by the movement of the hair cells of the cochlea are picked up by the **vestibuloacoustic nerve (cranial nerve VIII).** This nerve has two primary divisions: The **vestibular division** is concerned with body equilibrium, and the **auditory division** is concerned with hearing. The neural function of the auditory nerve will be addressed in the Advanced Unit of this chapter.

Summary of the Basic Unit

- The four speech production mechanisms are respiration, phonation, resonation, and articulation.
- The auditory mechanism is essential to acquire, produce, and monitor speech production.
- Respiration provides the air supply necessary for speech. The diaphragm, the external and internal intercostals, and other minor muscles make up the muscular framework; the thoracic vertebrae, the sternum, the ribs, and the costal cartilages make up the bony framework; the respiratory passages include the trachea, the bronchial tubes, and the lungs. These are located within the thoracic cavity.
- Compared to quiet breathing, breathing for speech is more consciously monitored and adjusted to meet the continually changing demands of speech.
- The phonatory system (i.e., the larynx) is responsible for producing a sound or voice that can eventually be modified to create voiced consonants and vowels; the thyroid, cricoid, epiglottis, arytenoids, corniculates, and cuneiforms form the cartilaginous framework of the larynx; the intrinsic muscles of the larynx help produce voice, while the extrinsic muscles primarily provide a supportive framework for the larynx.
- The Bernoulli effect and the myoelastic-aerodynamic theory of phonation can explain closing and opening of the vocal folds for voice production.
- The voiced and unvoiced sounds produced by the respiratory and phonatory systems resonate in the pharynx, oral cavity, and nasal cavity.
- Nasal sounds /m/, /n/, and /ŋ/ are resonated in the nasal cavity; non-nasal (oral) sounds are primarily resonated in the oral cavity.
- The velum moves in an upward and backward position to assist in velopharyngeal closure for non-nasal sounds.
- Articulation is the molding of the airstream into recognizable speech sounds by several structures in the mouth; the tongue, lips, velum, and mandible are the movable, or dynamic, articulators; the alveolar ridge, hard palate, and teeth are the immovable, or static, articulators.
- The auditory mechanism allows human beings to learn speech and language initially and to monitor verbal output on a constant basis; its three peripheral divisions

are the outer ear, middle ear, and inner ear; the tympanic membrane, ossicular chain, cochlea, and oval window are its crucial structures.

• The mechanical vibrations from the middle ear are converted to electrical energy in the inner ear. This electrical information is picked up by the vestibuloacoustic nerve in each ear and transmitted to the primary auditory cortex in the cerebral hemispheres.

Advanced Unit: The Neuroanatomical Bases of Speech Production

The anatomical structures of speech production reviewed in the Basic Unit would be ineffective without the organization and regulation of the central nervous system. Therefore, to fully appreciate the complexity of speech production, it is necessary to understand the nervous system, which initiates, integrates, coordinates, and regulates all the movements necessary for the production of sounds, words, and sentences. An ability that is so often taken for granted—talking—can quickly be lost or impaired if the nervous system is damaged.

We can offer only a general review of the basic neuromotor structures involved in speech production, but several excellent sources for details of the neuroanatomy and neurophysiology of speech production can be consulted (Bhatnagar, 2012; Fuller, Pimentel, & Peregoy, 2011; Hixon et al., 2013; Kent, 1997; Raphael et al., 2011; Seikel, Drumright, & Seikel, 2014; Seikel, King, & Drumright, 2010; Webb & Adler, 2007).

Major Divisions of the Nervous System

The anatomy of the human nervous system is subdivided into the central and the peripheral nervous systems. Both control speech production. The **central nervous system** (CNS) is made up of the brain and the spinal cord. The brain is inside the cranium (skull), and the spinal cord is surrounded by the spinal column (backbone). The **peripheral nervous system** consists of the various cranial and spinal nerves that serve as the final common pathway in carrying messages to and from the central nervous system (brain and spinal cord). This complex system's building blocks are the nerve cells.

Structural Units of the Nervous System: Neurons

Neurons (nerve cells) are the basic building blocks in the CNS and are responsible for receiving, transmitting, and synthesizing information. The three major parts of a neuron are the cell body, dendrites, and a single axon. The **cell body** (soma) is made up of the nucleus and surrounding cytoplasm. The **nucleus** is the controlling center of the neuron. **Cytoplasm** is a water-based substance that surrounds the nucleus and helps metabolize protein essential for the maintenance and growth of the nerve cell. Extending from the cytoplasmic material are many dendrites and a single axon. **Dendrites** are receptive (afferent) processes that transmit neural impulses generated from other nerve cells to the cell body; **axons** are motor (efferent) processes that transmit information away from the cell body to other nerve cells. The neural messages conveyed from one nerve cell to another through these specialized extensions can be inhibitory or excitatory. The shape and size of neurons differ, depending on their locations and specialized functions. A basic neuron and its varieties are shown in Figure 2.13.

At its terminal end, the axon divides into several small branches called **axon terminals,** which are covered with **end buttons,** or **terminal knobs;** these minuscule protuberances release an important chemical called a neurotransmitter. A protective and insulating material known as **myelin** covers the length of the axon. The term **nerve fiber** is sometimes used in reference to an axon and its **myelin sheath.** Axons can communicate with various targets, including a muscle, a gland, and other nerve cells.

Transmission of Neural Impulses

Within the brain, neural impulses typically travel from the cell body of one neuron via its axon to the cell body of another neuron through its dendrites. Either the tip of an axon

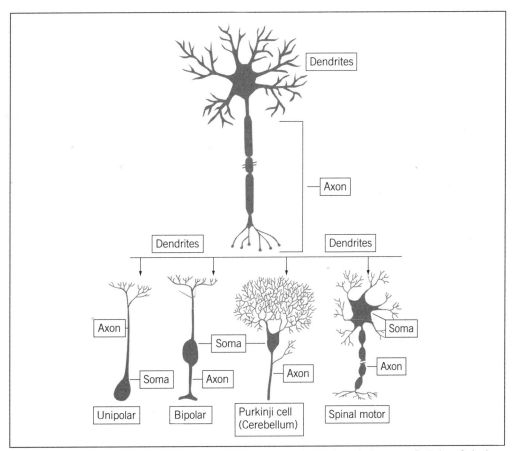

Figure 2.13. Varieties of neurons. *Note.* From *An Advanced Review of Speech–Language Pathology,* 3rd ed. (p. 29), by C. Roseberry-McKibbin and M. N. Hegde, 2011, Austin, TX: PRO-ED. Copyright 2011 by PRO-ED, Inc. Reprinted with permission.

(terminal knob) of one nerve cell makes close contact with a dendrite of another, or the terminal knob of an axon makes contact with the cell body. The axons of one neuron and the dendrites of another do not actually touch during the transmission of neural information (hence, a *close contact*). At the end of an axon, the neural impulse "jumps" across a microscopic space called a synapse (synaptic junction) to the dendrites of another neuron.

The **synapse** consists of the terminal knob of one neuron, the receptive site of another neuron, and the **synaptic cleft (space)** between the two. The terminal (synaptic) knobs of an axon contain and release a chemical substance called a **neurotransmitter**, which activates the **receptive sites** of the neuron and helps generate the electrical nerve impulses necessary for stimulation of the nerve cell body.

Central Nervous System

The five major components of the brain are the (1) cerebrum, (2) basal ganglia, (3) thalamus, (4) cerebellum, and (5) brain stem. These anatomical divisions have specific functions, but all the parts of the nervous system are integrated to allow human beings to think, write, read, walk, dance, and, most important for our purposes, *talk* without difficulty.

Cerebrum

The cerebrum, the largest and most important structure of the human body for speech, initiates the voluntary motor movements for the production of sounds and words. It is made up of billions of nerve cells, which are densely packed within the cranium. The **cerebral cortex**, its highly convoluted outermost surface, is organized in six layers, each consisting of different cell types. The cortex has its ridges **(gyri)** and more shallow **sulci** or deeper **fissures** (valleys). The cerebrum consists of two **cerebral hemispheres**, which are nearly identical in appearance but different in function and are connected by the **corpus callosum**—a thick bundle of myelinated fibers that maintains communication between the two hemispheres. A large, deep, central **longitudinal fissure** divides the left and right cerebral hemispheres.

Each cerebral hemisphere controls the opposite side of the body, which is described as **contralateral motor control.** For almost 95% of the population, speech and language are left lateralized, although the right hemisphere is involved with prosodic features and aspects of social communication.

Each cerebral hemisphere is anatomically divided into four major lobes: frontal, temporal, parietal, and occipital. The lobes are named after the major bones of the skull, and various sulci and fissures create the boundaries between them. Figure 2.14 illustrates the four lobes of the cerebral cortex and the important sulci that create their boundaries.

Frontal Lobe

The **central sulcus** (the **fissure of Rolando**), a deep cortical valley, is the boundary between the frontal lobe and the parietal lobe. The major portion of the frontal lobe is in front of the central sulcus; a smaller, inferior section lies above the lateral fissure, also known as the Sylvian fissure. The frontal lobe is the largest of all lobes, occupying about one-third of the cerebral hemisphere.

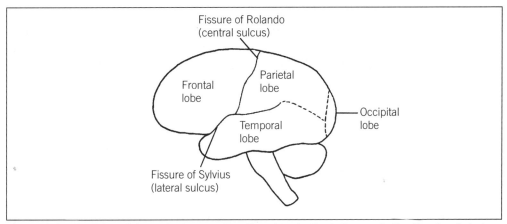

Figure 2.14. The lobes of the cerebral cortex. *Note.* From *Introduction to Communicative Disorders*, 3rd ed. (p. 83), by M. N. Hegde, 2001, Austin, TX: PRO-ED. Copyright 2001 by PRO-ED, Inc. Reprinted with permission.

The **primary motor cortex** is located on the precentral gyrus and controls voluntary movements in the opposite side of the body. All the muscles of the body, including those of speech production, are connected to the primary motor cortex through descending motor nerve cells. A large area of the primary motor cortex controls the lips, jaw, tongue, and larynx (see Figure 2.15), compared to how much of it controls other body structures. Damage to the lower third of the primary motor cortex may result in impaired movement of the articulators.

The **premotor cortex** (the **supplementary motor cortex**) lies just anterior to the precentral sulcus, a fissure situated in front of the primary motor cortex. This area may help plan complex and skilled motor movements such as playing the piano and producing propositional speech.

Another motor planning center for speech is **Broca's area,** located in the lower section of the frontal lobe just anterior to the portion of the primary motor cortex that controls jaw, lip, tongue, and laryngeal movements. This section is the **inferior frontal gyrus.**

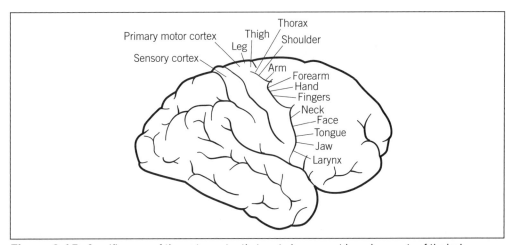

Figure 2.15. Specific areas of the motor cortex that control movement in various parts of the body.

Broca's area is important for the production of fluent and well-articulated speech. It is found in the cerebral hemisphere dominant for language (the left hemisphere for most people). Damage to Broca's area in the dominant hemisphere may lead to speech production problems. Broca's area and other areas important for speech and hearing are illustrated in Figure 2.16.

Temporal Lobe

Roughly shaped like a thumb, the temporal lobe is situated below the frontal and parietal lobes. The lateral fissure demarcates its superior boundary, and an imaginary inferior extension of the parieto-occipital sulcus posteriorly separates it from the occipital lobe. It contains three prominent gyri: superior (the first), middle (the second), and inferior temporal (the third). The temporal lobe also houses important areas for speech, language, and hearing.

The **primary auditory area** or **cortex** is situated on the superior temporal gyrus (see Figure 2.16). Posterior to the primary auditory cortex is the auditory association area. The collective term **Heschl's gyri** refers to the transverse convolutions that make up the primary auditory cortex and the auditory association cortex (Bhatnagar, 2012). The primary auditory cortex receives auditory stimuli from the vestibuloacoustic nerve bilaterally, and the auditory association area synthesizes it. The auditory association area is concerned with the analysis of speech sounds for the recognition of whole words and sentences.

The **auditory association** area in the language-dominant hemisphere is called **Wernicke's area,** located in the posterior superior portion of the first temporal gyrus in the left hemisphere. It is a relatively large area believed to help humans both understand and formulate speech and language.

Parietal Lobe

The parietal lobe, concerned primarily with somatic sensory experience, lies posterior to the frontal lobe and superior to the temporal lobe. It integrates contralateral body sensations such as pain, touch, temperature, and pressure. The parietal lobe also houses the

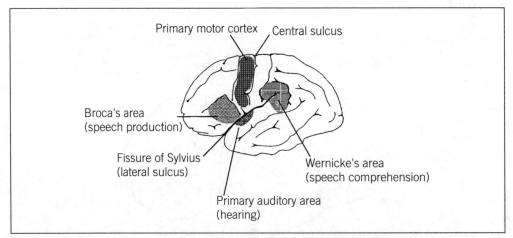

Figure 2.16. The major speech, language, and hearing areas of the brain. *Note.* From *Introduction to Communicative Disorders*, 3rd ed. (p. 84), by M. N. Hegde, 2001, Austin, TX: PRO-ED. Copyright 2001 by PRO-ED, Inc. Reprinted with permission.

supramarginal gyrus and the **angular gyrus,** which are relevant for speech and language. Damage to these areas in the language-dominant hemisphere may lead to problems with word finding, reading, and writing.

Occipital Lobe

The occipital lobe is located posterior to the parietal lobe and superior to the cerebellum and makes up the most posterior portion of the cerebrum. It is primarily concerned with vision.

Basal Ganglia

The **basal ganglia,** buried deep in the cerebral hemispheres, are **subcortical** structures of gray matter. They are a point of intercommunication for various neurological subsystems and consist of at least three nuclear masses: the caudate nucleus, putamen, and globus pallidus. Sometimes these are collectively termed the **corpus striatum** (Webb & Adler, 2007). Figure 2.17 illustrates the basal ganglia and their individual components.

Functionally, the basal ganglia are part of the *extrapyramidal system*, a system that helps modify and regulate cortically initiated motor movements, including speech. A structure that is functionally related to—although not anatomically part of—the basal ganglia is the **substantia nigra,** which is a part of the extrapyramidal system. Because motor movements are not directly controlled in the basal ganglia, the extrapyramidal system is an indirect activation system. It indirectly affects motor movements related to posture, automatic movements, and skilled motor movements by communicating with the cerebral cortex via other subcortical structures (e.g., the thalamus).

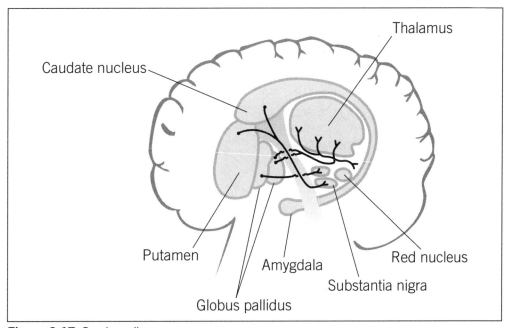

Figure 2.17. Basal ganglia.

Basal ganglia lesions may cause the following movement disorders:

- *Involuntary motor movements*—bizarre postures and unusual movements that cannot be brought under voluntary control (e.g., tremors, jerking, writhing, and flailing)
- *Hyperkinesia*—excessive involuntary movements (e.g., chorea, athetosis)
- *Hypokinesia*—involuntary movements that are characterized by too few movements
- *Bradykinesia*—slowness of movements and movements that have limited range of motion
- *Altered posture*—typically, a stooped or other abnormal posture
- *Changes in body tone*—either hypertonicity (too much tone) or hypotonicity (too little tone)
- *Dysarthria*—hypokinetic dysarthria, a motor speech disorder typically associated with Parkinson's disease, or hyperkinetic dysarthria, associated with various etiologies (e.g., Huntington's disease)

Cerebellum

The cerebellum sits below the occipital lobe of the cerebrum and just behind the brain stem (see Figure 2.18). It does not initiate or integrate motor movements but coordinates body posture, balance, and such fine and skilled motor movements as talking, running, typing, writing, dancing, and playing the piano.

By monitoring sensory inputs to the brain and motor outputs to the muscles, the cerebellum makes needed adjustments. For example, when a person is about to lift a box that seems heavy, the cerebellum regulates the cortically initiated outgoing motor movement so that range of motion, force, and strength are adequate to effectively accomplish the task.

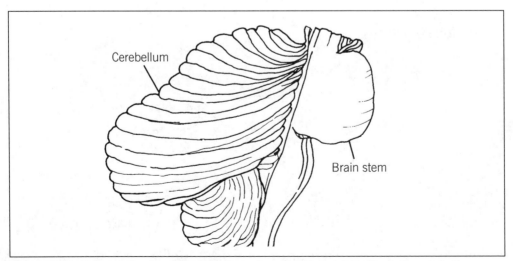

Figure 2.18. The cerebellum in relation to the brain stem. *Note.* From *Introduction to Communicative Disorders*, 4th ed. (p. 124), by M. N. Hegde, 2010, Austin, TX: PRO-ED. Copyright 2010 by PRO-ED, Inc. Reprinted with permission.

Damage to the cerebellum may lead to various impairments, such as the following:

- *Ataxia*—a general term that means incoordination of motor movements
- *Dysdiadochokinesia*—difficulty performing rapid alternating muscle movements
- *Dysmetria*—difficulty gauging the range, velocity, and strength required for a specific movement, causing both overshooting and undershooting of the target movement
- *Intention tremor*—involuntary movement typically present when trying to accomplish a target movement; contrasted with the tremor due to basal ganglia damage, which occurs at rest
- *Disequilibrium*—balance problems that predominantly involve the legs; a drunk-like unsteady gait; a compensatory *broad-based gait*, in which the feet are wide apart
- *Nystagmus*—rapid, oscillating movements of the pupil of the eye; the movements may be vertical, horizontal, or rotary
- *Ataxic dysarthria*—a motor speech disorder present with some but not all cerebellar lesions

Brain Stem

The **brain stem**, the oldest part of the brain from an evolutionary standpoint, is a diagonally oriented structure that connects the brain with the spinal cord through the diencephalon. It also serves as a bridge between the cerebellum and all other central nervous system structures (i.e., cerebrum, basal ganglia, thalamus, and spinal cord). The midbrain, pons, and medulla make up the brain stem, which also contains the *reticular formation, cranial nerve nuclei*, and *longitudinal fiber tracts*. The brain stem controls such life-supporting functions as breathing, swallowing, and regulating heartbeats. The parts of the brain stem are illustrated in Figure 2.19.

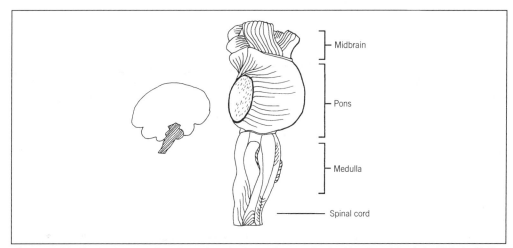

Figure 2.19. The brain stem. *Note.* From *Introduction to Communicative Disorders*, 4th ed. (p. 122), by M. N. Hegde, 2010, Austin, TX: PRO-ED. Copyright 2010 by PRO-ED, Inc. Reprinted with permission.

Midbrain

The midbrain (**mesencephalon**), is the most superior portion of the brain stem, residing below the diencephalon and above the pons. Its **superior peduncles** connect the brain stem to the cerebellum. The substantia nigra, a cellular structure connected in function to the basal ganglia, runs the vertical length of the midbrain at the level of the peduncles. The midbrain also contains the **corpora quadrigemina,** made up of the paired **inferior** and **superior colliculi**. The **inferior colliculi** relay auditory neural impulses from the ear to the auditory cortex, and the **superior colliculi** help in reflex control of oculomotor movements.

Pons

The **pons** (bridge), with a bulging appearance on its anterior surface, is located just below the midbrain. Along with the midbrain, it serves as a connection point between various cerebral structures and the cerebellum through the **middle** and **inferior peduncles.** The pons contains numerous descending motor fibers, and it houses various cranial nerve nuclei important for speech production (e.g., the facial nerve).

Medulla

Also called the **medulla oblongata,** the medulla is the most inferior portion of the brain stem. This cone-shaped structure is important for speech production because it contains numerous descending fibers that carry motor information to several cranial nerve nuclei. It also contains the motor fibers that descend to the spinal cord for innervation of the spinal nerves. The cranial nerves whose nuclei lie within the medulla are the vestibulocochlear, glossopharyngeal, vagus, accessory, and hypoglossal nerves.

Connecting Fibers

The connecting fibers (myelinated axonal fibers) of the central nervous system may promote inter- or intrahemispheric communication. They form the **medullary** center of the brain, and its nerve fibers may be projection, association, or commissural (Bhatnagar, 2012).

Projection Fibers

Projection fibers run in a vertical direction and establish connections between the cortex and subcortical structures such as the basal ganglia, the cerebellum, the brain stem, and the spinal cord. Some of these fibers carry sensory information, and others carry motor information. The motor projection fibers mostly originate in the primary motor and premotor areas in the frontal lobe and form the upper motor neuron system of the pyramidal tract (described later). The sensory projection fibers transmit **cutaneous** and **proprioceptive** information from the skin and joints and project them to various primary sensory areas in the cortex.

Association Fibers

Association fibers interconnect various areas of the cortex within each hemisphere. Some association fibers are short and connect gyri that are adjacent to each other (within the same lobe), while others are relatively long and connect distant cortical areas (between lobes). A long bundle of association fibers important for speech is the **arcuate fasciculus,** which connects Wernicke's area with Broca's area. Theoretically, a lesion to the arcuate fasciculus disconnects these cortical areas and may lead to **conduction aphasia.** Other short association fibers help connect the auditory cortex to Wernicke's area within the temporal lobe and the primary motor cortex to Broca's area within the frontal lobe.

Commissural Fibers

Commissural fibers in the brain run horizontally and help interconnect the two hemispheres. Among the several commissural pathways that interconnect the cortical areas in both hemispheres, the **corpus callosum** is the most important.

Peripheral Nervous System

The **peripheral nervous system** includes three types of nerves that are located outside the skull or spinal column: the cranial nerves, the spinal nerves, and the peripheral autonomic nerves. Peripheral nerves carry sensory information originating in various peripheral organs to the brain, while motor nerves transmit motor nerve impulses originating in the brain to the muscles, glands, and organs in the body.

The autonomic nerves help control many involuntary functions of the body. Those nerves are not summarized here.

Cranial Nerves

The cranial nerves originate from the brain stem and exit the base of the skull through small apertures called **foramina.** They **innervate** various muscles, including those of the head, neck, face, larynx, pharynx, tongue, and some glands. The cranial nerves are part of the lower motor neuron system of the corticobulbar tract of the pyramidal system (discussed later). Several of the cranial nerves are essential for speech production, while others serve senses such as vision, audition, smell, and taste. The cranial nerves can be sensory, motor, or both (mixed). There are 12 pairs of cranial nerves, which are named according to function and numbered in the sequence in which they exit the brain, in relation to the height in the brain at their point of exit. Table 2.2 outlines the 12 cranial nerves according to their name, Roman numeral, CNS (central nervous system) level, and basic function.

The first two cranial nerves, *olfactory* (I) and *optic* (II), are sensory (for smell and vision, respectively). The cranial nerves III *(oculomotor)*, IV *(trochlear)*, and VI *(abducens)* are motor and are responsible for eye movements. The remaining cranial nerves are related to speech or hearing and are listed in the following section. Cranial nerves V, VI, VII, and VIII originate in the pons; IX, X, XI, and XII exit from the medulla oblongata.

Cranial Nerves for Speech

The trigeminal nerve (V) is both sensory and motor, hence mixed in function. Its motor fibers innervate various muscles of the jaw, tensor tympani, tensor veli palatini, mylohyoid, and the anterior belly of the digastric muscle. The sensory fibers are made up of three

Table 2.2

THE CRANIAL NERVES AND THEIR FUNCTIONS

Nerve Number	Name	CNS Level	General Function
I	Olfactory	Telencephalon	Sensory: Sense of smell
II	Optic	Diencephalon	Sensory: Sense of vision
III	Oculomotor	Midbrain	Motor: Eye movements, pupillary constriction
IV	Trochlear	Midbrain	Motor: Eye movements
V	Trigeminal	Mid pons	Sensory: Ophthalmic & maxillary areas of the face Motor: Mandibular musculature
VI	Abducens	Inferior pons	Motor: Eye movements
VII	Facial	Pons-medulla junction	Motor: Facial expression, stapedial reflex, elevation of hyoid bone Other efferent: Lacrimation, salivation
VIII	Vestibulocochlear (auditory)	Pons-medulla junction	Sensory: Balance and hearing
IX	Glossopharyngeal	Medulla	Sensory: Tongue, pharynx, tonsils Motor: Pharyngeal musculature
X	Vagus	Medulla	Sensory: Viscera of neck, thorax, abdomen Motor: Larynx, pharynx, soft palate
XI	Spinal accessory (accessory)	Medulla	Motor: Strap muscles of neck
XII	Hypoglossal	Medulla	Motor: Tongue

branches: mandibular, maxillary, and ophthalmic. The mandibular branch is sensory to the tongue, mandible, lower teeth, lower lip, part of the cheek, and part of the external ear. The maxillary branch is sensory to the upper lip, maxilla, upper teeth, upper cheek area, palate, and maxillary sinus. The ophthalmic nerve is sensory to the forehead, eyes, and nose. Perhaps you have had some experience with the effect of temporary anesthetization of the trigeminal nerve during a visit to the dentist.

The facial nerve (VII) is also a mixed nerve. The motor fibers innervate various muscles important for speech production (articulation) and facial expression, including orbicularis oris, zygomatic, buccinator, orbicularis oculi, platysma, stylohyoid, stapedius, the posterior belly of the digastric, and various labial muscles. The sensory fibers (in the anterior two-thirds of the tongue) are partly responsible for taste.

The vestibulocochlear nerve (VIII), also known as the auditory nerve, is sensory for hearing and balance and has two branches: the *vestibular* and the *auditory*. The auditory branch carries sensory information from the cochlear in the inner ear to the brain (the primary auditory cortex). The vestibular branch helps maintain balance or equilibrium.

The glossopharyngeal nerve (IX) is mixed. Its motor fibers innervate the stylopharyngeus, a pharyngeal muscle that contributes to the elevation of the pharynx and the larynx. The stylopharyngeal movements aid swallowing function. The sensory fibers help process taste information from the posterior third of the tongue and provides general sensation to the pharynx, soft palate, faucial pillars, tonsils, ear canal, and tympanic cavity.

The vagus nerve (X) is also mixed. Its three branches, the **pharyngeal, recurrent laryngeal, and superior laryngeal,** have a wide and wandering distribution in the body. The nerve conveys sensory information from the larynx, pharynx, trachea, heart, and digestive system. Its motor fibers supply the heart, lungs, and digestive system, as well as the muscles of the pharynx, soft palate, and intrinsic muscles of the larynx.

The spinal accessory, or simply accessory, nerve (XI) is a motor nerve; it is both a cranial and a spinal nerve. Some of its fibers originate in the brain stem, while others originate in the spinal cord. As with the vagus nerve, its cranial fibers innervate the uvula and levator veli palatini (muscles of the soft palate). The spinal root supplies the sternocleidomastoid and trapezius muscles, which assist in turning, tilting, and thrusting the head forward.

The hypoglossal nerve (XII) is a motor nerve that primarily innervates the muscles of the tongue. It supplies all the intrinsic muscles of the tongue and three extrinsic tongue muscles: the genioglossus, hyoglossus, and styloglossus. Together, the intrinsic and extrinsic muscles of the tongue are responsible for various tongue movements important for speech production, as well as swallowing.

Spinal Nerves

Thirty-one pairs of spinal nerves emerge from the spinal cord through the afferent (sensory) and efferent (motor) roots. The afferent root is on the dorsal surface of the spinal cord (the part of the spinal cord that faces toward the back). The efferent root is on the spinal cord's ventral surface (the portion facing toward the abdomen). The 31 pairs are named cervical, thoracic, lumbar, sacral, and coccygeal, after the region of the spinal cord to which they are attached; they are numbered in sequence:

- 8 pairs of cervical spinal nerves, numbered C1–C8
- 12 pairs of thoracic spinal nerves, numbered T1–T12
- 5 pairs of lumbar spinal nerves, numbered L1–L5
- 5 pairs of sacral spinal nerves, numbered S1–S5
- 1 pair of coccygeal spinal nerves, numbered C1 (not to be confused with the cervical 1 spinal nerve)

Spinal nerves are all mixed. They carry sensory information from peripheral receptors to the CNS. and transmit motor information from the CNS to the muscles. Although not all spinal nerves are directly implicated in speech production, some contribute to it greatly through innervation of the respiratory musculature. For example, the diaphragm (an important muscle of inhalation) is innervated by the motor branches of the C3–C5 spinal nerves (phrenic nerves). Several other respiratory muscles are innervated by the thoracic spinal nerves (e.g., the internal and external intercostals). The file "Muscles and Nerves Involved in the Production of English Consonants" on the CD that accompanies this book provides a detailed review of the musculature associated with the production of all English consonants and their cranial or spinal nerve supply.

Neuromotor Control of Speech

How do all the structures described so far interconnect to initiate, regulate, coordinate, and synthesize speech and language? In this section we will give a brief overview of the integrative function of these structures, so that the dynamic neuromotor control of speech can be understood. The production of speech requires the action of various systems or mechanisms at five major levels: (1) cerebral cortex, (2) subcortical nuclei, (3) brain stem, (4) cerebellum, and (5) spinal cord. For clinical purposes, the integration of these systems is more commonly divided into the pyramidal system, the extrapyramidal system, and the cerebellar system.

Cerebral Initiation

We will begin by imagining that a person is having a conversation with someone and has just been asked a question. The sensory information of hearing a question is transmitted from the cochlea in the inner ear to the primary auditory cortex in the temporal lobe via the vestibulocochlear nerve (cranial nerve VIII). You may recall that the auditory cortex perceives spoken information. The information perceived by the auditory cortex is then transmitted to the auditory language association area (Wernicke's area), where the meaning of the words is thought to be understood. When a response to the question heard is imminent, the choice of words is thought to be formulated in Wernicke's area and transmitted to Broca's area through a long bundle of association fibers, theoretically the **arcuate fasciculus.**

Broca's area, located in the inferior frontal gyrus of the frontal lobe, receives the information and then plans the patterns of skilled movements necessary for speech production. The supplementary motor cortex is believed to also have some effect on motor planning.

The motor movements planned in Broca's area and the supplementary motor cortex are then transmitted to the primary motor cortex, specifically the lower third of the precentral gyrus in the frontal lobe, through short association fibers. The parts of the motor cortex that mediate the movements of the speech muscles (i.e., the tongue, lips, soft palate, face, and larynx) send out neural impulses through long projection fibers. The projection nerve fibers continue their vertical path through the **internal capsule,** an area of concentrated and compact projection fibers near the brain stem, and communicate with the nuclei for cranial nerves V, VII, IX, X, XI, and XII located in the brain stem.

The cranial nerves exit the skull to innervate the muscles of the face, tongue, soft palate, pharynx, and larynx for the movements necessary for speech. The respiratory muscles involved in speech production are innervated by the spinal nerves in the spinal cord, not the cranial nerves. It is important to note that the movements initiated at a cortical level are further regulated, integrated, fine tuned, and coordinated through subcortical structures such as the basal ganglia and the cerebellum.

As noted in an earlier section, the cerebellar system coordinates and regulates neural impulses; as such the system is also involved in speech production. We can now begin our discussion of the pyramidal and extrapyramidal systems.

Pyramidal System

The excitatory pyramidal system is the direct motor activation pathway, primarily responsible for facilitating voluntary movement of the muscles, including those for speech (Bhatnagar, 2012; Duffy, 2005; Webb & Adler, 2007). The nerve fiber tract of the pyramidal system courses from the cerebral cortex to the spinal cord and brain stem to eventually supply the muscles of the head, neck, and limbs (e.g., legs, arms, toes, fingers, etc.). The voluntary movements necessary for speech production are initiated at the primary motor cortex in the lower third of the precentral gyrus.

The pyramidal system consists of the **corticospinal** and the **corticobulbar tracts.** *Tracts* refers to a bundle of nerve fibers running through the central nervous system. The pyramidal system and its two tracts are a group of myelinated nerve fibers carrying neural impulses. Although the corticospinal and corticobulbar tracts are part of one system, they are addressed separately to promote easier understanding. The *projection fibers* of both tracts originate in the cerebral cortex; however, the point of termination for their neural messages influences their classification.

The nerve fibers of the **corticospinal tract** descend from the motor cortex of each hemisphere through the internal capsule. They continue to travel vertically through the midbrain and pons, and at the level of the medulla approximately 85% to 90% of the fibers cross over (**decussate**). The decussated fibers enter the spinal cord to communicate with the spinal nerves at various levels. Finally, the spinal nerves exit the **neuraxis** through the **vertebrae foramina** along the spinal column to innervate the muscles of the trunk and limbs.

Because of the high level of crossover at the medulla, the left side of the body is typically controlled by nerve fibers that originate in the right cerebral cortex, and vice versa. A person who has a stroke in the left cerebral hemisphere and has right-sided hemiparesis best illustrates the concept of contralateral motor control.

The **corticobulbar tract** is critical for speech production. Its fibers control all voluntary movements of the speech muscles except the respiratory muscles. Like the fibers of the corticospinal tract, the fibers of the corticobulbar tract primarily originate in the motor cortex and descend in a vertical fashion through the internal capsule; they then run along with the fibers of the corticospinal tract. However, the fibers of the corticobulbar tract terminate at the motor nuclei of the cranial nerves (III–XII) in the brain stem. Their point of decussation is at the level of the brain stem where they terminate. For example, the fibers that terminate at the motor nuclei of the facial nerve (VII) decussate in the medulla, whereas fibers that terminate at the motor nuclei of the trigeminal nerve decussate in the pons. The cranial nerves for speech then exit the skull through small foramina and inner-vate the muscles of the face, lips, tongue, soft palate, pharynx, and larynx for the formation of sounds and words. Figure 2.20 shows a broad sketch of the pyramidal (direct) motor activation system.

The corticospinal and corticobulbar tracts have been further subdivided into **lower** and **upper motor neurons** (Duffy, 2005). This division is of clinical significance because of the varying symptoms associated with lower versus upper motor neuron damage.

The nerve fibers that originate in the cerebral cortex and descend to the ventral horns of the spinal cord and those that terminate at the cranial nerve nuclei in the brain stem are all considered upper motor neurons. This means that the upper motor neurons do not exit the neuraxis; they stay within the CNS (Bhatnagar, 2012; Duffy, 2005; Webb & Adler, 2007). Technically, upper motor neurons include the pathways of both the pyramidal and extrapyramidal systems. However, the term is most frequently used in reference to the mo-tor neurons of the pyramidal system.

The lower motor neurons include nerve fibers that in fact exit the neuraxis (brain or spinal cord) and communicate with the cranial and spinal nerves—peripheral nerves—for innervation of the muscles. By definition, the lower motor neurons are part of the periph-eral nervous system. The lower motor neurons are the final route by which centrally medi-ated neural impulses are communicated to the peripheral muscles. Lower motor neuron activity causes muscular movements.

Because the pyramidal tracts control discrete skilled movements, damage to this sys-tem causes a general weakness and slowness of movements, including movements of the

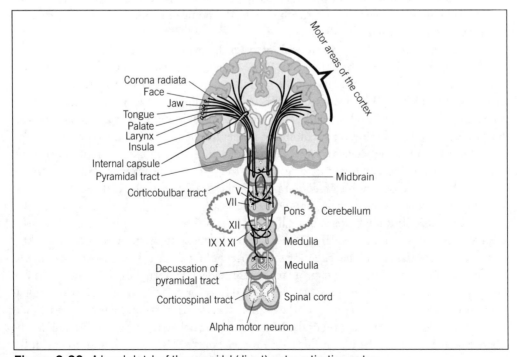

Figure 2.20. A broad sketch of the pyramidal (direct) motor activation system.

lips, the tongue, and the soft palate. The severity of symptoms may depend on whether the damage is limited to one side (unilateral) or affects both sides (bilateral) and whether the tracts of the extrapyramidal system also are involved. Patients are likely to show a mild form of articulation disorder, known as *unilateral upper motor neuron dysarthria*, if the damage is unilateral and limited to the upper motor neurons. However, the speech disorder may be more serious if both the pyramidal and extrapyramidal tracts are damaged, causing a form of dysarthria called *spastic dysarthria*. **Spasticity** is excessive tone of the muscles, resulting in muscle movements that are abrupt, jerky, rigid, slow, and labored; the head may be drawn back and rotated to one side of the body. Because of the involvement of both motor systems, patients may show slowness and weakness along with increased tone and associated motor disorders. See the Advanced Unit in Chapter 6 for details on various forms of dysarthria.

Extrapyramidal System

The **extrapyramidal system** is so named because its motor tracts are not part of the pyramidal system. The extrapyramidal system includes such *subcortical* nuclei as the basal ganglia, subthalamus, substantia nigra, red nucleus, and various pathways that interconnect them. The extrapyramidal system is an indirect activation system, as opposed to the pyramidal, which has a more direct connection with the lower motor neurons. It interacts with various motor systems in the nervous system before exerting an influence on the lower motor neurons. The indirect (extrapyramidal) system is shown in Figure 2.21.

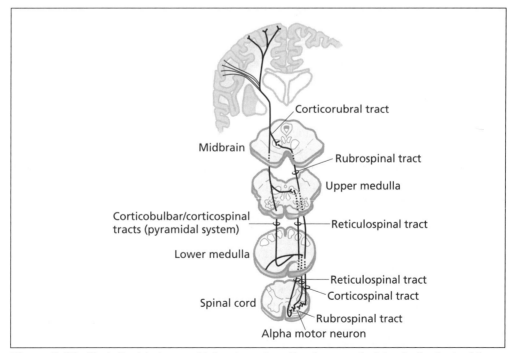

Figure 2.21. The indirect (extrapyramidal) motor system. Also shown are the intermingling tracts of the direct system (corticobulbar/corticospinal).

The neuronal activity of this motor system, like that of the pyramidal system, begins in the cerebral cortex and ultimately exerts an influence on the lower motor neurons. Note that the final result of the lower motor neurons is voluntary muscular movement. The extrapyramidal system helps regulate this movement and assists in the maintenance of posture and tone.

Even though the pathways of the extrapyramidal system are indirect, in contrast to the direct pathway of the pyramidal tract, the tracts of the two systems mingle at certain points, as shown in Figure 2.21; eventually, the nerve impulses from both systems take a common path to reach the muscles. The long axons of the corticospinal tract make only one synapse with the spinal nerves via the motor nuclei in the spinal cord. In the case of the corticobulbar tract, the synapse is with the cranial nerves via the cranial nerve nuclei at different levels of the brain stem. This type of connection is **monosynaptic.**

The extrapyramidal tract, on the other hand, is **polysynaptic.** It makes many synaptic connections before impulses reach the lower motor neuron to affect regulated and coordinated muscular movement. The effect of the extrapyramidal system on muscular movement is primarily **inhibitory** rather than **facilitatory,** as in the pyramidal (or direct) system.

Functionally, the pyramidal and extrapyramidal systems are difficult to separate. The separation is more clinical in nature because of the effect that each has on muscular movement. Damage to the pyramidal system results in different clinical symptoms, as compared to damage to the extrapyramidal system.

Because of the emergence of involuntary movements when the extrapyramidal system is damaged, it is assumed that this system (in normal conditions) regulates muscle tone, suppresses unnecessary movements, and reduces extraneous motor activity associated with automatic movements. It is also thought to regulate some coarse and stereotyped movements.

The motor disturbances of the extrapyramidal system are usually classified as "involuntary movement disorders." The most commonly used technical term for these movement disorders is *dyskinesia* (*dys* = "disorder," and *kinesis* = "movement"). *Hyperkinesia* is a form of dyskinesia characterized by too much or excessive movement, which can be slow or fast. *Hypokinesia* is too little movement or a limited range of movement. *Bradykinesia* is slow movements.

Several specific types of dyskinesias have been identified (Bhatnagar, 2012; Duffy, 2005). *Tremors*, for instance, are purposeless hyperkinetic movements that are rhythmic, oscillatory, and involuntary. Tremors in muscles at rest are found in **Parkinson's disease.** *Chorea* refers to quick, random, hyperkinetic movements that may also involve the speech muscles. *Hyperkinetic chorea* is a symptom of **Huntington's disease.** *Athetosis* is slow, irregular, coarse, writhing, or squirming movements, especially in the face, neck, and trunk. Such movements interfere with the fine and controlled movements of the tongue, larynx, soft palate, pharynx, and respiratory mechanism. *Dystonia* is characterized by slow, bizarre, and often writhing, twisting, and turning movements; dysarthria may result if the speech musculature is affected. *Myoclonus* is an abrupt, brief, almost lightning-like muscular contraction found most commonly in the limbs and trunk, but it may also occur in the facial, mandibular, lingual, and pharyngeal muscles. Finally, *orofacial dyskinesia*, or *tardive dyskinesia*, is characterized by bizarre movements limited to the mouth, face, jaw, and tongue. There is grimacing, pursing of the mouth and lips, and writhing of the tongue. These movements may affect articulation of speech.

It is important to note that medical professionals do not use the term *hypokinesia* to refer to the limitation in movement resulting from lesions of the pyramidal tract (upper and lower motor neuron system). The terms *hemiplegia*, *quadriplegia*, and *paraplegia* are used instead.

Theories of Speech Production

So far, we have considered various anatomic and neuroanatomic mechanisms necessary to produce speech. This advanced unit concludes with a brief account of theories that seek to explain how these mechanisms work to produce speech.

A **theory** is an explanation of a phenomenon. However, explanations of speech production are more like **models**, in that they envision a simplified and limited view of the phenomenon to understand it, while usually a scientific theory is more comprehensive. A phenomenon as complex as speech production may be broken down into its various components; a model then tries to represent aspects of these components. Models may be built with the help of computers. By inputting what they know about a phenomenon, scientists let the computer construct a model whose behavior may be changed by changing the input (assumptions) put into the computer. The model's output (behavior) may then be compared to human behavior. If, under analogous conditions, the model's behavior matches human behavior, the model is regarded as a good approximation to human behavior.

A **model** is essentially a theoretical attempt, albeit on a smaller or simplified scale. All speech production explanations, whether called theories or models, tend to include many assumptions, some testable, others not. Models tend to be even more speculative than theories. Nonetheless, most discussions of speech production theories often use the terms *models* and *theories* interchangeably; we do the same here.

To study a simplified aspect of speech production, several models take into consideration only one or two aspects of speech. One model may address only the breathing mechanism and the aerodynamics involved in speech production. Another may address only the phonatory system and phonetic speech production. Other models may include only the articulatory movements of the speech mechanism or only the vocal tract dynamics that shape the pharyngeal, oral, and nasal cavities. Some articulatory models may concentrate on timing of movements, others on spatial gestures inherent to articulation. Models concerned with feedback (**servosystem models**) of speech performance or **motor control mechanisms (schemes)** also have been popular. Still others address either how only consonants are produced or how only vowels are produced (Behrman, 2012; Raphael et al., 2011). There are plenty of hybrid models that include features from multiple models (Kent, Adams, & Turner, 1996; Raphael et al., 2011). There is no comprehensive, generally accepted theory that includes all speech production mechanisms and variables; a glaring omission in most, if not all, existing theories is the environmental variables that we do know affect speech production.

The multiple and contrasting models generally make similar assumptions about speech and face the same problems that need to be resolved (Kent, 1997). A fundamental assumption of linguists is that speech is a complex skill that contains many smaller structural elements that need to be put together in a rapid succession. All linguistic theories are essentially structural theories. For instance, most, if not all, linguists (including phonologists) who explain speech production assume that speech and language contain structures that need to be serially ordered. Phonemes, syllables, words, phrases, and sentences are the structural units of this serially ordered skill, which is executed with amazing rapidity.

Another assumption of structural theorists is that speech production is extremely complex because of the various neuroanatomic structures and neurophysiological functions that must be evoked to produce it. In teaching speech production, it is generally not possible to instruct a child to contract all the muscles, invoke all the processes (e.g., respiration, phonation, resonation, and articulation), select only the movements necessary from a wide range of possible movements, and combine and coordinate all the selected targets and movements. Therefore, linguists assume that there must be some basic and broad instruction that, when given, starts a complex chain of events resulting in speech.

A detailed description of the multiple theories (models) that try to explain how speech is produced is outside the scope of this chapter. For relatively simplified presentations, see other sources (Behrman, 2012; Hixon et al., 2013; Raphael et al., 2011). The purpose here is to sketch only the general outlines of selected models of speech production.

Feedback and Feedforward Models

Fairbanks's 1954 model of speech production is one of the oldest and the first of the closed-loop feedback models. Closed-loop machines receive feedback on their own performance and adjust further output, just as a thermostat does. Open-loop machines do not receive feedback and keep performing as programmed. In the 1950s, self-regulating feedback mechanisms were becoming widely used in mechanics, and many scientists began to apply such mechanical models to human behaviors. Very much like a machine capable of receiving feedback on its own performance, Fairbanks's speech production model included (1) a storage buffer, which holds in its memory the utterance to be produced; (2) a motor production control unit that can incite or regulate the respiratory, phonatory, articulatory, and resonatory mechanisms; (3) a feedback unit that receives auditory, tactile, and proprioceptive information; (4) a comparison input that receives information from the feedback unit; and (5) a mixing unit that receives error messages from the comparison unit. The feedback loop is completed when the mixer feeds error messages to the motor production unit for necessary adjustments (Fairbanks, 1954).

Accepted for many years, the feedback model is no longer considered valid because various kinds of feedback disruptions may not have significant negative effects on speech. (However, see the next section about a more recent theory that assigns some role to feedback; Abbs, 1996; Gracco, 1990.) For instance, speech production remains largely intact under a trigeminal nerve block, topical anesthesia, noise-induced auditory masking, and delayed auditory feedback (Kent, Martin, & Sufit, 1990). Feedback often may be slower than needed for speech production at the normal rate. Although feedback may play a role in correcting occasional errors in speech, it does not seem to play a major role in continuous speech production. Therefore, the conclusion is that there is no strong evidence to suggest that continuous feedback of any kind (e.g., auditory, proprioceptive, tactile) is essential to maintaining speech production; disruption in feedback of the kinds studied results in quick compensation by the speaker, thus reducing errors in speech production (Raphael et al.,

2011). Consequently, the model shifted to a *feedforward* concept. Some feedforward models include feedback as a component, however.

One feedforward model that includes feedback mechanisms is that of Gracco (1990), who postulated that (1) feedback of sensory information associated with speech production helps evaluate execution and intended articulation (speech goal) and (2) a feedforward mechanism helps make necessary adjustments in the system to better receive imminent signals. In essence, feedforward information better readies the peripheral speech systems to receive and execute speech movements so that the speech goals are achieved more efficiently than without such feedforward. In most feedforward models, the act of speaking involves making adjustments to the peripheral articulatory mechanism itself, not at the higher level of planning that would require a delayed response, because it has to wait for the production to take place, receive feedback, and then make changes. This theory, however, is subject to the same limitations as any other theory based on feedback; *feedforward* is even more speculative than feedback.

Acoustic Theory of Speech Production

A classic theory, the acoustic theory of speech production was proposed by Fant in 1960, based on international research on speech physiology. It is also known as the **source-filter theory** of speech production because of the two critical concepts that are its centerpiece: a *sound source* and a *resonating filter*. The larynx is the source of sound, and the supraglottal vocal tract is the resonator. As shown in Figure 2.8, the main resonating cavities include the pharyngeal, oral, and nasal (when coupled with the oral) cavities. In this theory and its various calculations of resonant frequencies of speech sounds (especially the vowels), the vocal tract is considered analogous to a tube with resonant properties. The tube is open at one end (the oral end, or the lips) and closed at the other (the glottal end) when the vocal folds approximate. In essence, closed vocal folds and various open mouth postures—as in the production of vowels—create a resonating tube. The speech sounds we hear are a product of both phonation at the level of the larynx and resonating modifications made by the supraglottal vocal tract. Because a resonator amplifies or diminishes selected frequencies, the resonating vocal tract is considered a *filter.*

The behavior of a resonator, or filter, is determined by its length and shape. The average adult male's vocal tract is about 17 cm long (Raphael et al., 2011). Movements of the tongue, lips, jaw, and velum change the shape of the human vocal tract. Therefore, the vocal tract is a resonator that is more dynamic than a musical instrument with fixed-size resonators. This dynamic resonator largely determines the *formants* (vocal tract resonances) of speech sounds. The first and lowest-frequency resonance has a wavelength four times the length of a tube closed at one end; this is the first formant (R1). First formants are largely determined by the size of the mouth opening in vowel production; the larger the mouth opening, the higher the frequency of R1. The second formant, which is three times the lowest resonant frequency (hence, 3R), is mostly determined by the size of the oral cavity; tongue movement, for example, will change the formant. The third formant, which is largely determined by the front versus back constriction of the vocal tract, is five times the lowest resonance (5R). It may be noticed that resonators that are closed at one end (e.g., the glottis) and open at the other (e.g., the lips) resonate only odd-numbered multiples of the lowest frequency; hence, we have R1, R3, and R5. These and other variables largely determine the quality of vowels that are finally heard by listeners.

This is an *acoustic* theory of speech production partly because the acoustic product (the speech that is produced and heard) *predicts* the features of the vocal tract that are necessary for that acoustic product to be realized; in other words, it is largely the characteristics of the vocal tract that determine the acoustic properties of speech sounds. Fant's measurements of the vocal tract cross-sectional area, the location of tongue constriction, and the degree of lip protrusions may be closely related to the different resonant characteristics of different vowel productions. To put it still differently, each vocal tract configuration (i.e., its shape and size) is closely correlated with the measured acoustic properties of specific speech sounds.

It is generally thought that the acoustic theory of speech better explains the production of vowels than the production of consonants (Hixon et al., 2013). Vowel and consonant productions have many similarities, including a source of sound and resonant modifications, an articulatory mechanism, and a common vocal tract with its many modifications. There are, however, important differences, too. While a single-tube (resonator) analogy is good for vowels, it is not good for all consonants. For example, production of nasal sounds is a two-tube resonant phenomenon (the coupled pharyngeal-oral and the nasal). Consequently, the acoustic result of such coupled (or *shunt*) tubes may be somewhat different from that of a single-tube resonator involved in vowel production. Moreover, the acoustic energy of vowels is at frequencies below 400 Hz, whereas the acoustic energy of some consonants (e.g., obstruents) is higher. Compared to consonants, vowels have wavelengths greater than the cross-sectional dimension of the vocal tract. While vowels have a single source of sound (the vocal folds), consonants have multiple sources (including friction noise created in the vocal tract). The source of vowels is complex periodic waves, whereas that of some consonants (e.g., obstruents again) have an aperiodic source (noise). Different classes of consonants evoke their own set of theoretical concepts; see other sources for details (Behrman, 2012; Hixon et al., 2013; Raphael et al., 2012).

Unlike many speculative models of speech production, the acoustic theory, especially as it is applied to vowel production, is based on empirical observations and measurements of physiological-phonetic features. It is based on well-supported physical phenomena (e.g., resonance). However, it is not clear whether it is a theory that *explains* speech production. It may very well describe how vowels are produced the way they are, with the acoustic properties they have, but may still not explain why people produce speech.

General Motor Program Models

A **motor program** specifies a sequence of movements to achieve a target response. In the present context, motor programs are prescribed and stored movement patterns necessary to produce various units or segments of speech; they may also be conceptualized as a set of neural commands that execute a pattern of movements involved in speech articulation (Behrman, 2012). The plan or program exists before the execution of speech, presumably stored in the brain. In producing speech, the speech system simply executes a ready-made plan of action (Kent et al., 1996). At each instance of an utterance, a program is invoked and speech is produced according to the pattern of movements stored in the program.

The construct of motor programs is thought to be essential in explaining speech production because online and continuous monitoring of speech would be too slow and inefficient a process; preexisting template-like programs may make it possible to produce utterances with the rapidity seen in normal speech production. Instead of initiating individual movements that form a sequence of sound (or word) production, a whole sequence may be invoked at once from an existing program. Generally, such motor programs are thought to involve an executive system (or level) that selects, organizes, and initiates complex sets of movements for particular instances of speech production and an effector system (or level) that helps perform the initiated motor plan through the actions of neuromuscular mechanisms (Behrman, 2012).

There are various versions of motor program models, some of which are free from feedback regulation of speech. These models postulate the existence of rigid programs that are not sensitive to sensory feedback on performance, because such feedback is unnecessary. Presumably, there would be no need for any corrections based on performance feedback. The programs contain detailed instructions on the movements necessary to produce speech. In essence, the programs are self-sufficient and need no experience or learning.

Other motor program models include a feedback mechanism because, without sensory feedback on how speech is being produced, errors in the execution of a motor program would not be corrected (Abbs, 1996; Gracco, 1990). Such models are a hybrid of motor program and feedback approaches to explaining speech production.

A broader view of motor programming requires the consideration of all central neural and peripheral neurophysiological systems involved in speech. Abbs (1996) suggests that speech generation requires the coordinated action of both the motor and sensory systems. Abbs presents a model that contains two mechanisms and a feedback unit. First, there are unobserved central mechanisms, which include the linguistic structure to be generated and a speech motor program unit. Second, there are indirectly observable peripheral mechanisms, which include the lower motor neuron pool and system response devices. The result of the actions of these two mechanisms is the speech movement output, which is mostly observable. Third, notwithstanding the criticism of the classic feedback models (e.g., Fairbanks's model), there is the afferent feedback mechanism, which feeds information on the movement output to the lower motor neuron pool, which communicates with the speech motor program, presumably resulting in adjustments or corrections.

Abbs (1996) cites evidence to show that when movements are interrupted (resulting in a motor output error), the primary motor cortex may be activated. Furthermore, when speech movements are physically interrupted (e.g., the movement of the jaw in producing bilabial sounds), compensatory actions result (e.g., greater movement of the lips to achieve closure). These observations suggest that the central motor system does monitor sensory inputs during speech and nonspeech movements.

Difficulties with motor program theories include the assumption of thousands of motor programs necessary to produce an infinite variety of utterances. Within the framework of cognitive theories, storing a vast number of motor programs would be challenging or impractical. Also, if all utterances are generated by existing motor templates, it would be difficult to produce novel utterances (Behrman, 2012). A more serious difficulty is that the motor programs are typically hypothesized but not directly tested or observed.

Connectionist and Spreading Activation Models

Students who have more than a casual interest in computers may have heard about *serial* and *parallel* processing. In computer language, serial processing involves a linear mechanism of handling information or instructions; one command is completed before another command is taken up for processing. Parallel processing, which is newer, is capable of simultaneous handling of multiple bits of information by mechanisms that exist in parallel. In parallel processing, also called *parallel distributed processing* (PDP), commands are processed and responded to in a faster manner than they are in serial processing. Some scientists believe that the basic concept of parallel processing applies to speech production. After all, speech requires quick processing of multiple kinds of information. To produce a sequence of sound patterns in as short a time as is evident, there must be parallel processing units that rapidly communicate with each other and thus efficiently produce an output (audible speech).

The speech production models that use the parallel processing concept are often described as *connectionist models.* Most connectionist models hypothesize the presence of information processing units that form an interconnected, close-knit network. How the information processing units are arranged depends on the particular model, as there are several connectionist models. The units may be arranged in layers or different configurations. This network is envisioned as a computational mechanism similar to what is found in computers. The network functions much like a computer program.

Kent et al. (1996) describe a typical connectionist system in which three kinds of units may be found: *output units, hidden units,* and *input units.* The system receives information from the input units. The hidden units help generate the output (speech) by creating an internal representation of what needs to be produced. It is thought that a direct connection between input and output units would create a system too simple to handle the complex skill of speech production. The task of generating much of the complex activity involved in speech production is assigned to the hidden units.

Units receive both excitatory and inhibitory signals. The *state* of a unit is the amount of activity or the signals it receives at any one time. Each unit also has a threshold of activity and carries a weight, which is roughly the memory capacity of a unit. The weight may be modified by experience. Feedback on performance helps modify the weight and threshold values of the units. The connectionist models are developed as an analogy to the central neural networks and the general working of the brain.

An extension of the connectionist model includes the assumption of spreading activation within the network of connected units. Dell (1986) postulated that in producing speech, all the features and syllables attached to a phoneme are automatically activated when that phoneme is activated. In other words, activation in one unit may spread to other relevant units, hence the term *spreading activation models.* Most assumptions of connectionist models are tested in *simulated* computer experiments.

Generally speaking, the connectionist models invoke speculative structures in the brain that are supposed to work like a computer's internal parts. All mechanical units are presumed to exist, but when some of them are presumed *hidden* somewhere, we have even more of an empirical problem of finding them.

Critical Evaluation of Speech Production Theories

Even a basic sketch of selected speech production models—such as the one attempted here—makes clear that much research needs to be done before a truly comprehensive understanding of speech production can emerge. Although speech scientists and experimental phoneticians have done much work on the behaviors of individual systems involved in speech (e.g., the laryngeal and the respiratory), an integrated view of speech production that takes into consideration all the peripheral and central neurophysiological systems is still lacking. The task is admittedly challenging because the parameters are many and each system is complex; when such complex systems work together, emergence of abstract organizational processes and additional complexities are inevitable (Abbs, 1996; Kent et al., 1996).

Most theories that seek to *explain* speech production are more speculative than those that try to *describe* it. For instance, the acoustic theory of vowel production describes how vowels are produced. The vocal tract dynamics, the resonating variables, the resulting acoustic properties are mostly measured and grounded in empirical observations. Consequently, we gain an understanding of the physiological process of producing vowels and the acoustic properties of what is produced with specific vocal tract configurations. However, the theory may fall short of explaining *why* vowels are produced. In fact, the larger question to be answered is: Why do people produce speech (and language)?

From a behavioral and clinical standpoint, two major problems in these and other such theories and models are evident. First, the models, except for the acoustic theory of speech production, are extremely mechanistic. Terms and assumptions of most models come from either the feedback mechanics of the pre-computer era or the information processors of the post-computer era. Fairbanks's (1954) thermostatic model of speech production included such mechanical units as *storage buffers, mixers, motor production control units, feedback control units,* and a *comparator.* The newer models add *production plants* and *feedforward controller units* to the list of presumed mechanical devices involved in speech production. Theories of this kind remind one of a speech production factory, set up on the lines of a food processing plant.

The motor programming models assume that the central nervous system has a program for actions, including speech production. Whether they are called *programs* or *schemata,* the assumption is that somehow plans are developed and stored somewhere in the brain. When the (generally unspecified) occasion for speech arises, the brain simply invokes the stored program or schema. Once again, the emphasis is on a mechanical process that initiates and ends an action according to the plan or schema.

Probably the most mechanistically speculative are the models based on computer processing of information. The idea that there is some limited and crude similarity between the architecture of computers and the architecture of the human brain has encouraged theorists to propose that the human brain works like a computer. Thus, we have *input units, output units, hidden units, serial processors,* and *parallel processors.* The mechanical devices that engineers have built into computers are imagined to exist in the brains of people.

Second, most speech production models ignore social and behavioral variables, without which audible and social speech production does not normally take place. That speech as a behavioral skill is acquired in social contexts does not seem to play any role in these models. Some models make room for experience or feedback, but such accommodations do not diminish the problem of ignored social and behavioral aspects of speech. Such accommodations are still a part of a mechanistic unit. Many models do not even adequately relate speech to language production (Kent et al., 1996). The models do not describe children learning to speak. Most models do not take into consideration such social-environmental and learning variables as (1) the stimulus conditions that prompt speech, (2) potential motivational variables that combine with stimulus conditions that lead to speech, (3) listeners' responses to speakers, (4) effects of listeners' responses on speech production, and (5) the interlocked interaction between listeners and speakers (Hegde, 2010c). Clinicians know that such listener–speaker interactions are the essence of communication, including speech production. A simplistic notion that there is a feedback unit that regulates speech production does not do justice to this complex pattern of social interaction.

Some theorists cite supportive evidence for their models generated through simulated computer experiments. But there is no assurance that this kind of evidence supports the existence of mechanical units postulated for human speech production. There are no independent warrants to support the model's assumed structures, processes, and units. Computer simulation may succeed in predicting speech patterns to some extent only because it is based on what is factually known about speech production. Most models of speech production are built on that knowledge; the assumptions fed into the computer to conduct a simulation experiment include what is known about speech production. It would be surprising if simulation experiments did not predict speech patterns that had been fed into the computer. That they do predict speech patterns is no evidence that structures similar to those in a computer exist in the brains of people. A related problem with computer analogies and simulations could be illustrated by the following quotation: "We leave it to the computer to learn what we have failed to understand. The computer might do the job but can it tell us how?" (Fant, 1989, p. 5).

In essence, in spite of the various limitations of models, the descriptions of speech production that they provide may appear plausible and may be the reason they survive. But there is no assurance that what they describe is how children and adults produce speech in social contexts. Progress may come when hypothetical and mechanical units are replaced with real neurophysiological variables coupled with environmental variables that are known to influence speech learning and production.

Summary of the Advanced Unit

- The human brain, weighing only about 3 pounds, controls all body functions.
- The nervous system is divided into the central and the peripheral nervous systems.
- Nerve cells, the most basic building blocks in the central nervous system, receive, transmit, and synthesize neural information.
- Each nerve cell consists of the cell body, several dendrites, and a single axon.

- Dendrites transmit impulses toward the cell body, while axons transmit impulses away from the cell body.

- Nerve cells communicate with one another at synaptic junctions by releasing neurotransmitters at such junctions.

- The brain is subdivided anatomically into five major components: cerebrum, basal ganglia, thalamus, cerebellum, and brain stem.

- The cerebrum is made up of two cerebral hemispheres, four primary lobes, and the cerebral cortex.

- The cerebral cortex houses several structures important for speech production, including the primary motor cortex, the supplementary motor cortex, Broca's area, Wernicke's area, and the primary auditory cortex.

- The basal ganglia are deep subcortical structures that play an important role in regulating the skilled motor movements necessary for speech.

- The cerebellum, while not initiating motor movements, helps monitor, regulate, and coordinate the speed, range, force, and strength of skilled motor movements, including speech.

- The brain stem is divided into the midbrain, pons, and medulla.

- Of the 12 pairs of cranial nerves, 7 are directly involved in speech production: trigeminal, facial, vestibuloacoustic, glossopharyngeal, accessory, vagus, and hypoglossal.

- The spinal nerves, which have a less direct role in speech production than the cranial nerves, supply several of the respiratory muscles, including the diaphragm, abdominals, and internal and external intercostals.

- Clinically, the central nervous system is often divided into the pyramidal, extrapyramidal, and cerebellar systems.

- The pyramidal system is a direct motor activation pathway; the extrapyramidal system is an indirect motor pathway.

- Some models of speech production (e.g., the laryngeal and the respiratory system) concentrate on individual systems of speech; others try to give a more comprehensive view of speech production.

- Feedback and feedforward models, the acoustic theory of speech production, motor program models, and connectionist and spreading activation models are among the conceptual and theoretical attempts seeking explanations of speech production.

- Most models of speech are mechanistic, involving many speculative mechanisms and processes, many borrowed from computer science. Neither linguistic nor phonetic theories generally address the social and behavioral variables that at least partly explain why people talk.

PHONETICS, PHONOLOGY, AND SPEECH SOUND DISORDERS

An educated southerner has no use for an r except at the beginning of a word.
—*Mark Twain,* Life on the Mississippi

Basic Unit: Basic Perspectives in Articulation and Phonology

Speech is a form of verbal behavior or verbal communication. Topographically, speech is a complex combination of sounds that help form words and sentences. Linguists, phoneticians, and phonologists study the ways sounds are produced, organized into observable or abstract patterns, and combined to form words in different languages. Speech–language pathologists (SLPs) have borrowed this information to study, analyze, diagnose, and treat speech sound disorders.

In this Basic Unit, we will address various aspects of sound production. For some readers, part of the information presented here will be a review of previous study, while other components may be more or less new. For those who do not have a background in the subject matter, the information is presented in a manner that is easy to follow and simple to integrate. This unit offers an overview of the following: (1) phonetics and speech sound disorders (SSDs), (2) dynamics of speech production, (3) phoneme classification systems, (4) the relation between phonetics and phonology, (5) SSDs in the natural linear phonological theory, and (6) SSDs in nonlinear phonological theories.

To preserve the simplicity of this unit, more technical and theoretical information will be addressed in the Advanced Unit of this chapter. Varied phonological theories will be introduced, and their clinical implications will be evaluated. The clinician's role in applying and testing theories advanced by linguists and theoretical phonologists will be considered.

Phonetics and Speech Sound Disorders

Phonetics is the study of physical, physiological, and acoustic variables associated with speech sound production. For an SLP, knowledge of phonetics is essential to make the most basic analysis of speech sounds and their disorders. To understand what happens when a sound is produced in error, one needs to know how sounds are typically produced; this information comes from phonetics.

Because different professionals are interested in answering different questions about sound production, several branches have evolved within phonetics, including (1) historical phonetics, (2) experimental phonetics, (3) articulatory or physiological phonetics, (4) acoustic phonetics, (5) perceptual phonetics, and (6) clinical or applied phonetics (Edwards, 2003; Shriberg & Kent, 2013; Small, 2012).

Historical phonetics is the study of how sounds change over time. No language's sounds are static, although they may seem so at any point in time. The way sounds are produced changes over time; new sounds may emerge, while some old sounds may disappear due to lack of use.

Experimental phonetics is the study of speech sound production; it analyzes physiological movements and acoustic properties with the help of laboratory instruments. One method developed by experimental phoneticians is speech synthesis, or the generation of speech-like sounds by a computer.

Articulatory, or physiological, phonetics concentrates on how a speaker produces speech sounds. The vocal tract and related anatomical structures are studied extensively to describe how the physiological systems work to produce speech sounds.

Acoustic phonetics is the study of the properties of sound waves as they travel from the vocal tract of a speaker to the ear of a listener. Related to the physics of sound, acoustic phonetics studies sound waves as generated by the vocal mechanism and articulated by the speaker.

Perceptual phonetics is the study of the judgments listeners make of the speech sounds they hear. This branch of phonetics makes an analysis of loudness, pitch, duration, and quality of speech sounds as perceived (judged) by listeners.

Finally, as the name implies, **clinical, or applied, phonetics** is the branch dedicated to practical application of the knowledge derived from experimental, articulatory, acoustic, and perceptual phonetics. A major concern of clinical phonetics is the study of speech disorders.

It is beyond the scope of this Basic Unit to expand on the very detailed information offered by the many branches of phonetic study. Rather, because students at this level would be expected to have gained this information in a phonetics course, our review will be limited to the aspects of phonetics essential in understanding the study of speech sound learning and speech sound disorders.

Phonemes and Allophones

The term *phonetics* is derived from the word *phone*, which is a generic term for any sound that can be produced by the vocal tract; a phone may or may not be a speech sound. However, in the study of speech production, a phone is typically considered a single speech sound. A **phoneme** is a family of phones or sounds perceived to belong to the same category by the listener. No speaker produces a phoneme in a single, static, invariable manner. From one instance to another, the same speaker may produce the same phoneme with slight variations. Different speakers also may produce the same phoneme differently. Therefore, a phoneme is defined as a group of sounds, each with subtle variations.

A variant or alternate form of a phoneme within a language is called an **allophone.** An allophone is a member of a particular phoneme family, not a distinct phoneme. Therefore, allophones do not change the meaning of a word. For example, in the word *tea*, the sound *t* in some contexts may be produced with tongue contact against the alveolar ridge, whereas in another context, it may be produced with a more forward contact against the upper front teeth, but in both cases, it is the word *tea* that is being produced. In the sentence "He has tea," the sound *t* may be produced with lingual-alveolar contact because the sound preceding the *t*, (/z/) is also produced with lingual-alveolar contact. However, in the sentence "I loathe tea," the *t* sound is produced with a more lingual-dental contact because the preceding /ð/ is produced **interdentally.** Such varied productions of a phoneme are **allophonic variations.** The occurrence of allophones is the direct result of the phonetic contexts that surround a phoneme. Try producing the two sentences interchangeably, and you will notice (feel) the subtle difference. The effects of phonetic context on phoneme articulation, causing such sound variations, is described later in this chapter under the heading "Dynamics of Speech Production."

Allophonic variations of a single phoneme may occur in free variation or complementary distribution. Allophones occur in **free variation** when they *can* be exchanged for one another in a certain phonetic context without affecting the word. In American English, allophones of /t/ can occur in free variation in word-final position. For example, in the word *bat*, the /t/ may be released with a small burst of air, or it may be unreleased if the tongue remains in position for a few seconds. The released production is transcribed [bætʰ], while the unreleased production of the same word is transcribed [bæt̚]. The diacritical markers [ʰ] and [̚] symbolize the aspirated and unreleased productions of a sound, respectively.

Some allophonic variants occur in specific places but not in others. Such allophones are said to be in **complementary distribution** because they *cannot* be exchanged for one another in specific phonetic contexts. For example, in American English /t/ has various allophonic variations that are context specific. In word-initial positions, /t/ is made with an aspirated release. However, when it is part of an /s/ cluster, it is unaspirated. The words *top* and *stop* would be transcribed [tʰap̚] and [st̚ap̚] if using **narrow phonetic transcription.** The use of narrow phonetic transcription helps to highlight the aspirated and unreleased allophonic variations of /t/ in the two words. That allophonic variants are in complementary distribution does not mean that if exchanged in certain phonetic contexts, the meaning of words would be affected. For example, if *top* is produced as [t̚ap̚] instead of [tʰap̚], the word may sound nonstandard, but the meaning remains unaffected (the listener will react the same). Such allophonic exchanges are not uncommon in people learning English as a second language or in children and adults using a nonmainstream dialect of American English.

Phonemes make a difference in morphemes. A **morpheme** is the minimal unit of meaning, the smallest unit of language carrying semantic interpretation. A **free morpheme** is a whole word that cannot be linguistically broken down into smaller units. **Bound morphemes** are word endings (suffixes) or beginnings (prefixes) that attach to a word (a free morpheme) to alter the meaning of that word. Although phonemes do not have any meaning in and of themselves, they can make a distinction between words such as *bit, sit, lit,* and *bit.* These words are all free morphemes and are contrasted by only one phoneme. Morphemes that are similar except for one phoneme are called **minimal pairs.** Using such minimal pairs, it can be determined whether a sound is a phoneme in a given language. For example, we know that *t* and *d* are two distinct phonemes in American English because they contrast word pairs such as *tie-die* and *ten-den*. The study of these sound differences in a language is called **phonemics** (Shriberg & Kent, 2013).

ACTIVITY

Define the following terms in your own words: *allophone, morpheme, bound morpheme, free morpheme, minimal pairs, phone, phoneme.*

Phonetic Transcription

The description of phonetics offered earlier included *written symbols* that represent sounds. In the study of sound production, speech–language pathology has adopted the symbols of the **International Phonetic Alphabet** (IPA) to represent the many phonemes of the English language.

The IPA was created in 1888 and was most recently revised in 2005. It was developed because orthographic spelling does not always represent how a sound is pronounced, thus creating confusion among professionals. For example, the /f/ in mainstream American English may be represented by the orthographic symbols "f" (*f*at), "ff" (pu*ff*iness), "ph" (*ph*ysician), or "gh" (lau*gh*ter). The different letters and letter combinations that can be used to represent the same phonemes are known as **allographs** (Shriberg & Kent, 2013).

To further complicate matters, any one allograph can represent different sounds and can also be silent. For example, the letter combination "*gh*" represents both the *f* sound in the word lau*gh*ter and the *g* sound in the word *gh*ost, and in the word si*gh*t it is silent. And we wonder why people learning English as a second language have difficulty mastering written English!

Speech–language pathologists generally use the symbols of the IPA to transcribe sound production. This allows for a consistent and mutually agreed upon system that decreases the confusion created by allographic variations. All students in speech–language pathology should be proficient in the use of the sound-symbol association of the IPA.

ACTIVITY

Transcribe the following orthographically written words using the phonetic symbols of the International Phonetic Alphabet: *computer, medicine, exercise, international, jogging, phonetics, vase, laughter, nose, program.*

The idealized or abstract description of a sound is transcribed according to the IPA and enclosed between slash marks or **virgules**, as in /t/. This is called **phonemic transcription** because the variations in actual phoneme production are not depicted. The sounds that are actually produced by an individual are transcribed and placed between brackets as in [t]; this is known as **phonetic transcription.** In most contexts, the word *phonetic* should be understood as an actual production of a speech sound by a speaker.

Brackets alone, however, fail to indicate exactly how a sound is produced. Therefore, the phonetic symbols enclosed by brackets may sometimes be further modified by special symbols called **diacritical markers.** For example, a dentalized production of /t/ would be transcribed as [t̪]. The mark placed under the [t̪] is the IPA symbol indicating the dentalized production of a phoneme. This detailed form of transcription is **narrow phonetic transcription**, as opposed to **broad phonetic transcription.**

Table 3.1 lists the phonetic symbols for the 25 American English consonants, 14 American English vowels, and 6 American English diphthongs and several orthographically written key words. Table 3.2 lists several diacritic markers believed to be important for our discussion as we proceed.

The broad phonetic transcription made possible by the standard IPA symbols may not be fully adequate to transcribe the varieties of speech sound errors children produce. IPA symbols are categorical, whereas the errors may be found on a continuum from fully correct to totally incorrect and something in between. Therefore, clinicians may need to do a narrow phonetic transcription with additional symbols that capture the different types of errors. Also, one may need some nonphonetic symbols or devices to characterize specific types of errors that fall in between the two extremes of correct/incorrect or those that sound somewhat in between two different sounds. See the Basic Unit of Chapter 6 under the heading "Limitations of Phonetic Transcription."

Dynamics of Speech Production

A comprehensive understanding of speech sound disorders requires a knowledge of the neuroanatomic and physiologic variables described in Chapter 2, as well as the basics of speech science, including the aerodynamic, acoustic, and suprasegmental aspects of speech production. Understanding how speech sounds change in connected speech in a phenomenon known as coarticulation is also needed (Behrman, 2012; Bhatnagar, 2012; Seikel, Drumright, & Seikel, 2014; Raphael et al., 2011). Assuming familiarity of these matters, we list the main terms for a quick review.

Aerodynamic Aspects of Speech Production

As a person begins to speak, a system of physiological valves effect changes in the volume and pressure of air flowing out of the lungs. The vibrations of the vocal folds, coupling and uncoupling of the nasal and oral cavities by the velopharyngeal mechanism, the constrictions of the oral cavity, and opening and closing of the lips modify the sound stream and help produce different kinds of speech sounds, as well as creating a variety of resonatory effects.

The subglottic air pressure increases when the vocal folds close, and the increased pressure then blows the vocal folds apart. Lip closure causes increased air pressure in the oral cavity, as well. Such a buildup of air pressure in the mouth helps produce various consonants, especially the pressure consonants, which include voiceless stops and fricatives. A puff of air forced out of the mouth may be articulated into such speech sounds as voiceless stops (e.g., /p/, /t/, and /k/). Incidentally, intraoral air pressure is greater in children than in adults.

Vocal fold vibration is necessary to produce voiced stops and fricatives. The vocal folds only approximate (do not fully close) and vibrate to produce voiced sounds. Voiced sounds are produced with less intraoral air pressure than voiceless sounds because only approximated folds allow loss of air pressure.

Table 3.1

PHONETIC SYMBOLS FOR ENGLISH CONSONANTS, VOWELS, AND DIPHTHONGS

Phonetic Symbol	Sample Allographic Representations	Phonetic Symbol	Sample Allographic Representations
Consonants		/j/	yellow, hallelujah, opinion
/b/	baby, rabbit	/r/	rabbit, marry, write, rhyme, Peace Corps
/p/	pan, pepper, hiccough	/l/	ladder, ball, island, funnel
/d/	do, ladder, begged, should	**Vowels**	
/t/	top, attack, talked, doubt, receipt, Thomas	/ɑ/	father, bought, mocking
/g/	get, egg, guest, ghost, vague	/æ/	cat, blast, jack, family
/k/	kitchen, actor, accustom, chemistry, boutique	/e/	mate, lake, vacation, relay
/m/	moon, hammer, tomb, phleghm, hymn, psalm	/ɛ/	better, elephant, exit, explain
/n/	not, dinner, know, gnat, pneumonia, mnemonic	/o/	boat, most, toast, tote
/ŋ/	bring, ink, tongue, anxious	/ɔ/	poor, caught, fawn, fought, want
/z/	zoo, buzzer, xylophone, his, asthma	/u/	moon, suitcase, true
/s/	say, assassin, psychiatrist, listen, cent	/i/	heat, piece, meek
/v/	valentine, savvy, wife's, Stephen	/ɪ/	pig, mitt, jingle, igloo
/f/	fan, affair, tough, telephone, half	/ʊ/	cook, put, rookie
/ð/	that, bathe	/ɚ/	batter, joker, color, maker
/θ/	tooth, thin	/ɝ/	purple, bird, dirty
/ʒ/	measure, azure, garage	/ə/	untie, extra
/ʃ/	ship, sugar, chef, mission, location	/ʌ/	cup, under, up, butter
/h/	hop, who	**Diphthongs**	
/dʒ/	job, judge, marriage, gem, exaggerate	/ai/	pipe, my, might, rite
/tʃ/	church, kitchen, nature, cello	/au/	cow, house, town, pout
/w/	when, win, one, quest, choir	/ɔu/	toil, boy, moist, loiter
/ʍ/	which, white (dialectical variations)	/je/	united, used, few, beautiful
		/ei/	vacation, take, face
		/ou/	loan, throne, phone

Table 3.2

DIACRITIC MARKERS AND PHONETIC SYMBOLS FOR SELECTED NON-ENGLISH SOUNDS

Diacritic Markers		Phonetic Symbols for Non-English Sounds	
[ˌ]	syllabic consonant	[ř]	voice alveolar trill
[˳]	partially devoiced	[χ]	voiceless velar fricative
[˯]	partially voiced	[ɣ]	voiced velar fricative
[..]	breathy	[ɸ]	voiceless bilabial fricative
[ʰ]	aspirated	[β]	voiced bilabial fricative
[⁼]	unaspirated	[ɲ]	palatal nasal
[˺]	unreleased	[λ]	palatal lateral approximant
[ ]	dentalized	[ʕ̃]	voiced pharyngeal stop
[˰]	lateralized	[ʕ̣]	unvoiced pharyngeal stop
[˜]	nasalized	[Δ]	posterior nasal fricative
[⃰]	nasal emission	[ʔ̥]	voiced mid-dorsum palatal stop
[͂]	denasalized	[3]	voiceless mid-dorsum palatal stop
[ˀ]	rounded vowel		
[ˤ]	unrounded vowel		
[͜]	labialized consonant		
[͝]	nonlabialized consonant		
[·]	lengthened		
[˃]	shortened		
[ˌ]	whistled		

Nasal sounds need only a minimal amount of intraoral air pressure, vocal fold vibration, and constricted oral cavity, as in the production of voiced stops. The velopharyngeal port is open to let the vibrating sound pass through the nasal cavity, adding nasal resonance.

Intraoral air pressure also is minimal for vowel productions, but the oral cavity is more open. English vowels, unless they are preceded or succeeded by a nasal consonant, do not have noticeable nasal resonance. Liquids and glides are articulated in a similar manner.

Several neural and physiological pathologies negatively affect the flow and pressure of air used to produce speech. For example, paralyzed vocal folds cannot approximate to build sufficient subglottic air pressure, causing excessive air leakage and resulting in a breathy voice. Similarly, inadequate velopharyngeal mechanism in clefts of the soft palate may cause undesirable nasal resonance in the production of oral sounds.

Acoustic Aspects of Speech

A branch of physics, **acoustics** is the scientific study of sound as a physical phenomenon. A physical force sets an object into vibration, which in turn creates waves of disturbance in the molecules of such elastic media as gases, liquids, and solid objects. The media then transmit the vibrations. Vocal folds vibrate to produce sound; the air molecules in the laryngeal, pharyngeal, nasal, and oral cavities transmit the sound. The laryngeal sound is also modified and articulated into speech sounds. All sounds, including speech sounds, are acoustic signals, with such physical properties as frequency, amplitude, and duration.

Frequency is the rate at which an object vibrates, measured in terms of the number of vibrations per unit of time, typically per second. A sound may be of a single frequency that repeats itself (**pure tone**) or a combination of different frequencies (**complex tones**), as found in speech sounds. The vibrations that constitute a complex tone may be **periodic** (with a pattern that repeats itself) or **aperiodic** (lacking a pattern). The **spectrum** of a sound describes a pattern of physical energy across a frequency range. Different speech sounds have different *spectra* that help us distinguish one sound from the other.

The frequency of vocal fold vibrations determines the **pitch** of speech sounds. English vowels, liquids, and glides have a range of low to mid frequencies; their pitch is in the same range. Nasals are in the low-frequency range. Strident fricatives and affricates (e.g., /s/, /z/, /ʃ/, and /tʃ/) are produced with high frequency, whereas stops as a class are produced within a wide range of frequency. The frequency range for alveolars is mid to high; for velars, it is mid range; and for bilabials, it is low.

Amplitude, or **intensity**, is the magnitude of vibration of a sound source. Greater magnitude means higher amplitude and greater loudness of sound as heard. Vowels are the most intense speech sounds. Among vowels, the low vowels are more intense than high vowels. Glides and liquids, though not as intense as vowels, are more intense than other classes of sounds. Strident fricatives, affricates, and nasals are of moderate intensity, whereas stops and nonstrident fricatives are among the least loud.

Duration is a measure of time during which vibrations are sustained. Speech sounds are sustained for relatively brief durations. Vowels have the longest duration of all speech sounds; some vowels may be as long as half a second, whereas others do not exceed 50 msec. Glides and liquids are of short to moderate duration, although the glides /w/ and /j/ are generally longer than the liquids /l/ and /r/. Strident fricatives and affricates have a moderate duration, whereas nonstrident fricatives have a short to moderate duration. Stridents are longer than other consonants, and fricatives are longer than affricates. Nasal sounds have short to moderate duration, whereas stop sounds have the shortest duration of all speech sounds.

Suprasegmental Aspects of Speech

Segmentals are consonants and vowels. Properties of speech associated with words, phrases, sentences, and continuous speech are **suprasegmentals,** also known as *prosodic features*. They include *pitch, stress, rate of speech*, and *juncture*.

Pitch is the variable sensory experience due to differing frequency of vocal fold vibration. Related to suprasegmentals, such falling and rising pitch variations in speech suggest differences in meaning. An utterance such as "She ate ten hamburgers," if produced with a falling intonation, means that it is a statement of observation, but the same utterance with a rising pitch may be a question. A mere analysis of the meaning of the words and the syntactic structure will not reveal which is the case. Pitch contours are described as the melody of a phrase, and changes in pitch contours are known as **intonation**. The emotional state of the speaker, the stress pattern employed, and the tongue position assumed in producing vowels determine the pitch contour. Generally, high vowels have a higher fundamental frequency (higher pitch). English is not a tonal language, and, therefore, words and syllables themselves are not produced with varying pitch levels to signal differences in meaning. In a tonal language, a single word produced with different pitches means different things.

Phonetic **stress** gives prominence to certain syllables within a sequence of syllables; it is a suprasegmental feature that works at the level of syllables. Within a syllable, the vowel segment is primarily stressed. In spoken English, higher pitch, longer vowel duration, and increased intensity, in that order, are important in producing stressed syllables (Fry, 1965). Stress also helps distinguish noun and verb forms of the same word. For example, the noun *convict* is produced with primary stress on the first syllable, whereas the verb *convict* is produced with stress on the second. The word *object* may mean "to protest" (verb) or "thing" (noun), depending on which syllable is stressed. When the stress shifts to the second syllable to indicate a verb, the first syllable is reduced to a schwa [ə]; therefore, stress affects articulation of specific sounds.

A form of stress that helps contrast two or more possibilities while emphasizing one of them is known as **contrastive stress.** A speaker who says, "Give me that *blue* pen," with an emphasis on the italicized word uses this type of contrastive stress. Different stress patterns create characteristic rhythms that are unique to languages, giving rise to a classification of languages into **stress-timed languages** (e.g., English, German, Russian, and Arabic), in which stressed syllables tend to be produced at regular intervals, and **syllable-timed languages** (e.g., French, Italian, Greek, Spanish, Turkish, and Hindi), in which syllables—not necessarily stress syllables—tend to be produced at regular intervals.

The numbers of words, syllables, or phonemes produced per second are the alternate measures of the **rate of speech.** Relatively faster or slower rates affect the prosodic features (suprasegmentals) of speech. Individuals differ in their rate of speech; generally, intelligibility may be lost to some extent as the rate increases. Increased speech rate may eliminate pauses in speech and decrease the duration of vowels and such longer consonants as fricatives. Reduction in the vowel duration is particularly striking in faster speech. For instance, the vowels /i/ and /e/ are reduced to /ɪ/, which may be further reduced to /ə/. Many other vowels also tend to be reduced to the schwa. In addition, some articulatory positions that are sustained at a normal or slower rate are missed at faster rates. Omitting certain articulatory positions while speaking faster than normal is called *undershooting*. The rate of articulation has clinical implications. In treating most speech disorders, a slower rate may be necessary. Speech rate is a major aspect of prosody. Speech at slower rates tends to be monotonous, softer, more deliberate, and less spontaneous.

Juncture helps make semantic or grammatical distinctions in speech and includes brief pauses in speech. Pauses help keep different grammatical clauses separate, so that the meaning of an utterance is not confused. For instance, "John, [pause] let us do it" is a request to John, whereas "John let us do it" is a statement of fact. Pauses also may be used to make lexical (semantic) distinctions. For instance, "greenhouse" is clearly different from "green house" because of the pause that splits the compound word into two separate words, signaling different meanings. Junctures may also involve pitch variations, which may be combined with brief pauses in speech. For instance, the pitch contour for "John" may be different (higher) in "John, let us do it" than in "John let us do it." A brief pause in speech may help draw listeners' attention.

Coarticulation of Speech Sounds

In connected speech, sounds are produced in words, and the words may be produced as a single utterance or as part of continuous speech. **Citation form** refers to an isolated and deliberate production of a word (or a phrase); the same word is produced somewhat differently in **connected speech**, because the individual sounds are then articulated differently. For example, in its citation form, /ð/ in the word "them" may be distinctly produced. But in such a phrase as "Catch them," the /ð/ may be reduced to "əm" as in [kætʃəm]. The change in this example is due to the difficulty in quickly moving from the voiceless /tʃ/ to the voiced /ð/. This illustrates **coarticulation**, which is the influence that sounds have on one another when linked together to make words, phrases, and sentences. In coarticulation, sounds may change or overlap (Small, 2012); slower and more deliberate speech may show fewer effects of coarticulation than more rapid or hurried speech.

A sound is affected by its **phonetic contexts**, especially by those sounds that immediately precede or follow it. Coarticulation changes the articulatory gestures themselves, resulting in allophonic variations of a phoneme. The same sound—for example, /k/—may be produced in a more forward position in the mouth while saying "kiss" but in a more backward position while saying "could," due to the influence of the following vowel in each of those two words. The lips may be more rounded in producing /s/ in the word "soup" but not so rounded in saying the word "sink." Another example is the production of /t/ in the words *tin* and *took*. In "tin," /t/ is followed by a front vowel and consonant, while in "took," it is followed by two back sounds. When producing "tin," the /t/ is made at the alveolar ridge, which is the textbook-defined point of constriction for that sound. However, the /t/ in "took" is produced with a slightly more retracted tongue position because of the back vowel and consonant that follow it. Regardless, the /t/ in both words is heard as /t/; the slightly different productions of the same sound in the two words are allophonic variations that do not affect the meaning.

Some phoneticians (MacKay, 1987) distinguish the terms *assimilation* and *coarticulation*. Others use them synonymously (Ohde & Sharf, 1992). If defined differently, **assimilation** results in a sound different from the target sound, as in *pomputer* for *computer*. It will be discussed further under the section on phonological patterns (processes). **Coarticulation,** on the other hand, results in an *allophonic variation* of the same sound.

Inventory of Sounds

Although a phoneme produced in isolation may not mean anything, it helps create meaningful words when combined with other phonemes. Phonemes also create meaningful contrasts in word pairs like *pop-mop, bat-fat,* and *shake-take* **(minimal pairs).** Therefore, phonemic contrasts have the potential to produce different morphemes and words. Each language has an inventory of sounds that its speakers learn to produce, and thus it becomes a part of their language repertoire.

While some phonemes are shared across languages, others are unique to a particular language. Reportedly, there are about 100 total phonemes used in the languages of the world (Shriberg & Kent, 2013). American English includes 24 consonants, 14 vowels, and 6 diphthongs. Several allophonic variations result from this large phonemic inventory, which help create the many **dialects** of American English. See Chapter 5 for more on ethnocultural and dialectical variations of English.

Morphophonemics

Morphophonemic rules specify how sounds are combined to form morphemes (meaningful units of a language). Free morphemes may be combined with bound morphemes (small elements of grammar that do not mean much when produced by themselves; e.g., the plural s morpheme). Sound alterations that result from the modification of free morphemes (e.g., words that can stand alone and still be meaningful) are called **morphophonemics.**

In American English there is a voicing morphophonemic rule according to which the English regular plural inflection /s/ is produced as /s/ if the word ends in a voiceless sound (e.g., *cups* and *hats*), but it is produced as /z/ if the word ends in a voiced sound (e.g., *dogz, bægz*). Similar rules apply to the regular past tense inflections, the possessive bound morpheme, and the regular third-person present tense.

Phonotactics

Phonotactic rules specify what combinations of sounds are possible or common in specific languages. Each language has phonotactic rules to combine speech sounds.

English words, for example, cannot be initiated with /ɛs + stop/ clusters, whereas Spanish has many words that begin with such clusters, such as "escuela [ɛskwɛla]" and "estoy [ɛstoi]." In English, the /ŋ/ sound can occur in the final and medial position of words but not in the initial position; the /b/ and /g/ sounds cannot be combined to initiate or terminate words.

Phoneme Classification

English phonemes are divided into two main categories: consonants and vowels. **Consonants** are phonemes produced by some narrowing or closing of the vocal tract. The closure may be complete, as in the production of /b/ and /k/, or partial, as in the formation of sounds like /f/ and /l/. Consonants produced in side-by-side combination are termed **clusters.** American English has a large set of **prevocalic** (before-vowel) and **postvocalic** (after-vowel) consonant clusters. The words *tree, break,* and *street* all contain prevocalic clusters, while *park, best,* and *help* have postvocalic clusters.

Unlike consonants, **vowels** are produced with a relatively open vocal tract configuration. In the production of vowels, the tongue does not make contact with any specific articulator for closure as it does with consonants. Vowels are further subdivided into simple vowels, pure vowels, and diphthongs. Pure vowels are also termed **monophthongs** (meaning *"single sounds"*), and they constitute most of the vowel system of American English (Lowe, 2012; Small, 2012). The terms *pure vowels* and *monophthongs* suggest a single articulatory position needed to produce them. **Diphthongs** (meaning *"two sounds"*) are made by the quick gliding of two simple vowels, so that they cannot be perceptually separated, as in the words *toy* and *bye*. Production of diphthongs needs two articulatory positions. Compared to pure vowels, diphthongs make up a much smaller set of sounds in American English.

Vowels and diphthongs are the carriers of syllables, while consonants and consonant clusters attach to vowels to form various syllable shapes. Because of their syllable-forming status, **vowels are also termed syllabics.** A few English consonants also can take on a syllabic nature, meaning that they can also form the nucleus for a syllable. These consonant syllabics include /m/, /n/, /l/, and /r/. The special diacritic marker /ˌ/ is used to differentiate the consonantal versus the syllabic property of these sounds. Following are examples of words containing these sounds as consonants and syllabics:

Sound	Consonant Property	Syllabic Property
/m/	/mæn/, /ləmɛnt/	/prizm̩/
/n/	/nɛkst/, /æntik/	/bʌtn̩/
/l/	/læmp/, /əlon/	/æpl̩/
/r/	/red/, /əraund/	/æftr̩/

Whereas vowels actually form a syllable or syllables in a word, consonants serve to initiate a syllable, terminate a syllable, or initiate *and* terminate a syllable. A syllable that ends in a vowel or diphthong is **open,** while one that ends in a consonant is **closed.** Such words as *my, key,* and *blue* are examples of open syllables; *stop, make,* and *took* are closed syllables.

Depending on how consonants and vowels are combined, various syllable shapes can be formed. Languages across the world have different sequencing rules dictating how consonants and vowels can be combined to form syllable shapes.

Consonants that precede a vowel are **prevocalic;** those that occur between vowels are **intervocalic;** and those that follow a vowel are **postvocalic.** Other terms used to describe the position of a sound are **initial, medial,** and **final.** *Initial* refers to a sound that is located at the beginning of a word, and *medial* and *final* denote sounds that are produced in the middle and at the end of a word, respectively. The terms are most commonly used in clinical practice.

The terms *initial* and *final* can be used to denote the position of sounds in both words and syllables. A sound may occur in the initial position of a syllable but not necessarily in the initial position of the word. For example, in the word "de-tec-tive," the first *t* is in the *medial* position of the word but in the *initial* position of the second syllable. The same is true for sounds in the final position. Sounds in syllable-initial and syllable-final positions are also termed syllable **releasing** and **arresting** sounds, respectively. Sounds that initiate a syllable are said to release the syllable, while those that terminate a syllable are said to arrest the syllable (Shriberg & Kent, 2013).

We have made several references to **syllables.** But what exactly is a syllable? Many of us can probably remember as children having to identify the number of syllables in words, a skill known as **syllabification.** In fact, the literature has shown that most first graders can correctly identify the number of syllables in a word (Owens, 2005). That most children and adults can accurately identify the number of syllables in words does not mean that they can define the term *syllable.*

We noted earlier that vowels are syllabics. That is because vowels alone can form words (e.g., *eye, awe, you*). Consonants alone cannot form syllables or words; consonants need vowels to form syllables or words. Therefore, vowels are the **nucleus** of syllables. In addition to a nucleus, a syllable also has an **onset** and a **coda.** *Nucleus* and *coda* are collectively known as **rhyme** (Gussmann, 2002; Yavas, 1998).

The *onset* component of a syllable is the consonant or consonant cluster that initiates it, while the rhyme is the remaining part. Within the rhyme, the vowel or diphthong that follows the initial consonant or cluster is the *nucleus.* The consonant or consonant cluster that follows the *nucleus* makes up the *coda.* For example, in the word *break,* the cluster *br* is the onset, the diphthong *ea* is the nucleus, and the final *k* is the coda. Together, the diphthong *ea* and the final *k* make up the rhyme. In American English, neither the onset nor the coda component is obligatory, since many words start or end with a vowel (e.g., *egg, in, act, see, you,* and *blue*).

Multisyllable words may have more than one onset, nucleus, and coda. Some may have more than one coda, while others may not contain a coda at all. The first syllable in a multisyllabic word may or may not have an onset. To illustrate this point, we will use the words *backpack, tomorrow,* and *entire.* The word *backpack* consists of two syllables: *back* and *pack.* Each of these syllables contains an onset, a nucleus, and a coda. The word *tomorrow* consists of three syllables: *to, mo,* and *rrow.* Each of its syllables has an onset and a nucleus, but there is no coda in *tomorrow,* because neither of its syllables ends in a consonant or consonant cluster. It should be noted that the *w* in the syllable *rrow* is only an orthographic consonant. Phonetically, the syllable ends in the vowel /o/. The word *entire* has two syllables: *en* and *tire.* The syllable *en* begins with the nucleus *e* and ends with the coda *n.* The syllable *tire* has an onset, a nucleus, and a coda.

....

ACTIVITY

Identify the onset, nucleus, and rhyme for each syllable in the following words: *joke* (1 syll), *today* (2 syll), *fun* (1 syll), *glasses* (2 syll), *art* (1 syll).

....

Consonant Production

Consonants have been traditionally described according to manner, place, and voicing dimensions. **Manner of articulation** indicates *how* the airstream that passes through the vocal tract is modified to form a consonant. **Place of articulation** indicates *where* along the vocal tract a constriction is formed to produce the consonant. **Voice** indicates *whether* the vocal folds are vibrating during the consonant's production. Table 3.3 represents the English consonants by place, manner, and voicing features.

Manner of Articulation

Classification of English consonants based on the manner of articulation yields the following categories: *stops, fricatives, affricates, nasals, glides,* and *liquids.* In the following descriptions, take note of the main feature of manner of articulation: different ways in which the airstream is modified to produce the different categories of sounds.

STOPS.

Stop consonants are formed by complete closure of the vocal tract at some point, so that the airflow ceases, or stops, and air pressure builds up behind the point of closure. The air pressure thus built up eventually is released and may produce a short burst of noise. Because of this audible burst of noise, stop consonants are also called stop plosives (*plosives* referring to the explosion of air upon its release), although the plosive phase does not occur in the production of all stop sounds or in all word positions. For example, many stop sounds in word-final position are unreleased and, thus, are not plosive in nature.

English stop consonants include /p/, /b/, /t/, /d/, /k/, and /g/. Although these sounds all share the same manner of production, they are produced in different places along the vocal tract. The airstream may be stopped by bilabial, alveolar, or velar closure—referring to the three places where closure may occur.

How Are Stops Produced?

1. A complete closure within the oral cavity to briefly stop airflow is the main mechanism by which stops are produced.

2. The obstructed stream of air and the built-up air pressure in the oral cavity are then suddenly released, resulting in a burst of noise.

3. Movements involved in producing stops are rapid, and the duration is short.

FRICATIVES.

Fricative sounds are so termed because of their hissing or turbulent quality, which results from the continuous forcing of air through a narrow constriction. Although all fricatives are noisy, the intensity of the noise depends on the sound's place of articulation. The fricatives are /s/, /z/, /f/, /v/, /θ/, /ð/, /ʃ/, /tʃ/, /ʒ/, and /ʤ/.

How Are Fricatives Produced?

1. Formation of a narrow or constricted channel through which air is forced is the main mechanism for producing fricatives.

Table 3.3

MANNER, PLACE, AND VOICING FEATURES OF ENGLISH CONSONANTS

Phoneme	Voicing	Manner	Place
/b/	voiced	stop	bilabial
/p/	voiceless	stop	bilabial
/d/	voiced	stop	alveolar
/t/	voiceless	stop	alveolar
/g/	voiced	stop	velar
/k/	voiceless	stop	velar
/m/	voiced	nasal	bilabial
/n/	voiced	nasal	alveolar
/ŋ/	voiced	nasal	velar
/z/	voiced	fricative	alveolar
/s/	voiceless	fricative	alveolar
/v/	voiced	fricative	labiodental
/f/	voiceless	fricative	labiodental
/ð/	voiced	fricative	linguadental
/θ/	voiceless	fricative	linguadental
/ʒ/	voiced	fricative	palatal
/ʃ/	voiceless	fricative	palatal
/h/	voiceless	fricative	glottal
/ʤ/	voiced	affricate	palatal
/tʃ/	voiceless	affricate	palatal
/w/	voiced	glide	velar/bilabial
/ʍ/	voiceless	fricative	glottal/bilabial
/j/	voiced	glide	palatal
/r/	voiced	liquid, rhotic	palatal
/l/	voiced	liquid, lateral	alveolar

2. The air that flows through the constricted space produces a frication noise.

3. The velopharyngeal port is closed during the production of fricatives.

AFFRICATES.

Affricate sounds have a stop and a fricative component. Although these sounds begin as stops, they are released as fricatives. There are only two affricates in the English language: /tʃ/ and /dʒ/.

How Are Affricates Produced?

1. The quick release of an obstructed airstream is the main mechanism for producing affricates.

2. The velopharyngeal port is closed during the production of affricates.

NASALS.

Nasals are produced by lowering the velum so that the velopharyngeal port is opened. Opening of the velopharyngeal port allows air vibrated by the vocal cords to enter the nasal cavity; this adds a nasal resonance to the consonants so produced. Only three consonants in English are produced with nasal resonance: /m/, /n/, and /ŋ/. However, in connected speech, oral sounds may become nasalized when they are surrounded by nasal sounds. For example, the vowel /æ/ in the word *cat* is fully resonated in the oral cavity, but in the word *man* it is nasalized because of the preceding and following nasal sounds. If you alternate between producing *cat* and *man*, while paying close attention to the vowel in the two words, you will notice the subtle difference.

How Are Nasals Produced?

1. A closed oral tract and an open velopharyngeal port are the main features of nasal sound production; nasals are produced like stops.

2. When the velopharyngeal port is open, nasal resonance is possible even if the oral closure is inadequate.

GLIDES.

Glides, also known as **semivowels**, are produced by a quick transitioning of the articulators as they move from a partly constricted state to a more open state for the vowel that follows. Glides are formed by a relatively unrestricted and transitory point of constriction in comparison to other consonants, particularly stops, fricatives, and affricates. Only two English sounds are glides: /w/ and /j/.

How Are Glides Produced?

1. A gliding motion of the articulators with a closed velopharyngeal port is the main feature of glide production.

2. Although constricted, the oral cavity is more open than during the production of consonants.

3. Glides are produced more like diphthongs.

Try saying the words *went* and *yam*, and you will notice the gradual gliding property as you progress from the glide consonant to the following vowel. You may also notice the more open point of constriction. Although some phoneticians consider /l/ and /r/ as glides, those are more commonly termed liquids.

LIQUIDS.

Unlike terms such as *stops* and *glides*, which suggest how certain sounds are produced, the term *liquid* bears no relation to how the two English liquids—/l/ and /r/—are produced. **Liquids** are sounds that are similar to glides and are often described as semivowels. Although their individual productions vary, /l/ and /r/ are both made with a vocal tract that is obstructed only slightly more than for vowels. Thus, these sounds are sometimes considered vowel-like consonants. The /l/ is also called a **lateral** because during its production the lateral, midsection part of the tongue is open, and air is thus directed through the sides of the tongue. The /r/, also termed **rhotic,** may be produced in various ways. Two of the most common ways are by (1) curling the tongue tip back slightly, so that it approximates but does not touch the alveolar ridge or palatal area, and (2) bunching or humping the tongue in the palatal area. An /r/ made by curling the tongue tip back is called a **retroflex** /r/, while one made by bunching and elevating the blade portion of the tongue is known as a **bunched** or **humped** /r/. The terms *lateral* and *rhotic* will be explained further in the section "Distinctive Features" below.

How Are Liquids Produced?

1. A closed velopharynx and a sustainable oral articulatory posture are the essence of producing liquids.

2. Though constricted, the oral passage is wider than it is during the production of other consonants.

Place of Articulation

As noted, place of articulation refers to the location in the vocal tract of the point of constriction (contact) for specific sounds. Note that this classification system considers the relationship between the primary articulators (e.g., the lips, teeth, tongue, and palates) that help shape the sounds. The following categories of English consonants are based on their place of contact (articulation): **bilabial, labiodental, linguadental (interdental), lingua-alveolar (alveolar), linguapalatal (palatal), linguavelar (velar),** and **glottal.**

The previously described manner of production is not sufficient for the identification of specific sounds. To help differentiate one sound from another, it is necessary to consider their place of articulation. For example, although /p/, /t/, and /k/ all share the same manner of production, they are made with different points of constriction. What follows is a description of English sounds according to their place of articulation, progressing from front to back.

BILABIALS.

These sounds are produced by pressing the two lips together, thus the term **bilabial**. The stops /b/ and /p/ and the nasal /m/ make up the bilabial sound class. The glide /w/ is also considered a bilabial, but it is not made by pressing the two lips together. Rather, /w/ is made by rounding the lips, while the tongue dorsum elevates toward the velum. Thus, /w/ is frequently categorized under two places of articulation, bilabial and **velar** (discussed later).

LABIODENTALS.

These sounds are formed by placing the lower edge of the upper incisors (teeth) on the upper portion of the lower lip. The contact between the upper incisors and the lower lip is very light, forming a narrow point of constriction. Only two English consonants, /f/ and /v/, are made with labiodental contact; they are both fricatives.

LINGUADENTALS.

Also termed **interdental**, linguadentals are made by protruding the tip of the tongue slightly between the cutting edges of the upper and lower front teeth. This forms a narrow constriction from which airflow is directed. For obvious reasons, the point of contact between the tongue and the teeth is light. Only two fricative consonants are linguadentals: /θ/ and /ð/.

LINGUA-ALVEOLARS (ALVEOLARS).

These sounds are produced by articulation of the tongue and the alveolar ridge and include /t/, /d/, /s/, /z/, /l/, and /n/. Although the tip of the tongue is raised, so that it makes contact with the alveolar ridge for all of these sounds, the type of contact varies according to the sound's manner of articulation.

For the stops /t/ and /d/, the tip of the tongue is placed firmly against the alveolar ridge, so that it completely impedes the flow of air for a short period of time. To produce the fricatives /s/ and /z/, the tip of the tongue is placed against the alveolar ridge, so that a narrow constriction is formed. This narrow constriction is shaped by a midline groove of the tongue that serves as a passageway for the escaping air.

The liquid lateral /l/ is produced by light contact of the tongue tip against the alveolar ridge for midline closure and lateral opening at both sides of the mouth. The air escapes through this lateral opening. Finally, /n/ is formed similarly to /t/ and /d/ in terms of place of articulation, with firm contact of the tongue tip against the alveolar ridge. The important distinction between the stops /t/ and /d/ and the nasal /n/ is their resonance. While /t/ and /d/ are fully resonated in the oral cavity, /n/ is produced with an open velopharyngeal port for nasal resonance.

LINGUAPALATALS (PALATALS).

Placement of the tongue blade against the hard palate forms the point of constriction for these sounds. The point of contact on the hard palate is typically just posterior to the alveolar ridge. The fricatives /ʃ/ and /ʒ/, the affricates /dʒ/ and /tʃ/, the liquid /r/, and the glide /j/ make up the palatal class according to place of articulation. The difference between these sounds is their manner of articulation. The consonants /ʃ/ and /ʒ/ are fricatives made with an intense noise, while /dʒ/ and /tʃ/ are affricates made with a stop and fricative component. The /r/ is a liquid, and /j/ is a glide.

LINGUAVELARS (VELARS).

Elevation of the tongue dorsum against the soft palate (velum) is the main feature of these sounds. The /k/, /g/, and /ŋ/ sounds form the velar class. Some definitions of velars include /w/ in this sound class because, as it is produced, the tongue elevates toward the soft palate. While /k/, /g/, and /ŋ/ are made with firm contact of the tongue against the velum, in the production of /w/ the tongue merely approximates the soft palate. The manner of production for these sounds varies: /k/ and /g/ are stops, /ŋ/ is a nasal, and /w/ is a glide.

GLOTTALS.
These are sounds made at the level of the glottis. In mainstream American English, /h/ is the only glottal consonant that has a phonemic property. Although the glottal stop [ʔ] is not a distinct phoneme of American English, it may occur as an allophonic variation of some stops in connected speech (Edwards, 2003). Words such as *button* [bʌʔn] and *cotton* [kaʔn̩] demonstrate the use of [ʔ] as an allophone of /t/. In this case, [ʔ] is an allophone and not a phoneme because it does not create a contrast in meaning. In other words, the meaning of *button* remains constant whether it is pronounced [bʌʔn] or [bʌtn]. The same is true for *cotton*. The glottal stop /ʔ/ is phonemic in some languages, such as Danish and Arabic (Edwards, 2003). Children with cleft palate speech often produce a glottal stop instead of **pressure consonants,** which include stops and fricatives.

Voicing

Voicing refers to the vibration of the vocal folds in the production of sounds. Sounds that are made while the vocal folds are vibrating are **voiced sounds,** and those made in the absence of vocal fold vibration are **unvoiced** or **voiceless sounds.** The voiced consonants of American English are /b/, /d/, /g/, /z/, /v/, /ð/, /ʒ/, /ʤ/, /m/, /n/, /ŋ/, /l/, /r/, /w/, and /j/. The voiceless sounds are /p/, /t/, /k/, /s/, /f/, /θ/, /ʃ/, /ʧ/, and /h/. Some sounds are identical in their manner of production and place of articulation and differ only in the voicing feature. These are known as **cognate pairs.** The cognate pairs of American English are /p-b/, /t-d/, /k-g/, /s-z/, /f-v/, /θ-ð/, /ʃ-ʒ/, and /ʧ-ʤ/.

Consonant Clusters

Consonants can be produced as singletons (alone) or in side-by-side combination with other consonants to form clusters. Consonant clusters occur in prevocalic and postvocalic word positions. American English contains many two- and three-member clusters, plus a few four-member clusters in the final position of words. Although the definition for clusters is not consistent from one source to another, we will use the term in reference to the contiguous combination of consonant sounds that precedes or follows a vowel within the same syllable. Consonant clusters are also known as **blends.** As with singleton consonants, clusters attach to vowels to create various syllable shapes. Table 3.4 shows examples of several clusters that occur in American English; several key words have been provided for each.

Distinctive Features

An alternative way of describing phonemes is by their distinctive features (Chomsky & Halle, 1968; Jakobson, Fant, & Halle, 1952; Jakobson & Halle, 1956). A **distinctive feature is an articulatory or acoustic parameter that according to its presence or absence helps define a phoneme.** Each phoneme is classified according to a cluster of distinctive features that are either present or absent.

Chomsky and Halle (1968) developed what is now a classic **binary system by which a phoneme (a consonant or vowel) is given a plus (+) value if a feature is present or a minus (–) value if the feature is absent.** An example of a distinctive feature is *round*, which refers to lip rounding in producing /r/ and /w/. Phonemes may share certain features, but each phoneme has a unique set of features that distinguishes it from all other phonemes. While

Table 3.4

SOME SYLLABLE-INITIATING AND SYLLABLE-TERMINATING CLUSTERS OF AMERICAN ENGLISH AND ALLOGRAPHIC REPRESENTATIONS

Consonant Cluster	Sample Allographic Representations	Consonant Cluster	Sample Allographic Representations
Syllable-Initiating		Syllable-Terminating	
kw-	quick, queen, quack, quantity	-mp	ramp, lamp, stomp
tw-	tweezers, twist, twang, twenty	-nt	ant, pleasant, count, plant
sw-	swim, sweat, swap, sweeten	-nd	hand, bend, fond, blind
pl-	play, plan, plastic, place	-ns	prince, cleanse
kl-	clown, clock, clap, clean	-rd	hard, guard, chard, lord
fl-	flag, flick, flounder, flack	-nz	lens, plans, buns
bl-	black, blast, blink, Blake	-ks	parks, lacks, plaques
gl-	glasses, gloat, glimpse, glad	-st	past, best, post, nest
sl-	slide, slap, slender, sleep	-kt	act, fact, deduct, induct
pr-	prize, present, practical, prepare	-ld	held, mold, peeled
br-	brown, brag, brain, bring	-rt	art, fort, mart, sort
tr-	truck, tree, train, trap	-ts	bets, mats, ports
dr-	drive, drink, drastic, dramatic	-rn	barn, torn, warn, horn
fr-	front, frog, frost, French	-rm	arm, farm, alarm, charm
ɵr-	through, threat, thrive	-lb	bulb
kr-	crown, crop, create, creep	-lp	pulp, help, gulp
gr-	green, gray, grass, gripe	-lt	halt, malt, fault
st-	stop, steel, steak, stork	-lf	self, golf, shelf
sp-	spot, sport, speak, Spanish	-lk	elk, milk
sk-	school, scar, score, Scott	-rst	burst, first
sn-	snake, snow, sniff, snack	-zd	buzzed, blazed
sm-	small, smile, smack, smudge	-rk	park, mark, fork
nj-	news, newsworthy, newcomer	-mz	arms, aims, stems
fj-	few, fugitive, fumes, future	-lz	balls, malls, steals
kj-	cute, coupon, accused	-gz	bugs, pegs

Table 3.4 (*continued*)

Consonant Cluster	Sample Allographic Representations	Consonant Cluster	Sample Allographic Representations
	Syllable-Initiating		Syllable-Terminating
mj-	music, amused, musician	-pt	opt, stopped, dropped
ʃr-	shrink, shriek, shrine	-ft	left, stuffed, lift
str-	stray, street, strong, strange	-rf	scarf
skw-	squander, squat, squint	-rv	starve, carve, swerve
spl-	splash, splendor, splint	-mpt	stomped, stamped
spr-	spray, sprint, sprinkle	-mps	lamps, cramps, blimps
skr-	scram, scream, screech	-nts	ants, pants, prints
		-ngz	strings
		-ngk	thank, bank, frank
		-ndz	hands, grounds

some phonemes vary by a large number of features, others may differ by only one or two features. For example, /s/ and /z/ share all the same distinctive features with the exception of voicing; /s/ has a (–) voice feature, and /z/ has a (+) voice feature.

Table 3.5 lists the distinctive features of English consonants according to Chomsky and Halle's binary system. Although this system initially appears different from the more traditional analysis of manner, place, and voicing (M-P-V), the two systems share various similarities. Although the terms may be somewhat different, most distinctive features have manner-place-voicing counterparts. For example, the distinctive features *strident* and *continuant* can be equated with the traditional phonetic term *fricative*, and the distinctive feature *interrupted* is comparable to the more traditional term *stop*.

Clinical application of the classic distinctive feature theory has faded since the onset of phonological theories and their applications in speech sound disorders. Nonetheless, it is important to understand the distinctive feature analysis because most of its features are now a part of the nonlinear phonological theories being advocated to SLPs; see under a later heading, "Speech Sound Disorders in Nonlinear Phonological Theories." For details, readers could consult Chomsky and Halle's original work and such clinical application studies as those by McReynolds and Engmann (1975) and McReynolds and Bennett (1992).

The 16 sets of binary features listed in Table 3.5 may be briefly described as follows:

1. **Vocalic.** Sounds made with no marked vocal tract constriction. All vowels are vocalic, but only the /l/ and /r/ consonants have this feature.

2. **Consonantal.** Sounds that have a marked constriction along the midline region of the vocal tract. Contrary to the traditional classification, Chomsky

Table 3.5

DISTINCTIVE FEATURES FOR CONSONANTS OF AMERICAN ENGLISH

Features	p	b	t	d	k	g	f	v	s	z	ʃ	ʒ	tʃ	dʒ	θ	ð	h	m	n	ŋ	l	r	w	j
Vocalic	−	−	−	−	−	−	−	−	−	−	−	−	−	−	−	−	−	−	−	−	+	+	−	−
Consonantal	+	+	+	+	+	+	+	+	+	+	+	+	+	+	+	+	+	−	+	+	+	+	−	−
High	−	−	−	−	+	+	−	−	−	−	+	+	+	+	−	−	−	−	−	+	−	−	+	+
Back	−	−	−	−	+	+	−	−	−	−	−	−	−	−	−	−	−	−	−	+	−	−	+	−
Low	−	−	−	−	−	−	−	−	−	−	−	−	−	−	−	−	+	−	−	−	−	−	−	−
Anterior	+	+	+	+	−	−	+	+	+	+	−	−	−	−	+	+	−	+	+	−	+	−	+	−
Coronal	−	−	+	+	−	−	−	−	+	+	+	+	+	+	+	+	−	−	+	−	+	+	−	−
Round	−	−	−	−	−	−	−	−	−	−	−	−	−	−	−	−	−	−	−	−	−	+	+	−
Tense	+	−	+	−	+	−	+	−	+	−	+	−	+	−	+	−	+	−	−	−	+	−	−	−
Continuant	−	−	−	−	−	−	+	+	+	+	+	+	−	−	+	+	+	−	−	−	+	+	+	+
Nasal	−	−	−	−	−	−	−	−	−	−	−	−	−	−	−	−	−	+	+	+	−	−	−	−
Strident	−	−	−	−	−	−	+	+	+	+	+	+	+	+	−	−	−	−	−	−	−	−	−	−
Sonorant	−	−	−	−	−	−	−	−	−	−	−	−	−	−	−	−	−	+	+	+	+	+	+	+
Interrupted	+	+	+	+	+	+	−	−	−	−	−	−	+	+	−	−	−	−	−	−	−	−	−	−
Lateral	−	−	−	−	−	−	−	−	−	−	−	−	−	−	−	−	−	−	−	−	+	−	−	−
Voiced	−	+	−	+	−	+	−	+	−	+	−	+	−	+	−	+	−	+	+	+	+	+	+	+

Note. From *The Sound Pattern of English,* by N. Chomsky and M. Halle, 1968, New York: Harper & Row.

and Halle rate /h/, /w/, and /j/ as (−) consonantal (not consonants). The remaining consonants have a (+) consonantal feature.

3. **High.** Sounds made with the tongue elevated above the neutral position required for the production of /ə/.

4. **Back.** Sounds made with the tongue retracted from the neutral position required for the production of /ə/.

5. **Low.** Sounds made with the tongue lowered from the neutral position of /ə/.

6. **Anterior.** Sounds made with a point of constriction located farther forward than that of the palatal /ʃ/.

7. **Coronal.** Sounds made with the tongue blade raised above the neutral position required for the production of /ə/.

8. **Round.** Sounds made with the lips rounded or protruded.

9. **Tense.** Sounds made with a relatively greater degree of muscle tension or contraction at the root of the tongue.

10. **Continuant.** Sounds made with an incomplete point of constriction. The flow of air is not entirely stopped at any point.

11. **Nasal.** Sounds that are resonated in the nasal cavity.

12. **Strident.** Sounds made by forcing the airstream through a small opening, resulting in the production of intense noise.

13. **Sonorant.** Sounds made by allowing the airstream to pass relatively unimpeded through the oral or nasal cavity.

14. **Interrupted.** Sounds produced by complete blockage of the airstream at their point of constriction.

15. **Lateral.** Sound made by placing the front of the tongue against the alveolar ridge (midline closure) and lowering the midsection of the tongue on both sides (lateral opening).

16. **Voice.** Sound produced with vibration of the vocal folds.

ACTIVITY

Identify the distinctive features of the following phonemes: /p/, /v/, /n/.

Other distinctive features that may be clinically useful include obstruent, sibilant, approximant, rhotic, and syllabic. Consonants that are made with a complete closure or narrow constriction of the oral cavity, so that the airstream is stopped or friction noise is produced, are collectively termed **obstruents;** these include the stops, fricatives, and affricates. **Sibilant** sounds are high-frequency sounds that have a more strident quality and longer duration than most other consonants. Sibilants include the fricatives and affricates /s/, /z/, /ʃ/, /ʒ/, /tʃ/, and /dʒ/. Glides and liquids are sometimes called **approximants** because of the approximating nature of the contact between the two articulators that help form them. Although they are certainly produced by the approximation of two articulators, the degree of contact is not nearly as closed as with stops, fricatives, and affricates (Ohde & Sharf, 1992). A sound with /r/ coloring is sometimes termed **rhotic;** this term may be used for the /r/ consonant and its various allophonic variations. Finally, **syllabics** are sounds that serve as a nucleus for a syllable; all vowels are syllabics, while most consonants are not. The consonants that can take on a syllabic property include the nasals /m/ and /n/ and the liquids /l/ and /r/.

Vowel Production

Tongue Position, Lip Rounding, and Tenseness Features

Vowel articulation is described according to (1) the position of the tongue, (2) the shape of the pharynx, (3) the shape of the lips, and (4) the muscular tension associated with vowel production. Unlike consonants, vowels are not characterized by the voicing feature, as all English vowels are voiced, unless whispered.

These features help distinguish all English vowels. A slight difference—in tongue height, for example—can create an important linguistic distinction between two sounds (e.g., /I/ and /i/). Word pairs like *bit-beat*, *mitt-meat*, and *fit-feet* vary by only one sound—their vowel. The vowel distinction can make the difference between a sentence that is logical (e.g., "I used my new mitt during last night's baseball game") and one that does not make much sense (e.g., "I used my new meat during last night's baseball game").

TONGUE POSITION AND SHAPE OF PHARYNX.

Two major tongue positions are tongue height (*high, mid,* or *low*) and tongue advancement (*front, central,* or *back*). High vowels are produced in the highest position possible, with the tongue close to the roof of the mouth. Low vowels, on the other hand, are produced with the tongue depressed in the mouth. Those in between the high and low dimensions are mid vowels. Tongue advancement or retraction for vowels is determined by comparing their production with the highest-front vowel /i/, the lowest-front vowel /æ/, the highest-back vowel /u/, and the lowest-back vowel /ɑ/. A **vowel quadrant** defines the four extreme points of vowel production: *high, low, front,* and *back.* This four-sided figure, with /i/, /u/, /æ/, and /ɑ/ at its extreme corners, has been used to categorize the production of all vowels into seven general categories according to tongue position: high-front, mid-front, low-front, mid-central, high-back, mid-back, and low-back.

- **High-front vowels: /i/ and /I/.** The /i/ is produced with the tongue in the highest and most forward position compared to other English vowels; /I/ is produced with the tongue in a slightly lower and more posterior position than /i/.

- **Mid-front vowels: /e/ and /ɛ/.** The /e/ is produced lower than the position required for the high vowels and slightly back from the position required for /I/. Some phoneticians call /ɛ/ a low-mid-front vowel (Ohde & Sharf, 1992).

- **Low-front vowel: /æ/.** Only the /æ/ is a low-front vowel, one of the lowest vowels in English. It is produced with the tongue lower and more posterior from the position required for /ɛ/.

- **Mid-central vowels: /ɝ/, /ɚ/, /ə/, and /ʌ/.** Although these are all mid-central, their place of production varies from one to another. The /ɝ/ is typically produced with the blade of the tongue bunched and raised toward the hard palate; the tongue height is about equal to that of /e/ and /I/, and it is retracted toward /o/. The /ɚ/ vowel, sometimes called a **schwa,** has the same point of production in the oral cavity as /ɝ/; however, in transcription it is used to represent the production of /ɝ/ in unstressed syllables—for example, in *barber* and *color* (Ohde & Sharf, 1992). The third mid-central vowel, /ə/, is made with the tongue lowered in relation to /ɝ/. This vowel is also known as an **unstressed schwa,** since it also occurs in unstressed syllables. The stressed counterpart of schwa is the /ʌ/ vowel. It is produced in a position close to /ə/, but the tongue is slightly more retracted toward /ɑ/.

- **High-back vowels: /u/ and /ʊ/.** The /u/ vowel is produced in the highest and most retracted position when compared to all English vowels, as in the words *soon, moon, blue.* The other high-back vowel, /ʊ/, is produced slightly lower and more forward than /u/ (Ohde & Sharf, 1992).

- **Mid-back vowels: /o/ and /ɔ/.** The /o/ vowel is produced slightly lower in the oral cavity in comparison to /u/. In relation to /o/, the /ɔ/ vowel has a slightly lower point of production.

- **Low-back vowel: /ɑ/.** The /ɑ/ vowel has the lowest and most retracted point of production of all vowels.

The *front-to-back* dimension of the position of the tongue has a direct effect on the **shape of the pharynx.** When the tongue is carried in a more forward position, the pharynx is enlarged, while a posterior placement of the tongue narrows the pharyngeal cavity. The different pharyngeal dimensions that result from varying tongue placement create the unique resonance characteristics of each vowel.

LIP ROUNDING.

The shape of the lips during the production of vowels may be described in terms of rounding. Vowels that are produced with the lips somewhat protruded, such as in the words *who*, *cook*, and *boat*, are categorized as **rounded.** Vowels that are produced with the lips in a more neutral or retracted position, as in the words *bet*, *hat*, *hot*, and *hey*, are called **unrounded.** Sometimes more descriptive terms, including *rounding, protrusion, retraction, spreading, eversion*, and *narrowing*, are used in reference to lip configuration (Shriberg & Kent, 2013). However, the terms *rounded* and *unrounded* are by far the most common, and the vowels in the two categories are as follows:

- **Rounded vowels:** /u/, *moon;* /ʊ/, *cook;* /o/, *boat;* /ɔ/, *caught;* /ɝ/, *bird*
- **Unrounded vowels:** /i/, *meet;* /I/, *bit;* /e/, *bake;* /ɛ/, *met;* /æ/, *hat;* /ɑ/, *pot;* /ɚ/, *butter;* /ə/, *untie;* /ʌ/, *up*

As shown in the examples, only the back vowels and the central vowel /ɝ/ are rounded, while all the front vowels and the central vowels /ɚ/, /ə/, and /ʌ/ are unrounded. Some phoneticians also categorize /ɝ/ as unrounded (Ohde & Sharf, 1992).

TENSENESS.

Although the exact level of muscular tension associated with vowels has not been experimentally confirmed (Shriberg & Kent, 2013), the terms **tense** and **lax** are often used to describe their production. Theoretically, the tense vowels are longer in duration and are produced with a higher degree of muscular tension, while the lax vowels are shorter and require less muscular effort. Shriberg and Kent (2013) suggest that the distinction *long-short* might be more appropriate, since some vowels are almost always short and others are almost always long. They also indicate that this dimension can be identified more easily under experimental conditions.

Tense vowels include /i/, /e/, /u/, /o/, /ɔ/, and /ɝ/. The lax vowels include /I/, /ɛ/, /æ/, /ʊ/, /ɑ/, /ɚ/, /ə/, and /ʌ/. Tense or long vowels can occur in open syllables—for example, *he, bay, Sue, toe*—and closed syllables—for example, *heat, bait, boot, bird*. Lax or short vowels can appear in stressed closed syllables—for example, *bit, bet, bat, book, pot, cup*—but not in stressed open syllables.

Distinctive Features of Vowels

As with consonants, vowels also may be described in terms of their distinctive features. Chomsky and Halle's (1968) binary +/– system for consonant production has also been applied to vowels. The following distinctive features have been used to describe vowels:

- *Vocalic*—sounds made without a marked constriction in the vocal tract. The level of constriction is not more than what is necessary for the production of /i/ and /u/. All vowels are vocalic.

- *Consonantal*—sounds made with a marked constriction along the midline region of the vocal tract. No vowels are consonantal.

- *Sonorant*—sounds produced as the airstream passes relatively unimpeded through the oral or nasal cavity. All vowels are sonorant.

- *Rhotic*—sounds made with an /r/ coloring. The mid-central vowels /ɜ/ and /ɚ/ are the only two vowels sharing the rhotic feature.

- *High*—sounds made with the tongue elevated above the neutral position required for the production of /ə/. The /i/, /I/, /u/, and /ʊ/ are all high vowels.

- *Low*—sounds made with the tongue lowered for the neutral position of /ə/. Only /æ/ and /ɑ/ share this distinctive feature.

- *Front*—sounds made with the tongue in a more forward position than that required for the production of /ə/. The vowels /i/, /I/, /e/, /ɛ/, and /æ/ are all front vowels.

- *Back*—sounds made with the tongue retracted from the neutral position required for the production of /ə/. Five American English vowels are back vowels: /ɑ/, /ɔ/, /o/, /u/, and /ʊ/.

- *Rounded*—sounds made with the lips rounded or protruded. The /ɜ/, /ɚ/, /ɔ/, /o/, /ʊ/, and /u/ vowels are rounded.

- *Tense*—sounds made with a relatively greater degree of muscle tension or contraction at the root of the tongue. The tense vowels are /i/, /e/, /ʌ/, /ɜ/, /o/, and /u/.

- *Voiced*—sounds produced with vibration of the vocal folds. All American English vowels are voiced.

Diphthongs

Sounds that have two places of articulation, with a gradual change from one place to the other during their production, are called **diphthongs**. They are a combination of two vowels forming a single phoneme and can be contrasted with **monophthongs**, or single sounds, which have a single primary place of production (Small, 2012). Diphthongs contain an initial and a final segment, which are also known as onglide and offglide segments, respectively. The *onglide* is the vowel that initiates the diphthong, and the *offglide* is the vowel to which it changes (Lowe, 2012). Diphthongs are represented phonetically by digraph symbols that highlight the initial and final elements. A phonetic mark known as a *ligature* is sometimes placed underneath the diphthong to highlight the unity of the onglide and offglide portions. Table 3.1 shows the phonetic symbols used for the diphthongs of American English, along with various key words.

Diphthongs serve the same function as pure vowels, in that they form the nucleus for a syllable (e.g., *boy* [bɔi], *bite* [baɪt], and *train* [treɪn]). In American English, diphthongs can be **phonemic** or **nonphonemic.** Diphthongs that cannot be reduced to pure vowels or monophthongs without changing the meaning of the words in which they occur are categorized as phonemic. The American English diphthongs that fall under this category are /aɪ/, /aʊ/, /ɔɪ/, and /ju/. Although /j/ was previously described as a consonant glide, this sound also has a vowel-like quality. Therefore, when it occurs side by side with /u/ as in the words *cue* [kju], *few* [fju], and *pew* [pju], it is considered the onglide component of the

/ju/ diphthong. The phonemic nature of /ai/, /au/, /ɔi/, and /ju/ can best be highlighted by contrasting words containing the onglide component of the diphthong as a pure vowel and words that contain the actual diphthong:

Contrast	Pure Vowel	Diphthong
/a—ai/	*pop*—/pap/	*pipe*—/paip/
/a—au/	*pot*—/pat/	*pout*—/paut/
/ɔ—ɔi/	*tall*—/tɔl/	*toil*—/tɔil/
/u—ju/	*coo*—/ku/	*cue*—/kju/

Only two American English diphthongs, /ei/ and /ou/, are nonphonemic, because they do not change word meanings when they are replaced by their pure vowel counterparts, /e/ and /o/. Whether a person says "take" as [teik] or [tok], it is perceived as the same word by the listener. Although /ju/ was described as a phonemic diphthong, in some instances it can be nonphonemic, meaning that it does not create a contrast in words made with the diphthong or its pure vowel counterpart. Examples of this are the words *coupon* and *news*. The meaning of these words does not change whether they are produced as [kjupɑn] or [kupɑn] and [njuz] or [nuz].

Diphthongs in which one of the stressed vowels combines with the schwa /ɚ/ are sometimes described as **rhotic** or **centering diphthongs**. This class of diphthongs includes /Iɚ/ as in *fear*, /ɛɚ/ as in *bear*, /ɑɚ/ as in *far*, and /ɔɚ/ as in *poor*. It should be noted, however, that these terms are not used consistently in speech–language pathology.

Phonetics and Phonology

As we saw in the previous section, phonetic analysis has resulted in the two broad categories of consonants and vowels; then sounds were categorized based on manner, place, and voicing features. These are the *phonetically based patterns of speech sounds*. This is an important point because there is an erroneous impression that *phonological* patterns of speech sounds were the first kinds of speech sound patterns found by phonologists.

Beginning with the onset of the generative grammar in the 1950s and 1960s, a newer, and more theoretically oriented, approach to studying speech sounds emerged. This approach, inherent to *phonology*, has had a long—somewhat obscure or neglected—history, but its modern thrust in the United States came from the works of Chomsky (1957) and Chomsky and Halle (1968). In the decades that followed, phonological analysis of speech sounds in both typical and atypical learners of their language began to be adopted by speech–language pathologists.

Phonology is the study of sound patterns found in all—as well as in particular—languages and the speakers' knowledge of those patterns. Although speakers' speech sound repertoire is its database, phonology is not particularly concerned with the mechanics of speech sound production; that is the domain of phonetics. While phonetics more directly studies aspects of speech production and perception, phonology studies speech sounds at a more abstract level of knowledge—the mental organization, underlying representation, processes, rules, and constraints that influence sound production. Phonology is heavily theoretical and abstract in its conceptualization of speech sounds; phonetics, on the other hand, deals with such observable variables as dynamic articulatory configurations (gestures) that produce different kinds of speech sounds with specific aerodynamic and acoustic properties. Arguably, phonetics is much more empirically grounded than phonology, because phonetic variables are observable, measurable, and modifiable through experimentation. The empirical data in phonological theories are often limited to catalogued sounds, sound patterns, and sequences in particular and general languages; the rest tends to be speculative. Unlike phonetics, phonology is concerned with the *knowledge* that supposedly underlies speech sound production; this knowledge may be a mental structure or representation that cannot be verified. Being more data based, phonetic descriptions of speech sounds are less controversial; being more speculative, phonological theories are controversial. Disagreements are more common in phonology, much less so in phonetics. New phonological theories emerge all the time, but that is not true of the less theoretical phonetics.

As Ohala (1997) and others have pointed out, there is a tendency among phonologists—especially among those who take the classic generative grammar approach—to disregard phonetics. Many phoneticians, who provide the data for phonologists to build their theories, believe that such a disregard is perilous to phonologists themselves (Pennington, 2007). Ohala (1997) states that without the support of phonetics and such other empirical disciplines as sociolinguistics, "phonology runs the risk of being a sterile, purely descriptive and taxonomic discipline" (p. 45).

Historically, as noted in Chapter 1, **disorders of articulation** covered all the speech sound disorders found in children. Errors were classified as substitutions, omissions (deletions), and distortions. No particular effort was made to group the errors into patterns, although patterns based on manner, place, and voicing could have been identified. Articulation disorders were rated for their severity, often as *mild*, *moderate*, and *severe*. Possibly, what later came to be called phonological disorders were included in the moderate and severe categories. For a brief time, *distinctive feature theory* (Chomsky & Halle, 1968) influenced the study of speech sound disorders and suggested analysis of error patterns based on those features.

The influence of the Chomskyan generative grammar and subsequent phonological theories began to shift the diagnostic and treatment criteria for speech sound disorders. Some speech sound production problems, considered purely motoric, were called articulation disorders, which included only a few errors, mostly distortions; these could be functional or organic (as in a child with a cleft palate), and they generally preserved phonemic contrasts (good speech intelligibility). **Phonological disorders,** on the other hand, were manifested by multiple errors that formed various patterns with lost phonemic contrasts and much reduced intelligibility and were presumably due to the operation of phonological processes (patterns), rules, or constraints. When a child says [do] for "go," substituting a more anteriorly articulated /d/ for the more posteriorly articulated /g/, in a process called *velar fronting*, the resulting word has lost its phonemic contrast, in the sense that the word's meaning is unclear.

A more recent shift, as mentioned previously, is the increasing use of the term *speech sound disorders* (SSDs) to include both articulation disorders and phonological disorders. Throughout this book, we use the term to mean both kinds of disorders. We define *speech sound disorders* simply as "clinically significant errors in articulating speech sounds." Obviously, such a definition makes no reference to potential etiologic factors; this is not because such factors are unimportant, but because it is not always possible to make a diagnosis on the basis of causes. When known and justified, causes should always be specified in individual cases. Furthermore, not all speech sound errors in children are disorders, as typical learners of a language make speech sound errors for varied durations of time. The errors have to be *clinically significant* to be called a disorder. Clinical significance is often determined on the basis of normative ranges established for sound mastery; however, there may be such other considerations as variations due to dialects and a different first language, academic performance including literacy skills, effects on personal and social life of the child, and so forth. Note that *clinically significant errors* are not restricted to deviant or atypical errors of the kind Dodd (2005, 2011) specifies as diagnostic criteria, although such special kinds of errors will always be noted and included in a diagnosed speech sound disorder.

As a background to our subsequent chapters, especially for those on assessment and treatment, we present the major phonological approaches to an analysis of speech sound disorders. Two of the several phonological approaches have gained recognition: the linear and the nonlinear approaches. Of the two, the linear approach of the natural phonological theory has been better established in speech–language pathology than the nonlinear approach. Phonological processes, phonological patterns, or error patterns of the linear approach continue to be used. The nonlinear approach, especially as embodied in the optimality theory, advocated to clinicians as superior to the linear approach since the mid-to-late 1990s (Barlow & Gierut, 1999; Bernhardt & Stoel-Gammon, 1994), has yet to gain widespread clinical application.

In the Advanced Unit of this chapter, we describe and critically evaluate select phonological theories that have had an effect on the assessment and treatment of speech sound disorders.

Speech Sound Disorders in the Natural Phonological Theory

Apart from the distinctive feature theory, with its brief duration of direct clinical application, Stampe's natural (and linear) phonological theory (Donegan & Stampe, 1979; Stampe, 1979) was the first to influence the study of SSDs in children. The theory described **phonological processes,** which are simplifications of adult sound productions that presumably affect entire classes of sounds. Processes are natural methods of speech sound production in typical speech sound–learning children, hence the name *natural phonology*. Phonological processes are based on phonetic limitations children experience when they are still learning to articulate their speech sounds. Each phonological process exemplifies a child's specific set of attempts to produce the adult model in a simplified manner. These attempts affect a class of sounds, and, therefore, a phonological process is also a pattern. For example, a 3-year-old child who has not yet acquired many fricative sounds may often substitute stops for these sounds, a phonological process known as ***stopping.*** In other words, the child simplifies the complex adult model by substituting sounds that are within his or her phonetic repertoire for those sounds that he or she has not yet learned to produce.

In recent years, there has been a preference for the term *phonological patterns* instead of *phonological processes*; however, when making a direct reference to the natural phonological theory, it is accurate to use the term *processes*, as that is what Stampe (1979) used.

Stampe's phonological processes are normal (natural) in typical speech learners, but they are a disorder when they persist beyond the age levels at which they typically disappear and correct productions begin to be mastered. When a normal or natural process of sound production is observed in a child who is expected to correctly articulate the sounds included in that process, the child is said to have a **phonological disorder**. When a phonological disorder is diagnosed, it means that what was previously a process is no longer natural. If a process is observed in an older child who should not be exhibiting that process, it is of clinical significance. When a natural process becomes clinically significant in a child who is supposed to have "outgrown" it, the process may be justifiably called a **phonological error pattern.** As described in Chapter 1, children who have a phonological disorder exhibit multiple error patterns and lose phonemic contrasts; as a consequence, their speech intelligibility is greatly reduced.

The natural phonological theory later came to be regarded as linear in its assumption, because the phoneme features in the theory are not organized into hierarchies. Hierarchical arrangement of features is a characteristic of nonlinear theories, as described in a later section.

Varying definitions of individual phonological processes (patterns) inundate the literature (Dean, Howell, Hill, & Waters, 1990; Grunwell, 1985; Ingram, 1981; Lowe, 1994, 2012; Miccio & Scarpino, 2011; Shriberg & Kwiatkowski, 1980; Stoel-Gammon & Dunn, 1985; Vihman, 1998). This can be confusing and frustrating for students who want to gain a basic understanding of phonological patterns. Our presentation of phonological patterns is relatively simplified, like those of Stoel-Gammon and Dunn (1985) and Lowe (1994, 2012). Consistent with the current preference, we describe them as phonological *patterns*, but we remind the reader that the original sources cited here describe them as *processes*. Because the patterns are those found in typical speech sound learners, they are not to be thought of as error patterns unless used in the speech analysis of a child with a diagnosis of an SSD.

Syllable Structure Patterns

Syllable structure patterns describe the sound changes that modify the syllabic structure of words as a child attempts to produce the adult target. These patterns include unstressed syllable deletion, reduplication, final consonant deletion, initial consonant deletion, cluster deletion, cluster substitution, and epenthesis. In syllable deletion, reduplication, and epenthesis, the number of syllables in a word is affected. In initial and final consonant deletion, cluster deletion, and cluster substitution, the syllable shape of the word is altered.

Unstressed Syllable Deletion (USD)

Unstressed or weak syllable deletion describes the omission of one or more syllables from a polysyllabic word. Although unstressed syllables are more often deleted, stressed syllables may also be deleted. Lowe (2012) prefers the term *syllable deletion* because in connected speech, "it is often difficult to determine the stress being placed on a particular syllable" (p. 13). Examples include the following:

[medo] for *tomato,*	[ɛfənt] for *elephant,*	[məs] for ***Christmas,***
[tɛfon] for *telephone,*	[nænə] for *banana*	[said] for ***outside***

ACTIVITY
Provide an example of the effects of syllable deletion on the following words: *popsicle, pencil, hamburger, computer, wagon.*

Reduplication (Redup)
Also called **doubling,** *reduplication* is the total or partial repetition of a syllable of a target word, resulting in the creation of a multisyllabic word form. Total reduplication occurs when the entire syllable is repeated (e.g., [baba] for *bottle*). Partial reduplication occurs when only part of the syllable is repeated (e.g., [babi] for *bottle*). Stoel-Gammon and Dunn (1985) state that syllable deletion is often accompanied by final consonant deletion in productions such as [kækæ] for "cat," in which the final /t/ is deleted first and then the syllable /kæ/ is totally reduplicated. Examples include the following:

[baba] for *bottle* (total)　　　[bada] for *bottle* (partial)

[dada] for *dog* (total)　　　[dadi] for *dog* (partial)

[tata] for *television* (total)　　　[tatu] for *television* (partial)

ACTIVITY
Provide an example of the effects of reduplication (both total reduplication and partial reduplication) on the following words: *hat, doll, shoe, book, hamburger.*

Diminutization (Dim)
Diminutization is the addition of /i/, or sometimes [Ci] (C = consonant), to the target word. Lowe (2012) describes diminutization as a special form of partial reduplication. Examples include the following:

[kʌpi] for *cup*　　　[dali] for *doll*　　　[hæti] for *hat*

[buki] for *book*　　　[papi] for *pencil*　　　[fofi] for *finger*

ACTIVITY
Provide an example of the effects of diminutization on the following words: *egg, coat, toe, food, cake.*

Epenthesis
Epenthesis is the insertion of an unstressed vowel, usually the schwa, /ə/, between two consonants. Typically, the vowel is inserted between two contiguous consonants that make up an initial cluster, as in [bəlu] for blue. Epenthesis can also occur when an unstressed vowel

is added after a final voiced stop (Stoel-Gammon & Dunn, 1985). Examples include the following:

[səpun] for *spoon*	[pəlet] for *plate*	[kəraun] for *crown*
[kʌpə] for *cup*	[bækə] for *back*	[lʊkə] for *look*

ACTIVITY

Provide an example of the effects of epenthesis on the following words: *clean, please, tree, leg, lamp.*

Final Consonant Deletion (FCD)

Final consonant deletion is characterized by omission of the final singleton consonant in a word, as well as deletion of all members of a final consonant cluster (Khan & Lewis, 1986; Stoel-Gammon & Dunn, 1985). It is important to note that the entire cluster must be deleted for this type of error to fall under the category of FCD. Considering this, [bɛ] for *best* would be considered FCD because the entire final cluster is deleted, but the production [bɛs] for the same target word would not, since only one member of the cluster is omitted. In essence, the deletion of a final consonant or final consonant cluster alters the syllable shape of the word, so that a word that should be closed is produced as an open-syllable word. A **closed-syllable word** is one that ends in a consonant or consonant cluster, whereas an **open-syllable word** ends in a vowel. To be considered a final consonant deletion, the word should end in an open syllable, not a consonant, even if other consonants are omitted. This error pattern is best described by stopping (to be discussed later) and syllable deletion. Examples of FCD include the following:

[bu] for *books*	[da] for *dog*	[hæ] for *hand*
[gu] for *good*	[karpɪ] for *carpet*	[wægɪ] for *wagon*

ACTIVITY

Provide an example of the effects of final consonant deletion on the following words: *jump, basket, keep, leg, stamp.*

Initial Consonant Deletion (ICD)

Initial consonant deletion, the omission of singleton consonants in the word-initial position, is rare in normal phonological development. However, it may be observed in some children, especially those who have a severe phonological disorder. Khan and Lewis (1986) consider omission of the *entire* initial cluster as an exemplar of ICD. Thus, [ek] for *break* would be considered an example of both total cluster reduction and initial consonant deletion, since all members of the cluster are deleted. However, the production [bek] for the same target would be considered partial cluster reduction, since only one member of the two-member cluster is deleted. If the syllable shape of the error is analyzed, it still begins with a consonant and thus cannot be considered an instance of ICD. This concept is easily understood if one remembers that, as in final consonant deletion, ICD alters the syllable shape of a word;

a word that should begin with a singleton consonant or consonant cluster now starts with a vowel. Examples of ICD include the following:

[on] for *phone*	[u] for *shoe*	[ap] for *stop*
[azɪt] for *closet*	[ɪndou] for *window*	[it] for *seat*

....

ACTIVITY

Provide an example of the effects of initial consonant deletion on the following words: *lake, please, fat, table, brown.*

....

Cluster Reduction (CR)

Cluster reduction is the deletion or substitution of some or all members of a cluster. Although cluster deletion and cluster substitution are often categorized under the same phonological process of cluster reduction, we agree with Lowe (2012) that they should be discussed separately to better highlight some of their important distinctions. Hodson and Paden (1991) use the term **consonant sequence reduction** to describe the "omission of one or more sound segments from two or more contiguous consonants" (p. 39). Although cluster reduction can occur in both initial and final clusters, Dean et al. (1990) consider deletion of final clusters as a rare or atypical process. A more inclusive term is **cluster simplification,** which highlights omissions or substitutions that in essence simplify the cluster or make it easier to produce.

CLUSTER DELETION.
Cluster deletion is the deletion of one or all members of a cluster; it may be total or partial. In total cluster reduction (TCR), all members of a cluster are deleted, whereas in partial cluster reduction (PCR), only some of the members of a cluster are deleted. In PCR, sound deletion often follows a general developmental pattern, in that the sound that is more difficult to produce or later developing is typically the one deleted. In phonological theories, the sound that is most difficult to produce within a cluster is often called the **marked member,** and the sound that is theoretically easier to make is considered the **unmarked member.** Stoel-Gammon and Dunn (1985, p. 38) describe some of the most common reduction patterns as follows:

1. Children attempting to produce a /stop + liquid/ cluster will typically delete the liquid (e.g., [gin] for *green*; [bed] for *bread*).
2. Children attempting to produce a /liquid + stop/ or /liquid + nasal/ postvocalic cluster usually delete the liquid (e.g., [pak] for *park*; [bon] for *born*).
3. Children attempting an /s + stop/ or /s + nasal/ cluster will typically delete the /s/ (e.g., [tov] for *stove*; [niz] for *sneeze*).

Further examples of cluster deletion include the following:

Total Cluster Reduction	Partial Cluster Reduction
[æg] for *flag*	[fæg] for *flag*

[ap] for *stop*	[tap] for *stop*
[et] for *straight*	[tet] for *straight*
[da] for *dark*	[dak] for *dark*
[pa] for *palm*	[pam] for *palm*

....

ACTIVITY

Provide an example of the effects of cluster deletion (both total cluster reduction and partial cluster reduction) on the following words: *drop, glue, strike, lamp, past.*

....

CLUSTER SUBSTITUTION.

Children learning to produce the sounds of their language often progress from cluster reduction to cluster substitution. Cluster substitution is the replacement of one or all members of a cluster by another sound. As in cluster reduction, the sound that is more difficult to produce or later develop is typically the one substituted (e.g., [bwed] for *bread* and [pwes] for *place*). Cluster substitution most often affects clusters that contain a liquid (Lowe, 2012). Stoel-Gammon and Dunn (1985) describe a pattern in which all members of the cluster are replaced by a sound that was not a member of the target cluster (e.g., [pag] for *frog*, [bov] for *stove*, [dit] for *street*).

....

ACTIVITY

Provide an example of the effects of cluster substitution on the following words: *drop, glue, strike, tree, grow.*

....

Substitution Patterns

In substitution pattern, one class of sounds is substituted for another class of sounds. The key concept is the sound *class* substitution. In the traditional sense of articulation disorders, the term *substitution* is used to indicate the replacement of one sound for another, as in the production of /f/ for /v/ or /p/ for /s/. In the phonological process sense, however, substitutions may affect not only one or two sounds, but several phonemes within one sound class. For example, a child's substitution of alveolar sounds (one sound class) for velar sounds (another sound class) is a phonological process **(velar fronting).**

Although many substitution processes have been described in the literature, we will summarize the following seven processes:

1. stopping
2. deaffrication
3. velar fronting
4. depalatalization
5. backing

6. liquid gliding

7. vocalization

Stopping

Stopping is most frequently defined as the substitution of stops for fricatives and affricates. Some think that stopping can affect fricatives, affricates, liquids, and glides (Lowe, 2012). Others, however, question the categorization of stops for affricates as stopping, since an affricate by definition already has a stop component (Hodson, 1986). Whether the definition is liberal or conservative, this process can affect many sounds, especially considering the high number of fricatives in American English. Stopping of fricatives is a common process in normal phonological development. Although stopping can occur in all word positions, it is most often observed in word-initial position. Examples (limited to fricatives and affricates) include the following:

[pæt] for *fat*	[tek] for *shake*
[pain] for *vine*	[top] for *sop*
[tɛr] for *chair*	[pu] for *zoo*
[dɑb] for *job*	[pʌm] for *thumb*

ACTIVITY

Provide an example of the effects of stopping on the following words: *suit, zipper, bus, cough, shoe.*

Deaffrication

Deaffrication is the replacement of an affricate by a stop or fricative; the target affricate is changed to a stop or a fricative. Some believe that deaffrication is the substitution of a fricative for an affricate. Because the affricate class includes only /ʧ/ and /ʤ/, this phonological process can affect only two sounds. Examples of deaffrication include the following:

[tɛr] for *chair*	[dɑb] for *job*
[sɑp] for *chop*	[dɪm] for *gym*
[karm] for *charm*	[zæn] for *Jan*

ACTIVITY

Provide an example of the effects of deaffrication on the following words: *chip, John, couch, page, chin.*

Velar Fronting

Velar fronting (VF) is the replacement of the velars /k/, /g/, and /ŋ/ by sounds that are made in a more anterior position, typically an alveolar stop. This process affects place of articulation. The more common substitutions are [t/k], [d/g], and [n/ŋ]; however, other substitutions can occur (e.g., [d/k], [k/ŋ]). Velar fronting may occur more commonly in word-initial than word-final position (Stoel-Gammon & Dunn, 1985). Examples of VF include the following:

[tɑp] for *cop*	[tʌp] for *cup*	[pæt] for *pack*
[dʌn] for *gun*	[do] for *go*	[bɛd] for *beg*
[rin] for *ring*	[tʌm] for *gum*	[dɪs] for *kiss*

ACTIVITY

Provide an example of the effects of velar fronting on the following words: *get, sing, kite, seek, fog.*

Depalatalization

Depalatalization (Dep) involves the substitution of an alveolar fricative for a palatal fricative; it may also include the replacement of an alveolar affricate for a palatal affricate (Stoel-Gammon & Dunn, 1985). In this type of substitution, /dz/ typically replaces /dʒ/, and /ts/ replaces /tʃ/. Although /dz/ and /ts/ are not considered American English phonemes, in our experience it is not unusual for children to replace the English affricates with these non-English sounds if they have /s/ and /z/ in their repertoire. Lowe (2012) considers any sound change that replaces a palatal with a non-palatal sound as an instance of depalatalization. Examples include the following:

[tɛk] for *check*	[dʌdz] for *judge*
[mætsɪz] for *matches*	[den] for *Jane*

ACTIVITY

Provide an example of the effects of depalatalization on the following words: *chew, edge, John, chop, chicken.*

Backing

Rare in normal development but observed in children with severe phonological disorders, *backing* is the opposite of velar fronting. Thus, it is the replacement of sounds that have an anterior point of constriction with posterior sounds. This process typically affects alveolar and palatal consonants. The most typical substitutions are [k/t], [g/d], and [ŋ/n], although others are possible. Some children may also substitute [h/s]. Examples of backing include the following:

[kɑp] for *top*	[gaɪm] for *dime*
[hop] for *soap*	[baɪk] for *bite*

ACTIVITY

Provide an example of the effects of backing on the following words: *chew, doll, shop, ten, so.*

Liquid Gliding

Liquid gliding (LG) is the substitution of a glide for a prevocalic liquid. This process affects the manner of articulation. The liquids /r/ and /l/ are typically replaced by the glides /w/ and /j/, respectively. The substitution pattern for /l/ is at times determined by the vowel following, so that /l/ is replaced by /j/ before front vowels and by /w/ elsewhere (Stoel-Gammon & Dunn, 1985). Examples of LG include the following:

[wæbit] for *rabbit*	[wiŋ] for *ring*
[wuk] for *look*	[jif] for *leaf*

Liquid gliding can also occur in consonant clusters that contain a liquid:

[bwɛd] for *bread*	[bwæk] for *black*
[gwin] for *green*	[gwæs] for *glass*

....

ACTIVITY

Provide an example of the effects of liquid gliding on the following: *let, red, right, brake, laugh.*

....

Lowe (2012) describes another form of gliding called *fricative gliding*, in which a fricative is replaced by a liquid or a glide. Examples include [ju] for *shoe*, [lʌ] for *the*, [jup] for *soup*, and [lop] for *soap*. Fricative gliding does not occur as frequently as liquid gliding.

Vocalization

Vocalization (Voc), also called *vowelization*, is the substitution of a vowel for a syllabic liquid (Stoel-Gammon & Dunn, 1985). This process can also affect syllabic nasals (Lowe, 2012). Replacement of mid-central vowels /ɚ/ and /ɝ/ by /ə/ or any other vowel is also considered vocalization. This may seem a bit contradictory, since the sound affected and the resulting sound are both vowels. However, this is a common way of categorizing such error patterns. The most common replacements are [o] or [u] for a syllabic liquid. Examples of vocalization include the following:

[sɪmpo] for *simple*	[kwækə] for *cracker*
[ebu] for *able*	[pepo] for *paper*
[tebo] for *table*	[boθde] for *birthday*

Stoel-Gammon and Dunn (1985) and Hodson and Paden (1983) suggest that vocalization can also affect postvocalic liquids (liquids that occur after a vowel). Postvocalic liquids are considered consonants rather than syllabics. Typically, the postvocalic liquid is deleted, so that the syllable or word ends in a vowel. For words that end in postvocalic liquids, this pattern can technically also fall under the category of *final consonant deletion*. However, when children demonstrate a pattern of vocalization of syllabics, the replacement of a vowel for postvocalic liquids is most often categorized under vocalization rather than final consonant deletion. In our experience, it is not unusual for children to demonstrate vocalization of postvocalic liquids in the absence of true final consonant deletion. Examples of vocalization of postvocalic liquids include the following:

[kɑ] for *car*   [bo] for *bowl*

[bɑni] for Barney   [tɛu] for *tell*

··

ACTIVITY

Provide an example of the effects of vocalization on the following words: *hair, together, able, ball, car.*

··

Assimilation Patterns

You may recall from an earlier section that **assimilation** refers to the phenomenon by which one sound changes to resemble another sound, particularly its neighboring sound. A sound may be articulated more like a preceding sound or a following one. In the context of phonological patterns, there has to be a sound that changes and a sound that causes the change for assimilation to occur (Lowe, 2012).

An assimilation pattern can affect a sound's manner of production, place of articulation, and voicing features. The name of a pattern specifies whether it is manner of articulation, place of production, or voicing that is affected. The most widely recognized types of assimilation include labial assimilation, velar assimilation, nasal assimilation, alveolar assimilation, prevocalic voicing, and postvocalic devoicing.

Labial Assimilation

In *labial assimilation*, a non-labial consonant becomes a labial because of the influence of another labial sound in a word. In most cases, labial assimilation may affect alveolar and palatal sounds (Stoel-Gammon & Dunn, 1985); however, any non-labial sound can be affected. The labial consonants that can affect other sounds include /b/, /p/, /m/, and /w/. Examples include the following:

[bʊb] for *book*   [pɛb] for *pen*   [wæp] for *wax*   [mɑb] for *moss*

Velar Assimilation

In *velar assimilation*, a non-velar sound is changed to a velar sound because of the influence of another velar in a word. Velar assimilation typically affects alveolar and palatal consonants. The velars that can influence the change are /k/, /g/, /ŋ/, and /w/. Examples include the following:

[kʌg] for *cup*   [gog] for *goat*   [kik] for *keep*   [wɪŋ] for *win*

Nasal Assimilation

In *nasal assimilation*, a non-nasal sound becomes a nasal because of the influence of another nasal in a word. The nasals that can influence this type of change are /m/, /n/, and /ŋ/. We previously included /m/ as a sound that could influence labial assimilation and /ŋ/ as a sound that could create velar assimilation. Note that in this case, the sound that changes becomes a nasal, not merely a labial or a back sound. In other words, the nasal affects a sound's manner of production. Examples include the following:

[mɑm] for *mop*   [non] for *nose*

[nɑŋ] for *long*   [maim] for *Mike*

Alveolar Assimilation

In *alveolar assimilation*, a non-alveolar sound is changed to an alveolar sound because of the influence of another alveolar in a word. Examples include the following:

[tɑt] for *toss*   [dod] for *door*

[sut] for *soup*   [lɪd] for *lip*

Prevocalic Voicing

In *prevocalic voicing*, a voiceless sound preceding a vowel (prevocalic) becomes voiced. The prevocalic sound that should be voiceless is likely taking on the voicing feature of the vowel that follows it. Stoel-Gammon and Dunn (1985) believe that prevocalic voicing can affect all obstruents, but of these, the most commonly affected are stops. Examples include the following:

[dɛn] for *ten*   [vait] for *fight*

[zut] for *suit*   [bai] for *pie*

Postvocalic Devoicing

In *postvocalic devoicing*, a voiced obstruent following a vowel (postvocalic) becomes voiceless or devoiced. Lowe (2012) states that the assimilation may be to the "voiceless feature of the following word boundary" (p. 37). This would explain why productions like [nos] for *nose* and [bait] for *bike* would still be considered postvocalic devoicing even though the target word does not contain any voiceless consonants that can influence this type of change. Examples of postvocalic devoicing include the following:

[pɪk] for *pig*   [sæt] for *sad*

[tʌk] for *tug*   [bis] for *bees*

The term **consonant harmony** is sometimes used in reference to assimilation processes that affect manner of production or place of articulation (i.e., labial assimilation, velar assimilation, nasal assimilation, and alveolar assimilation).

Assimilation can also be classified as progressive or regressive, depending on where the sound that changes is located in relation to the sound that causes the change. If the sound that changes *precedes* the sound that causes the change, the modification is **regressive** or **anticipatory assimilation.** If the sound that changes *follows* the sound that influences the change, the modification is **progressive assimilation.** In *regressive assimilation*, the characteristics of the sound influencing the change "regress" on to the sound that actually changed. An example of regressive assimilation is the production of [tot] for *coat*; the sound that changed, /k/, *preceded* the sound that influenced the change, /t/. In *progressive* *assimilation*, the characteristics of the sound causing the change "progress" to the changed sound. The production [bib] for *bean* is an example of progressive assimilation because the sound that changed, /n/, *followed* the sound that created the change, /b/.

Assimilation can be total or partial. In **total assimilation,** a sound that changes becomes identical to the sound that causes the change, while in **partial assimilation** the changed sound takes on just some of the characteristics of the sound effecting the change. Examples of total and partial assimilation include the following:

Type of Assimilation	Total	Partial
Velar assimilation	[kʌk] for *cup*	[kʌg] for *cup*
Nasal assimilation	[mɑm] for *mop*	[mɑn] for *mop*
Labial assimilation	[bʌb] for *bug*	[bʌp] for *bug*
Alveolar assimilation	[tɑt] for *top*	[tɑd] for *top*

To complicate matters more, assimilation has also been described as being **contiguous** or **noncontiguous.** In *contiguous assimilation*, the sound that changes and the sound that influences the change are adjacent to each other; there is no intervening sound between them. In *noncontiguous assimilation*, the changed sound and the sound that effects the change are separated by an int–ervening sound.

Speech Sound Disorders in Nonlinear Phonological Theories

An alternative to the natural linear phonological approach to SSDs is the nonlinear approach. There are several versions of nonlinear theories, and concepts have been borrowed and integrated from such theoretical variations as autosegmental, prosodic, metrical, and still other views. Some nonlinear theories, especially the feature geometry theory described in the Advanced Unit, include distinctive features. Goldsmith's (1979, 1990) autosegmental theory is an early version of nonlinear phonological theory. Optimality theory represents another influential nonlinear approach (McCarthy & Prince, 1993; Prince & Smolensky, 1993). Several investigators have introduced nonlinear theoretical concepts to SLPs (e.g., Barlow, 2001; Barlow & Gierut, 1999; Bernhardt, 1992; Bernhardt & Stemberger, 1998, 2000, 2011; Bernhardt & Stoel-Gammon, 1994; Dinnsen & Gierut, 2008, 2011; Gierut & Morrisette, 2005). These and other investigators have illustrated the application of nonlinear theories to assessment and treatment of SSDs. We describe and critically evaluate selected nonlinear phonological theories in the Advanced Unit of this chapter; in this section, we introduce its clinically relevant features.

Nonlinear theories generally do not appeal to phonological processes or patterns to account for variations or errors in speech sound productions. They claim not to use any rules at all, but various versions of nonlinear theories do use rules, whose operations are thought to explain speech sound errors. Compared to natural and linear theories, however, phonological rules of nonlinear theories are few. For example, in **optimality theory,** there are two major rules, which are called **constraints,** defined as restrictive rules on sound productions or their combinations. The theory proposes that all languages have two major constraints—the markedness constraint and the faithfulness constraint—which are in conflict with each other. The conflicts are resolved by the different rankings of the constraints in individual languages. Constraints are universal, whereas rankings are language specific. Languages differ only in the unique ways the constraints are ranked in them.

The **markedness constraint** specifies how common a feature is in the world's languages, as well as in a particular language; it is a relative concept based on the frequency with which a phonological structure occurs in a language and the ease with which children typically learn it. Although the terms *marked* and *unmarked* may be used to describe phonological features or structures, it is more accurate to think of *more marked* and *less marked*. Generally, sounds or sound combinations that occur **more frequently** in languages, and are learned sooner, are **less marked** than those that occur **less frequently** and are learned later. Sounds and sound combinations that occur less frequently across languages and are learned later are **more marked**. Speech sounds or sound combinations that do not occur at all in a given language are **fully marked**, whereas those that occur most commonly and invariably across languages are **fully unmarked**. Fully marked sounds pose the greatest difficulty for the child to master, if for some reason mastery of it is required (e.g., as in learning a foreign language). Fully unmarked phonological features are the easiest to learn and, therefore, are also called default features; when other options remain unspecified, *default features* tend to be produced. In this sense, markedness is an index of speech sound complexity; the more complex features are more marked than simpler features. Simpler features also occur more frequently in languages and are learned sooner than more complex features.

The **faithfulness constraint** specifies that the input and the output be identical. That is, the child should produce what is heard. Clinically, accuracy equals faithfulness. If the word is *cat* and the child says [cæt], then the child has met the faithfulness constraint (rule). If the child says [cæ] instead, the production violates the faithfulness rule. Faithfulness (correct production) is also described as *well formedness*. Speech sound errors violate the faithfulness rule, and correct productions adhere to it.

In all languages, markedness and faithfulness are in conflict with each other. While faithfulness requires that a production be accurate, the markedness rule makes it more or less difficult to be faithful. Speech sounds that are more marked in a child's language generate more errors, violating the faithfulness constraint. More marked features, though a part of the child's language, have a constraint against them. For example, final consonants do exist in English and need to be learned, but they are marked because of their increased difficulty; consonant clusters, although again a part of English, are even more marked than final single consonants. This means that there is a constraint against final consonants and an even stronger constraint against consonant clusters. The theory even posits that highly marked sounds and sound combinations are "banned" or "prohibited" in given languages. Unfortunately, children have to master the sounds that the theory bans. Children who manage to master a banned set of sounds or their combinations delight their parents, but the children will have displeased the markedness part of the theory by violating it, although they simultaneously will have pleased the faithfulness constraint by obeying it. This is what is meant by the statement that *all languages are a set of conflicting phonological constraints* (Dinnsen, 2008).

As noted before, differential ranking of the constraints helps resolve these conflicts. Constraints may be ranked relatively high or low. Constraints that are ranked low may be violated; those that are ranked high may not be. A constraint, for example, may require *COMPLEX, which means NO COMPLEX [features]; the asterisk indicates the null. This constraint bans clusters because of their markedness (complexity). But this constraint is ranked relatively low in English, because the language does contain clusters. The Fijian language, on the other hand, does not contain consonant clusters, and, therefore, the *COMPLEX constraint is ranked very high. The ban on clusters there is very strong; its violation is a serious matter and may in fact be described as a *fatal violation*. English-speaking children are allowed to violate the constraint against clusters by learning to articulate them, whereas Fijian children cannot violate it (Barlow & Gierut, 1999). It is not clear, however, why Fijian children face the fatal prospect of violating the *COMPLEX when they do not even have clusters in their language and hence are unlikely to struggle with their mastery. Similarly, it is not clear why English-speaking children face a constraint against clusters when their language has plenty of them and to learn a common feature of their language, they must violate a rule that applies to some other language that they are not trying to learn. It is additionally unclear why a feature that exists in a language should be banned first, degraded next, and finally "allowed."

According to optimality theory, an English-speaking child who correctly produces a consonant cluster that exists in the language (e.g., says [train] for *train*) is *violating* the markedness constraint *COMPLEX; this violation is good, because in English this constraint is ranked low, and lower-ranked constraints are good candidates for violation. On the other hand, the child who deletes a consonant (e.g., says [tain] for *train*) is *obeying* the same constraint. It should be noted, however, that the child who violates the *COMPLEX is nonetheless obeying the FAITH (faithfulness constraint) by having matched his or her output with the input. The child who reduces English clusters to singletons has a speech sound disorder, because the child, while obeying the lower-ranked *COMPLEX, is violating the higher-ranked FAITH; his or her output does not match the input. It should be clear to the reader that errors are due to certain constraints that are followed or violated, not phonological processes that operate (Barlow & Gierut, 1999). Therefore, rather than phonological processes being the bases for speech sound error analysis, this version of the nonlinear theory suggests a differential analysis of obeying or disobeying constraints (input-out match or mismatch). Disobeying higher-ranked constraints will cause speech sound problems. Disobeying lower-ranked constraints may not have the same effect; in fact, and in many cases, the lower-ranked constraints may have to be disobeyed, as the examples show.

Nonlinear theories also use such traditional phonetic-based features as voicing and place in their analysis of phonological disorders. Some sound features are described as *nodes*. There is the *laryngeal node* (for the voicing feature) and such place nodes as the *labial place node*, *coronal place node*, and *dorsal place node*. Speech sounds also may be described differently from the standard phonetic or phonological process-oriented descriptions. In the nonlinear theories, for instance, the *velars* /k/, /g/, and /ŋ/ are called **dorsals** (articulated with the body of the tongue), and the alveolars /t/, /d/, and /n/ are called **coronals** (articulated with the tip or the blade of the tongue). All speech sound features in nonlinear theories have an underlying (mental or cognitive) representation; they may or may not be correctly realized in articulation—resulting in speech sound errors. In the mental representation, redundant features or those that do not help distinguish one phoneme from another (noncontrastive) need not be specified, according to various theories of **underspecification** (Archangeli,

1988; Kiparsky, 1982; Steriade, 1987). For instance, all sonorants are voiced; therefore, if a sound is [+sonorant], then there is no need to specify [+voice] for the same sound in the mental representation. All elements (features, syllables, segments, etc.) in the underlying and surface representations may be **linked** or **delinked**. Linking is also called **spreading**, and delinking is also called **deletion**. See the bulleted list that follows for their clinical significance.

A few other examples and terms illustrate the general approach the nonlinear theories take in describing or explaining phonological disorders:

- **Final consonant deletion rule.** This is the same as the *final consonant deletion process* of the linear theory. In nonlinear theories, all errors are analyzed in terms of presumed mental representation of features. For example, if a child were to say [bʊ] for *book* even though he or she had the correct mental representation for the word, including the final /k/, realization of that mental representation as [bʊ] would be due to the *articulatory constraint against final consonants*. Some write this rule as *CODA (a prohibition against syllables being closed by consonants). This rule is justified on the assumption that open syllables (CV) are less marked than closed syllables (CVC). The child followed that constraint and deleted the final /k/, because *CODA is ranked higher than any FAITH; in other words, the child's mental representation of /k/ was **delinked** (deleted) from the surface realization.

- **Fronting.** In this error pattern, dorsal (traditional *velar*) /k/ and /g/ are replaced by coronals (alveolar stops). For example, a child might say [tɑp] instead of *cop* or [dʌn] instead of *gun*. Nonlinear theories assume that this error pattern occurs because dorsal features are more marked than coronal features, resulting in the constraint *DORSAL (no dorsal sounds). This rule is ranked higher than the FAITH, so the child's output does not match the input; instead, the child articulates the less marked coronals in place of the more marked dorsals. This phenomenon is also described as **linking** or **spreading**; the default coronals spread (or get linked) to dorsals.

- **Stopping.** In this error pattern, stops replace fricatives (and affricates, according to some). A child might say [pu] instead of *zoo* or [pum] instead of *thumb*. Nonlinear theory proposes that there is a markedness constraint against fricatives, *FRICATIVES (no fricatives), because fricatives are more marked than stops. The FAITH in this case is ranked lower, and thus the child violates it (input and output does not match).

- **Reduction.** This is the familiar *cluster reduction process* of the linear phonological theory. The child reduces a cluster to a single consonant (e.g., [bed] for *bread*; [pak] for *park*). Although there are various rules that could interact to produce different kinds of reduction, we will give a simple example with one major rule: *COMPLEX (no consonant clusters, which are more complex than singletons). Generally, the deleted consonant is more marked, hence more difficult to produce, than the consonants produced in the cluster.

- **Negative rules.** Some rules are negative and account for missing sounds. They are generally stated in the form *No _____. As illustrated, *COMPLEX means no complex productions such as consonant clusters, *CODA means no closing consonants, *FRICATIVES means no fricatives, and so forth. A negative rule may apply to a single sound, as in *s (which means avoid /s/).

- **Positive rules.** These unstarred rules account for the correct production of sounds; they dictate that the underlying (presumed) and surface (as produced) segments match. For example, MAX means the child should produce all the sounds in a word with no deletions. DEP also requires a complete production with no insertions; a violation of this low-ranked rule explains epenthesis (insertion of a schwa, as in [səpoon] for *spoon*). ONSET means a consonant must start the production of a syllable.

Concluding Remarks on Phonological Approaches to Speech Sound Disorders

Advocates of nonlinear approaches recommend it over the phonological process analysis of (linear) natural phonological theory (Barlow, 2001; Barlow & Gierut, 1999; Bernhardt, 1992; Bernhardt & Stemberger, 1998, 2000, 2011; Bernhardt & Stoel-Gammon, 1994; Dinnsen & Gierut, 2008, 2011; Gierut & Morrisette, 2005). No systematic survey of clinicians has been done to find out how widespread is the practice of nonlinear error analysis in the assessment and treatment of SSDs. Anecdotally, it seems that a phonological pattern (process) analysis is still popular with SLPs.

The main difficulty with all phonological approaches is their excessive concern with explaining SSDs with speculative mental devices. Phonologists' desire to develop grand theories that apply to all languages forces them to create theoretical bypasses like differential ranking of constraints that may be violated in specific languages. Most error patterns may be grouped on the basis of the traditional phonetic classification of speech sounds. They may be optionally grouped according to the natural phonological theory (phonological processes) or the nonlinear theory. Still, such concepts as single consonant deletions, cluster reductions, fronting, stopping, assimilation, and so forth are common to almost all kinds of analysis. Phonological patterns are more closely related to phonetic ease of production, although this fact is often lost in the overly theoretical discussions. Without its excess baggage of speculation, natural phonological theory is based on the empirical observation that some sounds are phonetically more difficult for children than others. Why it is not sufficient to say that children omit sounds that are difficult or that they substitute difficult-to-produce sounds with easier-to-produce sounds is a puzzle to those who are weary of speculative devices. It is possible that clinicians who use the phonological process analysis do not necessarily subscribe to the deeper theoretical concepts of natural phonological theory. The two most critical and unsupported assumptions of the natural theory are (1) that children already have adult-like phonological representations in their mind (or wherever they are supposed to be) and (2) that *innate* phonological processes simplify the speech sound production requirements. We are not sure that clinicians who do phonological process analysis necessarily believe in these assumptions of natural phonological theory. One can find patterns in speech sound errors without believing in any of these assumptions. A systematic survey of clinicians' practices may refute or support our conjecture that most practitioners do phonological process or pattern analysis on the assumption that the *processes are descriptions of children's patterns of articulatory simplifications,* with few or no additional assumptions. Most clinicians probably do not care whether children's articulatory simplifications are innate or something else; they probably are not seriously concerned about the mental representation of speech sounds or their features. For assessment and treatment of SSDs, issues of innateness and mental representations are immaterial. Clinicians have an urgency to teach the correct production of individual speech sounds, even when the errors are grouped on some basis.

The newer nonlinear theories may not have attracted clinicians to the extent the advocates had hoped for, because apparently the theories substitute new terms for old concepts and the rest is speculation. Many variations of nonlinear theories describe SSDs somewhat differently, with no agreement on basic terms to be used. Some nonlinear theories use such familiar concepts as manner-place-voice features but give them different names (e.g., laryngeal nodes, place nodes, etc.). Other theories use the distinctive features in their conceptual variations. The rest of the theoretical details about features and their hierarchies, autonomous roles, interactions, and so forth do not seem to the clinician of much practical significance. Nonlinear theorists seem to be more interested in explaining how the error patterns come about—for example, by universal constraints and their differential rankings in specific languages. Clinicians, as well as those who are skeptics of theoretical speculations, often do not understand why constraints other than those that are physiological or learning related exist at all. For example, some clinicians may wonder who bans clusters or final consonants and for what reasons. Nonetheless, clinicians who wish to use the nonlinear phonological approach to assessment and treatment of SSDs have now sufficient resources, which have been cited in this chapter.

Summary of the Basic Unit

- **Phonetics** is the study of physical, physiological, and acoustic variables associated with speech sound production.
- A **phoneme** is a family of sounds, and **allophones** are its varied productions.
- Phonemes help distinguish **morphemes** and create meaningful word contrasts.
- The **International Phonetic Alphabet** helps transcribe speech sounds.
- **Diacritical markers** are special symbols that help identify the precise production of a sound.
- The four main processes of speech production are respiration, phonation, resonation, and articulation.
- Connected speech is often influenced by the effects of **coarticulation, adaptation,** and **assimilation.**
- **Consonants** are sounds that are produced by a narrowing or closing of the vocal tract at some point and may be **prevocalic (initial), intervocalic (medial),** or **postvocalic (final).**
- **Vowels** are sounds produced with a relatively open vocal tract configuration.
- **Diphthongs** are a combination of two pure vowels produced by a quick gliding of the articulators.
- A **syllable** consists of **onset, nucleus,** and **coda;** the last two elements are called a **rime.**

- Consonants are categorized according to **place, manner,** and **voicing** features.
- **Distinctive features are** articulatory or acoustic parameters that are either present or absent in consonants and vowels.
- Consonants that occur in side-by-side combination within the same syllable are called **consonant clusters** or **blends.**
- Vowels are categorized according to **tongue position, lip rounding,** and **tenseness** features.
- **Phonology** is the study of sound patterns and the knowledge of those patterns found in all languages, as well as in particular languages.
- **Linear (natural) phonological theory** describes **phonological processes,** now often called **patterns,** that are a child's simplifications of adult models. Patterns may be grouped into **syllable structure, substitution,** and **assimilation processes.**
- **Nonlinear phonological theories** describe phonological disorders in terms of a conflict between such opposing and ranked constraints as markedness and faithfulness.

Advanced Unit: Phonological Theories and Speech Sound Disorders

This Advanced Unit is devoted to a description of theoretical concepts in phonology. We summarize linear and nonlinear phonological theories and offer a critical evaluation of such theories in light of clinical empiricism. Among the nonlinear theories, we highlight the currently popular optimality theory and point out its clinical significance. We also contrast phonetic and phonological theories. This section concludes with a brief discussion of the varied roles of the theoretician and the clinician.

Phonological Theories

Phonology as a study of speech sounds and their patterns is an old, even ancient, discipline. Its history goes back at least a few thousand years to the now classic work of Panini of the 5th century BC on the grammar of Sanskrit, the ancient language of India (Cardona, 1998; Shukla, 2006). Phonology as a study of sound patterns based on mental, cognitive, and innate structures, however, is a creation the 20th century. Phonology is concerned with the abstract sound systems of languages in general.

Phonetics is the classic and basic science of speech production. Phonetics is oriented to specific languages of the world, although some of its observations may be generalized to most if not all languages. Unlike phonology, phonetics is concerned with the physical act of sound production. Historically, developmental research on articulation was concerned with children's acquisition of individual phonemes. Traditional description of articulation disorders also was primarily concerned with the correctness of individual phoneme productions. Treatment of articulation disorders, in turn, emphasized techniques designed to remediate the production of individual phonemes.

Newer perspectives in the study of speech sound production emerged because of the influence of linguistic theories. Linguistic theories, propelled especially by the generative grammar theories, have asserted that a "mere" phonetic approach to speech sound production is inadequate. Beginning with distinctive feature theory, summarized in the previous unit, theories that are more abstract than the phonetic approach have been dominating the study of speech sounds and their disorders.

The Goals of Phonological Theories

More than the production of individual sounds in given languages, phonologists are keenly interested in the patterning of speech sounds across languages. What are the existing patterns of speech sounds in various languages? What kinds of knowledge underlie phonological competence? Is that knowledge innate or learned? What kinds of rules, processes, or constraints may be written for both patterns and changes in patterns? Two overriding questions that encompass all these concerns of phonologists are: (1) How are sound patterns of languages represented in the human mind? (2) How are speech productions, which are only surface structures, related to an underlying mental representation? These are the primary questions phonologists try to answer. Because phonologists ask questions that apply to languages in general, they hope that their answers will identify universal features of languages. In a nutshell then, the goal of linguistic and phonological theories is to find universal features and rules of languages, including phonological patterns and pattern changes that are represented in speakers' mental structures.

Speech–language pathologists have shown a keen interest in phonology as a subspecialty within linguistics and in phonological theories that explain sound patterns and changes. An important fact that does not receive much attention from speech–language pathologists is that phonetics also seeks to answer questions related to speech sound patterns of specific and general languages. Often, phonetic and phonological theories compete to explain the same speech sound pattern and change phenomena, although phonetics is less concerned with mental representations and underlying processes (Ohala, 1986, 1995, 1997, 2004, 2005). We will return to this issue in the section entitled "Phonetic Versus Phonological Theories."

In spite of a common search for universality and a universal knowledge of sound patterns, phonologists have proposed differing theories. We will briefly contrast the main features of the classical linear phonological theories with subsequently developed nonlinear theories.

Linear Phonological Theories

At least since the late 1990s, there have been two dominant types of phonological theories: linear and nonlinear. Linear theories include distinctive feature theory (Chomsky & Halle, 1968) and the subsequent theory of natural phonology (Donegan & Stampe, 1979; Stampe, 1979). The classical theories of phonology, especially those of distinctive features, assumed that segmental properties or features of a phoneme (e.g., vocalic, sonorant, low, nasal, voiced, etc.) are independent of each other. Segmentation is the process by which words are divided into smaller units. A segment may be a sound, a combination of sounds, or a unit that is smaller or more abstract than a sound, as, for example, the *sonorant quality* of a sound (Gussmann, 2002).

The standard or classic theories (e.g., Chomsky and Halle's 1968 theory of distinctive features) state that phoneme segments may act independently of each other and may combine with any other segment. There was no implication in the standard theories that features of a phoneme could be hierarchically organized. In the more recent literature (for details, see Ball & Kent, 1997; Yavas, 1998), the standard theories that suggest segments are a bundle of independent features or characteristics of a phoneme with no hierarchical organization are referred to as **linear phonological theories** (LPTs) or **multilinear theories.** In essence, LPTs propose that to understand phonological productions, one needs to distinguish the *mental representation* of a pattern of sounds (knowledge of sound patterns) from its *surface representations* (actual productions). These two levels of representation are interrelated by a set of transformational rules that help derive surface representation from the underlying mental representation. Rules, therefore, play an important role in classical (linear) theories, including the natural phonological theory. The linearity concept suggests that multiple rules are not applied simultaneously; instead, the rules are applied sequentially, one at a time. In essence, in the classical theory, phonological properties are linear strings of segments (Clements & Keyser, 1983; Stevens & Keyser, 1989), a view challenged by newer theories.

Natural (Linear) Phonological Theory

In an earlier section, we made a brief reference to Stampe's natural phonological theory (Donegan & Stampe, 1979; Stampe, 1979), often called *natural phonology*. When the distinctive feature analysis faded, natural phonological theory was the first phonological approach to influence the study of SSDs in children. Clinicians began to analyze children's error patterns in terms of **phonological processes,** which are simplifications of adult sound productions that presumably affect entire classes of sounds. In this section, we will continue to use word *processes* (as against currently preferred *patterns*) because that is the term used in the theory.

Theory of Phonological Processes

Stampe's (1979) natural phonological theory is a linear theory, like the classic generative theory of Chomsky and Halle (1968). The central concept of Stampe's theory that speech–language pathology has borrowed is that of *phonological processes.* These processes are based on the observation that there are common patterns of phonological acquisition across languages. Stampe believed these processes to be both universal and natural. They are natural in the sense that they reflect the "language-innocent phonetic limitations of the infant" (Donegan & Stampe, 1979, p. 126). The simplified articulation of speech sounds that characterize phonological processes furnish a child with some *interim pronunciations*, with which the child can communicate with parents and other family members. These simplified speech sound articulations will continue until the child's articulatory mechanism has matured fully and the correct production of speech sounds is mastered. Phonological processes are natural, as well, because they are not arbitrary or conventional rules; they are phonetically (physiologically) limiting variables. Processes reflect the needs and capacities of speakers, not socially imposed rules. As such, phonological processes are innately given mechanisms to simplify adult speech sound productions; they are *mental operations*. In essence, phonological processes are phonetically based; they are a response to the phonetic difficulties and physiological limitations of the infant.

The natural phonological theory proposes that children have the innately given adult phonological system; their underlying phonological or word representations are adult-like. Even though children have the adult system represented in them, they still cannot produce the sounds accurately because of their limited phonetic capacities. The innately given phonological processes help children simplify the adult models. This process continues until the sounds are mastered and the processes fade one by one.

Stampe's theory asserts that the phonological processes of sound deletions and substitutions found in typically developing children are not learned; rather, they are due to phonetic-physiologic limitations inherent to children's speech production mechanism. Errors found in typical language learners are not morphologically induced; they are phonetically induced. As children's articulatory mechanism becomes more proficient (more matured), the natural processes are suppressed and more correct sound forms replace them. If a child makes a speech sound error that is not due to phonetic (physiologic) limitations, the error may have been learned, however (Donegan & Stampe, 1979).

A phonological process is applied to a natural class of sounds. This means that a process affects all sounds that share a common articulatory difficulty. That is what is meant by the common statement that phonological processes result in a pattern of simplified speech sound production, or a pattern of errors beyond a certain age level. The natural theory further claims that a process changes only a single phonetic property to make the sound or sound sequence easier for a child to produce. The theory also suggests that multiple feature changes in sound substitutions are not due to natural processes but are learned.

The natural phonological theory recognizes that processes are subject to constraints. Obviously, a child does not need to *learn* a process; it is essentially what a child *has the ability to do* with speech sounds in a developmental sequence, given the physiological limitations. The child, for example, need not learn to delete final consonants; the deletion is due to the natural process of phonetic difficulty. On the other hand, the child needs to learn the constraint his or her language imposes on a process. The constraint in this example is that there are indeed final consonants in English; the child, therefore, eventually has to learn to produce final consonants.

The theory makes a distinction between a phonological process and a phonological rule. Processes are innate, unlearned, natural, and are due to the phonetic limitations a young child faces in producing adult speech patterns. Rules, on the other hand, are not innate, natural, or based on phonetic difficulties in producing sounds; and they possibly are learned. It is harder to devoice the plural morpheme /s/ when the preceding sound is voiced, as in the word *bugs*, though it can be devoiced with effort; voicing an unvoiced plural morpheme in such linguistic contexts is easy and natural. It is a phonetically determined change in the speech sound. On the other hand, the word *tomato* may just as easily be articulated as either [tometo] or [tomɑto]; which one is produced is a matter of social learning, presumably due to a learned dialectal rule, not a natural process. Rules may easily be violated by learning an alternative form of pronunciation; processes are harder to violate and require much effort if one were to try. Eventually, however, the simplification processes that children exhibit fade, and this fading is not a violation of the process but a *suppression* of it. Children suppress phonological processes as they master the correct production of sounds. Those who are unable to suppress their phonological process, and continue to simplify adult productions beyond certain age levels, have a speech sound disorder. The natural theory further assumes that phonological processes are not voluntary operations; they work at an unconscious mental level. On the other hand, a speaker might be aware of rules or might be made aware of them, as in second-language learning. Processes may be variable and not obligatory, but the rules are obligatory (Donegan & Stampe, 1979).

A variety of phonological processes have been described in the literature. Stampe's processes have been expanded and redefined by other investigators. Assessment procedures and standardized tests have been available to evaluate phonological processes in children. An often made claim is that it is sufficient to treat only a few speech sound errors within a pattern to eliminate all errors within that pattern. This predicted outcome has not always been demonstrated, and not all processes have been evaluated in treatment research. In the Basic Unit of this chapter, we described the most common processes clinicians use in analyzing speech sound disorders in children. Chapter 6 contains information on the assessment of phonological disorders in the diagnosis of speech sound disorders, and Chapters 7 and 8 contain treatment-related information.

Evaluation of Natural Phonological Theory

There is a significant gap between phonological clinical practice and research on phonological disorders. Several researchers have moved on from linear theories to nonlinear theories and now to multilinear theories (Barlow, 2001; Barlow & Gierut, 1999; Bernhardt & Stemberger, 1998, 2011; Bernhardt & Stoel-Gammon, 1994; Dinnsen & Gierut, 2008; Gierut & Morrisette, 2005; Rvachew & Brosseau-Lapré, 2012). There is no hard survey evidence on how many clinicians have adopted the newer nonlinear approaches, but it is likely that a majority have not; practitioners continue to analyze, when appropriate, phonological error patterns in assessing speech sound disorders in children. A few advantages of the phonological pattern analysis may have contributed to its continued popularity.

First, a relatively well-established status and the availability of phonological process assessment tools have facilitated continued error pattern analysis (e.g., Bankson & Bernthal, 1990a; Hodson, 2004; Lowe, 1995; Secord & Donohue, 2002). Second, Stampe's claim that typical learners of their own language make errors in producing speech sounds because of their immature articulatory system makes sense to most clinicians. It makes better common sense to say that errors are natural for children to make than to say that such errors are due to some deeper mental processes, as the nonlinear theories claim, as described in the following section. That children's errors are phonetic is a plausible hypothesis, as well. Third, the theory's claim that the speech sound errors of language-learners are due to physiological limitations also appears plausible. Clinicians find it acceptable to say that errors decline as speech sound production skills improve. Fourth, the phonological processes are seen as a practical way of grouping children's errors, even if there are limitations to the analysis. Error patterns, albeit inconsistent across children, help classify error types and bring some order to an otherwise bewildering bunch of errors, especially in the case of children with severe speech sound disorders. Fifth, a diagnosis of a speech sound disorder is relatively straightforward because there is information on the age ranges during which most of the phonological processes typically disappear. Processes that persist beyond the normative age levels are grounds for diagnosing a speech sound disorder. Sixth, error patterns, once established during assessment, help track treatment progress. After teaching a few phonemes within the pattern, the clinician can probe correct production of other phonemes in the pattern. Periodic probes and treatment trials, alternated appropriately, may make for an efficient treatment program. It was by repeatedly citing these advantages of a linear phonological analysis that its advocates vigorously recommended the natural processes analysis to clinicians originally.

Since the development of nonlinear theories, criticism of Stampe's natural phonological theory and the phonological processes therein has increased, however. Clinicians who are weary of embracing new theories remember that not too long ago, individual, sound-by-sound analysis of the traditional articulation disorders was just as vehemently criticized as inadequate by researchers, and a process or pattern analysis was recommended as far superior. Now pattern analysis is facing the same criticism from the nonlinear theorists. Criticisms vary across theorists, but most critics point out a few common limitations of the natural process approach, including the following:

• The validity and reliability with which the natural processes can be defined are questionable. There is no universal agreement on the definition of *processes* or *patterns*. The same error pattern may have different names; there is sometimes no agreement on what kinds of errors should be included in a pattern (e.g., refer to the definitions of *stopping* and *deaffrication* described in the Basic Unit). There also is no agreement on the number of natural processes. Some sources list far more than others. Shriberg and Kwiatkowski (1980) list 7 processes, whereas Ingram (1981) lists 27. Some clinical researchers create new processes that do not seem justified to others. For example, Hodson and Paden (1991) describe *stridency deletion* as a separate error pattern, which to others seems superfluous because the same error pattern can be subsumed under the more general *consonant deletion* (Ball, Muller, & Rutter, 2010).

• It is not clear within the theory how to handle unusual or atypical processes. Processes do not seem all that natural, in the sense that they may not be found in all, or even most, languages. They nonetheless exist, and the clinician needs to handle them. Initial consonant deletion, for example, is uncommon in English but not in French (Yavas, 1994). Some atypical processes may be unique to individual children, not shared by others in the same language community. Unusual patterns then attract new and ad hoc names that may not be consistent with the natural phonological theory (Ball et al., 2010).

• Vowel disorders, though generally ignored by most theories, cannot be adequately accounted for; there are no established processes for them. Reynolds (1990), based on his extensive study of vowel errors, has suggested that vowel errors may be classified as (1) lowering of mid-font vowels to /æ/; (2) fronting of low-back vowels to /æ/; and (3) diphthong reduction to monophthongs. Ball et al. (2010) suggest that this may be conceptually reduced to a substitution pattern.

• Not all kinds of errors may be classified into a pattern. For instance, distortions cannot be classified into any of the processes; they are relegated to a "simple" and "motoric" articulation disorder (see Chapter 1). A child's speech sound error that is more complex than the adult target (e.g., [ræk] for *yak*) cannot be classified into a pattern, because by definition, a pattern must simplify the adult production. Similarly, few errors, limited to one or two phonemes, cannot be a part of any pattern.

• How speech sounds are learned (or "acquired" in any other nonlearning framework) is not clear. According to the theory, children should "suppress" natural processes to master the correct production of sounds. Some clinicians find this an absurd proposition (Bernhardt & Stemberger, 1998), because it is equivalent to presuming that children can learn to walk only when they suppress a "falling down" process. The theory is inconsistent with how skills are mastered: According to Bernhardt and Stoel-Gammon (1994), skills are mastered by positive progression, not negative suppression.

• It is not evident that children "use" phonological processes to "simplify" the adult model. It should be noted, however, that Stampe (1979) did not claim that children consciously "use" phonological processes; in his theory, processes are unconscious mental operations. The controversial usage is often found in the clinical literature. It is improbable that children consciously and cognitively select certain sounds within one sound class to substitute for sounds within another sound class. It is the expert who analyzes children's production errors according to various phonological processes. As Grunwell (1997a) puts it, "The concept of phonological process in the clinical assessment of child speech is applied primarily as a ***descriptive device*** [emphasis added] that identifies or analyzes systematic patterns in children's pronunciations by comparison with the target adult pronunciations" (p. 47).

Those and other limitations of the natural phonological theory are magnified by nonlinear theorists. We suggested earlier several reasons clinicians continue to use the natural process analysis in spite of these criticisms. We might suggest one more possibility as our concluding remark. Clinicians do not concern themselves too seriously about most of the theoretical underpinnings of phonological patterns. Concentrating mostly on the one language they typically work with, they are not troubled by universal processes that may turn out to be not so universal, error patterns that do not fit the natural phonological theory, conflict between the underlying representation and surface realization, innate and unconsciously operating processes versus consciously applied learned rules, and so forth. Grunwell's (1997a) statement, quoted in the previous paragraph, agrees with our evaluation that clinicians are not especially concerned with the theoretical underpinnings of phonological processes. Ball et al. (2010) have written that clinicians may be using phonological processes as "just verbal labels of patterns in the data" (p. 134), implying a dissatisfaction with that clinical stance. Grunwell (1997b), however, does not see a problem with it. We suggest that patterns in the data, without the linguistic theoretical baggage, may be linked to treatment research to find empirically more valid speech sound patterns than those that are based on any of the deductive theories. We briefly describe this possibility in a later section of this chapter (see "The Clinician and the Theoretician").

Nonlinear Phonological Theories

Nonlinear theories question some of the assumptions of linear phonological theories. For one thing, these newer theories question the assumption of sequential (linear) organization of phoneme features. The newer theories also criticize LPTs for not adequately accounting for the effect of prosody on speech production or explain such phenomena as stress, tone, and intonation, which influence speech beyond the segmental levels. Standard LPTs even ignored the syllable, as the morpheme was presumed to be the basic phonological unit (Yavas, 1998). In essence, suprasegmentals are not effectively explained in LPTs.

Several **nonlinear phonological theories** (NPTs) challenge the assumption that segmental aspects of a phoneme are simply a bundle of independent and unorganized features that may freely combine with each other. These theories propose that segmental and suprasegmental aspects of phonemes (and speech) are organized into nonlinear tiers. Goldsmith (1979) is credited with authorship of the first nonlinear theory, which he called *autosegmental phonology*. Other NPTs include the *metric theory, feature geometry, optimality theory,* and *direct optimality theory*. Most of these theories are interrelated; some are branches of others, and newer theories attempt to improve on older ones. Given the theoretical disposition of phonologists, clinicians can expect the emergence of many newer theories. In more recent years, nonlinear theories have been expanded to such an extent that some now prefer the term *multilinear theories* to encompass them (Rvachew & Brosseau-Lapré, 2012).

As the scope of this chapter will not allow a detailed description of NPTs, we will briefly review some of the major concepts of those theories to highlight their distinguishing features. Although nonlinear theories vary in their assumptions, a few common features may be noted:

• In most NPTs, some sort of a hierarchy (as against linearity) helps organize segmental and suprasegmental phonological properties (units). Several theories or variations of theories propose somewhat different nonlinear hierarchies to organize phonological units.

• Mental and surface representations of LPTs are redefined as *input* and *output* representations in NPTs. Some nonlinear phonologists hypothesize a generator (GEN) and an evaluator (EVAL) reminiscent of Chomsky's (1957, 1965) language acquisition device or system (LAD or LAS). (See the next section, "Optimality Theory.") Based on an input representation for a word (essentially a sound pattern), the GEN produces a variety of potentially acceptable outputs (production possibilities). The EVAL then evaluates the generated possibilities in light of a set of ranked constraints.

• NPTs do not accept natural phonological processes as valid ways of understanding typical language learning, children's speech sound productions, or production errors. Nonlinear theorists claim to have abandoned rules and processes, though the claim is controversial.

• Instead of being rule based, NPTs are *constraint* based. It is the constraints that help determine what sounds or sound patterns get to be produced. Constraints are universal, and they help the EVAL to make judgments about the acceptability of various output options the GEN offers at any moment of imminent speech production. Constraints act much like rules, so the claim that NPTs dispense with rules is questionable.

- All NPTs are mentalistic. They all assume that there is a representation of the sound system in a child's mind.

- All NPTs presume that children have phonological knowledge—that is, that the children know the phonological rules, operations, and constraints. In essence, NPTs assume an underlying cognitive structure of phonological features.

- All NPTs assume some form of innateness or innate structure that is essential for phonological learning and production. Mentalism, cognitivism, and innateness go hand in hand in most NPTs.

- All NPTs assume some form of universal grammar or phonological structure. They propose that phonological constraints are universal in that they apply to all languages. This is consistent with the Chomskyan theory of universal grammar (UG).

What follows is an overview of optimality theory, a nonlinear theory that has been influential in both linguistics and speech–language pathology; of the NPTs, optimality theory has received much clinical attention. Subsequently, we will briefly mention other theories, followed by a critical evaluation of nonlinear theories in general.

Optimality Theory

Optimality theory is a currently popular version of NPT (Dekkers, van der Leeuw, & van der Weijer, 2000; Kager, 1999). Its origin is credited to Prince and Smolensky (1993) and McCarthy and Prince (1994). As is the case with most phonological theories, different versions of optimality theory (OT) have been proposed by different phonologists; they include *pure optimality theory* and *standard optimality theory* (Ellison, 2000). In addition, various minor and major modifications of OT exist (e.g., Bernhardt & Stemberger, 1998; Clements, 1995; Goldston, 1996). The versions of McCarthy and Prince (1994) and Prince and Smolensky (1993) seem to have received much attention and extended treatment (Kager, 1999; Dekkers et al., 2000). Some speech–language pathologists have found the OT and its variants useful in understanding phonological disorders, their assessment, and treatment (e.g., Barlow, 2001; Barlow & Gierut, 1999; Bernhardt & Stemberger, 1998). A contrasting description of different versions of the OT is not intended here. Instead, we will highlight its main concepts.

OT, just like the previous generative transformational grammar theory, is a theory of language capacity. The central notion of a set of universal grammar principles is common to both the traditional universal grammar (UG) and the OT. The concept of innate grammatical rules, though called constraints in OT, is also common to both. OT is different from UG, however, in postulating that while the innate constraints themselves are universal, they are ranked differently in different languages. Therefore, according to OT, a constraint ranked high in one language may be ranked low in another. In a comparison with UG, OT also substitutes (1) input representations for mental representations, (2) output representations for surface representations, and (3) grammatic (or phonologic) rules for constraints. OT postulates the existence of two mental mechanisms: The GEN generates a variety of output possibilities; the EVAL evaluates what is generated to select an optimal output, which eventually succeeds (gets produced).

Grammar is a different concept in OT from that in the Chomskyan LPTs. The rules of grammar (including phonological rules) in older theories were not violable. Any violation of rules would result in unacceptable output (e.g., agrammatic or phonologically deviant productions). In the OT, *constraints* replace the rules of earlier theories. The concept of constraints is not unique to OT, however. It is part of different theories, including Chomskyan theories of language, and often works the same as rules or filters that block certain outputs (de Lacy, 2006). Here we will be concerned with the concept as used in OT.

Though the constraints of OT specify the acceptable sound patterns or sequences of languages, they are *violable*. In fact, Kager (1999, p. 9) defined a *constraint* as a "structural requirement that may be either satisfied or violated by an output form." It has been observed that universal markedness constraints themselves are violated in certain grammars. That is, what is considered universal may be untrue for given grammars. What is new about OT's constraints is that they are a set of conflicting constraints. A language is defined in terms of those conflicting constraints.

There are two kinds of constraints that are in conflict with each other: *faithfulness constraints* and *markedness constraints*. These two constraints try to balance each other's opposing forces. The **faithfulness constraints** require a good match between output and input representations. In other words, when a child produces a word with a certain sequence of sounds, the production should match the underlying mental representation of that word (input). Generally, faithfulness constraints aim to achieve similarity between input and output. In simple terms, a faithful sound production is a correct production from the adult standard; the child's production is *faithful* to the adult model. When a child's production is not faithful, when it is different from the adult model, it is a mismatch. Mismatches may be grounds for diagnosing a phonological disorder.

Major faithfulness constraints include MAX, DEP, and IDENT; the IDENT constraint has several sub-rules mentioned in the following list:

MAX: The MAX faithfulness constraint stipulates *Do not delete any phonemes in a word*. Accordingly, a child who correctly produces all the sounds in a word adheres to this constraint, and a child who omits a phoneme in a word (e.g., says [bu] for *book*) violates this constraint. This type of production is described as a *deletion* process in natural (linear) phonology.

DEP: This constraint stipulates *Do not insert extraneous sounds into a word*. Accordingly, a child who correctly produces only the normally included sounds of a word adheres to this constraint, and a child who adds an extraneous sound (e.g., says [pəlet] for *plate*) violates this constraint. This type of production is described as an *epenthesis* process in natural (linear) phonology.

IDENT: This constraint stipulates *All corresponding segments should be identical*. It means that the input and output features should match. It has such sub-rules as ID[continuant], which stipulates that continuant sounds should not be changed to noncontinuant sounds; ID[feature], which stipulates that corresponding features must have identical voice, place, or manner features; and ID[laryngeal], which stipulates that voiced sounds should not be changed to unvoiced sounds. Violations of these constraints are typically described as various kinds of substitution processes in natural (nonlinear) phonology.

The concept of **markedness** is not unique to OT and dates back to the 1930s, when Trubetzkoy (1939/1969) and Jakobson (1941/1968) introduced it. It may be found in earlier versions of LPTs, including the **distinctive feature theory** (Chomsky & Halle, 1968) and the **natural phonological theory** (Stampe, 1979). It currently is not exclusive to a particular theory; it is now a mainstream linguistic concept (Haspelmath, 2006).

According to the classic meaning of the term, a phoneme is *marked* if a feature (e.g., voicing) is present in it; a phoneme that lacks the same feature is *unmarked*. For example, /g/ is marked for voicing (+ voice), whereas /k/ is unmarked (– voice) for the same feature. Unfortunately, the term has gained varied meanings over time. Generally, it suggests a gradient— more or less of some variable that applies to speech sounds. The gradient of markedness suggests two extremes on a continuum: marked versus unmarked. **Marked phonological features** are said to be (a) complex, (b) difficult to produce, (c) not natural (present in fewer languages), (d) infrequent in languages, (e) abnormal, (f) unpredictable, (g) acquired later, (h) language specific (unique to a given language), (i) perceptually weak (not easily perceived), and so forth. **Unmarked phonological features** are described in terms opposite to those that characterize marked features: (a) simple, (b) easy to produce, (c) natural (present in all or many languages), (d) frequently occurring in languages, (e) normal, (f) predictable, (g) acquired earlier by children, (h) universal (not language specific), (i) perceptually strong (easily perceived), and so forth (Haspelmath, 2006; Hume, 2004, 2011).

Observational studies have shown that some segments and segmental sequences are more frequently observed than others. For example, stops are found in almost all languages. Among the stops, voiceless stops are more common than voiced stops. The voiced/voiceless distinction also is common among languages. Voiceless fricatives are more common than voiced ones. Even among the voiceless fricatives, the dental-alveolar /s/ is found most frequently across the languages of the world. Most languages have two or three nasals at least; a language with a single nasal is unusual. It is claimed that all languages have the vowel /ɑ/. Front unrounded vowels (e.g., /i/) are found in more languages of the world than front rounded vowels (e.g., /y/). At the level of syllables, CV (consonant-vowel) is the most common structure. The more common a feature is across languages, the more natural it is; hence, the more unmarked it is. Generally, vowels, glides, nasals, and stops are unmarked and universal features of languages. Presumably, the child does not need "input" from the environment about unmarked features because he or she already "knows" about them.

It is claimed that unique, less natural, and marked features of language have to be learned with environmental input. For example, consonantal clusters in syllables along with final consonants would be marked. In addition to consonant clusters, fricatives, affricates, and liquids are regarded as marked properties of languages. Such marked properties need environmental assistance in order to be learned.

Developmental studies have suggested that relatively unmarked features are learned more easily or earlier than those that are marked and less natural; this is because unmarked features require less articulatory effort to produce, are acoustically less complex, and are perceptually clearer (Lowe, 1994; Toombs, Singh, & Hayden, 1981). For example, unmarked unrounded vowels are acquired sooner than marked rounded vowels. More natural (less marked) stops are acquired earlier than less natural stops. Markedness is reflected also in children's speech error patterns. Unrounding of rounded vowels, for instance, is more common than the reverse. Children with speech sound disorders tend to make fewer mistakes on more natural stops than on less natural stops. Children also master less marked syllable structures (i.e., CV) earlier than more marked syllable structures (e.g., CVC, CCV).

The presence and frequency of certain phonological processes (patterns) of the nonlinear theory may also be influenced by markedness (Yavas, 1998). For example, final consonant deletion, a common phonological process, creates the most unmarked open syllables. Another phonological process, the stopping of fricatives and affricates, also moves from the more marked (fricatives and affricates) to less marked (stops). In essence, many instances of articulatory error patterns tend to eliminate or diminish marked features and thus create less marked (more natural) segments.

Many markedness constraints are presumed to apply to the languages of the world (Dinnsen & Gierut, 2008). Commonly cited markedness constraints include *COMPLEX, *CODA, *FRICATIVES, and *LIQUIDS.

> *COMPLEX: This constraint stipulates *Do not produce clusters* (which are complex). Accordingly, a child who correctly produces an English word with clusters (e.g., *stop*) violates this constraint, and a child who reduces the cluster to a singleton (e.g., says [sop] or [top] for *stop*) adheres to this constraint. This type of production is described as a *cluster reduction* process in natural (linear) phonology.

> *CODA: This constraint stipulates *Do not produce final consonants* (no codas). Accordingly, a child who correctly produces final English consonants in a word (e.g., *cat*) violates this constraint, and a child who omits the final consonants (e.g., says [cæ] for *cat*) adheres to this constraint. This type of production is described as a *final consonant deletion* process in natural (linear) phonology.

> *FRICATIVES: This constraint stipulates *Do not produce fricatives.* Accordingly, a child who correctly produces English words with a fricative (e.g., *fat*) violates this constraint, and a child who substitutes another sound for the fricative (e.g., says [pæt] for *fat*) adheres to this constraint. This type of production is a part of the *stopping* process in natural (linear) phonology.

> *LIQUIDS: This constraint stipulates *Do not produce liquids.* Accordingly, a child who correctly produces English words with a liquid (e.g., *look*) violates this constraint, and a child who substitutes another sound for the liquid (e.g., says [wuk] for *look*) adheres to this constraint. This type of production is described as a *liquid gliding* process in natural (linear) phonology.

It is not possible to satisfy all constraints simultaneously, because they are in conflict with each other. One constraint, when fulfilled, may simultaneously violate another constraint. One constraint, when violated, may simultaneously satisfy another constraint. How to handle such conflicts among universal constraints has been a major theoretical problem for linguists (including phonologists). OT handles this problem by giving up the notion of *inviolable* universal constraints.

Instead of eliminating all conflicts among constraints, grammars must allow for minimal conflicts. In other words, grammars must allow for optimal output form, not necessarily an output that is expected to fulfill all constraints while violating none. An **optimal output form** is the one that "incurs the least serious violations of a set of conflicting constraints"

(Kager, 1999, p. 8). Therefore, the central concept of *optimality* is that the output (a child's production) is the *most optimal* or the best among the available choices the GEN generates, and is not necessarily correct output.

In OT, conflicts among various constraints are resolved not only by postulating that they are violable, but also by a unique ranking of universal constraints in each language. In the OT, the uniqueness of individual languages lies in their specific ranking of the same set of universal constraints. Kager (1999) believes that the grammar of one language may be derived from another language simply by re-ranking the constraints.

Whether an output is acceptable despite violating a constraint depends on the ranking of the constraints that have been violated or adhered to. For instance, the markedness constraint *COMPLEX dictates "No consonant clusters," because clusters are unique to certain languages and thus marked. Consonant singletons are unmarked and universal. Therefore, in languages that do not contain consonant clusters (e.g., Fijian), the *COMPLEX constraint ("no clusters") is ranked higher than it is in languages that do contain consonant clusters (e.g., English) (Barlow & Gierut, 1999). Consequently, the constraint *COMPLEX is rated lower in English than in Fijian. The constraint must be satisfied in Fijian but may be violated in English.

Another example will further illustrate the nature of constraints and adherence to or violation of them. One of the markedness and universal constraints is *Vowels must not be nasal*. Unfortunately for this universal constraint, some languages (e.g., several South Asian languages) have nasal vowels, whereas other languages (e.g., English) do not have them (except in assimilation). Therefore, *nasality* in vowels is marked, because the constraint doesn't operate in all languages. This means that the constraint against nasal vowels is ranked higher in English than in Kannada or Hindi (two languages of India that do have nasal vowels). The constraint may be violated in those languages, but it must be adhered to in English.

Each language tries to avoid violation of all constraints, but violation of higher-ranked constraints is more forcefully avoided than violation of lower-ranked constraints. In essence, only the lower-ranked constraints may be violated. Consequently, grammatical well formedness is considered a relative concept. There is greater **harmony** if constraint violations are few and violated constraints are lower ranked than constraints that are adhered to.

Generally, harmonic or optimal productions are those output forms (surface structures in the older theories) that are relatively consistent with the input forms (mental representations). For example, if a child's production of the word *telephone* matches that word's mental representation (which is presumably the way adults normally produce it), the production is harmonious. Note that the theory avoids the terms *correct productions, errors*, and so forth. How are the most harmonic (grammatically or phonetically more acceptable) productions achieved? How is the number of violations kept to a minimum? How are violations limited to lower-ranking constraints? Answers to these questions in OT lie in the GEN and EVAL mechanisms.

The process of realizing a harmonious (optimal) output that incurs the least number of serious constraint violations is postulated as follows: Given a particular input representation (e.g., the word *elephant*), GEN generates an infinite set of output candidates. The output candidates include both optimal (accurate or nearly so) and nonoptimal (less accurate or outright wrong) candidates. The EVAL then selects an output that violates the least number of constraints. EVAL also makes sure that violated constraints are less serious and ranked lower than those adhered to. In OT terms, the selected outputs are *optimal* and are winners and the nonselected outputs are losers (Teaser, 2000). Presumably, the winner gets produced. Figure 3.1 illustrates the workings of the GEN and EVAL as postulated in OT.

Clinical Implications of Optimality Theory

It is difficult to predict when a major shift from the linear to the nonlinear (or multilinear) approach will take place in the clinical practice of speech–language pathology. Before that shift takes place, there may even be a newer theory to catch up with.

The clinical implications of the nonlinear approach—OT in particular—have been explored in recent years (e.g., Barlow, 2001; Barlow & Gierut, 1999). As noted previously, most clinicians probably still use the standard phonological pattern analysis in grouping children's misarticulations. Clinicians also target the elimination of standard phonological patterns in treatment. Whether the implications of such nonlinear theories as OT will ever be followed in routine clinical practice is yet to be determined.

Some clinical researchers in speech–language pathology believe that OT offers significant advantages in understanding phonological acquisition and in planning treatment for phonological disorders (e.g., Barlow, 2001; Barlow & Gierut, 1999; Bernhardt & Stemberger, 2011; Bernhardt & Stoel-Gammon, 1994). Barlow and Gierut (1999) have pointed

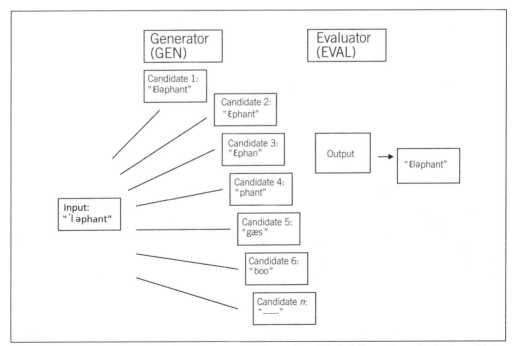

Figure 3.1. A diagram illustrating the input representation, a few of the infinite numbers of output candidates generated by GEN, and optimal output selected by EVAL. Note that the output candidate 1 is the most faithful, and others are less so to varying degrees. The evaluator selects the output that is most faithful and violates the least number of constraints.

out that the common phonological error patterns found in both typical and atypical speech sound learners may be understood in terms of conflicts between faithfulness and markedness constraints. Generally, markedness constraints (unique properties of a language) are higher ranked than faithfulness constraints (matching input and output representations). Also, in applying the OT to children's misarticulations, clinicians find themselves renaming the old phonological processes. Some examples of how OT may account for phonological error patterns found in children include the following (Barlow, 2001; Barlow & Gierut, 1999); starred items are markedness constraints, and unstarred items are faithfulness constraints:

- *Fronting*—The common substitutions are [t/k], [d/g], and [n/ŋ]. These substitutions are explained by the OT constraint *DORSAL, which prevents velar outputs. Consequently, coronal output (unmarked) surfaces instead of velar outputs.

- *Stopping*—In this process, stops are substituted for fricatives and affricates. Stops are unmarked; fricatives are marked. Therefore, the OT constraint *FRICATIVES, which prevents fricatives, causes the production of stops instead.

- *Final consonant deletion*—Open syllables (CV) are unmarked (universal), whereas closed syllables (CVC) are marked. Therefore, final consonant deletion is due to the markedness constraint *CODA (no final consonants).

- **MAX*—Consonant deletion (in any word position). *CODA is specific to final consonant deletion.

- **COMPLEX*—Cluster reduction. Clusters are more complex and are therefore marked; hence there is a constraint against them. This constraint prevents cluster productions and explains the error pattern, cluster deletions.

- *DEP*—A faithfulness constraint that specifies that input-output segments must match. This prevents any extraneous sound insertion, and its violation explains extraneous vowel insertions (e.g., [səwip] for sweep).

- *IDENT-FEATURE*—Another faithfulness constraint, this one specifies that input features should not be changed in the output. Violation of this constraint explains such error patterns as fronting of velars to alveolars, gliding of liquids, stopping of fricatives, prevocalic voicing, and final obstruent devoicing.

Sound patterns in all children, normally developing or exhibiting phonological disorders, are explained on the basis of a conflict between markedness and faithfulness constraints and the relative ranking of the constraints that conflict in individual cases. For instance, final consonant deletions by an English-speaking child occur because the markedness constraint *CODA outranks the faithfulness constraint MAX (no deletion). In English grammar, MAX is ranked higher than *CODA, so normal adult productions include final consonants. In essence, a child or any other speaker of English who deletes final consonants obeys *CODA (no final consonants) and ignores MAX (no deletions), whereas those who include final consonants do the opposite—they obey MAX and ignore *CODA. Cluster reduction in children is explained in a similar manner. Children who reduce clusters to singletons have in their grammar (input representation) *COMPLEX (no clusters) ranked higher than MAX (no deletion). Unfortunately for them, their language has the opposite ranking: MAX is ranked higher than *COMPLEX. Children exhibit *gliding* because, in their grammar, *LIQUIDS (no liquids) is ranked higher than IDENT-[consonantal] (don't change [consonantal]). In the grammar of children who exhibit *stopping* (the substitution of stops for fricatives as in [du] for *zoo*), the markedness constraint *FRICATIVES (no fricatives) dominates the faithfulness constraint. In each case, the ranking of the constraints in the adult grammar for the language is the opposite of the ranking in the child's grammar.

The essence of OT's clinical application is that if a child produces speech errors, the ranking of constraints in his or her input for the specific sounds in question is different from the ranking of the same constraints for the same sounds in the adult input. In other words, the child's grammar differs from the grammar of his or her language, hence the errors. With the grammar the child has, it would be a violation if the child did produce the sounds correctly (Barlow, 2001).

Other Nonlinear Theories

None of the other plentiful nonlinear theories have gained the kind of attention from clinical researchers that the optimality theory has; none have been clinically applied to any significant extent. Most of those theories are too abstract and speculative for clinicians, because each was designed to explain a small phonological-linguistic phenomenon that could not be handled by existing theories. Therefore, we will only briefly mention some of those whose key concepts are integrated into nonlinear theories in general.

Goldsmith (1979, 1990, 1999) developed the **autosegmental theory** to overcome the limitation of the standard generative theory (from Chomsky and Halle's *Sound Pattern of English*, 1968) in accounting for prosodic features and tonal languages. In a tonal language, meaning is changed by changing the pitch of the produced word; the same word, spoken with different pitches, signals different meanings. Goldsmith's theory was one of the first to postulate a hierarchy based on feet, syllables, and segments (Hayes, 1988). Such a hierarchy is also called a *tier* in the theory. The hierarchical organization of features distinguished Goldsmith's theory from the standard generative theory and promoted the concept of nonlinear phonological theories.

To account for tonal variations that signal differences in meaning, the autosegmental theory created a tier for the tones and placed it just above the sound segments. That suggested that the tones, not just the segments, determined the meaning of the words. The theory was subsequently extended to other phonological phenomena. A central concept of autosegmental theory is that phonemic features may operate independently in phonological rules or processes. That observation led Goldsmith (1979) to consider features as "autosegmental"—that is, operating autonomously. Thus, the name *autosegmental theory*.

A related theory, called the **metrical theory** (Goldsmith, 1990; Liberman, 1975; Liberman & Prince, 1977), pays particular attention to the syllable structures, stress patterns, and rhythms of speech. This theory was developed because the earlier generative (and linear) theories did not adequately explain stress patterns of languages. Chomsky and Halle (1968) assigned a + sign if stress was present on a vowel (and a – sign if absent), but the authors did not include the concept of stressed syllables, nor did they specify how many or which vowels in a word or utterance would be stressed. Chomsky and Halle also did not distinguish primary and secondary stresses (Ball et al., 2010). As explained in the Basic Unit, a syllable is described in terms of an onset and a rhyme. The rhyme, in turn, is described in terms of a nucleus and a coda. Thus, the onset, nucleus, and coda (the latter two constituting the rhyme) represent the basic structure of a syllable.

The *onset* of a syllable is the initial consonant or consonant cluster that launches a syllable. For instance, /fl/ launches the word *flute*, and /f/ launches the word *fan*. The onset may be absent, however, when the syllable is started with a vowel, as many words in English are. The *rhyme* is everything in a syllable except for the onset: The *nucleus* is the vowel or diphthong that follows the consonant, and the *coda* is the final consonant. For example, in the word *tap*, the onset is the /t/, the nucleus is the vowel /a/, and the coda is the final /p/. Both the onset and the coda may contain more than one sound. For example, in the word *strict*, /str/ is the onset and /kt/ is the coda.

In the metrical theory, rhythm involves alternating patterns of stress. When weak and strong syllables are produced in alternating positions, a unique rhyme is created. A rhyme may also be thought of as a timing unit called a **foot,** which consists of a stressed syllable and one or more unstressed syllables. While monosyllabic words have a single foot, some (but not all) disyllabic and polysyllabic words may have multiple feet. Multiple syllables that are stressed in a word may receive relatively more or less stress. That is, stress is a relative concept, in that among two stressed syllables, one stress may be relatively stronger than the other. Thus, syllables in a foot and feet in a word vary in strength. Such strength variations create the typical rhythm of speech. In the metrical theory, then, the syllable with its expanded structure is the main vehicle of prosodic features (the rhythm of speech).

In essence, according to the metrical theory, a word consists of such hierarchies (or tiers) as the foot, the syllable, the onset rhyme, and the CV before reaching the segmental level. These different tiers account for the prosodic effects of speech. As we shall see in the next paragraphs, other phonological theories have extended this type of hierarchical analysis to the segmental level, as well. Because the metrical theory deals with mostly the stress patterns in speech, its clinical application in assessing and treating speech sound disorders in children has been extremely limited (Ball et al., 2010).

Another nonlinear phonological theory, feature geometry, extends the concept of hierarchies to the segmental level. The **feature geometry** theory proposes that features of a segment also are hierarchically organized (Clements, 1985; Clements & Keyser, 1983; McCarthy, 1988). The term *geometry* suggests a hierarchical arrangement of features as against an unorganized bundle. Also, features may operate independently in phonological rules or processes, as postulated in the autosegmental theory. Therefore, feature geometry is typically a concept integrated into the autosegmental theory (Ball et al., 2010).

In organizing the segmental features and their combinations, the theory of feature geometry uses the anatomical structures used in speech production. The six articulators that create feature differences are the glottis, soft palate, lips, tongue blade, tongue body, and tongue root. Some feature specifications are entirely due to the action of an articulator. For instance, the feature [labial] is due to lip action, and the feature [nasal] is due to velopharyngeal action of opening. Other features are a function of several articulators. For instance, the features [consonantal] and [sonorant] are not limited to any one articulator and thus specify a category with no particular articulator. Features that are entirely due to an action of a single articulator are called **articulator bound,** and those that are produced with multiple articulators are called **articulator free.**

The articulator-free features are classified into two categories: the major class features and the stricture (or manner) features. The major class features include [consonantal] and [sonorant], and the stricture features include [continuant], [strident], and [lateral]. Among these, the [consonantal] and [sonorant] features are considered root features that give rise to major classes of sounds. The stricture or manner features are derived from the root features. Thus, a hierarchy of features is created instead of a bundle of unrelated features. Feature trees based on feature geometry show all related features in an organized manner. For instance, the specification of a terminal feature implies a particular articulator and all other higher features. For instance, consonants may be specified as *supralaryngeal,* which branches out into tongue root and soft palate on the one hand and oral place on the other. The oral place branches out into labial, coronal, and dorsal, each of which branches out into specific nodes. For instance, the dorsal branches out into [high], [low], and [back]. Thus, an articulator and its branching feature mechanisms are hierarchically organized (Halle, 1992; Yavas, 1998).

A concept used in feature geometry is that some features may dominate other features—again suggesting a geometric organization (Bernhardt & Stoel-Gammon, 1994). When referring to the dominant role some features play, the theory uses the term *nodes.* Nodes also help link higher and lower levels within the feature organization. Each level may also be considered a *tier.* At the very top of this geometric organization, there is the *root node,* which links a segment to the prosodic tier. Below the root node is the *laryngeal node.* The higher root node dominates the lower laryngeal node. The laryngeal node is dominant for the voiced segments of phonemes. Below the laryngeal node is the *place node,* which includes all oral characteristics of phonemes, although it is not associated with specific phoneme productions. Dominated by the root node, the place node dominates its own place nodes, which are associated with the actual articulators: the lips (*labial place node*), the tongue blade and tip (*coronal place node*), and the tongue dorsum (*dorsal place node*). The labial place node includes the labial sounds (/w/, /p/, /b/, /m/, /f/, /v/, and the rounded vowels). The coronal place node includes all the sounds made with the help of the tongue blade and tip (/t/, /d/, /s/, /z/, /ʒ/, /ʃ/, /tʃ/, /ʤ/, /ð/, /θ/, /r/, /l/, and /n/). The dorsal place node includes the velar sounds, made with the help of the tongue dorsum (/k/, /g/, and /ŋ/).

As this brief introduction suggests, the feature geometry theory's main concept is the geometric, sometimes independent, and hierarchical organization of features. The very notion of hierarchy includes the dominant and subordinate nature of features. The theory classifies the sounds much as they are classified in the traditional system of classification, although some terms may be new (*laryngeal* for *voiced* and *dorsal* for *velars*). As in the distinctive feature theory, pluses and minuses may be used to denote the presence and absence of features.

Phonetic Versus Phonological Theories

Phonologists acknowledge that their abstract phonological rules partly reflect physiological phonetic factors. As noted earlier, Stampe (1979) believed that natural phonological processes are due to phonetic (physiological) factors. Kager (1999) stated that "the systems of articulation and perception naturally impose limitations on which sounds (or sound sequences) should be favored" (p. 5). Nonetheless, he also stated that the "interactions of 'raw' phonetic factors" (p. 5) do not account for phonological systems. Phonologists thus see a need for formal, abstract, and universal rules or constraints that account for sound patterns.

Unlike most phonologists, some experimental phoneticians treat language universals, including phonological universals, as empirically determined phenomena (not innate and not due to a knowledge of a universal grammar of languages). For instance, Ohala (1980) suggests that there are only two reasons universal phonological patterns exist. First, many phonological patterns are caused by universal human constraints of "neurological, physiological, aerodynamic, anatomical, acoustic, auditory, or similar" (Ohala, 1980, p. 81) variables. Second, many phonological patterns exist because of sound changes (changes in pronunciation) over time. A person who accidentally mispronounces a word may lead others to copy that, thus leading to a sound change. It is known that, historically, patterns of sound productions change in given languages; changes are not linear across a given society, however. Different segments of a society may change the way certain sounds are produced, giving rise to dialects. The various American dialects are a case in point; certain sound changes that happened in the South did not happen in the East, North, or West, for example. Most phonological theories take note of phonetic factors, and some give them considerable attention (e.g., Archangeli & Pulleyblank, 1994). Nonetheless, phonologists generally either dismiss phonetic factors as inadequate in explaining phonological patterns (Kager, 1999) or treat them inadequately (Dekkers et al., 2000).

It is unfortunate that speech–language pathologists pay more attention to abstract phonological theories with little or no empirical content than to phonetic theories that are grounded in empirical data. The production of speech sounds—whether by typical or atypical learners—is possible only because of sophisticated anatomical, neurological, and physiological structures in humans. Even if we ignore the critical roles that learning and environmental variables play in the acquisition of speech sound productions, phonetics has made it abundantly clear that speech production is a biological as well as a physical event; if we pay due attention to learning related variables, speech production, in a more comprehensive account, is a biobehavioral event, as well. Learning variables may be more easily integrated with phonetic data than with phonological speculations. Teaching speech sounds to children with speech sound disorders (including phonological disorders) involves the manipulation of articulatory movements and learning variables. Clinical intervention hardly ever involves universal patterns, innate grammars, rules that apply to inputs and outputs, optimality constraints, GEN and EVAL, underlying representations, and so forth. Therefore, we would like to draw attention to some research and concepts that have received little attention in spite of being more relevant than the currently popular phonological theories to the clinical science of speech–language pathology.

Instrumental analysis of speech disorders is an important area of investigation that has challenged the typical claim that phonological disorders not associated with physical or physiological deficits "must result from breakdown at the cognitive level of linguistic knowledge and organization" (Grunwell, 1990, p. 5). It is now widely recognized that typical phonetic transcription of speech sound errors is inadequate to capture the topographic complexities of error productions. Transcriptions based on what the clinician hears may not capture subtle topographic features of the child's productions. An early study by Kornfeld

(1971) reported that even though in typical speech sound learning children's production of *grass* and *glass* were both heard as [gwas] and transcribed as such, a spectrographic analysis of those productions was different, suggesting production (phonetic) differences in what might be considered a phonological disorder. Kornfeld concluded that "adults do not always perceive distinctions that children make" (p. 462). Years later, Hewlett (1988) described the kind of contrasts inherent to error productions that cannot be heard but may be found on spectrographic traces as **covert contrast.** As reviewed by Gibbon (2002), more than 20 studies have now acoustically (instrumentally) measured covert contrasts for what is heard as phonemic errors or omissions; they might actually be phonetic errors or transient errors that may be corrected over time. For example, when the clinician cannot detect a difference between a /t/ and a /d/ and both are heard as [d]—a loss of phonemic contrast suggesting a phonological disorder—an acoustic analysis might show that [d] substituted for /t/ is different from [d] substituted for /g/ (Tyler, Figurski, & Langsdale, 1993). Similar covert contrasts have been demonstrated for voiced-voiceless sound substitutions and place of articulation for stops as well as fricatives (see Gibbon, 2002, and Munson, Edwards, Schellinger, Beckman, & Meyer, 2010, for review of studies). Covert contrast essentially shows that children's target and error productions have topographic differences. This clearly shows that what is interpreted as a phonological disorder might actually be a phonetic disorder. Kent (1997) has concluded that covert contrast implies only a "faulty phonetic implementation" (p. 265). Not surprisingly, supporters of phonological disorders interpret covert contrasts to mean that children who show them have relevant phonological knowledge, though they are not able to produce the contrasts in speech (Tyler et al., 1993). This is a curious claim because within the linguistic-phonological framework, phonological errors are thought to be due to a lack of phonological knowledge, but the covert contrast is interpreted as the presence of such knowledge, and yet the child is somehow assumed to be unable to produce the contrasts in spite of the knowledge that is expected to promote correct production. The main problem here is with the assumption of phonological knowledge; its presence or absence has no independent verification other than production. Phonological *knowledge* is an unwarranted assumption; we have only speech sound productions. As such, the entire concept of phonological disorders as conceptualized on a cognitive-linguistic basis may be questionable; as Gibbon concludes, covert contrast suggests "a phonetic deficit rather than a difficulty learning the underlying phonological rules of the language" (2007, p. 253).

A phonetic phenomenon called *undifferentiated gestures*, studied through **electropalatography (EPG),** also suggests that phonological disorders may be due to phonetic difficulties. EPG is an instrumental assessment of tongue and palatal contacts during speech production. An artificial hard palate is fabricated with embedded electrodes to fit a subject's palate; the electrodes send movement-related signals to a computer for viewing and analyzing data. EPG has been used in the study and treatment of motor speech disorders in adults (McAuliffe & Ward, 2006). Because the artificial palate has to be custom made for each speaker, the technique is expensive, is used mostly in research studies, and has not been used much in routine treatment of children with speech sound disorders (Dagenais, 1995). EPG studies have shown that instead of the orderly movements and tongue contacts found in normal speech production, children with speech sound disorders may exhibit **undifferentiated lingual gestures** (Gibbon, 1999). Such atypical tongue gestures may involve simultaneous anterior and posterior palatal contacts during the production of lingual sounds (e.g., /k/ or /d/). Those movements may be associated with both correct and incorrect production of phonemes. Again, phonetic transcriptions are unable to capture this phenomenon. If undifferentiated lingual gestures are documented in a substantial number of children diagnosed to have phonological disorders, the concept of phonological disorders will be further weakened, and phonetically based articulation disorders will be applicable to most children with speech sound disorders. History will repeat itself.

There is another theory that may be more relevant to SLP than the knowledge-and-constraint-based phonological theories. It is the **articulatory theory,** also known as **gestural theory,** a phonetic theory by its content but described also as a phonological theory. According to this theory, articulatory gestures, not necessarily phonemes or features, are the basic units of phonological analysis (Browman & Goldstein, 1986, 1992). A *gesture* is an actual articulatory movement or event that unfolds during speech production. It is a primitive phonological unit but is not the same as a feature or segment. Because gestures are real physiological actions, they are more concrete and measurable than abstract phonological representations. Gestures refer to the formation and release of articulatory constrictions and hence are primarily phonetic in nature. They may be described in terms of *tract variables.* A tract variable describes an articulator, a particular action of that articulator, a place in which that action takes place, and, when applicable, the degree of variability in that action. For example, *lip protrusion* is a tract variable involving the lips and the jaw; there is no degree of variability in the action associated with this variable. On the other hand, *tongue tip constriction* has a location as well as a variability degree of constriction; the articulators involved are the tongue tip, tongue body, and jaw. Other tract variables include *tongue body constrict location, tongue body constrict degree, velar constriction degree,* and *glottis constriction degree* (Browman & Goldstein, 1992). Articulatory gestures have durations, but they may overlap. The concept of gestural overlap accounts for contextual coarticulation or allophonic variation. More fluent and fast speech may be associated with a greater overlap of gestures than slower and more deliberate speech.

Unlike most abstract phonological theories, which concentrate on underlying representations and unobservable knowledge while ignoring how people talk, gestural theory does pay attention to the *act of talking.* The theory proposes that typical language-learning children store and retrieve their first words as patterns of articulatory routines that consist of discrete gestures, not as phoneme sequences. These early gestures are learned during the babbling stage and are gross approximations of adult gestures. Differentiation and coordination of these gestures are associated with more adult-like speech sound productions. In essence, articulatory gestures are the units from which words are formed (Browman & Goldstein, 1992).

Unfortunately, clinical application of gestural theory in treating speech sound disorders has been limited, although the theory does offer a method of analyzing speech sound disorders in light of articulatory movements instead of constraints or rules. One can question, however, whether any phonological theory has been applied in the *treatment* of speech sound disorders. Treatment of speech sound disorders has always been behavioral. The clinician has to teach the production of speech sounds, though they are initially analyzed, organized, and later theorized.

Evaluation of Phonological Theories

Speech–language pathologists are generally convinced of the usefulness of phonological theories. There is not much skepticism expressed about the relevance of phonological theories to a clinical and empirical discipline such as speech–language pathology. Most clinicians and clinical researchers believe that such theories offer powerful explanations of speech sound acquisition and organization (Barlow, 2001; Barlow & Gierut, 1999; Bernhardt & Stemberger, 2000; Smit, 2004; Williams, 2003). Therefore, the discipline is well aware of the widely advocated advantages of phonological theories. Their limitations, however, have received only scant attention.

Phonology sharply contrasts with speech–language pathology. While speech–language pathology is an empirical and clinical (applied) discipline that needs experimental methods to verify its treatment procedures, phonology is a taxonomic and speculative discipline. Experimental phoneticians (e.g., Ohala, 1986) have pointed out that phonologists rarely use experimental methods. Instead, phonologists are more interested in two overarching concepts: universality of grammar and innate knowledge of that grammar. Much of the controversy in phonological theories is due to this grand ambition among linguists to find *universal* rules, constraints, processes, representations, knowledge, and so forth. However, no sooner is a "universal" rule or constraint announced than an exception to it is found in some language. Such discoveries often lead to new rules rather than what scientists would expect: the abandonment of invalid rules. For example, at one point when innate phonological rules were determined to be universal and inviolable (cannot be violated), it was later found out that those rules are violated in certain languages. Instead of abandoning the concept of universal and inviolable rules, however, a new rule (now called a constraint) was formulated saying that *rules are violable.* A proper study of language variability, instead of an excessive concern with universal rules or constraints, would give a pause to theorists. Such a study also eventually identifies aspects that are more or less common among languages.

In newer theories, newer terms stand for the same old concepts. All are theories of language capacity as mental structures: The *deep* and *surface structures* of older theories are called *input* and *output representations* in newer theories. A phonological process was a *rule* previously but now is a *conflicting constraint.* Most of the changes and revisions in phonological theories are forced by some new observation—for example, that a certain rule, thought to be universal, is not universal.

The most troublesome feature of phonological theories is the pervasive and unobservable mentalism. In other words, everything that is important in language, according to phonologists, happens in a mental underground. Observable language productions are merely a reflection of an underlying mental structure or, as in OT, *input representation*; what speakers say is less important than what is inferred to exist in their minds, knowledge, or universal grammar. In most cases, phonological theories do not simplify the phenomena they seek to explain; they obscure them. As Ohala put it, "Explanation is, after all, reducing the unknown to the known, not to further unknown, uncertain, or unprovable entities" (1996, p. 262). It is a puzzle why speech–language pathologists, who, as empirical scientists, should be demanding observable and verifiable evidence, get attracted to obscure mentalism that reduces observable phenomena to something unobservable.

Another equally puzzling notion is that the child possesses phonological knowledge and that such knowledge is essential to acquiring the sound system of language. There is no evidence, however, that children acquire an abstract sound system; they learn to produce speech sounds that may have patterns based on response properties, which most likely are phonetic (physiological, acoustic, behavioral). The belief that to learn a complex response one should have knowledge of the complex mechanisms of that response has no empirical basis. The hypothesis of the necessity of phonological knowledge for speech sound learning is similar to a hypothesis that knowledge of the laws of physics is necessary for learning to ride a bicycle. As Ohala (2005) has put it, we eat, walk, see, and hear without consciously or unconsciously knowing about the physical constraints of those actions. He wrote, "Even a rock obeys the laws of physics without having to know them" (p. 38). Such concepts as phonological knowledge and innate constraints or rules do not explain speech sound productions or the patterns found in them. As Menn put it, "Calling a rule 'natural' or a constraint 'innate' is like calling a hurricane 'an act of God'; having said so, one knows no more than before about how to predict or to understand its causes" (2004, p. 68). A prior knowledge of a pattern is not necessary to learn behaviors that form a pattern; after learning a patterned behavior, knowledge of the pattern is not necessary to maintain the behavior.

Clinicians should understand phonological theories as well as critically evaluate them. From the standpoint of the assessment and treatment of SSDs, the current perspectives in phonology are excessively speculative. There is no compelling clinical advantage in speculating about innate rules, constraints, universal grammars, mental representations, hidden phonological knowledge, GEN and EVAL, and so forth. Ohala points out that "there may be no need for features, underspecification, autosegmental notation, feature geometry, or similar speculative devices" (2005, p. 35). Before the developmental and clinical implications of one approach are fully explored and explained to the clinicians, a new approach emerges. The emergence of a new approach devalues older approaches; currently, there is no unified theory that incorporates the useful features of all extant theories.

One gains the impression that changing perspectives indicates a significant step in scientific progress in the study of speech sounds and their patterns across languages. However, it is possible that different perspectives are parallel notions, not scientifically cumulative, and not equipped, therefore, to form a more comprehensive view of speech sounds produced in different languages. Many varied, conflicting, and competing theoretical models of speech sounds and their production indicate only that observations are still inadequate and theories are mostly premature. For example, the once widely accepted standard phonological feature theory did not account for prosody, a basic feature of speech. Most phonological theories have alternate forms and significant limitations on what they encompass, and none are universally accepted. Nonlinear phonological theories propose different hierarchies to organize segmental and suprasegmental features of speech, but there is no agreement on any hierarchical system. If the history of phonology and its effects on speech–language pathology is indicative of future developments, most of these theories will be modified or replaced before their clinical applications have been fully tested.

Finally, clinicians should make a clear distinction between theory and description. Most so-called theories of phonology are nothing more than attempts to improve upon the descriptive framework for phonological phenomena. As explanations of such phenomena they are highly suspect, however, because of their complete lack of independent support.

Therefore, clinicians need to develop certain critical standards with which to judge the usefulness or relevance of newer theories. A standard that must be fulfilled is that theories have empirical, not just logical or rational, content. If a theory is mostly formal, with no empirical content, then such a theory is not useful to a clinical science.

Explanatory Status of Phonological Concepts

The most relevant and perhaps the most troubling issue for clinicians is the explanatory status of phonological concepts, especially the concepts of naturalness and markedness, phonological rules and processes, and a child's presumed innate phonological knowledge. These are rational and formal concepts with no basis in the empirical experience of children learning their speech sounds.

The concepts of naturalness and markedness have come under heavy criticism in linguistics, but that is not reflected in speech–language pathology. The concepts are vague and lack empirical support; they have such multiple meanings as to be ineffective in any theory (Haspelmath, 2006; Hume, 2004, 2011); and they have limited usefulness, if any, in understanding different patterns of speech production and variations across languages. The basic idea that what is relatively more common across languages is natural (unmarked) is simply a taxonomic statement. It is only a *definition* of what one considers *natural* in speech. The idea does not explain anything, as definitions are not explanations. Furthermore, as Bernhardt and Stemberger (1998) have pointed out, there is no independent verification of naturalness and markedness; the concepts are circular. A process is natural because it is common, and it is common because it is natural. One way out of this circularity is the simpler notion that what is natural is easier to articulate, and what is marked is more difficult to articulate. Although articulatory difficulty poses measurement challenges, experimental phonetic studies have a chance to measure it. The notions of marked and unmarked, on the other hand, are immeasurable. Hume (2004) proposes that markedness can be reduced to the predictability of sounds and their patterns in given languages. This predictability is related to the language experience of speakers. Haspelmath (2006) believes that *markedness* is not a scientific term, as it stands for such commonsense notions as something more or less common; he suggests that the simpler concept of *phonetic difficulty* should replace that of markedness. He writes that "linguists can dispense with the term 'markedness' and many of the concepts that it has been used to express" (Haspelmath, 2006, p. 33). Blevins (2004, 2006), who advocates an evolutionary approach to understanding speech sound patterns, writes that language should be "viewed as a dynamic, probabilistic, evolving system—one which is ultimately grounded in the *physical realities of how we articulate* and perceive speech sounds" (2006, p. 158, emphasis added).

The taxonomic idea of naturalness and markedness is quickly expanded into an explanatory statement: What is natural is innate and does not require environmental input. That a frequently observed phenomenon is innate is an unwarranted assumption. Nothing in the frequency of a phenomenon suggests its causation. The cause of a phenomenon must be found independently of its frequency.

Can we assume that things that happen less frequently are less *natural* (however the term is defined) than those that occur more frequently? Most likely, we cannot. There are more species of insects than of hominids. Does that mean that insects are more natural than hominids? Furthermore, from a historical perspective, what is now more common could once have been less common, and vice versa.

The assumption that more frequently occurring behavioral events are innate, not in need of environmental assistance, is unwarranted. Similarly, the assumption that less frequently occurring behavioral events have no genetic basis and hence are entirely environmentally induced is also unwarranted. Therefore, the markedness theory is just another way of describing observed speech production phenomena. The theory has no explanatory power. For instance, the observation that children master CV structures earlier than CVC or CCV structures because the CV structure is more natural (occurs more frequently across languages) is no explanation. Such complex assertions are no better than a more down-to-earth statement that CV productions involve simpler articulatory movements than CVC or CCV productions and that simpler skills are acquired before more complex skills. The markedness concept is thus superfluous.

Phonological rules and processes often are stated in empirical terms. That is, a stated rule is said to capture a child's linguistic or verbal experience. For example, formal theorists often suggest that a child who does not produce consonants in word-final positions *follows the rule of final consonant deletion*. In the OT, the constraint *CODA (no final consonants) prohibits final consonants, and, obeying that prohibitory rule, children omit final consonants. Clinicians wonder, however, in what sense a child follows a phonological rule or obeys a constraint. Whether a speaker follows a rule or behavioral regularities simply give that impression is an important empirical issue. We will soon return to this issue.

Nonlinear phonological theories additionally assert that there are underlying abstract phonological *representations* for different phonemes, phonemic features, and their permissible combinations. Presumably, children keep these underlying phonological representations in their mind, brain, or somewhere else. Children who master their speech sounds are supposed to have correctly *realized* the underlying phonological representations. Children who make phonological errors are presumed to have failed in realizing those representations. Underlying representations, being unobservable, are tautologically inferred: The child who masters the sounds has realized the underlying representations, and the one who doesn't has not realized them correctly. The only evidence here is the successful or failed speech sound learning; there is no evidence of the underlying representations.

Most phonologists do not test their assumptions in experiments with human participants. They analyze language as though it is an autonomous machine. Some experimental phoneticians, on the other hand, have tried to put some phonological assumptions to the test. For example, Ohala (1986) tested the assumption that native speakers of English have a knowledge of the morphemic constituents of complex derived words even though the presumed stem is phonetically different from its form in other words (e.g., the morpheme *extrusion* consists of *extrude* plus *-ion*). The researchers trained linguistically naive participants to distinguish the base morpheme in complex derived words (e.g., *yellow* from *-ish* in *yellowish*) and then had the participants make similar judgments on such words as *skepticism*, *plasticity*, and *medicate*. A majority of respondents failed to show a generalized knowledge of the morphemic constituents of the complex derived words presented to them. These results and those of similar experiments (see Ohala, 1986) suggest that inferences about speakers' knowledge is precarious. The results also suggest that phonological (and grammatical) assumptions may be subjected to experimental testing—a practice that is rare among phonologists. Based on the results of his experiment, Ohala stated, "It is probably a mistake (without strong evidence) to make extravagant assumptions about the depth and detail of native speakers' knowledge of sound patterns in their language" (1986, p. 17).

An understanding of how phonological rules are formed gives us an insight into their empirical or formal status. Phonological rules are statements that describe (not explain) observed patterns of phonological behaviors. To give a simple example, when children do not produce certain phonemes in word-final positions, the observer captures this behavior by stating the rule of *final consonant deletion*. Does this mean then that the children somehow have discovered the rule of final consonant deletion and are following it? Or does this mean that someone has taught the children to follow the rule of final consonant deletion? Neither is likely, as observed patterns of behavior do not necessarily indicate that the people being observed are following a rule regarding that pattern. An even simpler question is Why would a child invent and follow a final consonant deletion rule? There is no answer in any of the linguistic theories.

There is an important distinction between *rule following* and *rule extraction*. **Rule following** is evident when a person's behavior meets the requirements of an explicitly stated rule, when the rule has been formally taught, and when the person can state the rule. Children who do not touch hot surfaces because they are taught not to are following a rule. Drivers follow traffic rules. Behaviors that follow rules are also known as *rule governed*. A behavior is **rule governed** only when it explicitly follows a rule that has been taught and that the person in question can state. Phonological rules are not taught to children, and they cannot state them; rules are unnecessary to learn speech sound productions. For example, the /mb/ sequence in English-speaking children is undocumented in word-initial positions not because children are told that the sequence is "banned" in English but simply because the children have not heard the sequence. Nobody, including the children's caregivers, knows anything about constraints that ban speech sounds. Although children on occasion do produce what they have not heard before, the simplest explanation of the absence of phonetic combinations that are nonexistent in a language is that the production of such combinations is not heard and, therefore, is not reinforced by the child's verbal community. Children do not persist with uncommon phoneme combinations simply because their verbal community does not support them.

While rule following, when it is the result of rule instruction, is a behavioral learning phenomenon, **rule extraction** is a scientific-analytic activity. Phonologists *extract* rules from regularities in the phonological productions of children. Extracted rules economically describe patterns of behaviors. They do not explain those patterned behaviors, nor are they part of a child's skills, knowledge, or abilities. Therefore, there is no compelling reason to drive the rules extracted from children's patterned speech–language productions back into their minds.

Linguistic rules, whether syntactic or phonologic, may be explicitly taught to speakers. Typically, students learn syntactic or phonologic rules only through explicit instruction. Speakers of foreign languages may learn rules and follow them. But even for speakers of foreign languages, explicit rule following may eventually fade into behaviors maintained by reinforcing contingencies as the speakers acquire native-like language skills.

In the newer nonlinear phonological theories, constraints are depicted as autonomous in-the-mind mechanical devices that say "no final consonants," "no deletions," "no fricatives," and so forth. It is hard to translate these formal and mechanistic concepts into the actions of children learning to speak their language or of children and adults interacting socially. A much more serious concern with the constraints of OT is why children would follow any hypothesized constraints. For example, why would an English-speaking child follow the constraint "no final consonants" when final consonants, which do not exist in some languages, do exist in English? Why would this child's grammar say "no fricatives" when English is full of them? Why would children who have articulation and phonological disorders have a grammar that is in clear conflict with the adult grammar? Moreover, why would the hypothetical GEN of the OT generate an infinite set of output candidates? Does a child, faced with the social conditions that are a stimulus for saying "Mom," think of *infinite* possibilities, including such totally unrelated and irrelevant utterances as "bom" or "Tom"? If the child does not think of them, what is the meaning of an infinite set of outputs being generated by a mechanism in his or her mind?

It is hard enough to explain why children misarticulate their speech sounds. But the speculation that children somehow have a deviant grammar is no explanation. Phonologists must face the task of explaining why some children have a deviant grammar in their minds.

Missing Empirical Variables

Reading phonological theories, one cannot imagine a child talking in social situations. One gets the impression that empirical variables are unimportant in learning to produce speech and language within a verbal community. Theories make no room for social interactions, environmental stimulus conditions, behavioral consequences for correct or incorrect speech productions (explicit or implicit reinforcement or corrective feedback from caregivers), ethnocultural variables and family environment, effects of education, socioeconomic variables, or neurophysiological conditions or limitations. Phonological theorists pay scant attention to such phonetic variables as aerodynamic factors, physical and acoustic influences, physiologic and motoric factors, or central neural mechanisms that are known to play important roles in speech learning and production. According to some phonologists, the child needs only a GEN and an EVAL and a system of ranked constraints to produce speech.

What about speech as social interaction? Under what environmental conditions is speech likely, and how may social reactions to speech alter the topography of speech? What about the effects of clinical treatment? Perhaps phonologists would encourage clinicians to assume that the goal of clinical work is to re-rank the wrongly ranked constraints in the child's mental representations, not to teach the production of specific sounds and patterns of sounds.

The Clinician and the Theoretician

A general misconception exists that there are linguistic or phonological treatment procedures. Whether it is the distinctive feature approach of the past or the phonological approach of the present, treatment involves only such procedures as showing a certain physical stimulus (e.g., a picture), asking a question (e.g., "What is this?"), modeling the correct response, and reinforcing the correct response or giving corrective feedback for the incorrect response. This is the typical behavioral treatment. Errors may have been analyzed as an articulation (phonetic) disorder with no pattern or as a phonological disorder with collapsed phonemic contrasts and error patterns. But the treatment has always involved, no matter how the disorder is theorized, teaching the production of specific phonemes. The results of such treatment studies may be interpreted in light of phonological knowledge, innate rules, or constraints adhered to or violated, but that does not change the fact that the production of phonemes is taught using the behavioral methods. One might claim that the linguistic interpretation of behavioral data is incongruous; the methods by which the data are generated are not consistent with the interpretation of the data. Even if untreated sounds within a pattern (e.g., final consonant deletion) are produced because other sounds were treated, one cannot claim that the theory of a phonological process or constraint re-ranking has been supported. Production of untreated phonemes that belong to a class is a matter of generalization, a learning variable, not a matter of presumed underlying knowledge and theoretical ranking.

Several lines of investigation, including covert contrasts, experimental phonetics, gestural phonological theories, and speech sound disorder treatment research suggest that the concept of phonological disorders may not be based on a solid foundation (Ball et al., 2010; Ohala, 2004, 2005). Phonological theories that assume that speech sound disorders are a problem of phonological knowledge have not been empirically supported, because the assumption can be neither supported nor rejected. If a sound is not in a child's inventory, it is assumed that there is no phonological knowledge of it; if the sound is there but produced inconsistently, it is assumed that the knowledge of it is incomplete; if there is covert contrast, it is assumed that there is knowledge of the sound but somehow production is incorrect. Such assumptions can never be proved false because they are presumed true no matter what the data show.

When phonological explanations are considered untenable, the only remaining explanation is that speech sound disorders are phonetic in nature. See Text Box 3.1 for more on the possibility that all speech sound disorders are phonetic.

A linguistic interpretation of behavioral treatment studies may be possible but does not necessarily show that nonlinguistic, behavioral interpretations are not valid. There is a need for controlled treatment studies in which the presumed power, usefulness, and application of phonological theories are tested, but they cannot be tested because their content is abstract and presumed.

Regarding the treatment of language and phonological disorders, a trend among linguistic theorists is to encourage clinicians to become more theory oriented in their clinical practices. Without theories, they contend, clinical work will lose direction or lack principle (Johnston, 1983; Schwartz, 1992). However, neither the clinician nor the clinical treatment researcher can afford theories that cannot be tested. Good treatment research is possible without theories, especially deductive linguistic theories, which propose theories first, hoping data will come next. Unfortunately, the theories sometimes get ingrained regardless of whether such data ever come.

Systematic treatment research is fully capable of finding speech sound patterns. For example, if final consonants are a response class (a pattern), their deletion is an error pattern. If the production of some sounds in that class are taught to a child who did not previously produce many final consonants, and if the probe data show generalized production of

---

Text Box 3.1. Could all speech sound disorders be phonetic?

Several lines of research, including *covert contrast,* reviewed in this chapter, suggest that all speech sound disorders may be phonetic in nature. Of course, most phonologists who claim that phonological disorders are a matter of deficient phonological knowledge deny this possibility. In their view, phonetic disorders are "mere" speech sound production problems. Most speech–language pathologists, too, believe that in some children, speech disorders are due to a lack of underlying knowledge or mental representations. But what evidence links typical and atypical speech production with different levels of underlying phonological knowledge? Some experimental phoneticians would argue that there is no evidence at all. Phonological knowledge is inferred from different patterns of speech sound production. If a child demonstrates a typical (normal or adult-like) speech sound pattern, it is inferred that the child has good phonological knowledge. If the pattern is deficient, the knowledge is deficient. In this line of thinking, there is no independent evidence of phonological knowledge; therefore, it does not explain phonological disorders. But even more critically, *the inference does not justify the diagnostic category of phonological disorder.* To justify that diagnosis, there should, first of all, be a method to measure phonological knowledge that is independent of speech sound production. Then *experimental* research should show the following: (1) When the independent measure of phonological knowledge is low, speech sound disorders result; (2) when the measure is high, speech sound productions are normal (typical); and (3) when phonological knowledge is raised in children, their speech sound errors disappear. Such evidence is currently nonexistent because there is no way to produce it. Phonological disorders are an inferred diagnostic entity with no independent verification. The so-called phonological disorder may be a severe form of articulation disorder. More than the counterarguments, treatment research supports the assertion that all speech sound disorders are phonetic: Phonological disorders are remediated only by teaching the production of individual speech sounds, not by raising children's phonological knowledge.

---

untreated and previously missing final consonants, the clinical researcher will have found a valid sound pattern. Final consonants that do not get generalized in replicated research probably form a different response class. Systematic research and replication are capable of establishing response classes based on experimental evidence. This inductive method (data first, theory later) is superior to the rationalist, deductive theories whose assumptions are untestable. Although data to refute them cannot be produced, their longevity is limited only by a newer deductive theory.

Summary of the Advanced Unit

- **Phonological theories** seek to explain universal sound patterns and the underlying phonological knowledge that speakers possess.

- The two types of phonological theories are the linear and the nonlinear. **Linear theories** propose a bundle of unorganized sound features, whereas **nonlinear theories** propose that the features are hierarchically organized.

- Stampe's linear, natural phonological theory proposes that **phonological processes** are innate and phonetically based; children simplify adult productions that they cannot yet articulate.

- Of the several nonlinear theories, the **optimality theory** has received much research attention. This theory explains speech sound disorders in terms of constraints that are adhered to or violated and are common to all languages.

- **Markedness** and **faithfulness** are the two main constraints of OT, and they conflict with each other; their conflict is resolved by a differential ranking in the languages.

- **Marked** features are natural, simple, common in languages, and acquired earlier than **unmarked** features.

- The autosegmental theory proposes that features may interact with each other or function autonomously; the related **metric theory** includes a hierarchy of features based on feet, syllables, and segments and pays particular attention to syllable structure and stress patterns.

- The **feature geometry theory** proposes that hierarchically organized features are based on the six anatomical structures of speech production: the glottis, soft palate, lips, tongue blade, tongue body, and tongue root.

- **Phonetic theories,** critical of phonological theories, propose that speech sound patterns are grounded in articulatory (anatomic-physiological) constraints.

- **Covert contrast** implies that misarticulations may still involve some discriminated response topographies, thus questioning the assumption of phonological disorders as separate from phonetic disorders.

- **Articulatory (gestural) theory** suggests that articulatory movements are the basic units of analysis (not phonemes or features).

- Phonological theories are excessively concerned with underlying and abstract knowledge, restraints, rules, universal patterns, and constraints whose clinical relevance is limited; they are often **devoid of empirical content**; instead of explaining speech sound productions or disorders, they mystify them. They ignore **learning variables,** without which speech sound acquisition cannot take place.

- **Experimental treatment research** may be the best way to find patterns based on the generalized production of untreated phonemes. A more valid theory may emerge from this inductive approach (data first, theory later) than the linguistic-deductive approach (theory first, data later or sometimes never).

TYPICAL LEARNING OF SPEECH SOUNDS: NORMS, PATTERNS, AND THEORIES

Communication is the name of the game.

—*Andy Rooney*

Basic Unit: Typical Learning of Speech Sounds: From Infancy Through the Early School Years

Children continually fascinate adults with the new skills they learn daily. An impressive accomplishment is the child's learning of speech sounds and sound combinations to form words. Parents and significant others view the production of the first word as a major achievement that is celebrated and remembered. This event typically earns a spot in the child's "milestones" scrapbook. The acquisition of speech sounds and their patterns, which allow a child to verbalize his or her first words, is a complex learning process that begins in infancy and proceeds through the early school years. Many experts in child development, developmental linguistics, and speech–language pathology have studied this acquisition process. Such intensive study is important for the speech–language pathologist because an SLP needs to distinguish normal from impaired speech sound learning (SSL) to determine whether a diagnosis of speech sound disorder (SSD) is appropriate.

This Basic Unit will describe the stages of typical SSL from infancy through the early school years. Approximate ages for the various stages of SSL will be provided. Although a developmental approach is taken, individual variability in SSL will be emphasized. The existence of individual differences in communicative development is now well established (Davis & MacNeilage, 1995; Stoel-Gammon, 1985; Stoel-Gammon & Cooper, 1981; Vihman, 1998). In addition, we summarize the research on variables that may be related to SSL in children.

In the Advanced Unit of this chapter, we describe and evaluate (1) methodological and theoretical issues in speech perception and discrimination research, (2) theories of articulation and phonological development, and (3) issues in researching variables that affect SSL.

Prelinguistic Development

The term *prelinguistic* refers mostly to infant vocalizations and infant speech perception. It implies that sound productions at that level are not entirely linguistic because the child does not produce them to achieve desired effects on the caretakers or other listeners. In essence, linguistic researchers believe that an infant's sounds or sound combinations often lack a specific referent and communicative intent, especially in the very early stages. We prefer the term *prelinguistic* over *nonlinguistic*, because the prefix *pre-* means "before," whereas *non-* means "not" or "absent." Therefore, vocalizations during the infant stage are considered "before" true language rather than "not" language altogether. This important distinction is highlighted because research suggests a positive relationship between early infant vocalizations and the later development of adult-based words—which parents often recognize (Locke, 1983; Oller, 1980; Oller, Weiman, Doyle, & Ross, 1976; Stark, 1978, 1979, 1980; Stoel-Gammon & Cooper, 1981; Vihman, 1998; Vihman, Macken, Miller, Simmons, & Miller, 1985). It is important to note that although infants may not produce prelinguistic vocalizations to affect their caretakers, the caretakers respond to them in various ways and are thus affected.

Speech–language pathologists working with infants and toddlers must determine whether an infant judged to be at risk for a communication disorder is on the proper course of speech and language learning. To make such a determination, the SLP must have a basic understanding of what is typically expected in an infant at varying stages of communication development. Some believe that an infant's perception of speech spoken in the environment may be the foundation for soon-to-be-learned communication skills. We will begin with what we know about how infants perceive speech.

Infant Speech Perception

Perception, as well as production, of speech sounds requires learning. But what exactly does the word *perception* refer to? The basic dictionary meaning of *perception* is "becoming aware of something through the senses"; the term is derived from the Latin verb *percipere*, which means "to seize" something. When people *perceive* something, they are said to have *seized* it, a prescientific term that means the same as *grasp* (as in *grasping* something someone says). Infants neither *seize* nor *grasp* speech sounds. Generally, perception is an unobservable mental event. As we will see in the Advanced Unit of this chapter, behavioral scientists would rather limit themselves to observable actions (Schlinger, 2010). Although SLPs are urged to consider alternative views of speech perception, what follows is the more traditional account, along with a critical evaluation of it in the Advanced Unit. In the discussion of perception that follows, we emphasize the observable responses of the infant.

Simply put, **speech perception** is understanding spoken speech (Kent, 1997b; Raphael et al., 2011). *Infant speech perception* pertains to an infant's understanding of speech. But how do we know that an infant perceives or understands speech? We can know only by looking at the kind of response the infant gives to sounds and their patterns. Most parents know that infants respond to patterns of sound stimuli. Researchers, though, have been interested in finding the youngest age at which infants can be said to perceive speech. Once that is known, the next question is whether infants perceive speech stimuli without learning, leading to the assumption that the knowledge is innate, or the skill is one that children learn. Several researchers have sought to answer such questions, and the study of infant speech perception broadened in the early 1970s. Since that time, a vast number of investigations have been conducted, resulting in abundant information on infant speech perception

(Houston, 2011). A related area of investigation is auditory development, with an emphasis on sound localization and auditory discrimination skills in infants (Houston, 2005).

Sound Localization and Auditory Discrimination in the Newborn

Research has shown that infants can localize sound by an eye movement or a head turn toward the source of the sound. Infants as young as 2 to 7 days old have been found to turn in the direction of a rattling noise 75% of the time (Muir & Field, 1979). This response from the newborn is not as astonishing as it may seem, because infants' hearing is well developed by about the 25th week of gestation (Birnholz & Benacerraf, 1983; Elliot & Elliot, 1964; Johansson, Wendenburg, & Westin, 1964; Kuczwara, Brinholz, & Klodd, 1984). Newborn infants have been hearing sounds for approximately 4 months prior to their birth. This means that infants begin to hear speech sounds in utero (see Houston, 2005, 2011, for a review of studies); however, because of the attenuation of external sounds that reach the developing fetus by the mother's body, mostly low-frequency sounds are heard. Whispered speech does not reach the fetus and, thus, is not reinforcing to the newborn, but low-frequency speech that passes through the maternal abdominal wall is (see Spence & Freeman, 1996, for a review). Fetuses also can hear the intonation and rhythm of the ambient (surrounding) language, called the *suprasegmentals* (Houston, 2011). Some studies have shown that newborn infants can discriminate between varied pure-tone frequencies (Bridger, 1961), intensities (Bartoshuk, 1964), durations (Spring & Dale, 1975), and white noise levels (Bench, 1969).

Infants prefer human speech to other noises, which is relevant for learning speech (Eisenberg, 1976; Jensen, Williams, & Bzoch, 1975; Shultz & Vouloumanos, 2010). Even more relevant is the finding that a child as young as 3 days old can discriminate his or her mother's voice from the voices of other women (DeCasper & Fifer, 1980). Infants as young as 19 to 72 hours find the maternal voice reinforcing to them; that is, they respond with increasing frequency to the maternal voice (Spence & Freeman, 1996). Furthermore, DeCasper and Spence (1986) found that an infant prefers a passage that his or her mother read aloud while she was pregnant over speech passages that she had not read aloud during that time. Newborn infants also respond better to verbal stimuli from the mother's language than to stimuli from a foreign language (Moon, Cooper, & Fifer, 1993).

Speech Perception

The infant's tendencies to localize sound, prefer the human voice to non-human noises, respond differentially to the mother's voice, discriminate frequency and loudness levels, and react to the rhythm and intonation of the ambient language are all quite remarkable skills. The importance of these phenomena is that the infant's response to speech sounds can predict language development in the second year of life (Tsao, Liu, & Kuhl, 2004).

Discriminating among classes of speech sounds is a complex skill. Because infants cannot speak, how do we study their differential reactions to different speech sounds? Two classical methods used to find an answer to this question involve high-amplitude sucking and visually reinforced head turns (Eimas, Siqueland, Jusczyk, & Vigorito, 1971; Kuhl, 1987). The sucking response is excellent for studying speech perception in infants because the rate of sucking usually changes when a new stimulus (such as a different sound) is introduced. The high-amplitude sucking method is used with very young infants (from birth to about 5 months old) because of its conditionability in such infants. With older infants, the visually reinforced head turn method is used.

In the **high-amplitude sucking method,** infants in two groups, one experimental and the other control, are allowed to suck on a pacifier attached to a pressure transducer. Initially, a baseline of this non-nutritional sucking rate is established. When the sucking rate is stabilized, the experimenter presents a repeating speech stimulus (e.g., the syllable *pa pa pa*). There may be an increase in the infant's sucking rate as a result of this reinforcing sound stimulus, presented contingent on sucking. However, with repeated presentation of the stimulus, the sucking rate levels off and then begins to decrease because of adaptation to the stimulus. Following that adaptation, the infants in the experimental group are presented with a different sound stimulus (e.g., the syllable *ba ba ba*), while those in the control group continue to hear the same sound. An increase in the sucking rate of the infants in the experimental group while the rate of sucking in the control group stabilizes or decreases is taken to mean that the infants in the experimental group distinguished the new sound from the old.

The **visually reinforced head turn method** exploits the tendency of an infant to turn toward a sound (sound localization) and reinforces that behavior visually. A reliable head turn response is evident in infants as young as 5 to 6 months old. During the experiment, an infant's attention is held by a researcher or assistant manipulating a toy within the infant's visual field. The experimenter then presents a repeated speech stimulus (e.g., the syllable *va va va*) through a loudspeaker. The infant turns his or her head toward the speaker at first but soon gets adapted to the sound and keeps looking at the toy being manipulated. The experimenter then presents a different speech sound stimulus (e.g., the syllable *sa sa sa*). If the infant promptly turns toward the speaker when the stimulus is changed from *va va va* to *sa sa sa*, the head turn is immediately reinforced by by placing a Plexiglas box housing an animated and lighted toy in front of the loudspeaker. *Control trials* (e.g., the continued and repeated presentation of *va*) and *change trials* (e.g., the new stimulus *sa*) are alternated a few times to see if the infant reliably turns toward the reinforcing box when the change trials are presented but not when the control trials are presented. If so, it is concluded that the infant discriminated ("perceived") the two sets of syllables (Eilers, 1980; Kuhl, 1987).

Neurophysiological methods are additional, more recent methods of studying speech perception. These include the recording of event-related potentials (ERPs) and functional magnetic resonance imaging (fMRI). In the ERP procedure, the electrical activity of the brain in response to various speech stimuli is recorded through electrodes placed on the skull (scalp). In fMRI, changes in the cerebral blood flow are measured as different kinds of stimuli—speech sounds in this case—are presented (Dehaene-Lambertz, Hertz-Pannier, & Dubois, 2006; Dehaene-Lambertz, Hertz-Pannier, Dubois, & Dehaene, 2008). It should be noted that under these procedures, the infant need not give a specific behavioral response.

There are many studies on infant speech perception (see Eilers & Minifie, 1975; Eilers, Wilson, & Moore, 1977; Eimas et al., 1971; Morse, 1972; see also Miller, Kent, & Atal, 1991, for a collection of papers; and Eilers, 1980; Gerken & Aslin, 2005; Houston, 2005, 2011; Jusczyk & Luce, 2002, for reviews of studies). Additional studies with varied methods have been concerned with infants' perception and discrimination of pitch contours (Morse,

1972), syllable stress levels (Spring & Dale, 1975), sounds produced at different places of articulation (Eimas, 1974), voice onset times (Eimas et al., 1971), and utterances from the infants' native language contrasted with utterances from foreign languages (Mehler et al., 1988). The results of more recent neurophysiological studies have shed light on the relation between auditory stimuli and cerebral regional responses, as summarized later.

There is a good deal of consistency among findings, although some discrepant findings have been reported in certain areas. Generally speaking, studies have shown that infants can be conditioned to respond differently to different sounds and syllables at a very young age; in fact, infants who are only 4 days old have been so conditioned. It should be noted that while most investigators and textbook writers report that *infants have an ability to discriminate between speech sounds*, we prefer to report that *infants can be taught or conditioned to discriminate between speech sounds by positive reinforcement*, as the methods used in the studies are methods of learning and conditioning—mostly operant conditioning, in which a particular response (e.g., an increased rate of non-nutritional sucking or a head turn toward a sound source) is quickly and consistently reinforced. Newborns do not simply discriminate with no prior exposure (for example, intrauterine exposure to the mother's voice) or learning experiences, as in the visually reinforced head turn and high-amplitude sucking experiments. This generally ignored issue of exposure and learning is addressed in the Advanced Unit of this chapter.

The many studies on infant speech perception, taken as a whole, have generally shown the following:

- Very young infants can be taught to make fine distinctions among speech sounds.

- Infants as young as 6 months can be taught to discriminate distinctions in pitch contours.

- Infants can be taught to discriminate among syllable stress levels.

- Infants can be conditioned to discriminate sounds produced at different places of articulation.

- Infants can be taught to discriminate varied voice onset times.

- Infants as young as 1 month can be conditioned to discriminate between [pa] and [ba].

- Infants as young as 2 months can be conditioned to discriminate between [ba] and [ga].

- Infants between 2 and 3 months can be conditioned to discriminate between [ra] and [la].

- Infants between 1 and 4 months can be conditioned to discriminate between [sa] and [va] and [sa] and [ʃa].

- Infants between 1 and 4 months can be conditioned to discriminate the vowel contrasts [u] and [i] and [a] and [ɪ], as well as [pa] and [pi].

- Infants between 6 and 8 months can be conditioned to discriminate between [sa] and [za].

- Infants 6 months old may be taught to discriminate some initial consonant clusters (e.g., [sta] from [ska]).

- Infants between 14 and 18 weeks can be more readily conditioned to discriminate between phonetically similar pairs (e.g., [pi] and [pu]) than between phonetically dissimilar pairs (e.g., [pi] and [ka]).

- Infants can generalize their learned discrimination to syllables or sounds produced by different speakers (e.g., if conditioned to discriminate syllables produced by a male speaker, they could discriminate the same syllables produced by a female speaker or a child speaker).

- Infants up to 8 months can be conditioned to discriminate speech sounds that are not used in their native language (e.g., infants with an English-speaking background will discriminate sounds found in Asian or African languages that are absent in English; similarly, Asian and African infants discriminate English sounds that are nonexistent in their languages).

- As infants reach 12 months of age or so, it becomes increasingly more difficult to condition them to discriminate sounds not used in their native language. This is not a universal tendency, however; some infants may continue to discriminate certain kinds of sound contrasts not found in their language (especially contrasts based on place of articulation).

- By age 2 years, most infants can reliably respond to differences in phonemes—leading to the often cited conclusions that they are *perceiving phonemes categorically and the phoneme boundaries are now adult-like.*

- Infants as young as 4 days old can discriminate utterances (not specific speech sounds) from their own language from those of an unfamiliar language.

- Individual differences are significant in speech perception.

In terms of sound classes, studies have shown that 6-month-olds may be taught to discriminate the following:

- stop consonant voicing contrasts
- stops from glides
- stops, nasals, affricates, and fricatives from each other
- liquids
- nasal from oral vowels and among oral vowels
  Studies also have shown the following:
- Infants as old as 12 to 14 months *cannot* be readily conditioned to discriminate between [θa] and [fa].
- Infants between 1 and 4 months *cannot* be readily conditioned to discriminate between [sa] and [za].
- Young infants *cannot* be readily conditioned to discriminate between [fi] and [θi].

- Young infants *cannot* be readily conditioned to discriminate between stops used in multisyllabic productions with relatively short syllable durations (e.g., [ataba] versus [atapa]).

- Up to 50% of infants cannot be conditioned at all, and repeated attempts to condition them will make them fussy or restless.

Studies of brain structures and functions have shown the following:

- Brain structural asymmetry (larger left than right side) is evident early in life.

- Processing of phonetic elements may be evident in the left temporal cortex as early as 3 months of age.

- During the first year, auditory stimuli cause blood flow in the left language regions (i.e., the inferior frontal and superior temporal regions) to increase more than in the right cortical areas; increased EPRs in the language areas also may be noted.

- Infant brain regions involved in speech and language are similar to those regions in adult brains.

....

ACTIVITY

Briefly describe the three main procedures to study infant speech discrimination.

....

Theoretical explanations of infant speech perception have undergone some changes over time. The classic explanation, which still has a significant number of adherents, is that infants have an innate ability to discriminate speech sounds. Subsequent researchers have modified this in many ways, and some even reject it as invalid. Furthermore, speech perception study methods and their conclusions are inconsistent. We will discuss these theoretical and methodological issues in the Advanced Unit.

Infant Speech Production

In the not-so-distant past, true speech sound learning was thought to begin with the production of the child's first meaningful words. The production of the "first word" was viewed as the child's initial step toward the acquisition of adult-like speech. A division of *prelinguistic* and *linguistic* development was common in the literature. Linguistic development was thought to begin with the first words, and anything the infant did with the vocal apparatus prior to this was *pre*linguistic. Therefore, most of the pioneering articulation developmental studies sampled children between 2 and 8 years old who were already producing words (and sentences).

However, the study of the speech or vocal skills of infants before they produce their first words began to flourish in the late 1970s and early 1980s (e.g., Oller, 1980; Oller et al., 1976; Stark, 1978, 1979, 1980). Research since that time has done away with the notion that vocal behaviors prior to the one-word stage are unimportant and bear no relationship to the development of meaningful speech (and language); such vocal behaviors may indeed be the building blocks of later speech and language skills.

Research on infant vocal behaviors has identified several interrelated stages that eventually lead to clearly identifiable speech sound and word productions. Investigators differ somewhat in describing these stages. Nonetheless, there is substantial agreement on the types of vocal behaviors infants produce and the broad sequence in which they learn those behaviors (Oller, 2000). The sequence in which infants learn to produce the sounds and words of their language is often divided into smoothly merging or even overlapping stages.

Infant Speech Learning Stages

A newborn's primary method of communication with the adult world is through crying and fussing. A few months after birth, the infant begins to produce vocal behaviors that are like consonant-vowel and vowel-consonant combinations, with adult-like intonations. Historically, distinct infant vocal productions were divided into two general categories: (1) **reflexive vocalizations**—automatic responses reflecting the physical state of the infant, including crying, coughing, burping, and hiccupping; and (2) **nonreflexive vocalizations**—"voluntary" productions, including cooing, babbling, and playful screaming and yelling (Oller, 1980; Stark, 1980). These categories, however, have come under revision in recent years (Oller, 2000; Oller & Griebel, 2008).

In 1980 Oller advanced several specific stages that mark the acquisition of articulation and phonological skills during the first year of speech development. These stages have been revised or refined over the years (Oller, 2000; Oller & Griebel, 2008). According to Oller, the initial vocalizations of infants cannot be transcribed into adult vocalizations of sounds and syllables; any attempt to "shoe horn" infant vocalizations into adult syllabic or segmental categories obscures the true nature of those vocalizations. He introduced the term *infraphonological* to describe an infant's initial vocalizations; he called such vocalizations *protophones*. **Protophones** are beginning or earlier forms of sounds that are related to the better-formed sounds and syllables infants produce later. These infraphonological skills of infants serve as *infrastructures* for speech sound development (Oller, 2000). A distinction between infraphonological productions and canonical babbling is this: **Infraphonological skills** are early infant vocalizations that are not recognizable as adult sounds or syllables; **canonical babbling,** on the other hand, refers to infant vocalizations that include adult-like sounds and syllables.

Oller's (1980, 2000) stages are widely used in describing infant speech learning and development. Some overlap in vocalizations exists from one stage to another; however, each new stage is characterized by vocal behaviors not observed in the previous stage. The ages at which the stages of infant speech production are said to occur must be viewed as approximate and may differ from one infant to another. What follows is Oller's 2000 classification, as well as Oller and Griebel's 2008 elaboration:

Infraphonological Stage 1: Phonation—From Birth to 2 Months

- Reflexive vocalizations such as crying, fussing, coughing, sneezing, and burping may be common, but speech-like sounds are rare.

- Vocalizations resembling vowels predominate, but they are protophones, more appropriately called *quasivowels*, which infants produce in a resting (relaxed) position, with little oral resonance and no lip-rounding or other articulatory postures. They are due to smooth, normal phonation with no within-utterance breaks. They are observed when the infant is alone or attended; they are neither stimulus bound nor emotional, and their function is ambiguous.

Infraphonological Stage 2: Primitive Articulation—From 1 to 4 Months

• New sounds, in the form of squeals and growls, appear.

• Movements of the vocal tract begin in both solitary conditions and face-to-face interactions. Vocalizations get elaborated to include primitive articulation, causing elaboration of quasivowels into longer or shorter durations, softer or louder ones, and with glottal and breathing interruptions within those productions. Infants 5 to 6 weeks old may breathe in some extra air before producing quasivowels.

• Goos, also called *coos*, appears at this stage; a **goo** is a variable form of protophone (vocalization) in which the phonation is interrupted, due largely to the tongue dorsum coming in contact with the throat or palate. The term *goo* refers primarily to vocalizations produced at the back of the oral cavity. Because the tongue movements involved in gooing are seemingly uncoordinated, the resulting articulation is considered *primitive*.

• Stage 2 vocalizations and variable quasivowels are built upon Stage 1 vocalizations.

Infraphonological Stage 3: Expansion—From 3 to 8 Months

• This stage is characterized as a period of vocal play and exploration, resulting in many new sounds and variability in their pitch, amplitude, duration, and vocal quality. Vocalizations of different pitch or quality may rhythmically alternate. Certain vocalizations may be heard repeatedly.

• Squeals, growls, yells, and vowel-like sounds (called *full vowels*) may be produced. Contrasted with the at-rest vocalization of the previous stages, during full-vowel productions the vocal tract is fully open, resulting in good resonation. The infant may exhibit different vocal postures in this stage.

• Infants may also blow through their tightly closed lips, resulting in protophones called raspberries (bilabial or lingualabial trills). Infants produce sounds with the vocal tract open and closed, such movements often being very slow, resulting in a type of vocalization called *marginal babbling* or *marginal syllables*. Marginal babbling includes protophones that are consonant-like and vowel-like but are not like adult consonants or vowels because of variability in the timing, resonance, or loudness properties. Variability is the most distinguishing feature of marginal babbling.

• Vocalizations of this stage, including full vowels, are not phonemes or allophones, even though they are fully resonant; they do not have the phonetic features of adult productions. They are the precursors to more adult-like sounds to be learned later.

Infraphonological Stage 4: Canonical Babbling—From 5 to 10 Months

• A stage most parents take note of in their babies, **canonical babbling** involves well-timed vocal tract opening and closing, normal phonation, and repetitive patterns.

Canonical babbles that include CV syllables are most speech-like and are often misinterpreted as such; there is no evidence that these babbles function as speech does. The oral movements are smoother and more rapid than in the previous stages, and the sounds are more constricted and resonated, so that they now resemble true consonants and vowels.

• The CV syllables become longer and may be *reduplicated* (hence, **reduplicated babbling**), so that syllable sequences such as [baba], [kaka], and [tata] result. For parents, CV reduplicated syllables that resemble [mama] and [dada] are of prime importance (for obvious reasons), although they are not produced for the same reason an older infant produces [mama] or [dada]. The infant may produce canonical syllables when alone, when looking at the family dog (as reported by one of our colleagues in reference to her own son's production of [mama] at 7 months), when looking at a toy, or when looking at the mother or father. Instead of producing canonical syllables to draw attention and care, infants may produce nonverbal gestures or undifferentiated vocalizations.

• Along with reduplication, the infant may produce **variegated babbles**, vocalizations in which the consonantal and vocalic elements keep changing. The infant may combine a variety of CV sequences, resulting in productions such as [madaga], [putika], and [tikadi].

• The infant's phonetic repertoire, although limited, may consist of stops, nasals, glides, and the lax vowels /ɛ/, /ɪ/, and /ʌ/.

• The production of back sounds (velars) declines sharply, while the production of front sounds (alveolars and bilabials) increases.

• Canonical syllables are essential to form the words of a language, though they are not the starting point of language because all previous stages help to achieve this stage. Canonical syllable productions precede conventional word productions.

The Integrative Stage: Onset of Speech

Oller (2000) also describes a final integrative stage, though not necessarily as a fifth stage in infant speech development. This final stage may last until the infant is 18 months old and may include a child's first meaningful words. A notable feature of this stage is that canonical babbling and meaningful words may coexist in it; in fact, the two forms may be combined to create what has been described as **jargon** (meaningful words combined with nonmeaningful babbled sounds). In this stage, infants also may produce **gibberish**, which is sequenced but nonmeaningful syllables produced with adult-like prosody. Because of the varied intonation patterns and adult-like prosody of infant speech in this stage, parents often gain the impression that the infant is producing whole sentences to make statements, issue commands, and ask questions (Davis, MacNeilage, Matyear, & Powell, 2000). An 18-month-old pretending to talk on the phone, rapidly producing a meaningless string of syllables, but with proper intonation patterns, offers a good example of gibberish.

Infants at the end of this stage begin to combine well-formed syllables to create new syllables. Their vocal mechanism will have grown to be a flexible apparatus. The coexistence of babbling and real words highlights how continuous speech development is—from the infraphonological phonation stage through subsequent stages and the production of real words.

....

ACTIVITY

Briefly describe the four *infraphonological* stages.

....

From Babbling to Speech Sounds

Jakobson (1968) hypothesized that (1) babbling is a random series of vocalizations with no order or regularity and is not related to later speech or language learning; (2) infants' babbling includes the sounds of all languages; and (3) phoneme acquisition follows a universal, invariable order. As Velleman and Vihman (2007) put it, "All of these hypotheses have been rejected on empirical grounds" (p. 25). Jakobson asserted that there is a *discontinuity* between infant babbling and initial speech sound learning because the child typically undergoes a period of silence between the end of the babbling period and development of the first real words. Oller (2000) thinks that the randomness of babbling and the discontinuity between babbling and later speech are myths that have never had any support.

Extensive infant speech research done since the 1970s, culminating in the stages of speech learning of the kind just summarized, contradicts Jakobson's theory and supports the conclusions that babbling is systematic vocal behavior and that there is a natural logic in its progression toward meaningful speech (Oller, 2000). The overlapping infraphonological stages that Oller and other researchers have found are based on much empirical observation of infants (Oller, 2000; Rvachew & Brosseau-Lapré, 2012). Studies have shown that although there are individual differences, most children continue to babble for approximately 3 to 4 months even after the appearance of the first "true" word (Stoel-Gammon & Dunn, 1985). In addition, it is evident that the speech sound patterns of babbling and meaningful speech share similar syllable types and phonetic repertoires (Stoel-Gammon & Cooper, 1981, 1984; Stoel-Gammon, 1985; Vihman et al., 1985). Furthermore, there is evidence to show that both the quantity and the quality of infant vocalizations (babbling) are related to later language development (McCune & Vihman, 2001; Nathani, Ertmer, & Stark, 2006; among others). Oller (2000) reports as well that infants whose canonical babbling is delayed until 10 months or later may be at risk for speech and language problems. Therefore, the previously described infraphonological stages clearly suggest that infants' early and later vocal productions are the rudimentary behaviors from which speech sounds are shaped.

Incidentally, the generally held assumption that babbling-like behavior is not found in animals has been found to be invalid. Vocal behaviors with many human infant babbling characteristics have been documented in pygmy marmoset, a South African monkey (Elowson, Snowdon, & Lazaro-Perea, 1998). However, as Oller (2000) and Skinner (1957) suggest, evolution of a highly flexible and adaptable vocal apparatus has made human speech and language as complex as they are. The flexible human vocal mechanism has made it more sensitive to environmental reinforcement contingencies that play a major role in learning to produce speech sounds and language (Skinner, 1957).

Another questionable assumption has been that infants babble all of the sounds of English or all of the possible speech sounds. In reviewing a large number of studies of infants from English-speaking environments, infants from other linguistic environments, deaf infants, and infants with Down syndrome, Locke (1983) found very little support for that assumption. He found that infants babble only a small set of sounds. Therefore, it is likely that infant babbling is an important behavior that expands into later speech sound production skills (Majorano & D'Odorico, 2011).

SOUNDS AND SYLLABLE SHAPES OF BABBLING.

The sounds and syllables of infant babbling have been investigated by various researchers (Davis & MacNeilage, 1995; Fisichelli, 1950; Irwin, 1947a, 1947b, 1948, 1952; Irwin & Chen, 1946; Locke, 1983; Oller et al., 1976; Pierce & Hanna, 1974; Pollock & Berni, 2003; Stoel-Gammon & Cooper, 1981, 1984; Vihman et al., 1985). As these references suggest, infant speech development has been investigated for more than 60 years.

VOWELS.

To find out what vowel-like sounds children at the end of their variegated babbling stage typically produce, Bauman-Waengler (1994) compared Irwin's (1948) data with those of a more current study conducted by Kent and Bauer (1985). Some differences and similarities were noted in the two sets of data. The rank order of the six most prevalent vowels, according to Irwin's (1948) study, was /ɛ/, /ɪ/, /ʌ/, /ʊ/, /ɑ/, /u/. Kent and Bauer (1985) reported a somewhat different rank order: /ʌ/, /ɛ/, /æ/, /ɑ/, /ʊ/. Although the rank order varied somewhat, at least four sounds remained constant as the most prevalent across the two studies: /ɛ/, /ʌ/, /ɑ/, /ʊ/.

A longitudinal study by Davis and MacNeilage (1995) of six infants from monolingual English-speaking homes (three males, three females) revealed much individual variability in the production of vowels or vowel-like sounds, as well as some general trends. Davis and MacNeilage analyzed the vowel data according to tongue height and tongue advancement dimensions. In relation to tongue height, the vowels were grouped into *high* (/i/, /ɪ/, /u/, /ʊ/), *mid* (/e/, /ɛ/, /ʌ/, /ə/, /ɔ/, /o/), and *low* (/æ/, /a/). For tongue advancement, the vowels were categorized as *front* (/i/, /ɪ/, /e/, /ɛ/, /æ/), *mid* (/a/, /ʌ/, /ə/), and *back* (/u/, /ʊ/, /ə/, /o/).

According to the tongue height dimension, mid vowels, particularly /ʌ/, /ə/, and /ɛ/, predominated in three subjects, while high vowels, particularly /u/, /ʊ/, and /ɪ/, predominated in the remaining three subjects. In relation to tongue advancement, front vowels, particularly /ɛ/, /æ/, and /ɪ/, predominated in four subjects, and the mid vowels /a/, /ʌ/, and /ə/ predominated in the remaining two subjects. If the vowels produced by this infant group are analyzed according to tongue height and advancement combined, the most commonly used vowels in the canonical babbling period were /ʌ/, /ə/, /ɛ/, /u/, /ʊ/, /ɪ/, and /æ/. Overall, these data are in agreement with those of Irwin (1948) and Kent and Bauer (1985). Pollock and Berni (2003) have reported that vowel production mastery is generally achieved by 36 months. Therefore, vowel errors beyond 36 months of age signal a speech sound disorder.

CONSONANTS.

What consonant-like sounds have been documented to be the most frequent in the late babbling period? Locke (1983) reviewed the major studies—Irwin (1947a, 1947b), Fisichelli (1950), and Pierce and Hanna (1974)—to answer this question. He noted that in those three studies, /h/, /d/, /b/, /m/, /t/, /w/, and /j/ were reported as the most frequently occurring consonant-like sounds. Furthermore, 12 sounds—/h/, /d/, /b/, /m/, /t/, /g/, /s/, /w/, /n/, /k/, /j/, and /p/—accounted for between 92% and 97% of the total sounds produced by 11- to

12-month-old infants across the three studies. The less frequently occurring consonant-like sounds were transcribed as /v/, /ʒ/, /f/, /θ/, /ð/, /i/, /ŋ/, /tʃ/, /dʒ/, and /r/, which occurred approximately 3% to 6% of the time across the three studies.

Davis and MacNeilage's (1995) study on the production of consonants during the canonical babbling period showed much individual variation among the infants; however, some overall trends were identified. The most frequently produced consonants according to place of articulation were labials (/b/, /m/, /w/), alveolars (/d/, /n/), and velars (/g/, /ŋ/). However, labials and alveolars occurred with a higher frequency than did velars. Considering manner of production, oral stops occurred with the highest level of frequency, followed by nasals and glides. Although Davis and MacNeilage did not report on voicing dimensions, their data suggest that voiced consonants occurred most frequently.

SYLLABLE SHAPES.

According to Oller (1980, 2000), the combination of consonant-like and vowel-like sounds begins during the Expansion Stage, at about 3 to 8 months. During the later babbling period, open syllables or syllables ending in a vowel are the most frequently occurring syllable shapes. Kent and Bauer (1985) found that V, CV, VCV, and CVCV syllable structures accounted for approximately 94% of all syllables produced at the end of the babbling period. Closed syllables (syllables ending in a consonant), though observed, were limited in the repertoire of the infant at this stage of development.

....

ACTIVITY

Setting individual differences aside, identify the most frequently occurring consonants, vowels, and syllable shapes during the late babbling period.

....

Transition From Babbling to Meaningful Speech

The transition from babbling to meaningful speech is an important milestone in learning to produce the sounds of speech. The child then moves from the preverbal to the verbal and finally to the phonological stage. Although the infant has made an amazing transition from vegetative crying and fussing to producing vocalizations resembling vowels or consonants in a very short period of time, the process of learning to produce the speech sounds of the surrounding language has really just begun.

A child's first productions that resemble words have frequently been labeled *proto-words* (Menn, 1975). **Protowords,** also known as *vocables* (Ferguson, 1978), *phonetically consistent forms* (Dore, Franklin, Miller, & Ramer, 1976), *invented words* (Locke, 1983), and *quasi-words* (Stoel-Gammon & Cooper, 1984), are vocalizations that an infant consistently produces under specified stimulus conditions.

These sounds or sound combinations "function" as words for the infant, even though they are not based on the adult model and are not true words. Adults often react to the infant sound combinations as though they were specific words, even when they are not (see Text Box 4.1). However, such infant sound combinations cannot be considered babbling, either, because they have some phonetic and semantic consistency (Stoel-Gammon & Dunn,

---

Text Box 4.1. "Functions" of utterances

We often read in books and articles that a certain utterance of a child *functions* as a syllable, word, phrase, or sentence, even though the utterance itself does not topographically match the adult production of the same. Thus, for example, a child says "wawa," and it functions the same as the word *water*. What is meant by this claim? Linguistically, it means that the child *intended* to say "water" but, because he or she could not, simplified it and said "wawa," an utterance possible for the child. Behaviorally, however, attributing such an intention to the mind of an infant or adult obscures the true nature of utterances. The child says "wawa" for water mostly because of an immature vocal mechanism and a phonetic repertoire that is still being learned. But what about the intention or function? If the child's production of "wawa" causes a caregiver to say, "Yes, that is water" or give the child some water to drink, the child is likely to repeat the utterance because of the reinforcement received. Intention or function in this sense is the effect of utterances on caregivers (or other people) who react to the child's utterance in specific ways. To say that the utterance "wawa" *functions* like the utterance "water" is to obscure the true nature of interactions in which certain forms of speech, though topographically different, are accepted, reinforced, and thus repeated. Therefore, we would rather say that utterances that do not topographically match those of adults may have the same effect as adult utterances of the same kind.

1985). Ferguson (1978) described protowords as "babbling-like sounds used meaningfully" (p. 281).

Protowords are frequently tied to a specific context and are often accompanied by a consistent gesture. These vocal productions have frequently been considered the link between babbling and adult-like speech. Four phonetic forms are frequently included in protowords: (1) single or repeated vowels, (2) syllabic nasals, (3) syllabic fricatives, and (4) single or repeated consonant-vowel syllables in which the consonant is a nasal or a stop (Ferguson, 1978; Halliday, 1975).

Carter (1974, 1979) studied the progression from protowords to real words in a single subject named David. Between the ages of 1 year 1 month and 1 year 2 months, David produced vocalizations that differed from babbling in that they had some phonetic consistency and were frequently accompanied by a gesture:

- [mm], [ma], [may], or [mə] when reaching for an object
- [la], [læ], [da], [dæ], or [də] when pointing to an object
- [hɪ], [hɪy], [he], [hə], or [hm] when giving or receiving an object

Carter (1974, 1979) suggested that these sound combinations accompanied by a gesture served as a foundation for the development of conventional (adult-based) words. Carter believed the following:

- The vocable /m + vowel/ accompanied by a reaching gesture leads to the acquisition of the words "more," "my," and "mine."
- The vocable /l + vowel/ or /d + vowel/ accompanied by a pointing gesture leads to the acquisition of words such as "look," "these," and "this."

- The vocable /h + vowel/ accompanied by a giving or receiving gesture leads to the acquisition of words such as "here," "where," and "have."

Carter's suggestions seem plausible because differential reinforcement from parents may help shape words from such sound combinations. It should be emphasized, however, that Carter's suggestions have not been confirmed by follow-up studies.

Ferguson (1978) proposed that infants develop about 12 vocables as they transition from babbling to the use of adult-based words. However, Stoel-Gammon and Cooper's (1984) study failed to support Ferguson's claim. Rather, their study with three subjects showed a wider variation among children. Stoel-Gammon and Cooper found that one subject used 13 vocables during the acquisition of 50 conventional words, while the other two subjects used only one vocable each during the same period. Generally, in phonological and language learning, individual differences hold, while claims of invariable patterns across children, though common among linguists, are often called into question.

Learning to Produce the First Words

Protowords mark the beginning of meaningful verbal productions in the speech of young children. Although they often are based on adult models, protowords do not match adult word productions.

What exactly constitutes a "true" word? Although an indisputable answer does not exist for this question, a general definition is available. A **true word** is what a child consistently produces in a particular stimulus context with a predictable consequence, such as a reaction from caregivers; it has a stable phonetic form, similar to adult word production. Topographic (formal) similarity to the adult phonetic forms distinguishes true words from protowords. A true word and its protoword may be consistently produced under similar stimulus conditions and have the same effect on listeners, such as caregivers and others (see Text Box 4.1); nonetheless, the protoword does not resemble the adult word. For example, a child may produce the phonetic form [lala] consistently when requesting a toy car and get the car from an adult; however, that production does not resemble an adult name for the object (i.e., "toy" or "car"). On the other hand, if a child says [ka] consistently when requesting a toy car (and gets it), the production would qualify as a true word because the child's production and the adult target are phonetically and partially similar, though not identical. It should be noted that the distinction is purely topographical—that is, based on the shape or the form of the response. Both the true word and the protoword have the same antecedent stimulus and may receive the same consequence (e.g., receiving the toy from an adult); in linguistic terms, they "function" similarly, but they have different forms. Therefore, we will simply refer to them as "protowords" or "words" (not "true words," which implies the existence of "false" words).

Studies of the phonetic configuration of early (adult-like) words have revealed common patterns in their overall form and the sounds that occur (Jakobson, 1968; Stoel-Gammon, 1984, 1985; Stoel-Gammon & Cooper, 1981; Winitz & Irwin, 1958). The early stage of word productions typically includes single syllables or fully or partially reduplicated syllables. (Closed syllables occur, but less commonly.) This pattern of syllable shapes was also noted during the latter stages of the babbling period. Speech sound production is generally characterized by stops, nasals, or glides. Fricatives occur much less frequently. Stops, nasals, and glides are speech sounds that are also characteristic of the late babbling period. These observations suggest that the production of a child's first words is influenced by the phonetic repertoire and syllable structure of the productions in the late babbling period. In other words, and to reiterate, there is behavioral continuity between babbling and early word forms (Stoel-Gammon, 1984, 1985; Vihman, Ferguson, & Elbert, 1986; Vihman et al., 1985).

An interesting occurrence that has been identified in the sound patterns of young children is the presence of *progressive idioms* and *regressive idioms* (Ferguson & Farwell, 1975; Moskowitz, 1973). Stoel-Gammon and Dunn (1985) refer to these as "advanced forms" and "frozen forms," respectively. **Progressive idioms,** or **advanced forms,** are advanced pronunciations in comparison to the child's current sound pattern or production of other words. Leopold (1947) offers one of the earliest examples of progressive idioms. He noted that his daughter Hildegarde produced the word "pretty" as [prəti] at 10 months old, a point at which she did not produce any other words with the initial cluster /pr/. Several months later, as Hildegarde's speech sound repertoire expanded, she produced "pretty" as [pɪti] or [bɪdi], which more closely matched her other word forms.

Regressive idioms, or **frozen forms,** are static or unchanging pronunciations of words despite a child's more advanced speech skills. That is, pronunciations that are less advanced in comparison to the adult target remain that way even when the child's speech sound repertoire becomes more sophisticated. Older children who continue to call their pets or family members truncated or simplified names provide examples. Read Text Box 4.2 for a personal example.

....

ACTIVITY

Define the following terms in your own words and give an example for each: *marginal babbling, reduplicated babbling, variegated babbling, canonical babbling, protoword, true word, progressive idiom, regressive idiom.*

....

Text Box 4.2. Regressive idioms? They could do better.

The first author's nickname probably developed as a regressive idiom. Although her name is Adriana [e.dri.a.na], some of her immediate family members still call her Nani [na.ni]. When she asked how such a nickname developed, her mother said that when Adriana was very young, a cousin of her age called her Nana [na·na] because she could not pronounce Adriana's long name. Because the cousin continued to call her that even as they got older, others picked it up, modified it a little, and followed suit.

The cousin's production of [na·na] for [e·dri·a·na] probably resulted from use of the phonological pattern of *syllable deletion* and *total reduplication*. Something that began as a developmentally appropriate simplification process continued even as the cousin's speech sound repertoire expanded, because "Nana" more than likely became her name for Adriana.

Learning to Produce Individual Sounds and Sound Patterns

Around their second birthday, children more consistently produce words and begin to combine words into simple phrases. They have progressed from the infraphonological stages to the production of protowords and their first adult-like words. This progression is not linear, however, because children often produce, as noted before, a combination of variegated babbling, jargon, protowords, and words simultaneously, especially during the first 50-word stage.

By the time children are 2 years old, their phonetic and lexical repertoires have increased dramatically as they continue to make progress in acquiring an adult-like speech sound pattern. At this point, the frequency of variegated babbling, jargon, and protowords decreases, while that of words increases. Children's words become phonetically more systematic, and as a result, the adult targets are more readily identifiable.

Several studies have been conducted on the acquisition of speech sounds during the preschool and early school-age years. Earlier studies tracked the sequence in which children acquire single speech sounds and the chronological ages at which they master their production. Later research traced the acquisition of distinctive features, and subsequent studies analyzed the systematic appearance and disappearance of phonological patterns (error patterns). Several investigators have analyzed the sequence in which children learn the more traditional sound patterns (e.g., sound patterns based on manner, place, and voicing features).

Single Phonemes

The acquisition of individual speech sounds in preschool and early school-age children has been extensively studied since the late 1930s. Several large-scale investigations have been conducted to gain a better understanding of the ages at which children can be expected to master certain speech sounds. Many of these now classic studies used the cross-sectional research method to derive group norms of speech sound production. Other studies used the longitudinal method to assess the phonological development of individual children.

Cross-Sectional Studies

In the **cross-sectional method,** researchers select a certain number of children from each of the age groups targeted in the study. An effort is made to obtain a group of children that reflects the socioeconomic distribution of the population as a whole. Because hearing and language problems have been associated with SSD, researchers tend to exclude children with a history of hearing loss or language disorder.

Once the group has been selected, each child's speech production is sampled by using various test stimuli. Typically, the child is asked to name a picture or an object representing the target sound in a single word. If the child cannot produce the target word upon picture or object presentation, the examiner may provide a model of the target production for the child to imitate. The degree of imitation permitted may vary from one study to another.

At each age level, the specific sounds mastered by the majority of children are determined. A criterion of *age of acquisition* or *age of mastery* is established for each sound. For example, a sound may be considered mastered when 90% of the children in a particular age group produced the sound correctly in the initial, medial, and final positions of words they were asked to say. Such a mastery criterion is consistently applied to all sounds tested in a given study.

Cross-sectional normative studies yield group data. Individual performance is not considered, and, typically, specific error types are not identified. The results provide information on the ages at which children may be expected to produce a sound correctly according to the adult standard. At least five major cross-sectional studies, the first published in 1931, are now considered classic (Arlt & Goodban, 1976; Poole, 1934; Prather, Hedrick, & Kern, 1975; Templin, 1957; Wellman, Case, Mengert, & Bradbury, 1931). In addition, Sander's 1972 reanalysis of the results of the Wellman et al. (1931) and Templin (1957) studies resulted in a slightly different set of norms, which are frequently cited in the literature. Another, smaller cross-sectional study, involving only two age groups (2-0 and 2-6 years) has been reported by Paynter and Petty (1974). Smit, Hand, Freilinger, Bernthal, and Bird (1990) have reported a large-scale study. In addition, two commonly used standardized tests offer information on ages of sound mastery in the form of standardized norms (Fudala, 2000; Goldman & Fristoe, 2000).

Normative studies are also available for other international dialects of English, including Canadian, British, Scottish, Irish, and Australian varieties (see McLeod, 2007, for summaries). McLeod is also a good source for speech sound acquisition in several international languages.

In her review of the classic studies, Smit (1986) noted some similarities in the subjects' ages and the sound-evoking procedures, but, because of methodological differences in data collection and analysis, the studies do not always agree on the age at which children master production of specific consonants. A primary methodological variability that may account for the difference in age of mastery is the use of differing mastery criteria. For example, some studies considered a consonant mastered when 90% of the study sample produced it correctly, whereas other studies considered it mastered when 75% of the sample did. Another variability in study methods is the word position in which phonemes were tested. Some studies tested phonemes only in two word positions—initial and medial—omitting the final position, while others tested them in all three positions.

Table 4.1 outlines the ages of mastery for speech sounds based on the five classic studies. Despite the differences previously mentioned, the results of each of the studies suggest that the acquisition of speech sounds is a relatively lengthy process. Some sounds are mastered quite early, while others continue to be misarticulated until the early elementary school years.

Fudala (2000) collected speech sound learning data to standardize the *Arizona Articulation Proficiency Scale–Third Edition* (Arizona-3). Her normative data are based on a sample of 5,500 children in the age range of 1 year 6 months through 18 years, living in 20 states in the United States, sampled on a nationwide basis. Fudala analyzed sound production in the initial and final positions of words and considered a sound mastered when 90% of the children in a given age group produced it correctly in a specific position.

Table 4.1

AGES OF CONSONANT MASTERY IN FIVE CLASSIC STUDIES

Consonant	Wellman et al. (1931) Age	Poole (1934) Age	Templin (1957) Age	Prather et al. (1975) Age	Arlt & Goodban (1976) Age
m	3	3½	3	2	3
n	3	4½	3	2	3
h	3	3½	3	2	3
p	4	3½	3	2	3
f	3	5½	3	2–4	3
w	3	3½	3	2–8	3
b	3	3½	—	2–8	3
ŋ	—	4½	3	2–8	3
j	4	4½	3½	2–4	—
k	4	4½	4	2–4	3
g	4	4½	4	2–4	3
l	4	6½	6	3–4	4
d	5	4½	4	2–4	3
t	5	4½	6	2–8	3
s	5	7½	4½	3	4
r	5	7½	4	3	5
tʃ	5	4½	—	3–8	4
v	5	6½	6	4	3½
z	5	7½	7	4	4
ʒ	6	6½	7	4	4
θ	—	7½	6	4	5
dʒ	—	7	4	4	—
ʃ	—	6½	4½	3–8	4½
ð	—	6½	7	4	5

Note. A dash indicates that data were not reported.

Goldman and Fristoe (2000) collected similar data to standardize their *Goldman-Fristoe Test of Articulation–Second Edition* (GFTA-2). They obtained a stratified national sample of 2,350 children in the age range of 2 through 21. With a mastery criterion of 85% of children producing a sound correctly at the earliest age, the authors reported the age of mastery for the total sample. To facilitate an easier comparison, we present the results of Fudala's and Goldman and Fristoe's normative research in a single table, Table 4.2.

As Table 4.2 shows, the mastery ages for most sounds reported by Fudala (2000) and Goldman and Fristoe (2000) are similar. A rough division of earlier and later learned sounds is sustained in both sets of data. Most early sounds are mastered by age 3; fewer new sounds are added during the fourth year, and later-learned sounds are mastered from age

Table 4.2

AGE OF MASTERY AS REPORTED IN TWO STANDARDIZED TESTS: ARIZONA-3 AND GFTA-2

Sound	Age of Mastery					
	Initial Position		Medial Position		Final Position	
	Arizona-3 (2000)	GFTA-2 (2000)	Arizona-3 (2000)	GFTA-2 (2000)	Arizona-3 (2000)	GFTA-2 (2000)
b	2	2		2	3	3
p	2	2		3	3	2
m	2	2		2	2	2
n	2	2		2	2.6	3
h	2	2		—	2	—
d	3	2		4	3	3
w	2.6	3			—	—
t	3	3		3	4	3
k	3	3		3	3	3
g	3	3		3	3	3
f	3	3		3	3	4
ŋ	—	—		3	4	5
j	4	5		—	—	—
ʃ	5.6	5		5	5.6	5
tʃ	5	5		5	6.6	5
l	5	5		5	5.6	5
dʒ	5	5		5	—	5
s	6	5		5	6	5
r	6	6		6	—	5
v	5	6		6	5	5
z	6	7		5	6	5
ð	5.6	7		7	—	—
θ	6.6	7		8	6.5	7

Note. The mastery criterion of Fudala's *Arizona Articulation Proficiency Test–Third Edition* (Arizona-3; 2000) was correct production by 90% of the sampled children; the test does not offer data on the medial position of words. The mastery criterion of Goldman and Fristoe's *Goldman-Fristoe Test of Articulation–Second Edition* (GFTA-2; 2000) was 85%. A dash indicates that data were not reported.

5 to 7. A difference of 12 months or more is found between the two sets of data for a few sounds (initial /d/, /j/, /s/, /v/, /z/, and /ð/; final /p/, /t/, /f/, /ŋ/, /s/, and /z/). One possibility for such discrepancy across test norms might be the actual individual differences in learning some of these sounds.

Smit et al. (1990) and Smit (1993a) provided normative information on the acquisition of speech sounds in a large number of children residing in Iowa and Nebraska. The studies sampled 997 children in the age range of 3 to 9 years. The authors developed and used an assessment instrument that tested all word-initial and word-final consonant singletons with the exception of /ʒ/ and word-final /ð/. They also assessed production of intervocalic /r/ and /l/, syllabic /l/, postvocalic /ɚ/, and several word-initial consonant clusters. Because they found a statistically significant difference on sound acquisition between boys and girls in the preschool age groups, their data were presented separately for males and females until age 7. Smit et al. used a mastery criterion of correct production by 75% of children, so that they could compare their data with those of Templin (1957). However, their recommended clinical age of mastery was correct production by 90% of children. In presenting Smit et al.'s data, we have applied the 90% acquisition criterion. Like Smit et al., Goldman and Fristoe (2000) offered separate norms for boys and girls. We show the normative data from both of these sources in a single table, Table 4.3, so that the gender differences found in the two studies may be easily compared.

Table 4.3 makes it clear that the gender difference in age of mastery is not marked for all the sounds and sound positions. The Smit et al. (1990) data reveal that the biggest difference between boys and girls occur with initial /tʃ/, initial /dʒ/, and initial /ð/. The differences favoring the girls (bolded in the table), amount to more than a year and up to two and a half years (/ð/ in the initial position). A six-month to one-year difference may be found for several sounds. The Goldman and Fristoe (2000; GFTA-2) data show smaller and likely clinically insignificant differences between the boys and girls for most sounds, though the small differences evident in the data favor girls. However, /s/ in the initial position and /z/ in the final position show a maximum difference of 3 years. Smit et al.'s data show no differences at all for those sounds in similar positions. In both studies, greater gender differences are found for late-learning sounds (e.g., /tʃ/, /dʒ/, /z/, /ð/).

A more recent small-scale, cross-sectional study of speech development was conducted by Bondarenko (2011). She studied 25 children in the age range of 2-0 to 2-11 years. Results were that by age 2 years, 75% of the children had mastered the consonant sounds /b/, /p/, /m/, /t/, /g/, /d/, /n/, /f/, /k/, /s/, /l/, /ŋ/, /w/, and /h/. None of the oldest children in the study (2 years 11 months) had mastered /z/, /dʒ/, /r/, /tʃ/, /ʃ/, /v/, or /θ/, suggesting their later acquisition (Bondarenko, 2011).

Generally, the classic studies of the 1930s and 1950s report later ages of sound acquisition for most of the early sounds (e.g., /m/, /n/, /h/, /p/, /w/, /b/ at age 3) when compared to more recent studies (the same sounds around age 2). Ages of mastery for most later-learned sounds are similar (or at least less dissimilar) across the classic and recent studies. An exception is in the results of Prather et al.'s 1975 study; ages of mastery for most sounds are lower than they are in the other classic studies shown in Table 4.1 and are closer to (or even lower than) those reported in more recent studies. Again, these discrepancies may be due to methodological differences discussed previously. As good clinical practice, we recommend that the more recent and updated information be used in diagnosing and treating speech sound disorders in children.

Longitudinal Studies

The **longitudinal method** is another way of studying speech sound learning in children. In this research method, investigators follow a few children for an extended period of time. Unlike cross-sectional investigators, longitudinal investigators repeatedly record

Table 4.3

GENDER DIFFERENCES IN THE MASTERY OF ENGLISH CONSONANTS

Sound	Age of Mastery							
	Smit et al. (1990)				GFTA-2 (2000)			
	Initial		Final		Initial		Final	
	Male	*Female*	*Male*	*Female*	*Male*	*Female*	*Male*	*Female*
b	≤3	3.6	≤3	≤3	2	2	3	3
p	3.6	3.6	≤3	≤3	2.6	2.6	3	2.6
m	≤3	≤3	≤3	3.6	2	2	3	2
n	≤3	3.6	≤3	3.6	2	2	3	3
h	≤3	≤3	—	—	2.6	2.6	—	—
d	≤3	≤3	3.6	≤3	2.6	2	4.6	3
t	3.6	≤3	4	4	3.6	3	4	2.6
k	4	3.6	≤3	≤3	3.6	4	4	3
g	4	3.6	≤3	4	4.6	4	4	4.6
f	3.6	3.6	5.6	5.6	4	3	4	3.6
w	≤3	≤3	—	—	3	3	—	—
ŋ	—	—	>9[a]	>9[a]	—	—	5	5
j	3.6	4	—	—	5	5	—	—
ʃ	7[a]	6	7[a]	6	6	5	6	5
tʃ	7[a]	**5.6**	7[a]	6	6	5	6	5
l	6	5	7[a]	6	6	4.6	7	5
dʒ	**6**	**4.6**	7[a]	6	5	5	6	5
s	9[a]	9[a]	9[a]	9[a]	**8**	**5**	5.6	5
r	8[a]	8[a]	8[a]	8[a]	6	7	5.6	6
v	5.6	4.6	5.6	4.6	7	6	5	4.6
z	9[a]	9[a]	>9[a]	>9[a]	8	7	**>8**	**5**
ð	7[a]	4.6	—	—	>8	7	—	—
θ	7[a]	**6**	7[a]	6	8	7	8	>8

Note. The mastery criterion was recalculated at 90% for the GFTA-2 (2000) data to make it more comparable to the data from Smit et al. (1990), which used the same criterion. Smit et al.'s youngest study group was 3.0 years, and GFTA-2's was 2.0. A dash indicates that data was not reported.

[a]Beginning with age 7, Smit et al.'s data are averages for boys and girls (separate mastery ages are not provided).

spontaneous speech samples from the same child to trace the development of speech sounds. Although longitudinal studies cannot provide norms, they do provide specific as well as detailed information on how children learn to produce individual speech sounds.

Stoel-Gammon performed such a study in 1985. She investigated the phonetic inventories of 34 children (19 boys and 15 girls) between the ages of 15 and 24 months. Using spontaneous speech samples, she investigated the range and type of consonantal phones children produced in meaningful speech. All children were 9 months old at the beginning of data collection. The samples were collected every 3 months at ages 9, 12, 15, 18, 21, and 24 months.

Although Stoel-Gammon collected data for both prelinguistic vocalizations and meaningful speech, she limited her analysis to the meaningful speech productions. Her criterion for *meaningful speech* was the spontaneous production of at least 10 identifiable words during a 1-hour recording session. Because children reached this criterion at different age levels, the number of children in the 15-, 18-, 21-, and 24-month age groups varied. At 15 months, only 7 children had reached the criterion, while at 18 and 21 months, 19 and 32 children had reached the criterion, respectively. At 24 months, only one child had not reached the meaningful speech criterion. This clearly highlights the reality of individual variability in the acquisition of speech and language skills.

Stoel-Gammon analyzed the data according to each child's phonetic repertoire in word-initial and word-final positions. Singleton phones were considered part of the child's repertoire when they occurred in a given position in at least two different words. Although individual variability was recorded, Stoel-Gammon reported that the early phonetic inventories in the initial position of words were primarily voiced anterior stops, nasals, and glides. By 24 months, voiceless stops, velars, and a few fricatives were included in the initial position. In the final position, the children's phonetic inventories consisted primarily of voiceless stops and alveolar consonants. Voiced stops tended to appear first in the initial position, while /t/ and /r/ appeared first in the final position. The following specific patterns were described in the study:

- At 15 months of age /b/, /d/, and /h/ in the initial position were in the inventories of 50% of the children; no sounds met the criterion in the final position.

- At 18 months of age /b/, /d/, /m/, /n/, /h/, and /w/ in the initial position were in the inventories of 50% of the children; /t/ was the only phone in the inventory of 50% of the children in the final position.

- At 21 months of age /b/, /t/, /d/, /m/, /n/, and /h/ in the initial position were in the inventories of 50% of the children; only /t/ and /n/ were in the inventories of 50% of the children in the final position.

- At 24 months of age /b/, /t/, /d/, /k/, /g/, /m/, /n/, /h/, /w/, /f/, and /s/ were in the inventories of 50% of the children; /p/, /t/, /k/, /n/, /r/, and /s/ were in the inventories of 50% of the children in the final position.

These results make it clear that the children's phonetic repertoire was significantly larger in the initial position of words. This is not surprising, because children at this age tend to use open-syllable words more often than closed-syllable words, where final consonants would be expected to occur. Also, the subjects' phonetic repertoire increased from a mean of 3.4 and 0.6 in word-initial and word-final positions, respectively, at 15 months to a mean of 9.5 and 5.7 at 24 months.

Stoel-Gammon's data, although demonstrating much individual variability, are comparable with some of the large-scale cross-sectional studies, in that they substantiated the early development of stops, nasals, and glides. Relative to the ages at which 50% of the subjects produced particular phones, this study is most comparable to Sander's (1972) and Fudala's (2000) information on phoneme mastery for children at 2 years of age.

Age Ranges for Speech Sound Learning

Probably the most significant aspect of speech sound development is the variability across children. If we select one sound in particular from Sander's (1972) data—/r/, for example—it becomes evident that the range of acquisition may extend over several years. Whereas the correct production of /r/ may be observed in 50% of 3-year-olds, the 90% mastery criterion is not reached until age 6. In general, the time span between the age of customary production (50% of children producing a sound correctly) and the age of mastery is greater for fricatives and affricates, especially for /s/ (Stoel-Gammon & Dunn, 1985). This underscores the idea that sound acquisition is a gradual process, and all children at particular age levels cannot be expected to adhere to a specific mastery criterion.

In recent years, much has been written about sounds that are acquired early, middle, and late (EML). The clinical importance of this classification of speech sounds is highlighted in some sources devoted to the treatment of the late eight sounds—a set of sounds mastered later than other sounds (e.g., Bleile, 2006). Shriberg (1993) suggested the EML classification of speech sounds on the basis of data collected on 64 children within the age range of 3 to 6 years who were diagnosed with speech delay. We have anecdotally noted that some, if not many, clinicians who use the EML classification believe it to be based on a large-scale normative study, which is not the case. Shriberg and his colleagues (Shriberg, Gruber, & Kwiatkowski, 1994; Shriberg & Kwiatkowski, 1994; Shriberg, Kwiatkowski, & Gruber, 1994) have used the following EML classification in their research on SSD:

- early sounds: [m, b, j, n, w, d, p, h]
- middle sounds: [t, ŋ, k, g, f, v, tʃ, ʤ]
- late sounds: [ʃ, θ, s, z, ð, l, r, ʒ]

To validate their EML classification of sounds, Shriberg and colleagues (Shriberg, Gruber, & Kwiatkowski, 1994; Shriberg & Kwiatkowski, 1994; Shriberg, Kwiatkowski, & Gruber, 1994) in the cited and other studies have compared their classification with the norms provided by Sander (1972) and others. A study by Fabiano-Smith and Goldstein (2010a) reported that in a group of 8 typically developing, monolingual, English-speaking children, only 16 of the 24 sounds were the same as in the EML categories. Advocates of this classification have frequently pointed out that of the 24 sounds (8 sounds in each of the three EML categories), 15 sounds (63%) agree with normative data; in other words, EML is validated against data that have been available for decades. Two potential limitations with this classification are that (1) a 63% agreement between normative studies and EML sound learning is not strong enough to justify it, and (2) if the EML data are thought to be nearly as good as the norms, clinicians might as well use the norms given in normative studies. The classification has only a limited clinical application. Whether the child's misarticulations are in the early, middle, or late category, they need to be assessed and treated.

Generally speaking, the finer the classification of speech sound learning according to age groups, the greater is the divergence across studies. This is mostly because of individual differences in children and methodological variations in studies. A more gross classification of sounds that are learned early and sounds that are learned late seems to agree more with the normative ages of mastery than the EML does. Table 4.4 shows the results of this classification. This two-tier classification may help in making clinical decisions, even though we think that all of the sounds that are misarticulated, and judged to be of clinical significance, need to be treated.

In her longitudinal study, Stoel-Gammon (1985) sampled the speech of 34 children in the age range of 15 to 24 months at 3-month intervals. Though the study is not normative, its results generally agree with the early sounds others report in normative studies. There is good agreement among the two major tests of articulation norms, the norms generated by Smit et al. (1990) and Sander's (1972) reanalysis of classic studies. The most notable disagreement is /j/; it could be either an early or a late sound. Another sound, /ŋ/, could also be either early or late.

The previously cited study by Bondarenko (2011) showed that by age 3, 75% of children may have mastered the consonant sounds /b/, /p/, /m/, /t/, /g/, /d/, /n/, /f/, /k/, /s/, /l/, / ŋ/, /w/, and /h/. Most of these sounds agree with the early sounds given in Table 4.4.

Another method of organizing speech sound learning chronologically is to group sounds based on some pattern. Place-manner-voice classification of speech sounds, for example, may provide a pattern to organize normative data. We will summarize such efforts in a later section, "Learning Speech Sound Patterns."

··

ACTIVITY

Identify the specified class of sounds: early sounds and late sounds.

··

Table 4.4

AGE RANGES FOR CONSONANT MASTERY

Early: 2 to 4 years

GFTA-2	p	b	m	n	h	d	t	k	g	f	w	ŋ		
Arizona-3	p	b	m	n	h	d	t	k	g	f	w	ŋ	j	
Smit et al. (1990) norms	p	b	m	n	h	d	t	k	g	f–	w		j	
Sander (1972) norms	p	b	m	n	h	d	t–	k	g	f	w		j	
Stoel-Gammon (1985)		b	m	n	h	d	t	k	g	f	w			s

Late: 5 to 7 years

GFTA-2	j	ʃ	tʃ	l	dʒ	s	r	v	z	ð	θ		
Arizona-3		ʃ	tʃ	l	dʒ	s	r	v	z	ð	θ	hw	
Smit et al. (1990) norms		ʃ	tʃ	l	dʒ	s	r	v	z	ð	θ	ŋ	–f
Sander (1972) norms		ʃ	tʃ	l	dʒ	s	r	v		ð	θ		

Note. GFTA-2 is the *Goldman-Fristoe Test of Articulation* (2nd ed.), by Goldman and Fristoe (2000); Arizona-3 is the *Arizona Articulation Proficiency Scale* (3rd ed.), by Fudala (2000). Smit et al. (1990) reported the latest age of acquisition for /ŋ/ at 9 years. GFTA-2 and Arizona-3 show it as an early sound. Stoel-Gammon's longitudinal study did not extend beyond age 2. Empty cells mean lack of data in a given study.

Consonant Clusters

Most classic cross-sectional studies did not offer norms on consonant clusters. Templin's (1957) study, however, did include norms on the mastery of initial and final consonant clusters as well as single consonants. As in single phonemes, consonant clusters were considered mastered when 75% of the sampled children correctly produced them. In addition, the *Goldman-Fristoe Test of Articulation–Second Edition* (GFTA-2; Goldman & Fristoe, 2000) offers norms for clusters in only the initial position, and the *Arizona Articulation Proficiency Scale–Third Edition* (Arizona-3; Fudala, 2000) provides norms for initial and final consonant clusters. The ages of mastery of clusters from these three sources are presented in Table 4.5.

Smit et al.'s previously described 1990 study and a subsequent publication (Smit, 1993b) also included data on the development of word-initial consonant clusters in 3- to 9-year-old children. Because of gender differences found in the study, their data were separately presented for male and female children for some early age groups. If their recommended clinical criterion of correct production by 90% of children is applied, the age of mastery of consonant clusters in the prevocalic positions would be as shown in Table 4.6.

An examination of the mastery ages for consonant clusters reveals significant discrepancies across the studies. At age 4, 75% of the sampled children in Templin's (1957) study had mastered 16 clusters in the initial and 12 clusters in the final position. Templin's findings revealed that by the age of 4-0, 75% of the children sampled correctly produced /s + stop/, /s + nasal/, /stop + liquid/ (except /gr/), and /stop + w/ initial clusters. Acquisition of sound classes was less predictable for the final clusters. Mastery for three-member clusters and clusters containing a fricative sound continued through the age of 8. Anthony, Boggle, Ingram, and McIsac's (1971) British study on the learning of consonant clusters generally agrees with Templin's (1957) data. Data from Goldman and Fristoe (2000), Fudala (2000), and Smit et al. (1990), however, show few or no clusters mastered by 4-year-olds. Most clusters are mastered by children 8 years of age and older in Smit et al.'s study. It should be noted that Fudala's Arizona-3 data are limited to just eight blends, all mastered at age 6.

McLeod, Doorn, and Reed (2001) studied consonant cluster learning in 16 Anglo-Australian 2-year-old children (2-0 to 2-11 years). An analysis of conversational speech, recorded monthly for 6 months, revealed that most 2-year-olds in the study produced at least some word-initial and word-final consonant clusters correctly, although there were children who produced none correctly. As expected, more correct cluster productions were noted on later observations. Word-initial /l/ and /s/ clusters were generally correct. Nasal clusters in word-final positions were often correct. Clusters involving /r/ were generally incorrect. At the initial observations, when the children were youngest, cluster reduction was more common; whereas at the later observations, cluster simplifications were more common. A noteworthy feature of this report is that the authors provided individual data on all 16 children (not just group means).

Greenlee (1973, 1974) reported two studies on cluster learning in children and described four learning stages. In the first stage, children omitted the entire cluster, a finding not supported by other studies (see Smit, 1993b, for a review of studies). In the second stage, children reduced clusters to single sounds, which finding is supported by other studies. Greenlee claimed that children omit the *marked* member (one unique to the language, not common across languages) of a cluster and retain the *unmarked* member (one common

Table 4.5

AGE   OF   MASTERY   OF   CONSONANT   CLUSTERS

Age	Initial Clusters			Final Clusters	
	Templin (1957)	Goldman & Fristoe (2000)	Fudala (2000)	Templin (1957)	Fudala (2000)
4-0	pl, bl, kl, gl, pr, br, tr, dr, kr, tw, kw, sm, sn, sp, st, sk	kw		mp, mpt, mps, ŋgk, lp, lt, rm, rt, rk, pt, ks, ft	
5-0	gr, fl, fr, str	bl		lb, lf, rd, rf, rn	
6-0	skw	br, dr, fr, gr, kr, tr, fl, gl, kl, pl, st	pl, tr, gr, st	lk, rb, rg, rθ, rdʒ, rst, rtʃ, nt, nd, nθ	ld, st, ts, ks
7-0	spl, spr, skr, sl, sw, ʃr, θr	sl, sp, sw		sk, st, kst, lθ, lz, dʒd	
8-0				kt, sp	

Note. A cluster is "mastered" when produced by 75% of the children sampled in the Templin (1957) study, 85% in Goldman and Fristoe (2000), and 90% in Fudala (2000). Goldman and Fristoe provided norms for only the initial position. The clusters are listed cumulatively; only newly mastered clusters are listed for each age.

Table 4.6

AGE   OF   MASTERY   OF   WORD-INITIAL   CONSONANT   CLUSTERS

Age	Male Group	Female Group
3-6	tw	
4-0		tw, kw
5-0		kl
5-6	kw	pl, fl
6-0	gl, kl, pl, bl	bl, gl
7-0	fl	
8-0	pr, br, tr, dr, kr, gr, fr	pr, br, tr, dr, kr, gr, fr
9-0	sp, st, skw, spl	sp, st, skw, spl
>9	sk, sm, sn, sw, sl, θr, spr, str, skr	sk, sm, sn, sw, sl, θr, spr, str, skr

Note. The mastery criterion is correct production by 90% of children sampled, according to Smit et al. (1990). Beginning with the 7-0 age group, the authors presented only the data averaged for males and females.

across languages); most other investigators have not looked into this possibility. If the claim is true, it may be because the unmarked (or less marked) sounds are phonetically easier to produce than the marked sounds. In the third stage, children substituted a sound for the marked sound that was previously omitted from the cluster. In the fourth stage, the full cluster mastery was evident.

Smit (1993b) made a comprehensive analysis of consonant cluster learning and error patterns found in the Iowa-Nebraska Articulation Norms Project data (Smit et al., 1990). She concluded the following: (1) In the initial stage of learning to produce clusters, children, even 2-year-olds, do not delete the total cluster, contradicting Greenlee's (1973, 1974) finding; (2) reducing the cluster to a single element is more common (e.g., [moke] for *smoke* but not *oke*), confirming Greenlee's results; and (3) three-element clusters may first be reduced to one, then to two, and finally produced correctly.

A few studies of American (Pollock, 2002; Pollock & Berni, 2003) and Australian (James, van Doorn, & McLeod, 2002; Waring, Fisher, & Atkin, 2001) children have offered data on percent consonant clusters correct (PCCC). Although studies do not fully agree, when the results of these and other studies (Greenlee, 1973; Smit, 1993b) are combined, some gross generalizations may be made:

- Two-year-olds may produce 20% to 32% of clusters correctly; word-final consonants may be more correct than word-initial consonants.

- Learning to produce the grammatical morphemes (e.g., the plural morpheme *s*, as in "books") tends to coincide with learning to produce clusters.

- Children more correctly produce two-element clusters before they begin to produce three-element clusters.

- Stop-consonant clusters (e.g., /pl/ and /bl/) may be mastered earlier than fricative-consonant clusters (e.g., /st/, /θr/).

- By the end of their third year, children may produce 86% of consonant clusters correctly.

- By the end of their seventh year, children may produce 95% to 98% of consonant clusters correctly.

- Correct production of some initial 3-phoneme clusters (e.g., skw, spr, str) may be achieved around age 9 (see Table 4.6).

Data on consonant cluster learning are limited and full of discrepancies. Further research is needed before any conclusive statements can be made on the learning of consonant clusters. As in the learning of single phonemes, longitudinal studies (e.g., Greenlee, 1974; Moskowitz, 1973) have revealed individual differences in the rate and order of consonant cluster learning. Thus, any set of normative data should be used with caution.

Vowels

The acquisition of vowels has been historically neglected, possibly because of the belief that English-speaking children acquire all of the English vowels by the age of 3 (Anthony et al., 1971; Templin, 1957) and that consonants are more important than vowels in speech intelligibility. Difficulties in transcribing vowels reliably have posed methodologic problems for investigators. Little information is available on the order and rate of vowel acquisition before the age of 3, a time in which children appear to learn many vowels.

Available evidence points out a difference in the learning patterns of consonants and vowels. The same early consonants that appear in babble are also the ones that are produced in the first few words—and more accurately than those that are not produced in the babbling stage. On the other hand, vowels found in babble may not be found in early words, and early vowels may often be incorrect in later meaningful speech (see Stoel-Gammon & Pollock, 2011, for a good recent review of vowel development and disorders).

A series of studies reported in Irwin and Wong (1983) summarized speech sound learning in children between the ages of 18 and 72 months. A total of 100 children participated in the study, with 10 males and 10 females in each of the following age groups: 18 months, 2 years, 3 years, 4 years, and 6 years. A total of five investigators collected the data, one per age group, and the same data collection and analysis procedures were used for all groups. These studies lend support to the common notion that vowels develop quite early. By the age of 3, individual children and the total group of 20 produced all of the vowels and diphthongs with 99% to 100% accuracy. At 2 years of age, all vowels and diphthongs were produced with at least 80% accuracy, with the exception of /ɚ/ and /ɝ/. At 18 months of age, only /ɑ/, /u/, /i/, /ʌ/ were produced with at least 70% accuracy; the same vowels were produced by 15-month-olds in a study by Selby, Robb, and Gilbert (2000). The latter study also showed that by 2 years of age, children had most of the vowels in their speech repertoire. Vowel production accuracy, however, is not achieved until about 3 years of age (Pollock, 2002).

Fudala (2000), in the *Arizona Articulation Proficiency Scale–Third Edition*, also offers normative information on the acquisition of vowels. If we apply to those data a criterion of 90% of children in a given age group exhibiting mastery of a speech sound, we find that all of the target vowels and diphthongs developed quite early, mostly between the second and third years. Exceptions to this were the mid-central vowels /ɝ/ and /ɚ/ and the rhotic diphthongs /ɪɚ/, /ɛɚ/, /oɚ/, and /aɚ/, which were mastered between 6 and 7 years. The youngest age group, 1-6 to 1-11, reached the mastery criterion of 90% of the following vowels and diphthongs: /ə/, /ʌ/, /ɛ/, /a/, /æ/, /ɔ/, /ɪ/, /i/, /ʊ/, /u/, /ou/, /ai/, /ei/, and /au/. The actual percentage of children in the youngest age group producing each of these vowels correctly ranged from 97.7 to 100. In summary, most vowels and diphthongs are mastered very early, with the exception of rhotic vowels and diphthongs. This helps explain why the vowelization phonological pattern, or substitution of /a/, /u/, and /ou/ for /ɝ/ and /ɚ/, persists for several years.

Vowel errors are difficult to classify and to get agreement on among researchers. Errors may be found across all parameters of vowel production: errors of backing or fronting, raising or lowering, tensing or laxing, rounding or unrounding (Pollock, 2002). In general, however, vowel errors in children with SSDs are less common than consonant errors. Some, but not all, children with severe SSDs may produce some vowels incorrectly. Children with SSDs are more likely to incorrectly produce diphthongs, mid-front vowels, and lax vowels (Pollock, Meeks, Stepherson, & Berni, 2004). Vowel errors in children with SSDs may be similar to those found in younger children who are typical learners. Cross-linguistic evidence suggests that vowel errors may be related to the number and complexity of vowels in a language (Goldstein & Pollock, 2000; Stoel-Gammon & Pollock, 2011). Children speaking a language with fewer and simpler vowels (e.g., Spanish) may be more accurate in their vowel production than those who speak a language with many and complex vowels (e.g., Swedish or Cantonese).

Common Consonant Error Types

What types of errors can be expected to occur on specific sounds or particular sound classes? Several investigators have tried to answer this question (e.g., Bassi, 1983; Bricker, 1967; Dyson, 1986; Hare, 1983; Irwin & Wong, 1983; Macken & Barton, 1980; Olmsted, 1971; Singh & Frank, 1972; Smit, 1993a, 1993b; Snow, 1963). The following list provides the common error types; by and large, errors on fricatives are the most common:

Nasals

- denasalization of /m/ and /n/ (the replacement of a nasal consonant by a non-nasal sound made in the same place of articulation, such as [doz] for *nose*)
- [m] or [ŋ] substituted for final /n/
- [n] substituted for final /ŋ/; also, an addition of a velar stop

Glides

- deletion of /w/, /j/, and /hw/
- substitution of [w], [d], [h], or [l] for /j/

Stops

- deaspiration of initial voiceless stops (also known as initial consonant voicing or the replacement of a voiced for a voiceless consonant)
- fronting of initial velars to alveolars (common and affects initial stops more often than final stops)
- deletion of final stops (less common for velars than for labial or alveolar stops)

Liquids

- substitution of [w] for initial /l/ and /r/
- deletion of initial liquids
- substitution of a rounded vowel and schwa for final /l/ and /r/
- deletion of final /l/ and /r/

Labial and Dental Fricatives

- substitution of stops for fricatives, primarily initial fricatives
- substitution of [f] for /θ/
- substitution of [b] for initial and final /v/
- substitution of fricatives for other fricatives (e.g., [f] for /v/ and [f] for /θ/)
- substitution of a fricative [s, f] for initial /θ/ and substitution of a stop [d] for its voiced cognate /ð/

Alveolar and Palatal Fricatives and Affricates

- deletion of final fricatives /s/, /z/, /ʃ/
- stopping of fricatives and affricates in the youngest age groups, primarily in the initial position

- devoicing of final /z/ and /dʒ/, can also affect initial /z/
- depalatalization of initial and final palatals /ʃ/, /tʃ/, /dʒ/ (manner of production)
- deaffrication of initial and final /tʃ/
- stopping of initial /s/
- dental distortions of /s/ (dental and interdental variants, including /θ/ and /ð/)

Consonant Clusters

- tendency for obstruent + /w/ clusters to be reduced to the obstruent
- tendency for obstruent + /l/ clusters to be reduced to the obstruent (or to another obstruent substituting for the target)—except /fl/ cluster tends to be reduced to an approximant [w]
- tendency for obstruent + /r/ clusters to be reduced to the obstruent (the remaining obstruent sometimes being a substitute for the clustered obstruent)
- tendency for clusters made up of /s/ + consonant to be reduced to the [w], nasal, or stop component of the cluster

Three major error patterns can be expected on three-member clusters:

1. When children reduce the cluster to a single element, they usually retain the stop or a stop substitute.
2. When children reduce the cluster to two elements, a wide variety of errors can be expected, although the most common one is the preservation of a stop at the appropriate place of articulation together with the **approximant** (or its substitute).
3. When all three members are preserved, the /s/ and the approximant (especially /r/) become vulnerable to errors that are typical for that consonant, such as dentalized [s] and [w] for /r/.

Learning Speech Sound Patterns

Historically, researchers have described age ranges for the acquisition of individual phonemes. In that method of analysis, patterns of development have not been well represented. As patterns of correct and incorrect productions have received increasing attention in the past several years, researchers have looked at patterns of sound production in terms of sound classes, distinctive features, and phonological processes or patterns.

Mastery of Sound Classes

Despite some differences in ages of sound mastery in many of the cross-sectional studies, a pattern of sound class acquisition may be noted. The order of acquisition based on the manner-place-voice speech sound classification has been somewhat more stable than randomly selected individual sounds. For example, nasals, stops, and glides are mastered earlier, followed by liquids, fricatives, and affricates. Mastery of sound classes overlaps across age groups. A general sequence is as follows:

- *Nasal consonants* are among the earliest to develop; /m/ and /n/ are mastered quite early, at about age 3, whereas /ŋ/ is mastered a bit later, at between 3 and 4 years of age.

- *Stops* are acquired early, with /p/ and /b/ being the earliest mastered within this sound class, between 2 and 3 years of age. There is no specific order of acquisition for the alveolar stops /t/ and /d/ or the velar stops /k/ and /g/. Great individual variation has been noted in the acquisition of the alveolar and velar stops; some children develop /t/ and /d/ prior to /k/ and /g/ and vice versa. In her study on the acquisition of velars by 2-year-old children, Dyson (1986) found that final velars are acquired before initial velars.

- *Glides* are learned relatively early. The /w/ is mastered by around 2 years, while /j/ is mastered at around 3 years of age.

- *Fricatives, affricates,* and *liquids* are the later-developing sound classes, although there is much variation in the acquisition of individual sounds within each class. The *fricative* sound class is quite large, containing nine consonants: /h/, /s/, /z/, /f/, /v/, /ʃ/, /ʒ/, /θ/, /ð/. The affricate /tʃ/ and /dʒ/ and liquid /l/ and /r/ sound classes have only two sounds each. Among the fricatives, /h/ and /f/ are among the earliest mastered, at around 3 to 4 years. The remaining fricatives are mastered somewhat later, between the ages of 4 and 6. The fricatives /ʒ/, /θ/, and /ð/ tend to be mastered the latest by most children. The *affricates* /tʃ/ and /dʒ/ are both mastered at about 6 years old. The *liquids* /l/ and /r/ are also mastered quite late, at approximately 6 years old. Errors of /l/ and /r/ are not uncommon among preschool and early school-age children (Irwin & Wong, 1983; Kenney & Prather, 1986; Olmsted, 1971).

Mastery of Distinctive Features

A child's articulation and phonological learning has also been described according to the acquisition of distinctive features (Menyuk, 1968; Prather et al., 1975; Singh, 1976). As defined in Chapter 2, **distinctive features** are articulatory or acoustic characteristics that are present or absent in a particular phoneme or group of phonemes.

Research or clinical application of distinctive features has waned in recent decades. In one of the earliest studies, Menyuk (1968) analyzed the presence of some distinctive features in spontaneous speech samples of American preschool children between the ages of 2½ and 5 years. Analyzing the percentage of sounds with specific features that children produced at varying ages, Menyuk rank-ordered the selected distinctive features from earliest to latest mastery:

1. + *nasal*—sounds resonated in the nasal cavity
2. + *grave*—sounds produced at the very front
3. + *voice*—sounds produced with vibration of the vocal folds
4. + *diffuse*—sounds made at the very back
5. + *strident*—sounds made by forcing the airstream through a small opening, resulting in the production of intense noise

6. + *continuant*—sounds made with an incomplete point of constriction, thus without stopping the flow of air entirely at any point

Prather et al. (1975), analyzing consonant acquisition in children 2 to 4 years of age, found a rank order of acquisition that was similar to Menyuk's, with the exception of the continuant and strident features. Their order of acquisition was as follows: + nasal, + grave, + diffuse, + voice, + continuant, and + strident.

Phonological Patterns in Typical Speech Sound Learners

In Chapter 3 we defined phonological patterns (PPs) as systematic sound changes that affect classes of sounds and the syllable structure of words. Terminological changes for the same phenomena are common in speech–language pathology; *phonological patterns* is currently preferred, but the term *phonological processes* was used in the not-too-distant past, and some continue to use that term. Some prefer to call PPs *error patterns*, for, indeed, they are errors from the standpoint of typical adult speech. In this book we generally use the terms *phonological patterns* and *error patterns*, but we use the term *processes* when we make a specific reference to authors or sources that have used that term in the past. *Phonological processes* is still the accurate term when the reference is to Stampe's (1969, 1979) theory of natural phonology.

The difference between speech sound learning and PPs found in young children should be clear. It may be said that children *learn to produce speech sounds*, as described in the previous sections. It is not accurate, however, to say that children learn to produce phonological patterns, as these are simplified productions that the child is capable of at given points. They may be naturally occurring errors in speech sound learning, as Stampe (1969, 1979) suggested. As children become progressively more proficient in their production of speech sounds, their error patterns decrease. In this sense, a decrease in the error patterns is simply a consequence of correct learning of speech sound production. It is not correct to say that error patterns are unlearned, because it is difficult to claim that errors were learned in the first place. As the correct sound patterns are *acquired*, error patterns are *shed*. Throughout this section we describe the rough timelines when phonological error patterns decline or disappear. Clinical concerns emerge when certain error patterns persist beyond certain specific ages.

The PPs that have been found to occur in the speech of typically learning children and those with phonological disorders have been categorized according to syllable structure patterns, substitution patterns, and assimilation patterns (Ingram, 1976; Lowe, 1994; Stoel-Gammon & Dunn, 1985):

Syllable Structure Patterns

- final consonant deletion (omission of final consonants; e.g., [bu] for *books*)
- cluster reduction (omission of consonants in clusters; e.g., [top] for *stop*)
- unstressed syllable deletion (omission of weak syllables; e.g., [medo] for *tomato*)
- reduplication (doubling of a syllable; e.g., [wawa] for *water*)
- epenthesis (insertion of an unstressed vowel; e.g., [səpun] for *spoon*)

Substitution Patterns

- stopping (substitution of stops for fricatives or affricates; e.g., [tun] for *sun*)
- liquid gliding (substitution of a glide for a liquid; e.g., [wæbit] for *rabbit*)
- vocalization (substitution of a vowel for a syllabic liquid; e.g., [pepo] for *paper*)
- depalatalization (substitution of an alveolar fricative for a palatal fricative; e.g., [fis] for *fish*)
- velar fronting (substitution of alveolars for velars; e.g., [rin] for *ring*)
- deaffrication (substitution of fricatives for affricates; e.g., [ʃɛr] for *chair*)

Assimilation Patterns

- labial assimilation (a non-labial consonant changed into a labial; e.g., [bʊb] for *book*)
- velar assimilation (a non-velar changed into a velar; e.g., [kʌg] for *cup*)
- nasal assimilation (a non-nasal changed into a nasal; e.g., [mɑm] for *mop*)
- voicing assimilation (a voiceless sound changed to a voiced; e.g., [dɛn] for *ten*— or a voiced sound changed to a voiceless sound; e.g., [pit] for *pig*)

The most widespread patterns found in typical speech sound learners include final consonant deletion, cluster reduction, unstressed syllable deletion, stopping, fronting, and liquid gliding (Grunwell, 1987; Ingram, 1976; Stoel-Gammon & Dunn, 1985). These patterns may be found in the speech of nearly all children.

Although certain patterns occur more frequently in typical learners, limited and often contradictory information exists on the initial appearance, productive duration, and suppression timelines of PPs. The different age levels at which the patterns are first observed and are eventually eliminated are not clearly identified for all the patterns. Different researchers' information is not directly comparable because of differing criteria used to conclude that a pattern is occurring. Also, different studies define the same or similar pattern differently, which makes direct comparisons difficult. With these limitations, we will provide a chronological review of the information available on the use of PPs in children who are typical learners of speech sounds.

Grunwell (1982) offered a chronology of gradual disappearance of the phonological patterns in typical speech sound learners. She outlined these "simplifying processes" as weak syllable deletion, final consonant deletion, reduplication, consonant harmony, cluster reduction, stopping, fronting, gliding, and context-sensitive voicing. Her analysis shows that, generally, most PPs are absent by age 5 or so. Patterns that disappear before age 3 include reduplication, stopping of /f/ and /s/, and context-sensitive voicing; those that last the longest include weak syllable deletion, stopping of /θ/ and /ð/ (substituting them with a stop, such as /t/), and gliding (substituting /w/ for /r/). The normative trends in sound acquisition help us to understand some of these timelines for error pattern elimination. For instance, sounds that get replaced are learned later; sounds that replace others are mastered earlier. For example, in the stopping error of [du] for *zoo*, the child substitutes the not yet mastered /z/ with already mastered /d/; in the stopping error of [tʌn] for *sun*, the child produces /t/ in the existing repertoire in place of the /s/ that is not in the repertoire.

In their study, Hodson and Paden (1981) noted that the PPs known to affect intelligibility the most in young children were rarely exhibited by the sixty 4- to 5-year-old typical speech sound learners with good intelligibility. Hodson and Paden suggested that by that age, speech sound production approximated the adult model. They did note devoicing of final obstruents, substitution of anterior strident phonemes for non-strident interdentals, liquid deviations, tongue protrusions, depalatalization, nasal assimilation, labial assimilation, velar assimilation, and metathesis in varying numbers of children. However, those deviations were judged not to greatly affect the children's intelligibility. Unfortunately, Hodson and Paden did not report the total number of instances a process was exhibited by each group or each child, or the actual percentage of occurrence for each process.

Dyson and Paden (1983) investigated elimination of the following five PPs in 40 children: gliding, cluster reduction, fronting, stopping, and final consonant deletion. Using 36 words to provide an opportunity for these five patterns to occur, they tested the children at 3-week intervals beginning at 2 years and ending 7 months later. Throughout the study, the patterns were ordered from most to least frequently occurring. During the initial testing, the order for the frequency of occurrence was as follows: gliding, cluster reduction, fronting, stopping, and final consonant deletion. During the last testing, at the age of 2 years 7 months, the order remained the same. However, at that point, Dyson and Paden found that final consonant deletion was almost completely eliminated, fronting and stopping were infrequent, and gliding and cluster reduction were still common.

Lowe, Knutson, and Monson (1985) studied the incidence of fronting in 1,048 preschool children between the ages of 2 years 7 months and 4 years 6 months. They observed fronting in 6% of the study participants and noted that velar fronting was more common than palatal fronting. They also noted that palatal fronting did not occur in the absence of velar fronting. Lowe et al. stated that fronting occurred infrequently after the age of 3 years 6 months.

Haelsig and Madison (1986) investigated the occurrence of 16 PPs in 50 children. The children were divided into five 6-month age groupings, resulting in 10 children in each of the following age groups: 3-0, 3-6, 4-0, 4-6, and 5-0. The authors used the *Phonological Process Analysis* (Weiner, 1979) to identify the error patterns the children exhibited. If we apply the McReynolds and Elbert (1981a) criteria to qualify as a process, a specific phonological process must have a possibility of occurring four times and be produced at least 20% of the time. The Haelsig and Madison results may be summarized as shown in Table 4.7. As can be seen in the table, the 3-year-olds exhibited more patterns than the 4-year-olds. A 20% occurrence was not evident for any process in 5-year-olds. The investigators did note individual variation across the subjects and the five age groups, and they acknowledged that the sample size in this study was limited.

Preisser, Hodson, and Paden (1988) reported average percentages of occurrence for eight PPs in 60 typically developing children divided into three age groups of 3-month age ranges: 1-6 to 1-9, 1-10 to 2-1, 2-2 to 2-5. Preisser et al. classified the PPs according to omissions and class deficiencies. Omissions included cluster reduction, postvocalic and prevocalic obstruent omission, and syllable reduction. Class deficiencies included liquid deviation, stridency deletion, velar deviation, and nasal/glide deviation. Using McReynolds and Elbert's (1981a) 20% criterion, the youngest age group, 1-6 to 1-9, used all of the patterns at a significant level, with the exception of prevocalic obstruent omission, which occurred

Table 4.7

PERCENTAGE   OF   OCCURRENCE   OF   PHONOLOGICAL   PROCESSES
IN CHILDREN 3-0 TO 5-0

Chronological Age Group	3-0	3-6	4-0	4-6	5-0
Phonological Process	Mean Percentage of Occurrence				
Deletion of final consonants	22	15	6	10	5
Weak-syllable deletion	38	31	26	28	13
Stopping	14	21	8	6	0
Glottal replacement	38	31	7	8	8
Liquid gliding	48	55	23	13	0
Vocalization	21	41	28	6	1
Alveolar assimilation	8	25	8	2	2
Labial assimilation	30	14	14	4	2

Note. From "A Study of Phonological Processes Exhibited by 3-, 4-, and 5-Year-Old Children," by P. C. Haelsig and C. L. Madison, 1986, *Language, Speech, and Hearing Services in the Schools, 17,* pp. 107–114. Adapted with permission.

an average of 14% of the time. By the oldest age group, 2-2 to 2-5, only liquid deviation, stridency deletion, and cluster reduction occurred at a significant level.

Roberts, Burchinal, and Foote (1990) conducted a study of phonological skills in children between 2 years 5 months and 8 years by testing them at varying times throughout the course of their study. As the researchers followed the children's development, they noted a noticeable decline in the use of PPs between the ages of 2 years 5 months and 4 years. Roberts et al. reported that by age 4, only cluster reduction, liquid gliding, and deaffrication had an occurrence level of at least 20%.

Stoel-Gammon and Dunn (1985) divided PPs according to those that were likely to disappear by 3 years and those that would be expected to persist beyond the age of 3; this division is summarized below, and the results of previously reviewed studies generally support it.

Patterns That Disappear by Age 3:

- unstressed syllable deletion
- final consonant deletion
- doubling
- diminutization
- velar fronting
- consonant assimilation
- reduplication

Patterns That Persist Beyond Age 3:

- prevocalic voicing
- epenthesis

- vocalization
- stopping
- depalatalization
- final devoicing

Based on the results of several studies (Grunwell, 1987; Khan & Lewis, 2002; Lowe, 2012; Smit, 1993b, 2004), it is possible to offer more specific suggestions on the decline or disappearance of individual patterns (see Table 4.8). These suggestions apply to at least 75% of children in the specified age groups, and individual differences are always noteworthy. In diagnosing a phonological disorder in a child, clinicians may use these suggestions, as well as those offered by Stoel-Gammon and Dunn (1985) listed previously.

ACTIVITY

Define phonological patterns and give an example of each from the three main categories.

Table 4.8

LIKELY AGES AT WHICH PHONOLOGICAL PATTERNS DISAPPEAR

Pattern	Likely Age of Disappearance
Denasalization	2.6
Assimilations	3
Affrication	3
Context-sensitive voicing change	3
Final consonant deletion	3
Fronting of initial velar singles	4
Deaffrication	4
De-rhotacization	4
Cluster reduction (without /s/)	4
Depalatalization of final singles	4.6
Depalatalization of initial singles	5
Alveolarization	5
Final devoicing	5
Cluster reduction (with /s/)	5
Labialization	6
Initial voicing	6
Gliding of initial liquids	7
Vocalization of prevocalic liquids	7
Epenthesis	8
Consonant cluster substitution	9

Note. Information is based on multiple studies and is suggestive; individual differences are significant.

Clinical Use of Speech Sound Norms

How do clinicians use normative information in making clinical decisions? Evaluating the various normative studies can be a daunting task. In making clinical decisions, the clinician should consider the following:

- the variability of norms across studies
- gross and general patterns still found in studies
- individual differences that get masked in group norms
- guidelines the clinician is expected to adhere to in work settings (e.g., a policy established in the school district for diagnosing an SSD and qualifying a child for treatment)
- selection of target phonemes based on norms, child-specific considerations (e.g., academic needs), coexisting problems (e.g., a more serious language problem that needs immediate attention), or, most likely, a combination of these and other factors

We address the issue of selecting target phonemes for treatment in Chapter 7. See Text Box 4.3 for some interesting issues and comments about speech sound learning and clinical decision making.

Text Box 4.3. How do we use normative information in clinical decision making?

Many clinicians may believe that norms are a solid and reliable means of diagnosing a speech sound disorder and selecting treatment targets. But that belief is not entirely valid. Difficulties with norms include the following:

Norms are an artificial statistical attempt to eliminate the true individual differences and variability that exist in children.

Norms specify that 75% or 90% of children sampled have mastered a specific sound at a given age level, but the individual child may not be one of those 75% or 90% of the children sampled in the studies.

Clinicians assess and treat individual children, not a statistically "normalized" group of children.

For some sounds, the age of mastery varies greatly among studies (e.g., depending on the study, /s/ may be mastered at 3.6 years or 8 years; /r/ may be mastered at 4.6 or 8).

There is no invariable (universal) order in which speech sounds are acquired.

It is not necessary to treat all earlier acquired sounds in error before treating later acquired sounds.

Norms are only one possible rough guide in selecting treatment targets.

Other child-specific variables may be even more important than norms (see Chapter 7 for details).

See the online article "Confusion About Speech Sound Norms and Their Use" at http://poti .wikispaces.com/file/view/confusion+about+speech+sound+norms+and+their+use.pdf for a critical view of norms and their usefulness by Gregory Lof.

Speech Intelligibility

Several variables affect speech intelligibility. It is well known that familiarity with a child's speech is a significant factor in intelligibility, as all parents seem to have a near-perfect understanding of their young children's speech, though it may be indecipherable to strangers. In one study, strangers understood only 50% of 2-year-olds' speech (Coplan & Gleason, 1988). Knowledge of the topic of conversation also may aid intelligibility. From a clinical standpoint, though, simplifying PPs, along with the incorrect use of individual phonemes, will undoubtedly be the most important variables affecting a child's speech intelligibility. As the child masters progressively more individual phonemes and discards various PPs, speech intelligibility improves.

How intelligible can we expect children to be in the normal course of development? Villman and Greenlee's (1987) study with ten 3-year-old children revealed an average level of intelligibility of 73% for that age group. It should be noted, however, that the range was quite broad, from 54% to 80%. Gordon-Brannan (1994) reported a mean percentage of intelligibility of 93% for 4-year-old children, with a range of 73% to 100%. The range of intelligibility reported by these studies highlights the prevalence of individual variability among children.

Roulstone, Loader, Northstone, Beveridge, and the ALSPAC Team's (2002) study involving 1,127 children who were 2 years old found that most children were intelligible to their parents. Only 12.7% of parents found their children difficult to understand, and 2.1% of parents reported that they could rarely understand their children. Flipsen's (2006) study has special clinical relevance, as most clinicians transcribe children's speech samples recorded during assessment. He demonstrated that 88% to 100% of the words 3- to 4-year-olds produce may be transcribable (intelligible). By age 5, 98% of the words may be transcribable.

Anecdotal data, clinical experience, and parental reports support the notion that by 5 years of age, typically developing children are nearly 100% understandable. However, that a child is understood 90% to 100% of the time does not suggest that the child has "perfect" speech. It simply means that the child is understood most of the time despite the possible presence of some developmentally appropriate misarticulations. This is because speech intelligibility is not a sole function of articulation; it is partly determined by the context of speech, the topic, child familiarity, knowledge of typical speech sound errors children make, and so forth. Speech intelligibility is likely to vary from child to child according to his or her articulation and phonological skills. What follows is a set of rough guidelines that clinicians may use with discretion:

Easy Reference for Speech Intelligibility Expectations

Age	Intelligibility Level
19–24 months	25% to 50%
2–3 years	50% to 75%
4–5 years	75% to 90%
5+ years	90% to 100% (a few articulation errors may persist)

Variables Related to Speech Sound Learning

As the review of information included so far suggests, there is a wealth of normative information on the acquisition of speech sounds. A more complete understanding of speech requires a description of variables that may be causal for, or at least correlated with, the normal or impaired learning of speech sounds. In this section, we summarize the research findings on factors that may affect the speech sound leaning process.

Researched variables associated with the acquisition of speech sounds and articulatory performance may be grouped under (1) anatomic, neurological, and physiological variables; (2) motor skills; (3) hearing loss; (4) auditory discrimination; (5) oral sensation; (6) language skills; (7) personal characteristics; (8) genetic factors; and (9) tongue thrust.

Speech Anatomic Variables

Because speech production is a neuromotor event, researchers have investigated oral and neural anatomic factors that may affect the acquisition of speech sounds and general articulatory proficiency. It is well known that the structural integrity of the speech mechanism is essential to normal speech production. Variables that negatively affect speech production also could affect children's learning of speech sounds.

The anatomic structures that affect the learning and production of speech sounds include the lips, teeth, tongue, hard palate, and soft palate. Abnormality in these structures could negatively affect the acquisition and production of speech sounds. Muscular weakness, deficient neural control of muscles involved in speech production, and growth deficiencies in the oral and facial structures may all cause difficulty learning the speech sounds.

When abnormalities do exist in the speech mechanism, they vary greatly across children and adults. In some speakers, the abnormality may be minimal; in others, it may be gross. Such variations could produce wide-ranging effects on speech sound acquisition. Therefore, it is important to consider the degree of abnormality, not just its presence or absence. Among the major speech or speech-related structures researched, the following are significant:

- **Lips.** Important articulators of speech sounds, the lips come in contact with each other with varying degrees of pressure and force in producing the bilabial sounds (/p/, /b/, and /m/). The consonants /w/ and /hw/ and several vowels require lip rounding. Structural abnormalities that prevent the approximation of lips or lip rounding may be related to delayed speech sound acquisition or impaired production. Lip size, strength, and mobility typically vary across individuals, and such variations do not cause speech sound learning difficulties (Fairbanks & Green, 1950). Only gross structural anomalies, such as those found in a cleft of the upper lip, may affect speech sound learning (in such cases, adequate surgical treatment, done early, generally prevents speech sound learning problems).

- **Teeth.** Among the different classes of sounds, teeth are significantly involved in the production of labiodental /f/ and /v/ and linguadental phonemes /θ/ and /ð/). Teeth also are important in the production of alveolars /s/ and /z/, in that an airstream is directed over the upper incisors. Teeth may be missing, they may be malpositioned, or the two dental arches may be misaligned. Of these, misalignment of the dental arches, known as *malocclusion*, has received much research attention. Malocclusions are classified as Class I, II, or III. In a **Class I malocclusion,** the dental arches are generally aligned, but a few individual teeth are misaligned. In a **Class II malocclusion,** the lower jaw is receded, and the upper jaw is protruded. In a **Class III malocclusion,** the lower jaw is protruded, and the upper jaw is receded. The normal occlusion and Class II and III malocclusions are shown in Figure 4.1. Malocclusions may be found in individuals who exhibit normal articulation, as well as in those who exhibit SSDs. Even though they are slightly more common in individuals who have SSDs, *dental arch malocclusions themselves do not invariably cause articulation disorders.* Most individuals learn to produce speech sounds correctly in spite of such deviations by using compensatory strategies. Similarly, missing teeth, too, *are neither sufficient nor necessary to cause SSDs, even though they may be associated with a slightly higher frequency of misarticulations.*

....

ACTIVITY

Determine which type of malocclusion is most likely in a child with a receded lower jaw, a child with a protruded upper jaw, and a child with missing or misaligned teeth.

....

- **Tongue.** Although the tongue is the most important of the articulators, there is relatively little research on how its size, shape, and mobility affect the acquisition of speech sounds. A variable that has been researched to some extent is **ankyloglossia,** which is a short lingual frenum. Although an extremely short frenum may be associated with SSDs, it is not a factor in a majority of children who misarticulate. Within the limits of normal variation, tongue strength is not a factor in the rate of speech or reading (Neel & Palmer, 2012). Several investigators have studied the consequences of glossectomy for speech intelligibility (e.g., Leonard, 1994; Skelly, Spector, Donaldson, Brodeur, & Paletta, 1971). **Glossectomy** is the total or partial surgical removal of a diseased (e.g., cancerous) tongue. Some adults and children who undergo glossectomy may retain surprisingly

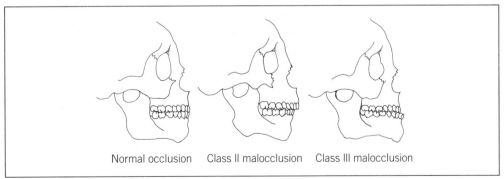

Normal occlusion   Class II malocclusion   Class III malocclusion

Figure 4.1. Normal occlusion of the dental arches contrasted with Class II and Class III forms of malocclusion. *Note.* From *Introduction to Communicative Disorders*, 4th ed. (p. 113), by M. N. Hegde, 2010, Austin, TX: PRO-ED. Copyright 2010 by PRO-ED, Inc. Reprinted with permission.

good articulation, suggesting that a radically altered tongue is capable of a range of fine movements necessary for producing intelligible speech. Adults whose tongue has been partially surgically removed may still produce intelligible speech, though there may be errors of articulation, especially in producing fricatives and plosives (Leonard, 1994). Generally, normal anatomic variations and surgical alterations of the tongue produce *limited effects on articulation and intelligibility because of various compensatory strategies the speakers learn, to limit the negative effects.* This conclusion underscores the dynamic adaptability of the tongue.

- **Hard Palate.** Limited research done in the past suggests that normal variations in the structural dimensions of the hard palate (e.g., its width, length, height) are of no consequence (Fairbanks & Lintner, 1951). However, clefts of the palate, if not surgically closed, can be expected to affect speech sound production. Clefts of the hard palate are initially closed within the first two years of life, with no significant or permanent effects on articulation. Therefore, clefts have not been a significant variable in misarticulations in children. If a cancerous hard palate is surgically removed, totally or partially, speech intelligibility is severely affected. However, such patients are fitted with a palatal prosthesis to close the opening between the oral and nasal cavities. Such prosthetic devices help improve speech intelligibility.

- **Soft Palate.** The soft palate, or velum, is a part of the velopharyngeal mechanism, which is important in articulation and resonance. It couples and uncouples the oral and nasal cavities. Closure of the velopharyngeal port is necessary to prevent unwanted nasal resonance on oral sounds, to maintain desirable oral resonance, and to build intraoral air pressure to produce certain consonants, known as **pressure consonants.** These include fricatives (e.g., /s/, /f/, /z/), stops (e.g., /b/, /g/, /t/, /k/), and affricates (e.g., /ʤ/ and /tʃ/). **Velopharyngeal inadequacy,** difficulty in closing the nasal port for the production of oral sounds, results in *hypernasality* on oral sounds and nasal emission (audible air leakage through the nose). It also results in the production of pressure consonants that are weak, imprecise, or unclear. The speaker tends to compensate for the velopharyngeal inadequacy by producing consonants in unusual ways. A common articulatory pattern is to shift the production of consonants to the posterior portion of the oral cavity. Major substitutions that result from compensatory articulation include the following (Bzoch, 2004; Kummer, 2014):

    - substitution of such stops as /p/, /b/, /t/, and /d/ with the **glottal stop,** which is produced by a stoppage and sudden release of air at the level of the glottis
    - substitution of linguavelar stops /k/ and /g/ with a **pharyngeal stop,** which is produced by making a pharyngeal contact by the base of the tongue
    - substitution of fricatives and affricates with **pharyngeal fricatives,** which are produced by lingual-pharyngeal contact with an unusual lingual configuration
    - substitution of sibilants with **velar fricatives,** which are produced in the back velar region and sound like distorted /k/ or /g/

○ substitution of stops /t/, /d/, /k/, and /g/ with **mid-dorsum palatal stops,** which are produced in the same manner the glide /j/ is produced

....

ACTIVITY

Define the following terms in your own words: *ankyloglossia, glossectomy, pressure consonants, velopharyngeal inadequacy, nasal emission, neurological factors.*

....

Neurophysiological Variables

Speech production may be negatively affected if neural control of the muscles of speech is impaired. If the peripheral or central nervous system controlling the speech mechanism is damaged, muscles of speech may be weak, uncoordinated, or paralyzed. If such pathologies exist during the years of speech and language acquisition, specific speech sound learning may be impaired. If such neural damage occurs in adults, the typically acquired and produced speech characteristics may be lost or impaired to varying degrees.

A speech disorder associated with central or peripheral nervous system damage is called **dysarthria.** Weakened, uncoordinated, or paralyzed speech muscles cause a variety of speech problems in both adults and children. Dysarthria and its varieties in children are described in the Advanced Unit of Chapter 6.

Speech disorders also can result from central nervous system damage when the peripheral neuromuscular mechanism is normal but the speech motor programming areas, including Broca's area, and the supplemental motor area are damaged. This disorder in children is called **childhood apraxia of speech** (CAS) and is described in the Advanced Unit of Chapter 6.

Cerebral palsy is a nonprogressive neuromotor disorder in children that in many cases causes communication problems, including articulatory problems. Cerebral palsy is typically congenital, although the brain injury that causes it may be sustained anytime up to age 16. The speech disorders associated with cerebral palsy are described as **developmental dysarthria,** described in the Advanced Unit of Chapter 6.

Motor Skills

That the motor skills of speakers with SSDs may be less proficient than those of normal speakers has an intuitive appeal because speech is a neuromotor task. Therefore, researchers have explored the relationship between two kinds of motor skills: general motor skills and orofacial motor skills. Research has generally discredited the notion that compared to those with normal articulation, children with articulation disorders are less proficient in such general motor tasks as finger tapping, ball tossing, or other kinds of gross or fine motor skills.

Motor skills executed by orofacial structures have generally yielded evidence that is somewhat inconsistent though suggestive of some deficiency in children who misarticulate. A common clinical procedure in articulation assessment is to ask the child to produce a string of syllables as rapidly as possible. The most popular task is to have the child first repeat /pʌ/, /tʌ/, and /kʌ/ in isolation, and then repeat /pʌtə/, /tʌkə/, /pʌkə/, and finally /pʌtəkə/. In each case, the clinician counts the number of syllables rapidly produced in a given unit of time, usually 10 or 15 seconds. Alternatively, the clinician can measure the time it takes for the client to repeat a certain number of syllables. The rapid rate of alternating syllable repetition is known as the **diadochokinetic rate.** The diagnostic use of this procedure is described in the Basic Unit of Chapter 6.

Children attain the adult diadochokinetic rates variably, between the ages of 9 and 15. Generally, children with articulation disorders are likely to have slower than normal diadochokinetic rates. However, children with misarticulations with normal diadochokinetic rates are frequently seen in speech clinics. Therefore, a slower diadochokinetic rate is not a necessary factor in SSDs. Consequently, the clinical and theoretical significance of slower diadochokinetic rates in children with SSDs is not clear.

Hearing Loss

It is well established that normal hearing is essential to unimpaired acquisition of speech sounds and oral language. The child who cannot hear the spoken language of his or her verbal community, or hears it inadequately, does not typically acquire the oral language. Two to three percent of school-age children may have a hearing impairment that exceeds 25 dB HL (Lundeen, 1991).

Normal hearing is essential for oral speech and language acquisition for two reasons. First, normal hearing makes the child aware of the speech and language spoken in his or her surroundings. It is difficult, if not impossible, to learn what is not heard, seen, or felt. Oral speech and language need to be heard. Second, normal hearing makes it possible to monitor one's own production of speech and language as it is being learned. This monitoring is essential to progressively better approximate adult productions. Hearing one's own speech, the child can self-monitor and further refine his or her productions. Without the benefit of hearing one's own speech, the child would be unable to self-monitor.

The terms **hearing impairment** and **hearing loss** mean that there is a hearing problem. Technically, it means that the auditory thresholds exceed 25 dB HL in the case of adults and 15 dB HL in the case of children. *Hard of hearing*, on the other hand, is a diagnostically more specific term. A person who is hard of hearing has residual hearing that can assist in speech–language acquisition, comprehension, and production. A hard-of-hearing person is aware of normal conversational speech but may need amplification (e.g., a hearing aid). The term *deaf* also is diagnostically specific. A deaf person is unaware of normal conversation and is not able to use hearing for speech–language acquisition, comprehension, and production.

Whether hearing impairment affects the acquisition of speech sounds and if it does, to what extent, depend on several factors. An important factor is the age of onset. Hearing loss may be **congenital,** which means that it was present at the time of birth, or **acquired,** which means that the onset was subsequent to birth. Generally, the earlier the onset of the hearing loss, the greater the effects on speech and language acquisition.

Another important factor is the severity of the hearing loss. **Hearing acuity,** which means how well a person hears, is measured in terms of decibels (dB). The **range of normal**

hearing varies from 0 dB HL to 15 dB HL in children and from 0 dB HL to 25 dB HL in adults. Even a slight hearing loss, frequently associated with middle ear infections, may cause speech and language delay. Therefore, the upper limit of normal hearing in children is considered to be 15 dB HL. Typically, the severity of hearing loss is classified as follows:

- slight impairment: 16 to 25 dB HL
- mild impairment: 26 to 40 dB HL
- moderate impairment: 41 to 70 dB HL
- severe impairment: 71 to 90 dB HL
- profound impairment: 91+ dB HL

Severity of hearing loss is related to the type of loss. Sensorineural hearing impairment tends to be more severe than conductive hearing loss. **Sensorineural loss** is associated with pathology in the inner ear or the neural pathways that carry auditory messages to the brain. **Conductive hearing loss** is associated with pathologies in the outer and the middle ear; the inner ear and the auditory pathways are normal. Generally, sensorineural hearing loss tends to be more severe than conductive loss. In any case, if the hearing loss is significant for the frequencies of speech (500 to 4000 Hz), a greater effect on speech and language acquisition is to be expected.

Still another factor related to hearing impairment and speech sound acquisition is the age at which clinical services are initiated and the quality of such services. The earlier the age at which comprehensive, intensive, and regular oral-aural (speech) rehabilitation services are initiated, the lower the negative effects on speech sound acquisition and production.

Children with a significant degree of hearing loss are likely to exhibit a variety of speech problems (Calvert, 1982; Dunn & Newton, 1986; Levitt & Stromberg, 1983). The speech problems such children tend to exhibit include the following:

- omit final and initial consonants, and omit /s/ more consistently
- produce final consonants too weakly
- substitute voiced consonants for voiceless consonants, nasal sounds for oral sounds, one vowel for another, and diphthongs for vowels and vowels for diphthongs
- produce distorted sounds; may produce stops and fricatives with too little or too much force
- produce vowels with imprecision, indefiniteness, and often with excessive duration
- shorten the first or second vowel in diphthongs
- produce speech with marked hypernasality, especially in vowels
- insert unnecessary vowels between consonants (e.g., [səlow] for *slow*)
- inappropriately release final consonants (e.g., *mop*^{h} for mop)

- speak at a lower rate (presumably because of longer duration of consonants and vowels)

- pause more frequently

- show slower articulatory transitions

- use inappropriate stress on syllables

- exhibit a harsh and breathy voice

- speak with a pitch that is too high or too low

- exhibit inappropriate prosodic features

People who become deaf after acquiring speech and language tend to omit or distort sounds that are produced with low intensity and high frequency. These include /s/, /ʃ/, /tʃ/, /f/, and /θ/ (Calvert, 1982). In many cases, such people produce consonants in the final position of words with very little force. Consequently, listeners may not hear them.

Children who experience **repeated middle ear infections** (otitis media) that result in hearing loss exceeding 20 db HL run an increased risk for speech and language problems. Otitis media with no or insignificant hearing loss (less than 20 db HL) poses minimal or no risk, although studies have produced some conflicting evidence, as reviewed in Shriberg, Friel-Patti, Flipsen, and Brown (2000) and Shriberg, Thielke, et al. (2000).

··

ACTIVITY

Define the following terms in your own words: *congenital hearing loss, acquired hearing loss, sensorineural hearing loss, conductive hearing loss, hard of hearing, deaf.*

··

Auditory Discrimination (Perception) of Speech Sounds

A variable often researched for its relation to speech sound production problems is known as auditory discrimination of speech sounds (Winitz, 1984) and more recently has been described as perception of sounds (Rvachew, 2007; Rvachew & Brosseau-Lapré, 2010). Auditory discrimination is tested in various ways. In some studies, children with misarticulations have been asked to listen to pairs of words or nonsense syllables and say whether the elements in a pair were the same or different. In these studies, no attempts were made to present sounds that the children themselves misarticulated. Such studies, conducted since the 1930s, have produced contradictory findings. Some suggested that children with articulatory production problems also had difficulty making judgments about sounds they heard. Other studies failed to replicate those findings, suggesting that despite a problem in speech sound production, children may correctly judge the sounds they hear (see Winitz, 1984, for reviews of these studies). All clinicians and caregivers know that, regardless of whether misarticulating children can hear the difference between any two phonemes, they rarely get confused in real-word communication.

Some investigators have wondered whether a more consistent relationship between articulatory production and auditory discrimination would emerge if children were asked to discriminate between correct and incorrect productions of sounds they themselves mis-articulated. In studies using this method, the examiner would provide examples of correct productions and incorrect productions that reflected a child's error. In a study that involved 131 children with misarticulations, Locke (1980a) reported that 70% of those children could discriminate between the correct and incorrect productions of sounds they misar-ticulated. Similar findings have been reported by other investigators (e.g., Eilers & Oller, 1976). We will consider a more definitive method of clinically determining the relation between discrimination and production in the Basic Unit of Chapter 7.

Evidently, most children can discriminate between correct and incorrect produc-tions; therefore, auditory discrimination does not seem to be a strong variable related to production problems in most children. In those who do have both production and discrim-ination (perception) problems, there is no evidence to conclude with certainty that the dis-crimination problem causes the production problems. They may be coexisting problems. Nonetheless, clinicians spend time on teaching auditory discrimination between speech sounds or speech errors and target productions. As we will see in Chapter 8, the traditional approach (Van Riper, 1939; Van Riper & Emerick, 1984) includes discrimination training (ear training), and the cycles approach includes "auditory bombardment," in which a child listens to lists of words containing the target sounds or patterns. Other clinicians include discrimination training mostly on theoretical grounds (Rvachew & Brosseau-Lapré, 2012). We will revisit this issue in the Basic Unit of Chapter 8.

Oral Sensation

There has been some speculation as to whether children with reduced oral kinesthetic sensation may be prone to difficulty in learning to articulate speech sounds. *Kinesthetic sensation* is awareness of muscle movement and position. If this sensation is defective, it may be difficult for the child to position and move the oral articulators. Research on this topic is based on that possibility.

Various kinds of stimuli applied to selected oral structures, especially the tongue, may be used to test oral sensation in children with and without SSDs. Small plastic objects of various three-dimensional forms placed on the tongue for identification, with no visual information, help assess **oral form recognition.** The study participants may be asked to point to the correct one of a number of drawings of objects to identify the shape of the ob-ject in the mouth. Also, the tongue may be stimulated at two points to assess what is known as **two-point sensory discrimination.** Finally, the mouth may be **anesthetized** to study the effects of **sensory deprivation** in articulation.

Research on oral sensation has not produced strong or unequivocal evidence to sug-gest that children with SSDs have deficient oral form recognition. While some evidence suggests that some children with misarticulation may have poorer oral form discrimina-tion skills (Ringel, House, Burk, Dolinsky, & Scott, 1970), other evidence suggests that the skills are the same in children with and without misarticulations (Arndt, Elbert, & Shelton, 1970). Even if children do have some oral sensation limitations, there is no as-surance that they are the causes of SSDs or that intervention for oral sensation should be a part of treatment for speech disorders. Neurologically impaired adults with poor oral form recognition skills and poor two-point discrimination may retain good articulation skills (McDonald & Angst, 1970). Also, there is no evidence that typical children or adults depend on an awareness of oral muscle movement and position to articulate speech sounds. Most speakers generally are unaware of the specific position and movement of speech muscles as they produce simple or complex speech (Netsell, 1986).

Studies of anesthetization have been done only on adults, however, so their relevance to children with or without speech sound problems is not clear. Generally, the studies of adults have indicated that when the mouth is anesthetized, there is a general increase in misarticulations and a specific increase in misarticulations of fricatives and affricates (Gammon, Smith, Daniloff, & Kim, 1971; Prosek & House, 1975). Nonetheless, the speech remains mostly intelligible. If the speech is impaired under experimentally reduced oral sensation in adults (or even in children), the inference that articulation disorders in children may be related to reduced oral sensation or that oral sensation should be a treatment target is unwarranted.

Language Skills

Language is a larger system or set of skills that subsumes articulation. Speech sounds are building blocks of language. Therefore, researchers have wondered whether articulation and phonological disorders necessarily imply a language disorder and whether a language disorder similarly implies articulation or phonological disorders.

To study the relation between language and SSDs, researchers have typically analyzed the coexistence of the two sets of disorders in children. SSDs and language disorders may coexist in up to 50% of preschool children (Tyler, Lewis, Haskill, & Tolbert, 2002). Various studies suggest that 35% to 75% of children with phonological disorders may have language disorders, and roughly the same number of children with specific language impairment may have an SSD (see Fey et al., 1994; Rescorla & Lee, 2001; Shriberg & Kwiatowski, 1994; Tyler & Watterson, 1991, for reviews of studies). In a small sample study of 12 children, Bauman-Waengler (2011) reported the coexistence of SSDs and language disorders in 9 children (75%). A smaller percentage of children with SSDs (10% to 40%) also may have language comprehension problems (Shriberg & Kwiatkowski, 1994). Children with severe SSDs are more likely to exhibit a concomitant language disorder (Lewis, Ekelman, & Aram, 1989). Obviously, language impairments and SSDs do not coexist in all children who have one or the other problem. Therefore, each can be independent of the other. Nonetheless, there seems to be a strong tendency toward an association between language impairments and phonological disorders.

Genetic research also suggests that SSDs and language impairments (LIs), along with reading disorders (RDs), are comorbid (associated) conditions. SSDs and language impairments may coexist in 11–15% of 6-year-olds and 40–60% of preschoolers (Shriberg et al., 2005). Some researchers believe that LIs, RDs, and SSDs may be genetically linked, with a common set of genes responsible for the phenotype of all three kinds of disorders (see Lewis et al., 2006, for a review and evaluation of pertinent studies and genetic hypotheses).

Children with significant SSDs may use less complex language, shorter utterances, and incomplete sentences. Speech sound errors of some children with SSDs and language problems may increase when they are asked to produce progressively more complex sentence structures (e.g., longer, passive, complex, or compound sentences) or words with a greater number of syllables (longer words). When syntactic complexity is combined with syllabic complexity, a greater increase may be evident in errors of articulation (Panagos, Quine, & Klich, 1979).

Some investigators have tried to assess the relationship between language disorders and SSDs by treating one or the other to see if the untreated disorder improves without intervention. The results are somewhat conflicting but generally indicate that what is treated (language or articulation) tends to improve more than what is not treated, suggesting that the best clinical strategy is to independently treat both kinds of disorders (Fey et al., 1994; Tyler et al., 2002). We will have more on treating concurrent speech and language disorders in the Advanced Unit of Chapter 8.

Whether literacy skills (reading and writing) and articulation skills are related has been a more recent concern. A definite relation may be expected if SSDs are also associated with significant language impairment; we noted earlier that RDs are a comorbid condition with SSDs (Lewis & Freebairn-Farr, 1991). Literacy and related skills (e.g., phonological awareness) are discussed in the context of SSDs in Chapter 9.

Personal Characteristics

Certain personal characteristics of children, especially age, gender, intelligence, and "personality" (of both children and their parents), have been researched for their possible differential association with articulation disorders. Most are weak variables and of limited clinical significance; therefore, we mention them only briefly below:

- That **age** is a significant factor in articulation learning is a generally accepted notion among speech–language pathologists. Normative data, as reviewed earlier in this chapter, indicate that between the ages of 4 and 6 years, most typically developing children will have articulatory skills that resemble those of adults, although improvements may be noted until age 8. Both neurophysiological maturation of the articulators and continued learning may account for this age effect. Age in and of itself cannot be a variable that leads to better performance in any skill, including articulatory skill.

- **Gender** is another classic variable associated with articulation and phonological disorders. Research since the 1920s, including a study done in the 1990s (Smit et al., 1990), has shown that girls master sounds sooner than do boys. The difference, however, is typically small and statistically insignificant. Survey research since the 1930s also has shown that articulation disorders are more common in boys than in girls. A familial aggregation study has shown that females have reduced risk for developing SSD (Lewis et al., 2007).

- **Intelligence** is another personal characteristic that researchers have studied in the past by correlating I.Q. scores or results of speech samples with articulation proficiency. Research, limited in recent years, has fairly consistently shown that I.Q. scores within the normal limits are not highly correlated with scores on articulation tests (Winitz, 1969). Children whose I.Q. falls below 70, however, have shown a higher prevalence of articulation disorders. Generally speaking, the lower the I.Q., the higher the prevalence and frequency of articulatory problems; nonetheless, compared to children with normal intelligence, those with intellectual disabilities learn the sounds in the same sequence, though at a slower rate and with some variability (Roberts et al., 2005). In addition, children with developmental disabilities show a preponderance of consonant deletions and generally inconsistent errors (Shriberg & Widder, 1990).

• The **personalities** of children who misarticulate and the personalities of their parents have been of interest to several researchers. A decade of earlier research into this poorly defined and highly questionable mentalistic construct has not produced anything of clinical or theoretical significance (Bloch & Goodstein, 1971). More recent research has hinted that children with misarticulations may be "too sensitive" (emotionally hurt more easily than those without articulation disorders; Shriberg & Kwiatkowski, 1994). Generally, unknown replicability and questionable clinical relevance of findings beset the research on personality of either the child with misarticulations or the parents of such children.

• The **socioeconomic status** of families has provoked some research, on the assumption that it might influence speech sound learning in children. In several studies, parents' occupational status was correlated with their children's articulatory proficiency. Reviewing cumulative research evidence on this topic, Winitz (1969) concluded that although a slightly greater number of misarticulating children belong to lower socioeconomic levels than the upper levels, children in all socioeconomic strata are capable of learning their speech sounds in their typical home environments. Any difference in the prevalence of speech sound errors in children of parents in lower versus upper socioeconomic levels may disappear by the time the children enter school or soon thereafter (Templin, 1957). Subsequent studies have shown that infants of mothers belonging to lower socioeconomic status may begin to babble on schedule, but their vocalizations may be fewer than those found in infants of upper socioeconomic classes (Oller, Eilers, Basinger, Steffens, & Urbano, 1995; Oller, Eilers, Steffens, Lynch, & Urbano, 1994). Data from Smit (1993a, 1993b) suggest, however, that socioeconomic status is not significantly associated with SSD.

• **Birth order and the number of siblings** and their influence on articulation have interested researchers since the 1950s. It is often stated that the first born and the only child in a family both have better articulation skills than the second born and those with siblings. Data to support this claim are weak; in one study, teachers' ratings were used to assess children's articulatory proficiency (Koch, 1956). There are data to contradict the claim that number of siblings and articulatory proficiency are related (Wellman et al., 1931). We need better studies.

Genetic Factors

Genetic research on SSD has been concerned with a higher **familial prevalence**, or *familial aggregation*, of SSD and a search for specific genes through molecular analysis (Newbury & Monaco, 2010). A familial prevalence of a disorder that is higher than that in the general population means that a person with a given disorder is likely to have blood relatives with the same disorder. Shriberg and Kwiatkowski (1994) have reported that among a group of 62 children with articulation disorders, 39% had one other family member and 17% more than one family member with SSD. Up to 40% of brothers of a child with SSD may be affected, whereas the same rate for sisters was 19.4% in one study; mothers and fathers were equally affected at 18.2% and 18.3%, respectively (Lewis, 1992). Another familial aggregation study has suggested that if one family member has SSD, the odds for a second family member to have the same disorder are nearly double the odds faced by a child with no family history (Lewis et al., 2007). Twin studies also generally have indicated that the concordance rate (the chance that both twins will have the same disorder) is higher for identical twins than for fraternal twins or ordinary siblings (see Lewis, 2010, for a review of studies).

Other research has shown that when compared to siblings of children with normal articulation, siblings of children who misarticulate tend to perform more poorly on measures of articulation (Lewis et al., 1989). Furthermore, children of persons with a history of articulation disorders perform more poorly on tests of articulation than those whose parents have normal articulation skills (Felsenfeld, McGue, & Broen, 1995). These differential prevalence data of the general population versus families with at least one case of SSD suggest the influence of genetic variables, although they do not effectively rule out the influence of shared environmental factors.

Molecular analysis seeks to find genes that may be responsible for a given disease or disorder. So far, the search for genes that may be causal to SSD has not been as fruitful as it has been for dyslexia (reading disorders, RD). Several studies that have sought a molecular analysis have failed to distinguish children with LI (language impairments), RD, or SSD; the study participants often had all three or a combination of some (Lewis et al., 2006; Stein et al., 2004). Research suggests that certain chromosomes seem to be worth exploring, however. These include chromosome 3 and possibly chromosomes 1, 6, and 15; abnormalities on these chromosomes may often be associated with both SSD and RD (Lewis et al., 2006; Stein et al., 2004). The challenge, however, has been to find a gene that may be responsible for SSD with no comorbid conditions (such as LI and RD). A previously much publicized "speech gene" (SPCH1), eventually named *FOXP2*, on chromosome 7 (7q31) turned out to be not particularly relevant to SSD in the absence of other disabilities; the gene is now thought to play a role in the development of a constellation of disabilities, including severe language problems, childhood apraxia of speech and other speech impairments, intellectual disabilities, reading problems, and so forth. *FOXP2* mutations are rare, and therefore cannot account for SSD in the majority of children (Lewis et al., 2006).

Genetic researchers suggest that SSD is a multifactorial disorder with multiple phenotypes (manifestations or symptom complexes) and possibly of a heterogeneous causation, involving multiple genes. Genes involved may affect other skills or underlying processes that may influence speech sound (and language) learning. Evidence suggests that the genetic influence is broad, rather than narrowly focused on speech sound learning (Lewis, 2010). Researchers well recognize the influence of multiple factors, including the environmental: "Genes do not lead directly to phenotypes. Instead, genetic, cellular, anatomical, and environmental conditions interact to produce an SSD phenotype" (Lewis et al., 2006, p. 1305). A certain number of children with SSD have neither a familial aggregation nor a known genetic basis for the disorder. In such children, learning is thought to play an important role in the disorder's etiology, but that, too, is likely to interact with other variables. Some of the environmental risks include gender (being male), low maternal education, low socioeconomic status, and middle ear infections with effusion (Campbell et al., 2003; Shriberg et al., 2005).

Research on familial aggregation and a possible genetic basis of SSD has led to classifications of SSD into several subtypes. See Chapter 1 for an overview of subclassifications of SSD and their clinical implications.

Tongue Thrust

An issue that generated some controversy in the past because of its hypothesized relation to SSD is tongue thrust, also known as *reverse swallow* or *infantile swallow*. It is a form of oral myofunctional disorder. **Tongue thrust** refers to a certain manner of swallowing and tongue placement in the oral cavity during rest, not to the thrusting of the tongue against the frontal teeth, as the term implies. Children younger than 5 years of age typically carry their relatively large tongue more anteriorly than do older children and adults. As the oral cavity is enlarged, the tongue is carried more typically (in a relatively posterior position). In essence, tongue thrust is common and normal in children below 5 years of age.

Tongue thrust is characterized by (1) a forward gesture of the tongue during swallowing, so that the tip of the tongue is in contact with the lower lip; (2) the forward carriage of the tongue in the oral cavity in such a way as to keep the tongue tip against or between the anterior teeth while the mandible is slightly open; or (3) fronting of the tongue during speech so that the tongue is between or against the anterior teeth while the mandible is slightly open (R. Mason & Proffit, 1974). A child may exhibit one or more of these characteristics. The effect on dentition and speech will depend on whether one or more characteristics are present.

Tongue thrust may be functional (behavioral) or due to such organic conditions as enlarged tonsils. Behavioral tongue thrusting is not associated with any structural abnormalities. Organic conditions that cause tongue thrusting are enlarged adenoids and tonsils that partially block the posterior airway passage (American Speech-Language-Hearing Association [ASHA], 1989; R. Mason, 1988).

An anterior resting posture of the tongue in the oral cavity may affect the individual placement of teeth. However, when the anterior tongue carriage is combined with tongue thrust swallow, some children may develop patterns of malocclusions, although more evidence is needed to establish this relationship firmly.

In some children, tongue thrust swallow and forward tongue resting position may be associated with SSD. A lisp and distorted productions of /z/ and /l/ are common. Interdentalization of /t/, /d/, /n/, and /l/ has been reported as well (ASHA, 1989). Although tongue thrust itself may be corrected (Hanson, 1994), it is not clear whether such correction is warranted or direct treatment for correct production of speech sounds is sufficient. Newer, well-designed experimental studies are lacking.

The American Speech-Language-Hearing Association's (ASHA's) Preferred Practice Patterns on orofacial myofunctional disorders (ASHA, 2004) states that speech–language pathologists who are appropriately credentialed and trained may offer their services to clients who need them. In addition to that document, the reader is referred to ASHA (1991) for additional information and to ASHA's ad hoc committee report on the issue (ASHA, 1989). Treatment for tongue thrust is not provided in many public schools unless a child has an accompanying SSD.

Evaluation of Research on Speech Sound Learning

The question of what variables are related to children's speech sound learning is of both theoretical and clinical significance. If research clearly identifies causes of speech sound learning, clinicians may manipulate or change some of those variables in children with SSD. However, research on such variables presents numerous challenges to those who wish to draw a cause–effect conclusion.

Research has identified only a few variables that are of clinical and theoretical significance. Research on most of the variables is both dated and questionable on methodological grounds. Some of the research is dated possibly because contemporary investigators do not find the variables worth investigating. Research on such variables as oral form recognition; general motor skills; oral anesthetization; structural problems or dimension of the hard palate, lips, and teeth; general intelligence; and socioeconomic status have not illuminated the independent variables (potential causes) of speech sound learning. Nor has the research given new insight into treatment of speech sound disorders.

Correlation Versus Causation

A particular methodological limitation makes it difficult if not impossible to draw cause–effect conclusions regarding several researched variables related to speech sound learning. This limitation stems from the typical method of correlating one variable with another and then presuming causation. Causes can be determined only through experimentation, not correlation.

When two variables (e.g., articulation skills and intelligence; socioeconomic status and articulation skills) are simply measured and correlated, no variable is experimentally manipulated. Researchers have typically measured children's speech sound production along with another variable of interest. In some studies, two groups, one clinical (children with impaired articulation) and one normal are formed. Sometimes the group with normal skills is described as the control group and the one with problematic skills as the experimental group. However, there is no experimental manipulation in such studies and the terms *control group* and *experimental group* are misnomers.

Whether only one group (with SSD) or two groups (one with and one without SSD) are included, the previously reviewed studies on the variables associated with speech sound learning have measured some other variable presumably related to articulation. For example, socioeconomic status, intelligence, integrity of the speech mechanism, or some such may be measured. The results of the study are then correlated. If the correlation is positive and statistically significant, it is concluded that the two variables (e.g., articulation and socioeconomic status) are related. A conclusion often implied or even explicitly stated is that the variable, such as phonological awareness, correlated with articulation disorders, is a causal variable. In other words, among the correlated variables, one is identified as the cause (e.g., phonological awareness), and the other (e.g., speech sound production) as the effect.

That correlation does not necessarily imply causation is common knowledge. A significant positive or negative correlation means that the two factors vary together. A third and unobserved variable may be responsible for the observed covariation. For example, lower socioeconomic status, though correlated with articulatory skills, may have nothing to do with articulation. The parents with lower socioeconomic status also may have lower education. It may be the education of the parents that is causally related to articulation disorders in their children. Please note that this is only an *example* of an unobserved third variable that may be responsible for the observed covariation; it is *not* suggested here that parental educational status (or lower socioeconomic status of the family) is causally related to better or worse articulatory skills in children.

Some genetic researchers tend to overinterpret their findings, and the media often hail such findings as a cure-all. Early *FOXP2* researchers claimed to have discovered a "talking gene" (*SPCH1*), which was thought to be responsible for specific language impairment and autism. The claim was not supported by subsequent research (Hegde & Maul, 2006). Even though some genetic researchers have drawn strong conclusions that there is a genetic basis (cause) for SSD, the evidence is far from clear. Fifty percent or more of children with SSD do not have familial aggregation or an identified gene locus. Neither higher familial prevalence (aggregation) nor a higher concordance rate for identical twins brought up in the same home environment rules out the influence of environmental variables. Familial aggregation studies should show such aggregation in families that are different on such relevant variables as socioeconomic status, parental education and income, living conditions, and so forth. Twin researchers should study identical twins raised in different home environments; they should show that fraternal twins do not have higher concordance rates than ordinary siblings.

Because of the correlational method used in most studies, the only valid conclusion is that certain variables may be associated with articulatory acquisition and performance. The investigated variables may be causally related, but the data do not support that conclusion.

....

ACTIVITY
Briefly explain why correlation does not mean causation.

....

Summary of the Basic Unit

- Infants' sound productions are commonly referred to as **prelinguistic** vocalizations.

- **Infant speech perception** studies have shown that infants can localize sounds soon after birth and can discriminate between varied pure-tone frequencies and tone loudness and differing white noise levels.

- Infants have a greater interest in human speech than in other noises; an infant as young as 3 days can discriminate mother's voice from the voices of other females.

- Two methods have been used to study infant speech perception: **high-amplitude sucking method** and **visually reinforced head turn method**; results show that infants as young as a few days can be conditioned to discriminate certain speech sounds. Certain animals, too, can be taught to discriminate speech sounds, suggesting that such skills are not unique to human infants.

- Infant vocalizations have been divided into two major categories: **reflexive vocalizations** and **nonreflexive vocalizations.** More recent research suggests infraphonological and integrative categories; the four infraphonological stages include (1) **phonation,** (2) **primitive articulation,** (3) **expansion,** and (4) **canonical babbling,** which includes **reduplicated** and **variegated babbling;** the final **integrative stage** includes the onset of speech.

- **Babbling** and the onset of speech sounds are now considered a continuous process, with no break; infants babble only a small set of sounds and babble certain sounds more frequently than others

- Vowel mastery is achieved by 36 months.

- **Protowords** are an infant's consistent vocalizations absent a recognizable adult model; they are considered a link between babbling and adult-like speech.

- The first **true words** a child produces appear to be influenced by the phonetic repertoire and syllable structure of the productions of the late babbling period.

- **Progressive idioms** are words that have an advanced pronunciation in comparison to the child's current skills; **regressive idioms** are the child's static or unchanging pronunciations of certain words despite having more advanced phonological skills.

- Several **cross-sectional studies** have documented that nasals, stops, and glides tend to develop early, while fricatives, affricates, and liquids develop much later. Studies using the **longitudinal method** have shown individual differences in the acquisition of speech sounds.

- Other studies have assessed children's phonological development according to sound classes, **distinctive features,** and the disappearance of **PPs.**

- A child's **speech intelligibility** is affected by the misarticulation of sounds; 95% of a 3-year-old's speech may be intelligible, and by age 5, most of a child's speech is intelligible to strangers.

- Significant structural deviations (palatal clefts or impaired speech muscle control), not normal variations within those structures, may be associated with speech sound learning problems.

- Speech problems associated with central or peripheral nervous system damage are known as **dysarthria;** and those due to motor planning of speech gestures in the absence of neuromuscular impairments in children are called **childhood apraxia of speech (CAS).**

- Children with SSD have a slower diadochokinetic rate, although deficiencies in motor skills are neither necessary nor sufficient to produce articulatory problems.

- Normal hearing is essential for typical oral speech–language learning.

- SSD and **auditory discrimination** problems may coexist in some children.

- **Oral sensation** or **oral-form recognition** deficiencies do not account for SSD.

- Forty to eighty percent of children with SSD also may exhibit a language disorder.

- **Intelligence** may affect speech sound learning only if it is below normal.

- **Lower socioeconomic status** may be only a minor risk factor in speech sound learning problems.

- The familial prevalence of speech sound disorders is higher than that in the general population.

- **Tongue thrust** may be associated with articulation disorders.

- Most of the studies on the variables associated with speech sound learning have used the correlational method, which may only suggest, but not confirm, causes of such learning.

- To better understand the potential causes of SSDs, one needs to use the experimental method, which is not practical in most cases; however, researchers should at least separate the variables that are typically confounded (e.g., twinning and the common environment).

Advanced Unit: Research Issues and Theories

The Basic Unit of this chapter has summarized the information on speech sound learning and variables related to that learning. This Advanced Unit includes methodological and theoretical issues related to speech perception and discrimination. Subsequently, we will review theories of speech sound learning, concentrating mostly on the linguistic and behavioral explanations.

Methodological and Theoretical Issues in Speech Perception and Discrimination Research

Speech perception research poses both methodological and theoretical issues. Theoretical issues have been widely discussed in the literature, because advocates of different theories have been criticizing each other for decades. The methodological issues, however, have not received similar attention. Therefore, we will begin with an examination of the research methods used in infant speech perception that support a different interpretation than the one researchers typically make.

Methodological Issues: Conclusions Inconsistent With Methods

As noted in the Basic Unit, much of the research on the earliest stages of speech–language learning concerns speech perception in infants. Perception is a sensory experience and, as such, is a private event. Perception is measured by presenting a certain external stimulus and noting an overt response. However, investigators of perception tend to make inferences regarding what goes on inside the person who reacts to a stimulus. In this sense, perception is a presumed process that begins *within* an organism soon after a stimulus has been presented and ends when an overt response has been observed.

Researchers of early speech perception depended on a discriminated response from an infant. While the concept of *perception* comes from the classical sensory psychology, the concept of *discrimination* comes from the behavioral science of classical and operant conditioning. A discriminated response is a changed or different response when stimuli are changed. As a behavioral (learning) process, discrimination is an observable and measurable change in responses when stimuli are systematically changed under well-controlled experimental arrangements. SLPs are familiar with discrimination learning or training. The clinician who teaches a child to say *soup* but not *toup* when shown a particular stimulus is teaching discrimination. A point not often well appreciated is that speech perception researchers have combined the concepts and methods of behavioral science with those of sensory psychology. Consequently, some methodological and theoretical issues arise in research on infant speech perception and discrimination.

The two major methods used to study infant speech perception—the high-amplitude sucking method (HAS) and the visually reinforced head turn method (VRHT)—are essentially operant conditioning methods, in which some overt response to changes in speech stimuli is positively reinforced. In the HAS method, a new speech stimulus positively reinforces an increased sucking response. In the VRHT, a head turn response toward the loudspeaker that presents a new stimulus is positively reinforced by presentation of a lighted and animated toy.

It is important to note the difference between the two methods. In both methods, a new speech sound stimulus is a reinforcer. In the HAS method, the new speech sound stimulus increases the sucking response rate. In the VRHT method, the new sound stimulus evokes a head turn response, which is reinforced (increased) by an animated and lighted toy.

Initially, just the sucking response of infants was thought to provide an excellent means of studying auditory development (responses) and perhaps other behavioral development. The earliest studies on sucking behavior in infants were made in Russia in the late 1950s (see Moon & Fifer, 1990, for a brief review) and demonstrated that an infant's non-nutritional sucking behavior habituates (gradually reduces), and that it can then be increased by presenting a new auditory stimulus. Unfortunately, just measuring non-nutritional sucking behavior in infants did not prove productive in understanding any aspect of infant development. The method became productive only when used as an operant conditioning device. That is, the method began to produce useful information only when sucking behavior could be increased by reinforcing it or decreased by withholding reinforcement.

As summarized in the Basic Unit, investigators have come to the conclusion that infants *have an ability* to perceive certain speech sounds and to discriminate between certain classes of sounds. The results often are summarized by stating that *infants can perceive and discriminate speech sounds and categories of sounds.* Furthermore, investigators have debated whether this ability is innate, learned, or a combination. Some strongly believe that humans have a specific phonetic processing mechanism that is innate (Liberman, 1970) and is distinguished from the general auditory processing mechanisms. Others believe that speech perception skill in the infant may be a function of the general sensitivity of the auditory system to discontinuities in the sound stream.

Very few investigators recognize that learning and conditioning are the central parts of speech perception research (Jusczyk & Luce, 2002; Moon & Fifer, 1990). Lack of this recognition has led to claims regarding data that are incongruent with the methods by which those data are generated. The results of HAS and VRHT experiments do not forcefully demonstrate that *infants can perceive and discriminate speech sounds and their categories* without conditioning or some form of experimental manipulation. The results do not demonstrate any innate ability to discriminate speech sounds. If the speech discrimination ability were innately present in infants, there would be no need to systematically reinforce discriminated (different) responses to different speech stimuli. The results of speech perception studies most forcefully show that *infants can be readily conditioned* to respond differently to different speech stimuli. The studies are experiments in learning. In these experiments, infants have *learned* to reliably respond to speech stimuli. Therefore, an appropriate interpretation of speech perception research is that infants may be conditioned to discriminate certain sounds or syllable pairs at certain ages.

Theoretical Issues in Speech Perception: Learning Cannot Be Discounted

The finding that infants could be conditioned to make distinctions between speech sound contrasts has triggered researchers to ask whether infants have an innate ability to discriminate speech sounds or learn these skills after some initial exposure to language (Jusczyk & Luce, 2002). In an attempt to answer this question, Trehub (1976) conducted a study in which a group of Canadian infants were presented with native (English) and nonnative (Czech) sound contrasts. The infants were all part of English-speaking homes with no exposure to the Czech language, thus eliminating that language experience as a variable. The expectation would be that because of their exposure to English, the infants would do better discriminating English sound contrasts versus Czech sound contrasts.

Contrary to that expectation, Trehub found that the infants in her study discriminated between the two syllables containing the Czech sounds (i.e., [ʒa] and [řa]) just as well as they discriminated between those containing the English sounds (i.e., [pa] and [ba]). The results of this and other studies were originally interpreted to mean that infants have an innate ability to make fine discriminations between speech sounds (native and nonnative).

A second portion of Trehub's study lends support to the idea that the environment has a role in speech perception, however. In addition to presenting native and nonnative sound contrasts to infants, Trehub tested adult monolingual English-speaking subjects' discrimination between the two Czech sounds presented to the infant group. Although the infants could discriminate the two pairs of sound syllables (English and Czech) equally well, the adult subjects had a high degree of difficulty in discriminating the Czech sounds.

That it becomes progressively more difficult to discriminate between sound contrasts not found in the ambient language as infants grow older is further supported by Werker and Tees's (1984) study. They presented non-English sound pairs to infants between 6 and 8 months, 8 and 10 months, and 10 and 12 months old. Werker and Tees found that the youngest age group had little difficulty perceiving the difference between Hindi (a language of India) and Thompson (a Salish language spoken in Canada) sound contrasts. They further found that the 8- to 10-month-old group performed less well than the 6- to 8-month-old group and the 10- to 12-month-old group performed worse than the two younger groups. This indicated that infants' discrimination of non-native sound contrasts begins to deteriorate around 10 months and continues the downward trend as they get older. As infants learn more of the ambient language sound contrasts, learning to discriminate sounds of a language they do not hear becomes progressively more difficult (Best,

McRoberts, Lafleur, & Silver-Isenstadt, 1995). Furthermore, electrophysiological studies have shown some differential neural (brain) responses to different stimuli in older children and adults; such neural responses do not involve overt behavioral responses of discrimination, however. This suggests the influence of the language learning environment, not the presence of an innate mechanism of universal speech sound perception. As Rvachew and Brosseau-Lapré (2012) conclude, "Clearly, the [early sound contrast acquisition] process involves learning: the initial universalist view, whereby the phonetic categories were innately given at birth . . . is not tenable" (p. 101). There are many more studies than cited here, generally supporting this position (see Houston, 2005, 2011, for reviews). Also to be noted is that no study has shown that it is *impossible* to teach older children and adults to discriminate foreign sound contrasts. Anecdotally, adult second language learners can and do learn foreign sound contrasts, albeit with varying degrees of effort and precision.

Results of several other studies also have questioned the earlier interpretation of a specific speech decoder mechanism being innately available to infants. The often-made claim that infants can discriminate the sounds of all languages (suggesting a universal innate mechanism at work) has been shown to be incorrect; infants fail to discriminate not only many foreign language sound pairs, but also some of their own language vowel contrasts; in addition, some studies found that infants could not be conditioned to make certain kinds of speech discriminations. For example, Eilers and Minifie (1975) found that infants ages 1 to 4 months could not distinguish [sa] from [za], and Eilers et al. (1977) reported that infants as old as 12 to 14 months could not perceive the difference between [fa] and [θa]. Other studies have shown that discrimination between /f/ and /θ/ continues to be difficult even in children 3 to 4 years old (e.g., Locke, 1980a, 1980b). Moreover, a typically underreported and overlooked fact is that a full 50% of infants in studies on speech perception fail to learn the experimental tasks. Failure to condition half the participants is attributed to the infants' "fussiness" or uncooperative behavior. Incredible as it may seem to other scientists, data on infants who did not learn to discriminate speech sounds are routinely discarded, as revealed by Nittrouer (2001) and discussed by Rvachew and Brosseau-Lapré (2012). From the beginning, researchers should have reported the actual number of infants found to be conditionable and the number not conditionable in a given study. Nittrouer (2001), however, has demonstrated that bringing the same "fussy" (initially unconditionable) infants back for study on a different day and at a different time did not help. She found that infants who could not discriminate began to exhibit fussiness, whereas it was previously thought that their fussiness made conditioning difficult. Clinicians experience an analogous situation when they work with young children: When faced with a difficult treatment task, children exhibit uncooperative behavior. When this has been documented, uncooperative behavior is not the cause of treatment interruption but an effect of the selected treatment task. Based on a series of studies, Nittrouer (2002) has concluded that it is not innateness but experience with language that is responsible for speech perception. She further concludes that speech perception is not anything special at all; it is like the perception of any other task or skill. This skill improves over the first decade of life and perhaps beyond; it is not completed during infancy as early researchers had claimed. Such improvement can come only through sustained learning.

The hypothesis that humans have an innately given linguistic decoder that helps discriminate speech sounds early in infancy also implies that subhuman animals lack a linguistic decoder and, hence, would be incapable of speech perception (Liberman, 1970). To find out if that is true, attempts have been made to teach speech sound discrimination to several species of animals. The animals most frequently used for experiment are the chinchilla and gerbils, both rodents (Houston, 2011; Kuhl & Miller, 1978; Sinnott & Mosteller, 2007). The other animals used in speech sound perception experiments include dogs (Baru, 1975) and monkeys (Kuhl & Padden, 1983). A variety of operant conditioning experiments have been conducted with animal subjects (Burdick & Miller, 1973; Kuhl & Miller, 1978; Sinnott & Mosteller, 2007), including reinforcement of correct right or left motor response to different speech sound stimuli. Most experiments have succeeded in conditioning different responses to different speech sound stimuli, thus mounting a serious challenge to the hypothesis of an innate, speech-specific skill of human infants. Once trained with a set of speech stimuli, the animals tested have shown generalized responding when presented with similar stimuli or stimuli generated from different speakers, including male, female, and child speakers. Further evidence that speech discrimination is not unique comes from studies in which infants discriminated nonspeech sounds and noises (Jusczyk & Luce, 2002; Jusczyk, Rosner, Cutting, Foard, & Smith, 1977). Research evidence now clearly shows that learning to discriminate between speech sounds is not an exclusively human skill, nor is this skill a special province of speech because discrimination is a general skill related to learning (Baru, 1975; Burdick & Miller, 1975; Kuhl & Miller, 1975; Miller & Kuhl, 1976; Nittrouer, 2002). The evidence does not support the theory of a special speech-specific mechanism responsible for phonemic discriminations.

It has generally been thought that sensitivity to sound differences may be a general characteristic of the auditory system of many organisms, and speech perception in human and subhuman species is made possible by their auditory system. However, speech perception may not be entirely a skill based on audition. Studies have shown that infants, around the time they begin to babble, shift their gaze to the mouths of speakers around them. This suggests that the infants also rely on visual cues of speech directed to them (Lewkowicz & Hansen-Tift, 2012; see also Munhall & Johnson, 2012). Additional evidence that speech perception is not entirely an auditory phenomenon comes from deaf children who learn to discriminate speech sounds with the help of visual cues.

Speech perception research generally discounts individual differences to emphasize a universal innate mechanism of categorical speech perception and make claims that are not always supported by data (Rvachew & Brosseau-Lapré, 2012). If the studies are a test of an innate ability, they are so only in a trivial sense: that *infants have an ability to learn* to respond to speech sounds and respond differently to different speech sounds *when such responses are systematically reinforced.* Any kind of learning, in persons of all ages and members of all species, presupposes such a general ability to learn; hence, the notion of an *innate ability to learn* does not explain any kind of learning. It is now generally accepted that learning speech sound contrasts and maintaining those contrasts require environmental input or experience (see Houston, 2005, 2011, for a review of studies). In most speech perception research, environmental "input" and "language experience" are terms that obscure the important environmental variables—interaction with caregivers, stimulation, and positive reinforcement.

In essence, an appropriate interpretation of the results of infant speech perception and discrimination experiments requires a due consideration of the experimental methods used. The methods are those of operant conditioning; hence, the results most forcefully show that infants can be *taught* to discriminate among speech sounds. The methods used in the studies do not allow for a direct test of some innate ability.

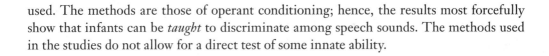

ACTIVITY

Is speech perception a learned skill or innate? Justify your answer.

Theories of Speech Sound Learning

A theory explains a phenomenon by finding its cause or causes. In technical terms, researchers need to specify the independent variables (causal factors) associated with the dependent variables (speech sound perception and production) in a systematic and organized manner. Such independent variables need to be isolated in experimental research. In the present context, researchers of speech sound mastery need to find out why it takes place, although the task is formidable.

In Chapter 3, we summarized specific phonological theories and critically evaluated them. As noted in that chapter, many linear and nonlinear phonological theories also seek to explain speech acquisition and production. We will not readdress specific phonological explanations of speech acquisition in this chapter. But the reader will find similarities between the linguistic explanations of speech sound acquisition summarized here and the phonological explanations summarized in the previous chapter.

Explanations of speech sound acquisition in children fall into two main groups: linguistic and behavioral. Linguistic explanations are offered by both linguists and psycholinguists (psychologists who specialize in linguistic studies), with occasional contributions from speech–language pathologists. Linguistic explanations are plentiful, popular, contradictory, and ever changing. Behavioral explanations are scarce, underappreciated, and misrepresented—dismissed in the literature of linguistics and speech–language pathology.

Linguistic Explanations

There is no single universally agreed upon linguistic theory of speech sound acquisition. This broad category also includes cognitive, neurolinguistic, computational (statistical), and other kinds of theories. Some are hybrid theories, including different kinds of models. New theories emerge in rapid succession. Disagreements among the proponents of different theories can be quite striking. The SLP may be left wondering what to accept.

Classic research on speech development was concerned mostly with the mastery of individual speech sounds. In explaining the acquisition of individual speech sounds, researchers investigated potential independent variables that might promote or impede the acquisition of individual sounds. This line of investigation predated the heavy influence of linguistic theories on research in speech–language pathology (Winitz, 1969). As reviewed in this chapter, such variables as oral anatomical structures, intelligence, and socioeconomic status were correlated with speech development. By and large, this line of investigation to find the potential independent variables of speech sound acquisition has been discouraging. No variables have been isolated in such a way as to explain speech sound acquisition. Most studies correlated one variable (e.g., dental abnormalities or low socioeconomic status) with speech sound acquisition. This method is incapable of finding the cause of any phenomenon. In recent years, this line of investigation has declined, with the possible exception of investigating socioeconomic status.

Subsequent explanations of speech sound acquisition have been linguistic in their orientation. These explanations are influenced by their assumptions about language. With some variations, linguists view language as a mental system of representations, patterns, rules, constraints, and ranking of constraints. These internal representations are thought to dictate speech and language production. Such mental representations are subsumed under an *innate universal knowledge* concept. The knowledge is of a universal grammar (UG). Therefore, most linguistic explanations of speech and language acquisition and production point to an innate knowledge of UG. A cardinal linguistic assumption is that what the child (or adult) says is unimportant except when it is viewed as a window to the speaker's internal representations, mental structures, grammatic or phonologic rules, constraints, innate devices, universal or innate knowledge, cognitive process, and such other inferred variables. Such inferred variables prompt certain kinds of questions. For example, linguistic theorists, having been less interested in how children learn speech sounds, tend to ask, How does a young child achieve the *mental representation* of the adult speech sound system? Being less concerned with how children learn to produce speech sounds of differing acoustic or other properties, they ask, How does a child *extract* relevant properties from the adult speech? Unlike the classical researchers, linguistic researchers have been more concerned with the acquisition of a phonological *system* than individual sounds. Unfortunately, linguistic theories on the nature of speech and language and inferred internal mechanisms that underlie their production have been an ever-changing scene. Therefore, at any one point, only a few historically significant theories may be sampled.

Jakobson's (1968) theory of phonological acquisition was one of the early linguistic explanations of speech sound acquisition. His views, described as the **hypothesis of discontinuity** between babbling and later speech acquisition, have been summarized in the Basic Unit of this chapter. Essentially, Jakobson proposed that speech sounds are not shaped out of early vocalizations found in the babbling stage. This view contrasted with the behavioral view that early vocalizations, including babbling, provide a foundation for later speech development (learning). Jakobson thought that early vocalization and babbling were random activities, and that speech sound acquisition follows a universal and innate pattern in which the distinctive features are acquired in a hierarchical manner. Just as the generative grammarians proposed that language unfolds within a predetermined, innate sequence, Jakobson proposed that the acquisition of distinctive features is an unfolding process. We noted earlier that Jakobson's hypothesis of discontinuity is now considered invalid.

Another influential explanation of articulatory and phonological development was proposed by Stampe (1969). His theory of **natural phonology** describes universal phonological processes evident in children's speech and considers these processes as innate mechanisms of simplifying adult productions (Donegan & Stampe, 1979; Stampe, 1969, 1979). Natural processes (e.g., cluster reduction or final consonant deletion) reflect limitations of the human speech production mechanism, as well as the universal patterns in phonological productions in all languages of the world.

The two most controversial aspects of the theory of natural phonology are (1) that processes are real mental operations going on in the mind of the child, and (2) that processes are innate. In simple terms, children know that they are using a phonological process and as they become more mature, they actively *suppress* those processes. That the processes or other operations are innate is a hypothesis common to most generative accounts of language (e.g., Chomsky, 1957, 1981; Chomsky & Halle, 1968; Stampe, 1969, 1979).

The natural phonology presumes that because of the innate processes, children correctly perceive speech sounds from the very beginning. They do not have unique phonological strategies; their strategies are both universal and accurate. Children's speech errors are only production problems, not perceptual problems. Children's task in phonological acquisition is to suppress natural tendencies to simplify adult models and thus achieve the adult phonological skills. This process is guided mostly by innate mechanisms. According to Stampe, children's erroneous patterns of production are *explained* on the basis of the innate, psychologically real processes (Yavas, 1998).

Some of the newer phonological theories, especially **nonlinear phonological theories** (see the Advanced Unit of Chapter 3 for a description), also make strong nativist assumptions about phonological acquisition that are similar to Chomsky's (1981) on language acquisition. Phonological acquisition is made possible because the child is born with a set of universal phonological principles or constraints (Bernhardt, 1994; Bernhardt & Stemberger, 2011). These innate principles provide a framework, like templates, that helps a child acquire a phonological system. Phonological input is decoded and encoded according to the innate templates. Universal principles or templates help categorize certain common features of language. For example, environmental input fits the template regarding the commonality of CV structure in all languages or of all languages having vowels. When certain phonological aspects of a child's language differ from the universal templates, the inputs of that language help set up new parameters. For example, a particular input from a specific language might help set up the parameter that the language has few or no final consonants or that the syllable stress patterns are unique (different from what is specified in the template).

A different set of theories incorporate a **cognitive model** (Ferguson, 1978, 1986; Macken & Ferguson, 1983; Menn, 1983). Cognitive theorists believe that children test hypotheses about PPs they hear and test them against what they know about those patterns. That belief is supported by several kinds of observational data, including the following: First, a child's identifiable initial words are different for different children. It seems that each child has a preference for certain early words. For example, a child might prefer only two-syllable words starting with a particular consonant such as a stop or a nasal. Cognitive theorists interpret this to mean that children select certain unique strategies to master phonological skills. Second, children seem to have unique ways of simplifying complex or polysyllabic adult forms. Cognitive theorists find this to be a tendency to explore different ways of producing a difficult word. Third, children may show a tendency to *initially* use a correct word form with an adult phonemic sequence and *later* revert to a more simplified form. The typical example given is that of a child who first produces the word *pretty* correctly and later incorrectly produces the same word as [bɪdi]. Researchers have observed that the initial correct productions do not match the child's overall phonological skills, but the subsequent incorrect productions do. This phenomenon is known as *phonological regression* and is interpreted as evidence that the child is testing certain hypotheses about adult phonological forms.

Theorists disagree as to whether children initially learn phonemic sequences or whole words. While most theorists pay attention to the acquisition of *segments* (speech sounds with defined features) that children master, some theorists believe that children learn about phoneme contrasts only through word productions (and knowledge). Both the **prosodic theory** (Waterson, 1971) and the **word-based phonological theory** (Ferguson & Farwell, 1975) suggest that children pay attention to *words* as initial phonological learning units. These two theories state that children's acquisition of phonological skills begins with a mastery of certain initial words. In these theories, the early words are schemata of adult forms that include such common features as intonation and syllable structure. According to the prosodic or word-based phonological theories, children do not have a complete and accurate phonological system to begin with; instead, children have an imperfect perceptual production mechanism that is progressively refined to match the adult phonological system.

A distinction between **underlying phonological representations** and actual **realization in production** is common to many linguistic views of phonological development. Recent linguistic theories of phonological development propose that children have underlying phonological representations that change through development. Underlying phonological representations may be similar to the innate systems of linguistic knowledge attributed to children by generative linguists. When a nativist bias is not included, underlying representations mean remembered and cognitively stored forms of what the child hears in adult speech.

Different phonological theories propose different sorts of underlying phonological representations. Some theories presume that children's underlying representations are complete, in that all phonemes of language, their entire inventory of features, and their permissible combinations are already available. This is similar to transformational generative linguists' assertion that children have an innate UG—a complete and perfect knowledge of grammatical rules that applies to all the languages of the world. When children with a complete or universal phonological representation begin to experience a given language, they then delete what is redundant or irrelevant to their specific language. This means that a complete phonological underlying representation leads to a sequence of phonological development that proceeds from a general knowledge of a universal phonological system to that of a particular language (Yavas, 1998).

An alternative view of phonological representation is that it contains only universally specified minimal sets of contrastive features. These contrasts include [consonantal], [sonorant], and [continuant]. With this basic phonological equipment, children begin to receive linguistic input from their environment. Because of this input, children begin to add what is missing in their universally specified minimal sets of feature contrasts. Their underlying, minimal, and universal representation is thus expanded to include all the relevant features of their particular language. In this view, children progress from a set of simpler, minimal feature specifications to a more complex, comprehensive system (Yavas, 1998).

The more recent nonlinear theories propose that the underlying representations are constraints that are in conflict with each other. The conflict between the faithfulness and markedness constraints is resolved by an inherent ranking system. What were once non-violable rules have been rephrased as violable constraints that are innate; see Chapter 3 for more on this approach.

The phonological representations, whatever form they take, are internal, unobservable, and speculative. Postulating internal patterns to explain observed behavioral regularities is popular, but such inferred patterns do not explain observed regularities in speech sound production.

....

ACTIVITY

Define the following terms in your own words: *natural phonology, cognitive model, prosodic theory, word-based phonological theory.*

....

Behavioral Explanations

The behavioral view of speech (and language) learning generally takes the Skinnerian outlook. Nonbehavioral (cognitive/mentalistic) psychologists are often in agreement with linguists and in fact have carved out a specialty called *psycholinguistics.* The behavioral view, therefore, is an extension of the tenets of behaviorism (Skinner, 1957) to the study of speech and language. For at least three reasons, a comprehensive understanding of the behavioral view of speech–language development requires an orientation that is totally different from that of linguistics and cognitive psychology.

First, behavioral scientists use an entirely different paradigm of speech–language behaviors. They do not see speech and language as a mental system with cognitive or some kind of innate representations that underlie productions. Behavioral scientists do not ask how children acquire mental representations of the speech sounds they hear being produced around them. Instead, they ask, How do children learn different functional response classes of language? In a sense, behavioral analysis takes a whole-word, whole-utterance approach rather than a segmental or feature approach to speech and language; as we noted earlier, there is a whole-word approach to phonological phenomena in linguistics, albeit with a different theoretical underpinning. Unlike linguists, behavioral scientists see speech and language as verbal behavior that is similar to nonverbal behaviors. Both verbal and nonverbal behaviors are learned. Verbal behaviors are learned through the mediation (reinforcement) of a verbal community. Although verbal behavior has certain unique properties, it does not have a special status. Certain generative linguists of the Chomskyan orientation attribute special status to language by stating that it is the creation of a unique mental apparatus at the human level. Behavioral scientists consider *mental apparatus, faculty of language, universal knowledge, underlying representations, innate grammars, phonological knowledge,* and so forth to be rational concepts that lie outside the realm of natural science. Therefore, the differences between the behavioral and linguistic views are based on fundamental paradigmatic differences and are not just due to differences in certain assumptions and explanatory concepts.

Second, behavioral scientists are less inclined to explain a phenomenon based on data obtained from nonexperimental methods. Much of phonological development data (as well as language development data) are merely observational. Observational data do not rule out alternative hypotheses; hence, when used exclusively, they are inadequate to support any kind of theory. Some strong theoretical statements often are made based on observations of children's speech and language skills recorded over time (the longitudinal method) or recorded simultaneously at different age levels (the cross-sectional method). Questionable reliability of observations and potential investigator biases in recording the observations are problems in such investigations. Behavioral explanations often are based on experimental evidence in which some variable is systematically manipulated under controlled conditions and the effects of such manipulations are carefully noted (Hegde, 2003). Typically, such data on phonological development are limited, with the exception of research on infant speech perception. A growing body of experimental behavioral research is available on how children learn to produce Skinner's (1957) functionally different verbal behaviors (such as mands, tacts, intraverbals, and autoclitics; see Hegde, 2010c, for an overview).

Third, the behavioral analysis of speech–language and its learning is generally unknown to SLPs. Most students taking courses on language development and disorders, as well as those on speech sound disorders, do not receive adequate and accurate information on the behavioral view. Instead, students and professionals learn about it from its critics; textbooks and research articles typically provide some dated references to an inadequately described behavioral view, describe it from the standpoint of critics who have not understood it, and then summarily dismiss it.

Traditionally, the behavioral view described in various sources is that of Mowrer's 1960 theory, supplemented by Olmsted's 1971 theory. The basic idea in this view is that speech sounds are shaped out of babbling by environmental contingencies of positive reinforcement. During the course of the day, the infant receives much care from caretakers, usually the mother, in the form of feeding and changing. During such activities, the mother produces many vocalizations and even clearly articulated sequences of speech sounds (syllables and words). Such maternal productions are associated with activities that provide for the infant primary positive reinforcement (e.g., feeding) and negative reinforcement (e.g., elimination of discomfort when changed). In due course, maternal vocalizations and speech productions signal primary reinforcement for the infant. The infant's own babbling and other vocalizations acquire secondary reinforcement because of their similarity with the maternal vocalizations that are associated with primary reinforcement. The infant's babbling and other vocalizations, even if they begin as vocal play or random behaviors, are highly sensitive to environmental contingencies. For example, experimental studies on infant vocalizations have shown that babbling can be increased by contingent positive reinforcement (e.g., such social reinforcers as smiling, touch, and shaking a rattle) and decreased when such reinforcers are withdrawn (see McLaughlin, 2006, for a summary of studies). In essence, the interaction between the infant's initial vocal behaviors and the environmental events that help shape speech sounds is the essential feature of the classical behavioral view formulated by Mowrer.

Evidence fully supports the fundamental behavioral or learning-based assumption that infants' babbling provides a basis for shaping speech sounds. As noted previously, Jakobson's (1968) view that babbling is not systematically related to later speech sound acquisition has been rejected, not only by behavioral scientists, but also by most contemporary linguistically oriented researchers (Oller, 2000; Oller & Griebel, 2008; Rvachew

& Brosseau-Lapré, 2012). Even though much of the infant speech perception research has been conducted within a linguistic framework, the methods used have been behavioral, and the results themselves, as noted before, suggest that infants are sensitive to environmental contingencies of conditioning and learning. We noted earlier that in addition to developmental and observational data on babbling and infant vocalizations, babbling may be systematically increased with various kinds of social reinforcers presented in experimental conditions (see Goldstein, King, and West, 2003, for a brief review of studies). A study on operant conditioning of infant babbling concluded that "the infant's sounds were tightly linked to the behavior of the caregivers" (Goldstein et al., 2003, p. 8034) when the caregivers were trained to positively reinforce the infant's babbling. The authors further stated that babbling leads to specific speech sounds and eventually to social communication, because communication is heavily socially reinforced.

An often voiced criticism is that the behavioral view simply assumes that children imitate speech and learn patterns of speech production. No Skinnerian view has ever advanced imitation as the only and ultimate mechanism of speech and language learning. In the behavioral view, imitation, when it does occur, is only the beginning; it is the contingent consequences (mainly positive reinforcement) under specified stimulus conditions that teach and sustain speech, including imitated speech (see, for example, Goldstein et al., 2003; McLaughlin, 2010; Moerk, 1990). Twin studies have shown that caregivers who encourage imitation may promote language learning in identical twins (McEwen et al., 2007). Several other studies have shown that when the experimenters or mothers reinforce infant vocalizations by saying, "Hello, baby" or "Tsk, tsk," the infant vocalizations increase in frequency (Bloom, 1988; Bloom, Russell, & Wassenberg, 1987; Goldstein et al., 2003); there was no significant effect when the same reinforcers were presented noncontingently (presented somewhat randomly, not dependent on infant vocalizations). Furthermore, several investigators have shown that specifically built robots, with no prior experience with speech, may be taught to produce vowels and syllables by modeling and positive reinforcement (Howard & Messum, 2011; Yoshikawa, Asada, Hosada, & Koga, 2003). Another study involved a neural network model (a mechanical device) that could be taught to produce either voiced or voiceless sounds, depending on which production was reinforced (Warlaumont, Westermann, Buder, & Oller, 2013). These findings are consistent with the behavioral view that speech and language are learned through contingent consequences (Skinner, 1957; Hegde, 2010c). Clinicians, of course, know well that modeling by the clinician, imitation by the client, and positive reinforcement by the clinician are important in teaching speech and language skills to children. The extensive work of Moerk (1983, 1989, 1990, 1992, 1996, 2000) shows that language learning is largely aided by reinforcement and corrective feedback and that the parents informally teach language to their children.

Another related criticism of the behavioral view is that children cannot possibly learn speech and language as claimed by behavioral researchers because children do not receive enough direct instruction on how to produce speech sounds and grammatical elements of their language. Linguists believe that there is simply not enough information available about language for children to learn it; thus, there must be some innate knowledge. This view is known as the **poverty of the stimulus** hypothesis (Chomsky, 1957). As Pullum and Scholz (2002) have demonstrated, it is a hypothesis advanced and repeated without any empirical data to support it. The hypothesis asserts that, because there is a poverty of speech and language stimuli, speech and language skills are not explicitly taught, and therefore cannot be learned and must be due to an innate mechanism. Skinner (1957) never wrote that speech and language are explicitly taught the way teachers teach various subject matters in the classroom. Speech is learned naturally, through everyday interactions; but these interactions, when analyzed carefully, show that caregivers do model, correct, and reinforce speech productions in their children (Moerk, 1990, 2000). Reinforcement contingencies are inherent to everyday verbal interactions, including caregiver–infant interactions (Hegde, 2010c). Studies such as those cited here have shown that during mother–infant face-to-face interactions, imitation occurs once a minute, and it is the mother who often imitates the infant vocalizations. More important, mothers deliver "powerful and selective rewards" when their infant's behavior matches their own (E. Ray & Heyes, 2011). In addition, earlier research on motherese has clearly shown that adults do use certain strategies that promote speech–language learning in infants. Particularly relevant to the present context are such strategies as slower and more clearly articulated speech sounds when caregivers speak to infants and young children (Newport, Gleitman, & Gleitman, 1977; C. Snow, 1977; Stern, 1977).

Contrary to the nativist assertion that there is a poverty of stimulus (not enough in the environment to teach the child speech and language), E. Ray and Heyes (2011) describe the wealth of the stimulus for children. In a recent study (Julien & Munson, 2012), adults were asked first to listen to 2- to 3-year-olds' production of word-initial speech sounds and then to produce the same words as though they were responding to the children's productions. The authors found that the adults modified their productions to make them more accurate than the children's productions, suggesting a teaching and learning strategy inherent to natural adult–infant interactions.

Some cognitivists have been suggesting for sometime now that language is learned implicitly, not by *explicit tutoring*—a view that is consistent with the behavioral analysis. According to that view, infants and children learn their speech and language skills in natural environments through everyday interactions with their caregivers (Ellis, 2011). Ellis states that complex knowledge may be acquired through interaction but with no explicit tutoring. A variation of the implicit learning view is that children are able to learn sound sequences (and other aspects of language) based on the frequency with which the speech and language elements are present in the environment. Also known as the statistical learning approach, this view emphasizes that speech and language are learned skills, not innately determined (Saffran, 2003; Saffran, Newport, Aslin, Tunick, & Barrueco, 1997).

Another alternative linguistic view, generally known as the connectionist view, proposes that speech and language skills are learned through environmental interactions—although this view involves abstract (speculative) neural networks that manage the learning; the theory proposes that a training environment is required for learning to take place, and it rejects the notion of innate, domain-specific knowledge being necessary for speech and language learning (Westermann, Ruh, & Plunkett, 2009). Yet another cognitive-linguistic view, known as the usage-based theory of phonology and language (Bybee, 2001, 2006; Silverman, 2011; Tomasello, 2005), postulates that phonological (and other language) structures are learned because the child frequently hears the exemplars of utterances; the higher the frequency with which a child hears certain sound patterns, the greater the chance the child will learn to produce them—a view similar to the statistical learning of speech and language. Although usage-based theories do not explicitly suggest reinforcement contingencies, they are more data based than the Chomskyan generative theories, and they do emphasize natural interactions that promote speech learning.

Research on **language variability** is another line of investigation that has affirmed the role of environmental contingencies in teaching speech and language skills to children. While the generative nativists emphasized universal features and uniformity of language, **sociolinguistic** and **sociophonetic** approaches have drawn attention to language variability within and across children in the same culture and across cultures. The fact of language variability is prima facie evidence against a fixed innate structure that can only create relatively uniform surface forms. Indeed, speech–language variability alone has led to the provocative assertion that language universals (Evans & Levinson, 2009) and the attending concept of universal grammar (Christiansen & Chater, 2008) are both linguistic myths.

Still other critics who otherwise take a linguistic view find the popular phonological processes that are presumed to dictate erroneous sound productions in children illogical, unempirical, and even absurd (Ball et al., 2010; Bernhardt & Stemberger, 1998; Bernhardt & Stoel-Gammon, 1994). It is illogical to postulate an innate phonological process that forces a child to make speech sound errors. The postulated innate phonological process is unempirical because it is unobservable. Such processes are as absurd as positing that young children have a process for "falling down," which should be suppressed before they can learn to walk (Bernhardt & Stemberger, 1998). The hypothesis that error patterns in learning speech sounds or any other skills should be "suppressed" before learning the correct skill is not consistent with any kind of learning research. The child is supposed to "unlearn" final consonant deletion, for example. But how does a child unlearn something he or she does not do? One can possibly unlearn something he or she has learned to do, not something not done. Why should we postulate a cause (in this case, a process of consonant deletion) for something that does not exist? Is it not more sensible to say that the child learned to produce the final consonants? Errors decrease as correct responses increase; no learner "suppresses" errors. As Bernhardt and Stoel-Gammon (1994) put it, children learn progressively more complex speech skills; learning is positive and additive, not negative and subtractive. The way the process-based theories describe speech sound learning is akin to assuming that children are "little linguists" (Bernhardt & Stoel-Gammon, 1994, p. 125).

In essence, there are several lines of investigation both within and outside linguistics that justify the role of learning in speech–language acquisition. It is just the Chomskyan generative linguists and phonologists that refuse to see the accruing empirical evidence in favor of caregiver interactions that implicitly teach speech–language skills to children. As Saffran et al. (1997) conclude, "Language acquisition theorists have had a tendency to dismiss learning as a minor or theoretically uninteresting component. . . . The present approach [of incidental and statistical learning] takes learning seriously as a potential critical aspect of language acquisition" (p. 104).

As we noted, many investigators use such general terms as "environmental input" and "social interactions" as important variables in early speech sound imitation and learning. But what do these terms mean? How can they be operationalized? A closer examination of environmental input and infant–caregiver interactions supports a more precise behavioral formulation of variables that help informally teach speech sound production. Such an examination will reveal that infants' early vocal behaviors—later canonical babbling and subsequent production of consonants, syllables, and words—are all due to modeling, shaping, and positive reinforcement, which caregivers implicitly provide through their everyday interactions with the infants.

....

ACTIVITY

Define the following terms in your own words: *behavioral explanation, implicit learning, wealth of the stimulus, language variability, connectionist view.*

....

Summary of the Advanced Unit

- The two major methods of studying speech perception and discrimination in infants—high-amplitude sucking and visually reinforced head turn—are operant conditioning methods; therefore, their results show that infants can be taught to discriminate between speech sounds, not that such discrimination is innate.

- Jakobson's (1968) theory proposed that speech sound acquisition follows a universal and innate pattern in which the distinctive features of speech sounds are acquired in a hierarchical manner; his assumption that babbling is not the basis of speech sound learning has since been rejected.

- The theory of natural phonology proposes that natural phonological processes are innate and reflect limitations of the human speech production mechanism. Some of the newer phonological theories, especially nonlinear phonological theories, also suggest that phonological acquisition is made possible because the child is born with a set of universal phonological principles or constraints.

- Cognitive theorists propose that children actively test hypotheses regarding phonological constraints and systems and thus arrive at the adult system.

- The prosodic and whole-word phonological views suggest that *words*, not phonemes or features, are the initial learning units.

- The linguistic theories of phonological acquisition are varied but share certain common features that include an assumption of innateness of some basic patterns, a rejection of a strong role for environmental variables, assumptions about such cognitive patterns as hypothesis testing by infants, and a distinction between underlying phonological representations and phonetic realizations.

- The behavioral view of speech development is that teaching and learning are inherent to social interactions; babbling may be reinforced and increased; caregiver actions include modeling, imitation of infants' productions that modify such productions, positive reinforcement, and informal shaping of successively more complex forms of speech. Studies on babbling in infants, mechanical simulation of speech learning, statistical learning theory, implicit learning, connectionist views, usage-based phonological theories, and sociolinguistic and sociophonetic research support a significant role for learning in speech–language acquisition.

- Because phonological theories are varied, controversial, and ever changing, their clinical application is often premature.

CULTURE AND COMMUNICATION: BIDIALECTAL AND BILINGUAL CONSIDERATIONS

I speak Spanish to God, Italian to women, French to men, and German to my horse.

—*Charles V (Charles the Wise), 1337–1380*

Basic Unit: Ethnocultural Variables and Speech Sound Learning

Ethnicity, cultural background, and language are typically interrelated. Nonetheless, ethnocultural variations in such diverse societies as those of the United States may or may not include language variation. Many U.S.-born-and-raised children, especially those of the second generation of people who emigrated to the United States from other countries, may be ethnically heterogeneous but verbally (linguistically) homogeneous with the native English-speaking population in the United States. On the other hand, a certain number of U.S.-born children of parents who speak a language other than English, and older children who emigrated to the United States with parents whose primary language is other than English, may be both ethnically and verbally diverse from the majority population. In such cases, linguistic diversity is typically associated with bilingualism.

Ethnocultural variation and the attending verbal diversity are not limited to recent immigrants. Some U.S.-born, native English-speaking, monolingual persons may nevertheless be verbally diverse because of their ethnocultural diversity. African Americans who have lived in the United States for generations are a case in point. Their language (verbal) diversity is an element in their ethnocultural heritage. To some extent, such diversity may be evident in other ethnocultural groups who have lived in the United States for many generations. For example, although empirical studies are lacking, it is possible that Mexican, Japanese, Chinese, and East Indian people who have lived in the United States for generations may retain subtle verbal differences that are of no social or occupational consequence. To what extent, and after how many generations, the traces of ancestral verbal heritage fade in a new culture are interesting questions for empirical research.

It is obvious that ethnic background is not a necessary condition for language diversity. Diversity of verbal expressions can thrive within a single ethnic culture. In the genesis of verbal diversity, relative geographic isolation is a powerful variable. The same language, the same ethnic background, and even broadly the same culture can give rise to verbal diversity when there is overriding geographic separation. The varied dialects of world languages, spoken by otherwise relatively homogeneous populations, are a case in point. The many dialects of British English spoken in the United Kingdom and of American English spoken in the United States are familiar examples of verbal variations in the face of broad ethnocultural homogeneity.

Pronounced verbal diversity can pose significant challenges for educators, healthcare workers, human service professionals, and business people. Obvious or subtle shades of language variation are interwoven with a host of poorly understood variables related to family, society, and culture. Diversity may be pronounced in bilingual immigrant adults and children whose primary language is other than the dominant language of their adopted country. In the United States, immigrants whose first language is other than English tend to exhibit that pronounced language variation.

Verbal variations may be considerable in children who, even though born in the United States, are raised as bilingual speakers by bilingual parents or monolingual, non–English-speaking parents. The extent of variation may diminish, or in many cases be negligible, when children born in the United States are raised by English-speaking bilingual parents. The diversity may be minimal or of no consequence when children are raised as monolingual English speakers by English-speaking monolingual parents.

This chapter is written to help speech–language pathologists who assess speech sound disorders (as well as broader aspects of language) in children whose primary language is neither English nor the mainstream English, previously often referred to as *Standard English*. It is now recognized that there is no one standard form of English; American English has several dialects, none substandard. We use the term *mainstream English* when scientific (nonevaluative) comparison among different dialects is implied.

To make appropriate speech sound assessment and treatment decisions, clinicians need to know about a child's verbal and cultural background. They also need to acquire special expertise in assessing and treating children who speak any of the following:

- a language other than English (e.g., Spanish or Hmong)
- English as a second language acquired sometime after the acquisition of their primary language
- a dialectal variety of American English (e.g., African American English or a variation of mainstream English)
- a different form of English (e.g., Australian or South African English)

In principle, clinicians need to know the following:

- how a child's non-English primary language and sound pattern characteristics differ from those of English
- how the primary language affects learning of the second language
- how to determine whether there is a speech sound (and language) disorder in the child's first language, the second language, or both

Acquiring the needed knowledge can be a daunting task for clinicians. Language variation in the U.S. population has increased significantly and shows an escalating trend.

Clinicians in some states and regions of certain states face such enormous verbal diversity that the demand can be overwhelming. It is not uncommon for speech–language pathologists in certain public schools to face children who speak a dozen or more non-English primary languages.

It is sometimes implied that only speech–language pathologists of the mainstream culture face this problem, but, in fact, all speech–language pathologists face the problem of providing clinical services to children of diverse backgrounds. For example, a speech–language pathologist who is Hispanic American, African American, or Chinese American working in an American public school or health-care setting is liable to face the same problem. What should a Hispanic speech–language pathologist who speaks only Spanish and English do when a child's primary language is Russian? What should an African American speech–language pathologist do when a child's primary language is Hmong?

The answer cannot be that all speech–language pathologists should be multilingual. Therefore, there are no easy answers to these questions. Nonetheless, there are many steps speech–language pathologists can take and many professional skills they can learn to help children with varied language and culture. In this chapter, it is not possible to catalog all the phonological differences between the many languages that are now spoken in the United States; many such differences have not been adequately described. Descriptive research has mostly been concerned with speech sound acquisition and production in (1) African American English (AAE) or Black English, (2) some Native American languages, (3) some varieties of Spanish, and (4) certain Asian languages. There is more information on AAE and the Spanish language and its variations than on any other minority language spoken in the United States. We recognize that AAE is an English dialect, whereas Spanish, Mandarin, Hindi, and Native American Blackfoot are languages that when spoken as primary languages, may create secondary English dialects. Clinicians are primarily interested in how AAE and dialects influenced by other primary languages differ from more generally spoken English in the United States.

In this Basic Unit, we summarize the salient information available on children who speak AAE or a language other than English as their primary language. The main purpose is not to exhaustively list the phonological differences between English and other languages, but to illustrate the point that phonological differences across languages of interest must be understood. In addition, we summarize the basic professional dispositions and guidelines necessary to appropriately assess and treat children of ethnocultural diversity. In the Advanced Unit, we will discuss theoretical issues and clinical research issues.

African American English

A variety of terms, including *Black English* (Dillard, 1972), *Black English Vernacular, African American Vernacular English*, and simply *African American English*, have been suggested for the specific dialect of American English spoken by varying numbers of African American adults and children. The term *African American English* is consistent with the name used to describe the ethnic group with which it is predominantly identified; therefore, that term is preferred here (Battle, 2002; H. N. Seymour, 2004; van Keulen, Weddington, & Dubois, 1998).

Variations of American English include the General American Dialect, Eastern American Dialect, Southern American Dialect, and several other forms spoken in smaller regions of the country (Edwards, 2003; Garn-Nunn & Lynn, 2004). The General American Dialect (GAD) is so named because it is spoken in a relatively large geographic region—from the Great Lakes to the Pacific Seaboard (Edwards, 2003). It is also common to refer to GAD as Mainstream American English (MAE), again because it is spoken in a larger geographic region than the other dialects (Pearson, 2004). MAE is also spoken in areas where one of the other dialects is predominant. For instance, members of the broadcast media, including television and radio, in the southern states where the Southern American Dialect is dominant are likely to use MAE. It may be noted that the terms GAD and MAE both avoid the invalid notion that one dialectical form of American English is the standard for all speakers in the country.

African American English is a dialect of American English, although some have argued that it is a separate language (van Keulen et al., 1998). Because non–African American English and AAE share more features in common than those that distinguish them, it may be appropriate to consider AAE as a dialect of American English. Scholars, clinical professionals, and such professional organizations as the American Speech-Language-Hearing Association reject the historically held view that AAE is a substandard form of MAE.

The origin of African American English is not certain. It is thought that its potential origins include English spoken by Whites or such independent sources as Creole (Dillard, 1972). Geographically, AAE may have its origins in West Africa, where the Europeans visited for trade. Because the Europeans and Africans had no common language, a pidgin may have developed that served the needs of basic business communication. A **pidgin** is a simplified and limited system of verbal communication that develops out of necessity when two communities with no common language are forced by circumstances to communicate with each other. A pidgin may develop into a **Creole,** which is a more complex system of primary communication with its own phonological, semantic, syntactic, and pragmatic rules. A Creole then may be taught to children by their parents as the main or only means of communication. When parents teach a Creole to their children, it begins to pass from one generation to the next (Crystal, 1987; Dillard, 1972; Wolfram, 1994). Thus, African American English may have started as a pidgin in Africa and later become a Creole among Africans in North America. Also, the languages that Africans spoke before they were brought to North America may have affected their forced learning of English as a second language. The current forms of AAE may have evolved over time and with greater interaction with European American English.

Not all African Americans speak AAE. A few may speak it all the time, some may speak it most of the time, and some speak it only occasionally. Some African Americans do not speak it at all. Many who speak AAE also speak MAE and switch from AAE to MAE or vice versa, depending on the audience, a phenomenon known as *code switching.* AAE is not entirely limited to African Americans. Some rural southern Whites may use elements of AAE in their speech. Although all American dialects have evolved and changed in the past centuries, read Text Box 5.1 to understand how the distinguished American writer Mark Twain captured some of the American English dialects of his time, including a form of Southern American Dialect spoken mostly by rural White people. This dialect and AAE share many language and phonological features, evidence that AAE is not entirely a race-based dialect.

Text Box 5.1. Lessons in Huck Finn's English

Mark Twain's American classic *The Adventures of Huckleberry Finn* is a lesson in American dialects, including some unmistakable similarities between certain English dialects White people spoke and African American English (AAE). Twain wrote the book in more than four dialects, including the Missouri AAE, and "the extreme form of the backwoods South-Western dialect, the ordinary 'Pike-County' dialect; and four modified varieties of the last" (Twain, 1884/1986). Huck, a southwestern White teenager, and Jim, his African American adult companion, spoke with common expressions like the following:

- ain't no matter (also, *hain't* for *ain't*); I don't take no stock in dead people

- the widow she cried over me; Tom he made a sign

- she done it herself

- I warn't (for *I wasn't*)

- stars was shining; they was going to; we was; horses is

- carelessest, foolishest

- I dasn't (for *I don't*)

- I knowed mighty well; drownded man; I thinks; I rests; many thinks

- what you going to do?; nobody could a seen it

- learn me something

- no, says I; I says to myself; says they

- ornery (for *ordinary*)

- clumb over (for *climb over* or *climbed over*)

- set (for *sit*)

- resk it (for *risk it*)

- nuther (for *neither*)

- afeard (for *afraid*)

- suthin (for *something*)

- govment (for *government*)

- git (for *get*)

- p'fessor (for *professor*)

- sence (for *since*)

It is now well recognized that AAE has its own phonological, syntactic, semantic, and pragmatic rules. It has a distinct communication style. Many sources provide excellent descriptions of AAE characteristics, rules of usage, and communication style (Craig, Thompson, Washington, & Potter, 2003; Dillard, 1972; Hecht, Collier, & Ribeau, 1993; Kamhi, Pollock, & Harris, 1996; Pearson, Velleman, Bryant, & Charko, 2009; Roseberry-McKibbin, 2002; Stockman, 2010; van Keulen et al., 1998; Willis, 1992; Wolfram, 1994). The reader may consult these and other sources for a better understanding of African American culture, family, value systems, language and verbal behavior, and communication styles.

ACTIVITY

Describe at least five phonological features of Huck's speech that are the same as those in AAE.

Assessment of speech sound production skills in any child requires, in addition to other procedures, conducting an interview with the family and the child, recording a speech–language sample, and administering standardized or client-specific measures of language and speech. In essence, the clinician should arrange communicative situations to sample speech and language. Even if the concern is only to assess speech production in a given child, the clinician should know the characteristics and unique properties of the language of the child and the family. The communication style and interactional patterns of the families the clinician serves should be appreciated.

In this chapter, for the sake of brevity and special relevance, we will be concerned mostly with phonological aspects of AAE. However, a few critical features of language and communication style will be summarized, as well.

ACTIVITY

Describe the primary differences between a *pidgin* and a *Creole*.

African Americans have a rich linguistic tradition. They use language effectively, eloquently, and often colorfully. A distinct rhythm and a unique style of communication is part of the African American culture. Emotional and gestural expressions may enhance their communication to a greater extent than in some other ethnic groups. Their public behavior may be intense and expressive. African Americans may be more inclined to touch or make physical contact during conversation. While eye contact may be a form of verbal expression, rolling the eyes may be considered offensive. Children may not, out of respect for adults, maintain eye contact during conversation with adults.

Children telling stories may include personal judgments and evaluations. A child may prefer to refer to her mother as "momma" (not as "mother"); "momma" is viewed more positively.

Cultural heritage, family relationships, and mutual help and support are highly valued in African American society. Loyalty to family, respect for the elderly, and group efforts for the common good are cultural values. Persons who are not blood relatives may be considered part of the family because of their supportive role and the broader concept of a family. Children are highly valued, well supported, loved, and cared for and may be reared more authoritatively than in other cultural groups.

To analyze the speech sound production skills and potential problems an African American child may have, the clinician should take into consideration the language characteristics of African American English. Please see Table 5.1 for a summary of the major language characteristics of AAE.

Phonological Characteristics of AAE

Many phonological characteristics are common to both African American English and Mainstream American English. However, it is important to understand the unique phonological features of AAE, so that such features are not misinterpreted as phonological disorders (Craig et al., 2003).

All of the unique phonological features of AAE may not be found in all speakers of that dialect. Wolfram (1986) has shown that the presence of certain phonological features may depend on socioeconomic status. Compared to African Americans in lower socioeconomic classes, those in the middle and upper classes produce fewer phonological features of AAE. The number of years in school also may be a significant variable clinicians need to consider. For example, 94% to 100% of African American *preschool* children of low-income families living in large urban centers (e.g., Detroit) may speak AAE. On the other hand, older children in grade schools may speak both MAE and AAE (Craig & Washington, 2002; Washington & Craig, 1992). A few features, however, may be found in speakers of all socioeconomic classes and age groups, though with varying frequency. For example, omission of the postvocalic *r* in such words as *sister* (pronounced *sistə*) may be observed across socioeconomic classes. In contrast, the substitution of /f/ for /θ/ in such words as *bath*, pronounced as *baf*, common in middle and lower socioeconomic classes, is uncommon in upper middle and upper socioeconomic classes. Therefore, a lack of /f/ substitution for /θ/ may not suggest that an African American does not speak AAE; it may only mean that he or she belongs to a middle or upper class.

Geographic regions, too, make a difference in the way AAE is spoken. Washington and Craig (1992) reported that AAE spoken in a northern state, such as Michigan, may be different from AAE spoken in a southern state, such as Mississippi. On some tests of articulation, scoring adjustments to suit AAE were needed only for African American children living in Mississippi, but not in Michigan, according to the Cole and Taylor (1990) and Washington and Craig (1992) studies.

All consonants and vowels found in Mainstream American English are also found in African American English. The speech of many AAE speakers may not contain the /ð/, as it is substituted by /d/ in the word-initial position and by /v/ or /d/ in the word-medial and word-final positions. The /θ/ may be replaced by /t/ or /f/. Most AAE speakers reduce some diphthongs into single vowels, a phonological process known as **ungliding**. Generally, more consonants than vowels differ across AAE and MAE. Consonants in the word-medial and -final positions show greater differences than those in the initial positions.

The main features of AAE may be summarized as follows:

• **Absence (omission) of consonants.** A final nasal sound or an oral stop is more likely to be absent than other consonants. A final consonant in a word is likely to be absent

Table 5.1

MAJOR LANGUAGE CHARACTERISTICS OF AFRICAN AMERICAN ENGLISH

AAE Characteristics	MAE Statement	AAE Statement
Noun possessives may be omitted.	That's the woman's car. It's John's pencil.	That **the woman** car. It **John** pencil.
Noun plurals may be omitted.	He has two boxes of apples. She gives me 5 cents.	He got two **box** of **apple**. She give me 5 **cent**.
Third-person singular verb may be omitted.	She walks to school. The man works in his yard.	She **walk** to school. The man **work** in his yard.
Forms of *to be* (is, are) may be omitted.	She is a nice lady. They are going to a movie.	**She a** nice lady. **They going** to a movie.
Present tense *is* may be used regardless of person or number.	They are having fun. You are a smart man.	**They is** having fun. **You is** a smart man.
Person or number may not agree with past and present forms.	You are playing ball. They are having a picnic.	**You is** playing ball. They **is** having a picnic.
Present-tense forms of auxiliary *have* may be omitted.	I have been here for 2 hours. He has done it again.	**I been here** for 2 hours. **He done** it again.
Past-tense endings may be omitted.	He lived in California. She cracked the nut.	He **live** in California. She **crack** the nut.
Past-tense *was* may be used regardless of number and person.	They were shopping. You were helping me.	They **was** shopping. You **was** helping me.
Multiple negatives may be used to add emphasis to the negative meaning.	We don't have any more. I don't want any cake. I don't like broccoli.	We **don't** have **no more**. I **don't never** want **no** cake. I **don't never** like broccoli.
None may be substituted for *any*.	She doesn't want any.	She don't want **none**.
In perfective constructions, *been* may be used to indicate that an action took place in the past.	I had the mumps when I was 5. I knew her.	**I been had** the mumps when I was 5. **I been known** her.
Done may be combined with a past-tense form to indicate that an action was started and completed.	He fixed the stove. She tried to paint it.	He **done fixed** the stove. She **done tried** to paint it.
The form *be* may be used as the main verb.	Today she is working. We are singing.	Today **she be** working. **We be** singing.
Distributive *be* may be used to indicate actions and events over time.	He is often cheerful. She's kind sometimes.	**He be** cheerful. **She be** kind.
A pronoun may be used to restate the subject.	My brother surprised me. My dog has fleas.	My brother, **he** surprised me. My dog, **he** got fleas.
Them may be substituted for *those*.	Those cars are antiques. Where'd you get those books?	**Them cars,** they be antique. Where you get **them books**?
Future-tense *is* and *are* may be replaced by *gonna*.	She is going to help us. They are going to be there.	She **gonna** help us. They **gonna** be there.
At may be used at the end of *where* questions.	Where is the house? Where is the store?	Where is the house **at**? Where is the store **at**?
Additional auxiliaries may be used.	I might have done it.	**I might could have** done it.
Does may replace *do*.	She does funny things. It does make sense.	**She do** funny things. **It do** make sense.

Note. Adapted from *Multicultural Students With Special Language Needs* (Table 5.1, pp. 52–53), by C. Roseberry-McKibbin, 1995, Oceanside, CA: Academic Communication Associates. Copyright 1995 by Academic Communication Associates. Reprinted with permission. MAE = Mainstream American English; AAE = African American English.

if the following word begins with a consonant, as against a vowel (e.g., the /t/ in "best buy" is more likely to be omitted than the /t/ in "right on"). A consonant that serves a morphemic function is more likely to be absent if the meaning can still be clear (e.g., the omission of the plural *s* in such expressions as "two cup") (Stockman, 1996, 2010; Wolfram, 1994).

• **Consonant cluster reduction.** Clustered consonants in the initial positions are produced more often than those in the final position. There also are a few sound substitutions within initial clusters (see Table 5.2).

• **Unstressed syllable deletion.** In such words as *until* and *about*, the initial syllable may be markedly reduced or omitted altogether. Frequency of unstressed syllable deletion increases with age (Stockman, 1996). An unstressed syllable is more likely to be deleted if a single vowel forms the syllable shape (e.g., _away_), the preceding word ends in a vowel (e.g., _go_ *away*), or the word is a preposition or conjunction (e.g., _behind_ and _because_). On the other hand, the unstressed syllable is likely to be produced when the word is a noun, adjective, or verb (e.g., the initial syllable is produced in *begin* but may be deleted in *before*) and when the word has three syllables (e.g., the initial syllable is produced in *depression* but may be deleted in *divorce)* (Stockman, 1996).

Table 5.2 lists the major phonological characteristics of AAE.

In summary, AAE contains most of the same phonemes as MAE. A phoneme inventory is likely to show no or only a few differences between AAE and MAE. The phonemes, however, may be used differently in the two languages. Omissions and substitutions of sounds, often prominent in the word-medial and -final positions, give AAE its most characteristic feature. As we will see in subsequent sections, omission and substitution of phonemes are also a characteristic of speakers who use English as a second language.

Speech Sound Learning in Children Speaking AAE

Most of the classic studies on speech sound learning summarized in Chapter 4 have sampled mostly White American children. While the undersampling of African American (AA) children has been a problem in previous studies, only an adequate sampling of such children without evoking and analyzing AAE features of speech and language would not have been helpful, either. There is a great need for comprehensive studies on how AA children master the AAE sound patterns.

Progress has been made in recent years, however. Several studies are now available that shed light on the patterns of AAE speech sound learning, production, or both (Cole & Taylor, 1990; Craig et al., 2003; Craig & Washington, 2002, 2004; Craig, Washington, & Thompson, 2002; Kamhi et al., 1996; Pearson et al., 2009; Pruitt & Oetting, 2009; Stockman, 1996, 2008, 2010; Stockman, Karasinski, & Guillory, 2008; Thompson, Craig, & Washington, 2004; Washington & Craig, 1992, 2002; also see Stockman, 2010, for a review of studies to date). Investigators have used differing but acceptable methods. For instance, some investigators have compared AA children's articulatory performance with that of White children of similar age (Pearson et al., 2009; Stockman, 1996). To evoke speech sound productions, investigators have used pictorial stimuli, items of standardized tests of articulation, conversational speech, and oral reading samples. Phonological processes or individual sound productions have been analyzed.

Table 5.2

THE PHONOLOGICAL CHARACTERISTICS OF AFRICAN AMERICAN ENGLISH

AAE Phonologic Feature	MAE Examples	AAE Examples
/I/ lessening or omission	tool always	too' a'ways
/r/ lessening or omission	door mother protect	doah mudah p'otek
/f/ voiceless th substitution in word-final or -medial position	teeth both nothing	teef bof nufin'
/t/ voiceless th substitution in word-initial position	think thin	tink tin
/d/ voiced th substitution in word-initial and -medial positions	this brother	dis broder
/v/ voiced th substitution in word-final position	breathe smooth	breave smoov
Consonant-cluster reduction in initial and final positions	throw desk rest left wasp	thow des' res' lef' was'
Consonant substitutions within clusters	shred strike	sred skrike
Differing syllable stress patterns	guitar police July	gui tar po lice Ju ly
Modification of verbs ending in /k/	liked walked	li-tid wah-tid
Metathetic productions Devoicing of final voiced consonants	ask bed rug cab	aks bet ruk cap
Deletion of final consonants	bad good	ba' goo'
i/e substitution	pen ten	pin tin
b/v substitution	valentine vest	balentine bes'
Diphthong reduction (ungliding)	find oil	fahnd ol
n/g substitution	walking thing	walkin' thin'
Unstressed-syllable deletion	about remember	'bout 'member

Note. Characteristics may vary depending on variables such as geographic region. Adapted from *Multicultural Students With Special Language Needs* (Table 5.2, pp. 54–55), by C. Roseberry-McKibbin, 1995, Oceanside, CA: Academic Communication Associates. Copyright 1995 by Academic Communication Associates. Reprinted with permission. MAE = Mainstream American English; AAE = African American English.

In their study of 64 typically developing AA children in second through fifth grade, Craig and colleagues (2003) sampled oral reading and found that the sampled children produced all but one phonological feature characteristic of AAE. Analysis of children's reading samples revealed three dominating phonological patterns: monophthongization of diphthongs (e.g., [ɑr] for *our*), substitutions for /θ/ and /ð/, and consonant cluster reduction. Instead of /θ/ and /ð/, the sampled children produced /t/ and /d/ in prevocalic position and /f/, /t/, and /v/ in intervocalic and postvocalic positions. The Craig study also noted that when AA children's oral reading is sampled, morphosyntactic features (e.g., the production of *ain't*, multiple negations, lack of subject–verb agreement, omission of articles) may not be observed. Phonological patterns unique to AAE, though, are likely to be observed even in oral reading.

Studies of Craig and Washington (2002) and Craig, Washington, and Thompson (2002) profiled language production of African American children. Pearson et al. (2009) reported one of the largest studies based on a national sample that included both AA children and children who spoke MAE as their only or main dialect in the age range of 4-0 years to 12-11 years. The authors administered the Dialect Sensitive Language Test (H. N. Seymour, Roeper, & de Villiers, 2000) to 537 AA children and 317 children who spoke MAE. Using a 90% mastery criterion, Pearson et al. found that the interdental fricative /ð/ is the most contrastive single speech element that distinguishes AAE speech from that of MAE in children. More commonly, /ð/ is replaced by /d/, and /ð/ was among the latest developing sounds in AA children. AA children mastered the prevocalic /r/ in initial position as well as final positions within clusters (/rs/) relatively early. Also, compared to children who spoke MAE, AA children mastered relatively early the late-developing /s/ in both word-initial and -final positions and /z/ in word-final position.

Based on various studies, speech sound learning patterns in children who speak AAE may be summarized as follows:

- With the exception of /ð/, the sound inventories of AAE and MAE learners are comparable. Final consonant deletions may persist beyond the third grade, as they are features of AAE, not an error pattern (W. Haynes & Moran, 1989).

- Learners of AAE and MAE generally follow the same pattern of speech sound acquisition, except for more delayed acquisition of /ð/ but earlier acquisition of the prevocalic /r/, /rs/ clusters, /l/, and /z/ in final position by AAE learners.

- As expected, as they get older, both AAE and MAE learners master progressively more speech sounds correctly and evidence fewer phonological patterns.

- By age 2, AA children produce, in conversational speech, all 15 commonly occurring English consonants: /m/, /n/, /p/, /b/, /t/, /d/, /k/, /g/, /w/, /j/, /f/, /s/, /h/, /l/, and /r/ (Stockman, 2006, 2008). Final consonant deletions that characterize AAE may persist longer, however.

- By age 3, most AA children will have mastered obstruents plus sonorant initial-consonant clusters, including /br/, /pr/, /dr/, /tr/, /gr/, /kr/, /sl/, /sm/, /sn/, and so forth.

- By age 3-4 to 3-11, AA children may correctly produce up to 82% of consonants, and such productions may be consistent with the MAE patterns; by age 6, up to 98% of consonants may be correctly produced in single words.

- By ages 5 and 6, AA children may produce such later learned fricatives as /z/, /ʃ/, /tʃ/; most children by then also may produce the initial /l/ and /s/ blends.

- Global language learning patterns, too, are similar across children who speak AAE and those who speak MAE (Pearson, 2004).

- AA children of families at lower socioeconomic strata may exhibit more articulatory errors, but the same trend is true for all children in the same stratum.

In essence, evidence suggests that AA children who speak AAE acquire speech sound skills in the same manner as do children in other groups. Speech sound learning in AA children is susceptible to the same kinds of interference found in other children. For example, such variables as hearing impairment, intellectual disability, and neurological impairments may be expected to negatively affect speech sound learning in all children. The clinician should interpret all data relative to the speech sound production of AA children in the context of what is known about (1) articulatory proficiency in all children and (2) the characteristics of AAE. To date, no special or unique theory has been proposed to explain speech sound acquisition in AA children.

Assessment of Speech Sound Disorders in African American Children

African American children's speech contains more speech sound errors only when their speech samples are analyzed from the standpoint of MAE. Most of the errors are likely to be characteristics of AAE. Therefore, AA children's speech should be assessed in the context of AAE.

The speech sounds AA children tend to misarticulate are, for the most part, the same as those White children misarticulate. For example, in one study, of 10 consonants misarticulated, 8 were the same across the two ethnocultural groups (H. N. Seymour & Seymour, 1981). The same study also showed that sound substitutions may be common to children in the two ethnocultural groups. However, AA children tend to exhibit more omissions than do White children, mostly because such omissions are a feature of AAE. Provided that the special features of AAE are taken into consideration, the clinical evaluation of speech sounds for the two groups need not differ in any drastic manner (H. N. Seymour & Seymour, 1981).

A few standardized tests are available to assess speech sound disorders in AA children who speak AAE. Generally, it is inappropriate to use a standardized test in assessing a child from a minority group when that minority group was not sampled or not sampled adequately in the standardization process. Even more important, assessment of speech sound patterns in AA children requires not only an adequate sampling of those children, but also test items that reflect AAE. It should be emphasized that just sampling AA children is of no use when none of the test items are written for AAE.

Some of the commonly used tests of articulation may be highly biased against verbally diverse children, especially AA children. Some tests may give credit to the child if the item is dialect sensitive; for example, the third edition of the *Arizona Articulation Proficiency Scale* (Fudala, 2000) allows such credit for AAE. Washington and Craig (1992) have found that that test is appropriate for AA children, especially those living in a northern state (especially

Michigan). For such children, even the suggested scoring adjustment may not be needed. Washington and Craig caution, however, that the test may be biased against AA children living in the southern states of the U.S. Whether or not a test gives credit for a dialect-sensitive item, the clinician should. For example, an AA child's production of "*baf*" for *bath* should not signal an articulation disorder. The clinician should examine the test items for dialectal or language-specific variations that may be found in the child who is being assessed. It is clear that the procedure of giving credit to AA children for an AAE feature reduces the chances of wrongly diagnosing an articulation disorder in them (Cole & Taylor, 1990).

Giving credit for dialect-sensitive items on a standardized test is better than misinterpreting AAE speech sound features as disorders. Nonetheless, this strategy may not solve the basic problem (Laing, 2003; Stockman, 1996). When most items on a test for a given phoneme are dialect sensitive, giving credit for them may leave few or no items for making a judgment about that phoneme's production. Also, single-word articulation tests, regardless of dialect sensitivity, may produce erroneous data. For example, an AA child who has trouble producing certain consonants in isolated words may have no trouble producing the same consonants in continuous speech, especially when the target consonants precede a word that begins with a vowel (Stockman, 1996).

There are several assessment strategies that are alternatives to the traditional, standardized test–based method of assessing speech and language skills in children belonging to minority and specific dialectal groups (Hegde & Pomaville, 2013). Laing (2003), for instance, suggested an *alternate response mode (ARM)*, which requires a modified stimulus presentation to assess whether a missing final consonant is an AAE feature or a potential disorder that should be further probed. Similar to what is done in contextual testing of articulation (McDonald, 1964; Secord & Shine, 1997; see Chapter 6 for details), test word presentations designed to assess final consonant productions may be quickly followed by a word that starts with a vowel (e.g., *house—eyes*). When the target final consonant (/s/ in the example) is placed before a vowel (/e/), the consonant is not absent in AAE. The target stimuli may be drawn from such standardized tests as the *Goldman-Fristoe Test of Articulation* (Goldman & Fristoe, 2000) and combined with words that start with a vowel. Laing (2003) has shown that this modified procedure reduces the frequency of final consonant absences in AA children, thus minimizing the chances of overdiagnosing a speech sound disorder in an AA child.

Other alternative approaches are a part of *authentic assessment* (Udvari & Thousand, 1995). For instance, Seymour and colleagues (Ciolli & Seymour, 2004; Seymour, 2004; Seymour & Pearson, 2004) describe an alternative method for assessing the phonological skills of AA children. Their approach is based on the observation that MAE and AAE share features that contrast (differ) as well as features that do not contrast (coincide). As noted previously, absent consonant clusters and absent final consonants in AAE contrast with (differ from) the presence of consonants in clusters and word-final positions in MAE. Therefore, contrastive features are not a basis for making a diagnosis of an articulation or phonological disorder. An AA child who says "fas" for *fast* is producing an acceptable contrastive feature of AAE; it is not a basis for clinical diagnosis. On the other hand, if the same child were to produce "ret" instead of *rest* (also a matter of cluster reduction), a disorder (or a delay in some cases) may be suspected, because this type of cluster reduction is not contrastive; it is not a feature of AAE.

The concept of contrast also helps distinguish substitutions that are a part of AAE from those that may suggest a disorder. For example, an AA child who says *mouf* for *mouth* is likely exhibiting a contrastive feature of AAE; however, an AA child who says *mous* for *mouth* probably has a disorder, because such a substitution is not characteristic of AAE. This kind of analysis helps avoid a simplistic (and inappropriate) rule application that cluster reduction and final consonant absence are typical of AAE. The analysis helps make a differential evaluation of the kinds of cluster reductions that are contrastive versus those that are not. Seymour, Roeper, de Villiers, and de Villiers (2005) have published an assessment instrument called the *Diagnostic Evaluation of Language Variance–Norm Referenced* (DELV-Norm Referenced) and a screening test (Seymour, Roeper, de Villiers, & de Villiers, 2003) called the *Diagnostic Evaluation of Language Variation–Screening Test* (DELV-Screening Test). The two instruments include language and phonological assessments based on the contrastive and non-contrastive features of AAE and MAE.

Stockman (2006, 2008) has researched another dynamic and alternative method of diagnosing speech sound disorders in African American children. Her research specifies that production of the following 15 word-initial consonants constitutes the minimal competency core of the speech sound repertoire of AA children: /m/, /n/, /p/, /b/, /t/, /d/, /k/, /g/, /w/, /j/, /f/, /s/, /h/, /l/, and /r/. These are the most frequently occurring English consonants, and, as noted earlier, typically developing AA children produce them by age 2. Therefore, Stockman suggests that if an AA child does not produce these consonants in word-initial positions by 33 to 36 months, there is a reasonable justification for diagnosing a speech sound disorder. By making a retrospective analysis of speech data, Stockman demonstrated that the minimal competency core could distinguish AA children with speech sound disorders from those who were developing normally. This method is straightforward, well researched, and simple to use.

An alternative method that may supplant other, carefully selected procedures described so far is the *portfolio assessment* (DeFina, 1992). The portfolio assessment approach simply expands the database used to evaluate a child's speech and language skills. For instance, the clinician may select a child's handwriting samples and written assignments; taped interviews of parents, teachers, and peers; the child's language sample; written notes from the teacher about the child's speech and language skills; the child's story retell samples; and so forth (Hegde & Pomaville, 2013). These items, placed in the child's portfolio, may be updated periodically to assess change in the child's speech, language, and literacy skills. When combined with the results of other assessment procedures, the portfolio will help create a more complete picture of the child's skills and limitations that need clinical attention.

In assessing phonological skills, conversational speech offers some advantages over standardized tests. Conversational speech allows for the normal speech behavioral patterns to play their role. Stockman (1996) strongly recommends that the clinician sample a child's *ordinary* or *naturalistic* language productions. Ordinary language is exhibited in routine daily activities at home and in other naturalistic contexts. Conversational speech samples may be difficult to transcribe adequately, especially when the speech is unintelligible. One potential solution to this problem is to obtain a conversational speech sample as well as an oral reading sample (Craig et al., 2003). Each will help mitigate the limitations of the other.

Conversational speech will sample sound productions in various natural contexts, and the oral reading sample will reveal how the child produces printed target words.

Some clinicians may depend on parental or community input in determining whether a speech disorder exists in a child who speaks an unfamiliar dialect. Terrel, Arensberg, and Rosa (1992) suggest that a parent's speech may be considered a standard against which a child's speech and language skills may be evaluated. Some clinicians warn that if the parents or other caregivers do not think a child has a problem, the clinician should be extremely cautious in diagnosing one (Stockman, 1996).

An appropriate diagnosis of a speech sound disorder in children who speak AAE requires data collection from multiple sources, some of which may be unconventional. Careful selection of standardized tests based on the contrastive and non-contrastive features of AAE and MAE (Seymour et al., 2003); giving credit for dialect-sensitive items; analyzing the minimal competency core (Stockman, 2006, 2008); obtaining an extensive conversational speech sample, including naturalistic (ordinary) speech; carefully interviewing parents, teachers, peers, and other caregivers; comparing the child's speech to that of the caregivers; analyzing periodically updated portfolio items; and developing a good understanding of the culture and communication pattern of the child and the family help in making an appropriate diagnosis of a speech sound disorder. These guidelines do not apply if an AA child is not an AAE speaker and the family is concerned about the child's speech sound competence in MAE. In such cases, the speech sound disorder (or more likely a variation) is diagnosed within a more typical orientation.

Treatment of Speech Sound Disorders in African American Children

Treatment of speech sound disorders in African American children requires a discriminated approach. The variables to consider before a treatment plan is developed for an AA child with a properly diagnosed speech sound disorder include whether (1) the child is an AAE speaker or an MAE speaker, (2) the child and the family expect a mastery of speech sound patterns in AAE, MAE, or both, and (3) the educational demands suggest a particular treatment goal with which the caregivers agree. The context of treatment is AAE when the child is an AAE speaker, and it is MAE if the child is an MAE speaker. If the child speaks MAE exclusively, and the family prefers that the MAE speech sound pattern be the treatment target, then the clinician tailors the treatment goals as she or he would with any MAE-speaking child with a speech sound disorder. It is only when clinicians serve African American children and families that speak AAE that special considerations apply. Therefore, the following guidelines apply to children who speak AAE as their primary dialect and have a speech sound disorder in that dialect.

Because the speech sound inventory of AAE is, with a few exceptions, the same as that of MAE, all speech sounds of MAE can be potential treatment targets for children who speak AAE (Craig et al., 2003; Pearson et al., 2009; Stockman, 2006, 2008, 2010). However, specific AAE sound patterns and rules of usage should be considered in selecting treatment target words and in accepting productions as correct or incorrect during treatment. For example, an African American child's imitation of the clinician's modeled *bathtub* as *baftub* may be accepted as correct, unless the goal is to teach MAE. In essence, the acceptable, correct, and clinically reinforced productions will be based on the previously summarized patterns of articulatory behaviors that characterize AAE.

Stockman (1996) suggests that a priority system may be used in selecting treatment targets for AA children. Phonemes whose pattern of production is the same in MAE and AAE should be the first set of targets of intervention. Speech intelligibility of an AA child will improve greatly if phonemes that are produced in the same manner in both languages are taught first. Stockman suggests that the next set of phonemes to be taught should be those that the child does not produce or does not produce correctly within the patterns of AAE. Even when the clinical stimulus input is MAE, if the child gives responses that are consistent with AAE, the child should be reinforced. The example given earlier about clinician-modeled *bathtub* and child-imitated *baftub* is a case in point. Specific phonological error patterns targeted for intervention should be consistent with AAE patterns. For example, in targeting the elimination of final consonant deletion, only those phonetic contexts in which the final consonant is mandatory in AAE should be taught.

For many AAE-speaking children and their families, MAE speech sound patterns may be an acceptable goal. If clients face problems in social, academic, occupational, or other contexts because they speak AAE, the client or the parents may decide that acquiring the sound patterns of MAE is the goal. Stockman suggests that clinicians can legitimately offer clinical services when there is no speech impairment but there is a personal, social, or occupational handicap. Treatment offered in such cases would clearly be elective and comparable to any accent or dialect modification treatment that clients seek in clinical settings other than the public schools, where clinicians are legally and ethically prohibited from diagnosing a speech sound difference as a speech sound disorder.

Unless experimental treatment data or clinical data demonstrate otherwise, clinicians can assume that the basic treatment principles used in treating speech sound disorders will be effective in treating AA children, as well. Such treatment principles are described in Chapter 7. Procedural modifications to suit the client may be necessary, as it is in the case of all children with an ethnocultural background. For instance, stimulus materials selected for teaching phonemes should be client specific, unambiguous, and familiar in the child's environment. Reinforcing consequences used in treatment should be functional for the child.

General guidelines for treating children who belong to a minority ethnocultural group are summarized in a later section, "Working With Children Who Speak Varied English Dialects: General Guidelines."

Native American Languages

According to the 2010 census data (U.S. Bureau of the Census, 2010), about 5.2 million persons have identified themselves as Native Americans (including Alaska Natives), either exclusively or in combination with one or more races (http://www.census.gov). From 2000 to 2010, there was a 27% growth in this population, which constitutes 1.7% of the U.S. population. The majority—78%—live outside reservation areas. The rest live in American Indian and Alaska Native legal and statistical areas that include 324 reservations. Many school-age children do not live on reservations or with their parents; they live with non–Native American families so they can attend school (Robinson-Zanartu, 1996; Yates, 1987). Historically, this practice has estranged Native American children from their families and culture.

Native Americans overall belong to more than 500 separate tribal groups, each with a distinct culture and language. Each tribe has an autonomous government and deals with the U.S. federal government as an independent government. Native Americans are predominantly a young population: Half of all Native Americans are younger than 21 years of age. Although Native Americans live in all parts of the United States, about 50% of the population lives in the western states. They are most highly concentrated in Arizona, New Mexico, California, Oklahoma, and North Carolina.

Research on the speech and language characteristics of Native Americans is extremely limited. Detailed analyses of phonological characteristics of Native American languages are lacking. This is partly because of the variety of languages and dialects that are spoken by Native Americans in North, Central, and South America. The American Indian Web site *Native Languages of the Americas* (http://www.native-languages.org/languages.htm) lists approximately 800 Native American languages. Many sources suggest that there are at least 200 Native American languages in North America (Highwater, 1975).

Many Native Americans, especially the younger people, do not speak their native language. Only about 27% of Native Americans speak a language other than English at home (http://www.census.gov). It is estimated that only 50 Native American languages are spoken by more than 1,000 persons (Crystal, 1987); several are spoken by fewer than 10 (Krauss, n.d.). For example, Kiowa, a Tanoan language, is spoken by only 18 of the total population of 2,000 persons. Osage, a language of the Siouan family, had only 5 fluent— and aging—monolingual speakers out of a total population of 2,500 (http://www.sil.org/ ethnologue/countries.usa.html). Many younger people speak English primarily and have only a minimal understanding of their native language. Only 760,000 Native Americans in North America speak one of their 200 languages. Unfortunately, many Native American languages are extinct, and many more are on the verge of extinction.

The classification of Native American languages in North America is controversial. This may be due to the lack of exhaustive study of the many languages Native Americans speak. The estimated number of Native American language families varies from a high of 60 to a low of 3. Highwater's (1975) classification includes 8 language families: Algonquian, Iroquoian, Caddoan, Muskogean, Siouan, Penutian, Athabascan, and Uto-Aztecan. Greenberg's (1987) classification includes only Eskimo-Aleut, Na-Dine, and Amerindi. The American Indian Web site *Native Languages of the Americas* (http://www.native-languages .org/languages.htm) lists six families of Native American languages: Eskimo-Aleut, Algonkian-Wakashan, Nadene, Penutian, Hokan-Siouan, and Aztec-Tanoan. Varied spellings are common for some language family names (e.g., Na-Dine, Nadene; Algonquian, Algonkian).

The origin of the Native American language families is poorly understood. Native American people's geographic isolation and their widespread habitat, throughout the Western Hemisphere, may have been responsible for the variety of their languages. Experts have not found any genetic relationship among the families of Native American languages (Highwater, 1975). Therefore, whether it is appropriate to group these languages under a broad umbrella of Native American languages is not clear.

ACTIVITY

Give the following: the number of persons living in the United States who identify themselves as Native American, the number of separate tribal groups found in the United States, the number of Native American languages spoken in North America, the percentage of Native Americans in the United States who live in the western states, the number of Native Americans in North America who speak at least one of the many Native American languages.

Phonological Characteristics of Native American Languages

It is not possible to list the phonological characteristics of Native American languages, because of their variety. Most available sources give an overview of Native American phonological characteristics and highlight a few examples from different languages.

Native American languages have been undergoing significant changes, some more than others. For example, there is Old Blackfoot and New Blackfoot. In New Blackfoot, the glottal stop of Old Blackfoot is being replaced by a creaky voice, long segments, or both. New Blackfoot has reportedly lost the word-initial /w/ and /h/. In Old Blackfoot, vowels in the word-final positions or followed by [x] were devoiced. In the new version, vowels in the word-final positions are voiced normally. However, vowels are deleted when they are preceded by glides. Most vowels preceding [x] are voiceless. There are no diphthongs in Old Blackfoot, but they are emerging in New Blackfoot (http://www.native-languages.org/blackfoot.htm).

Blackfoot has no voiced non-sonorant consonants. There are no liquids, either. Most stops are released, not aspirated, and the length of consonants is contrastive. Blackfoot contains only three vowels: /i/, /o/, and /a/. However, those three vowels have 11 tense and lax allophonic variations. Vowel length is contrastive, but only the tense vowels have length as a feature.

It is not surprising that phonological properties of Native American languages vary greatly. Because the languages belong to different language families with little or no genetic linking, many may have independent origins. Some Native American languages have far fewer sounds than English. For example, the Arawakan language has only 17 phonemes (Welker, 1996). Nasalized vowels are a common feature of several Native American languages. To contrast meaning, vowels may be produced with a different pitch or tonal quality. In some languages, such as Navajo, vowel length distinguishes meaning. In other languages, vowels may be voiceless. The three vowels used in the Cheyenne language of the Algonquian family may all be either voiced or voiceless. Voiceless vowels are whispered (Leman, 1980).

Among the consonants, the glottal stop is one of the few sounds common to most Native American languages. Several Native American languages also have sounds that are produced in the posterior vocal tract. Glottalized consonants, which are produced with a glottal stop and in conjunction with another consonant, are common to several languages. For example, the word *ts'in* contains a glottal stop and means *bone*, whereas *tsin*, without such a stop, means *tree*. The /k/-like plosive sound /q/, which is produced in the uvular region (unlike the English /k/, which is produced at the velum), also is a common feature across several languages. In many Native American languages, /k/ and /q/ are contrastive

(Welker, 1996). Consonant clusters are few in Navajo, and no clusters occur in syllable-final position. Navajo has several sounds that are absent in English (Harris, 1998).

In some Native American languages (e.g., Cheyenne), /p/, /t/, and /k/ are always unaspirated. In some contexts, a /v/ may sound more like the English /w/. For example, in Cheyenne, a /v/ preceding /a/ or /o/ may sound like /w/, although native speakers will recognize it only as /v/.

Speech Sound Learning in Children Speaking Native American Languages

Reliable and systematic observations of speech sound learning in Native American children are lacking. This is partly because of the variety of Native American languages and the relatively few children and young people who speak them. Because of the paucity of data and the multitude of languages spoken, it is difficult to make generalized statements about Native American children's phonological skills, learning, and speech sound disorders. Clinicians should study the phonological characteristics of the individual child being served and refrain from making generalized statements about Native American languages.

Native American languages are alive mostly in older persons. Many children of Native Americans grow up speaking English and do not acquire their native language. For example, in one articulation screening study of the Papago Indian Reservation, the dominant language of 68% of children screened was English. Only 12% of the children spoke Papago as their dominant language at home. The remaining 20% spoke both Papago and English at home (Bayles & Harris, 1982). In Alaska, 17 of the 19 Native American languages are not transmitted to children; in Oklahoma, only 2 of 23 languages are transmitted to children (Crawford, 1995). Among the Navajo community, the number of children speaking only English more than doubled from the 1980s to the 1990s. In other communities, the change has been even more rapid, as the Navajo are known to be the most loyal to their language (Crawford, 1995). Such rapid change makes it especially difficult to study the development of Native American articulatory skills in children.

A few studies have looked at the English articulatory skills of Native Americans. Bayles and Harris (1982), who administered the *Goldman-Fristoe Test of Articulation* to Papago children, reported that 5% of the 583 children assessed had a speech sound disorder. The characteristics of Papago speech sound production were taken into consideration in scoring the children's responses. For example, the children were given credit for reduced aspiration and weak production of final consonants.

More systematic studies are needed before a description of speech sound acquisition of Native American languages can be offered. Studies should sample children who speak only their native language, as well as those who speak their native language and English.

Assessment of Speech Sound Disorders in Native American Children

Assessment of speech production skills in Native American children poses special challenges. Because Native American children's cultural and language backgrounds are so different from the mainstream American culture, Robinson-Zanartu (1996) asserts that most assessment tools are "irrelevant as valid indicators of Native American learning" (p. 379). To underscore the divergence of cultural experiences of Native American children, Robinson-Zanartu (1996, p. 379) cites the example of a child's response to the question "What is a neighbor?" The child replied, "Family or close friend." On a typical language test, this response would get a failing score, but it is rooted in a rich cultural tradition of extended family and social structure that is different from that of the mainstream American culture. It would be appropriate to score it as correct.

For the speech–language pathologist, assessment challenges are greatest when the child's primary language is a Native American language and the clinician lacks familiarity with it. Because speech–language pathologists who are themselves Native American are few or nonexistent in many clinical or educational facilities, it is likely that an assessment of Native American speech sound production will be extremely difficult for most speech–language pathologists. A few areas in the country (e.g., parts of the southwestern United States) tend to have specialists and resources available to assess children of Native American background. In most of the country, people with expertise in Native American phonology are few or nonexistent.

The problem is not immediately solved even when a speech–language pathologist of Native American heritage is available, because he or she may or may not speak the particular language of the child to be assessed. Because of the unusual diversity of Native American languages, clinicians in particular regions of the country need to develop resources on the language or languages of Native Americans living in their service area. Currently, various Web sites offer a variety of information on Native American languages. Much of the information is not specific to phonological or articulatory aspects of the languages described; but this may change, and clinicians need to monitor these sites to obtain the latest information. Even the sites that do not offer specific information on articulation and phonology do offer plenty of useful information on the Native American culture, language, customs, family, and community life.

In areas with sizable Native American populations, it is likely that the local university's linguistic department would have a specialist in Native American languages or in the particular language spoken in the region. Such a specialist can be a valuable resource. Clinicians who serve Native American children in their clinics should develop a working relationship with such a specialist if possible. There are a few excellent publications that may be of help to clinicians (Leap, 1993; Phillips, 1983; Robinson-Zanartu, 1996; Westby & Vining, 2002).

It was noted earlier that many Native American children acquire English as their dominant language; thus, most Native American children who need the services of a speech–language pathologist probably need one for English. In such cases, the clinicians need to assess the children's speech sound production skills in English. It is still necessary to understand the cultural background of the child and the Native American communication style (see Text Box 5.2 for a summary of the communication style). Clinicians also should follow the general guidelines in assessing children of varied ethnocultural heritage. See the section entitled "Working With Children Who Speak Varied English Dialects: General Guidelines."

If a Native American child speaks English as a second language, the clinician then has to treat the child as bilingual. With the help of resources on Native American language and culture that the clinician has developed, speech sound production skills in both the native

Text Box 5.2. A summary of the communication style of Native American people

- Respect is highly valued; one way of signifying respect for another person is to avoid eye contact with that person by looking down.

- Children's communication with adults is respectful and discreet. To show respect, little eye contact is made with adults. Making eye contact is viewed as a way of showing defiance or rudeness.

- Native American mothers, especially those in the Navajo population, may be silent with their infants.

- Most children are taught that one learns more by listening and observing than by speaking.

- Parents often feel that their children's auditory comprehension skills are more advanced than their expressive language skills.

- Speech, language, and hearing difficulties occur five times more frequently among Native Americans than in the general population.

- Children are generally discouraged from speaking the tribal language before they are capable of correct articulation. Opportunities for oral practice in the language may be limited.

- Before they begin using words, some children communicate primarily by pointing and gesturing for a long period of time.

- Among some western Apache Indians, children may be rebuked for "talking like a white man" if they speak English or talk too much in the village.

- Native American etiquette requires a lapse of time between the asking and answering of a question. Some Native Americans believe that an immediate answer to a question implies that the question was not worth thinking about.

- Children often do not answer a question unless they are confident that their answer is correct.

- Children do not express opinions on certain subjects because they believe they first need to earn the right to express such opinions.

- In many groups, it is considered inappropriate for a person to express strong feelings publicly.

language and English should be assessed. The bilingual child's dominant language may be either English or the native language.

The clinician should determine whether there is a speech sound disorder in the child's dominant language, in the secondary language, or in both. In determining whether there is a disorder in the Native American language, the clinician should know the phonological properties of that language. In determining whether there is a disorder in English, the clinician should credit the child for varied productions of sounds that are consistent with those in the native language. Some of the suggestions offered in the section on Spanish language in this chapter will be applicable in assessing children who speak a Native American language and English.

Treatment of Speech Sound Disorders in Native American Children

Assessment of a Native American child's speech sound production skills will help determine whether the child has a disorder in his or her monolingual Native American language or in monolingual English. In the case of a bilingual child, the assessment will help determine whether the child has a disorder in either the dominant language, the secondary language, or both. This kind of differential assessment is essential for planning treatment.

The kind of professional expertise necessary to assess a Native American child is also necessary to offer appropriate treatment. A monolingual English-speaking Native American child's speech sound disorder is treated in a way that is similar to treating a child who speaks only English. Cultural differences are still important to consider, however. For example, stimulus materials selected for treatment should be familiar to the child. Target words selected for speech sound training should be useful and prevalent in the child's home and school and sensitive to the child's culture. The child's and the family members' disposition toward speech disabilities, their cultural values about effective communication, and their educational goals should be a basis to plan for effective intervention.

If a child needs treatment in a Native American language, only a clinician who can speak the language can offer it. The clinician who does not speak the relevant language should act as the child's advocate and find appropriate referral sources.

If a Native American child who speaks English as a second language needs treatment in that language, the clinician should treat the child as he or she would a bilingual child or a child with an African American background. Treatment targets should be consistent with the Native American child's speech and language. For example, if in the child's native language certain consonants are *not* aspirated, the equivalent *aspirated* English sounds, if not aspirated, should still be acceptable. This rule may not hold, however, if the child and the family seek treatment with a goal of acquiring MAE. Then the acceptable productions would be the same as those set for a child whose language is MAE.

Spanish Language and Dialects

Children whose primary language is Spanish or who speak Spanish and English, with one of the two being a dominant language, are a significant number among minority ethnocultural groups. People whose primary language is a dialect of Spanish belong to different ethnocultural groups, often referred to by the term *Hispanic*. The term does not have ethnic or racial connotations; it refers only to an individual's Spanish background. Hispanics may be of different races; there are Black, brown, and White Hispanic persons. In more recent years, the use of the term *Latino* has been gaining acceptance, because the term *Hispanic* has colonial connotations of Spain's dominance over people in most parts of the Americas (Iglesias, 2002). In this chapter, the terms *Hispanic* and *Latino* are used interchangeably, as they are by the U.S. Census Bureau (http://www.census.gov).

Latinos, though they share a Spanish cultural or Spanish language heritage, are not a geographically or culturally homogeneous group; they are varied in the same way Asians are. People who speak a variety of Spanish outside Spain have a wide geographic distribution, spanning North, Central, and South America. Latinos of Mexican origin constitute the largest group in the United States. Other countries from which Hispanics hail include Puerto Rico, Cuba, Dominican Republic, Spain, Guatemala, El Salvador, Nicaragua, Costa Rica, Honduras, Panama, Colombia, Venezuela, Ecuador, Chile, Bolivia, Paraguay, Uruguay, and Argentina. Such a widespread geographic distribution of Hispanic peoples comes with varied culture, customs, language differences, and behavioral dispositions toward communication and its disorders.

Hispanics are a significant segment of the population in the United States; according to the 2010 census data, 50.5 million Hispanics live in the country, constituting 16% of the total U.S. population. Mexicans (63%), Puerto Ricans (9%), and Cubans (4%) add up to 76% of the Hispanics in the United States (http://www.census.gov).

Spanish is the second-most common language spoken in the United States. The different groups of Latinos in the country speak different varieties or dialects of Spanish. For example, the Spanish of the Mexican is different from the Spanish of the Bolivian, which is different from the Spanish of the Cuban. In essence, each geographic–cultural group speaks a different variety of Spanish. There are at least eight major dialects of American Spanish (Dalbor, 1980), named after their geographic locations: Mexican and Southwestern United States, Central American, Caribbean, Highlandian, Chilean, Southern Paraguayan, Uruguayan, and Argentinean. In the United States, Spanish of the Mexican, Puerto Rican, and Caribbean (especially Cuban) varieties are spoken most commonly.

Hispanic children may be monolingual English speakers, monolingual Spanish speakers, English–Spanish bilingual speakers with good fluency in both, or bilingual speakers with one dominant and one weak language. To assess and treat communication disorders in Latino children, clinicians should have a good understanding of their cultural and linguistic heritage. This chapter summarizes only phonological characteristics, development, assessment, and treatment of children with a Spanish linguistic background. Clinicians should consult other sources to gain a broader understanding of Latino people and their culture, language, and communication patterns (Brice, 2002; Brice & Brice, 2009; B. A. Goldstein, 1995, 2000, 2004; Iglesias, 2002; Kayser, 1995, 1998; Kohnert, 2007; Langdon & Cheng, 1992; Perez, 1994; Roseberry-McKibbin, 2002; Yavas & Goldstein, 1998; Zuniga, 1992).

To assess English articulatory skills in Latino children, clinicians need to know the major language characteristics of Spanish that influence English expressions. It is not possible to provide a detailed description of the Spanish language in this chapter; however, a brief summary of some major language differences found in children of Hispanic background is provided in Table 5.3.

Speech Sound Patterns of Spanish-Influenced English

Children whose primary language is Spanish but who speak English as their second language may exhibit Spanish phonological characteristics. A proper assessment of speech sound disorders in such children should take into consideration those variations in English articulation that are presumably due to the characteristics of Spanish, their first language.

The Spanish phonological system is somewhat simpler than that of English (Stockwell & Bowen, 1983). Both languages contain two glides (semivowels): /j/ and /w/. However, English has three times more vowels (15) than Spanish (5). The five Spanish vowels are /i/

Table 5.3

MAJOR LANGUAGE DIFFERENCES FOUND IN CHILDREN
OF HISPANIC BACKGROUND

Spanish Language Characteristics	Sample English Utterances
The adjective comes after the noun.	The house green. . .
s is often omitted in plurals and possessives.	The girl book is. . .
Past-tense -ed is often omitted.	We walk yesterday.
Double negatives are required.	I don't have no more.
Superiority is demonstrated by using mas (more).	This cake is more big.
The adverb often follows the verb.	He drives very fast his motorcycle.

Note. Adapted from *Multicultural Students With Special Language Needs* (Table 6.1, p. 67), by C. Roseberry-McKibbin, 1995, Oceanside, CA: Academic Communication Associates. Copyright 1995 by Academic Communication Associates. Reprinted with permission.

and /ɛ/ (front vowels) and /u/, /o/, and /a/ (back vowels). While English contains 24 consonants, general Spanish contains 18. The English consonants /v/, /θ/, /ð/, /z/, and /ʒ/ are absent in Spanish. Some of these consonants may be produced as allophonic variations of consonants that are present in Spanish. For example, a /d/ may be produced as /ð/. Some Spanish consonants, though comparable to English consonants, may be produced differently in the two languages. For example, many Spanish consonants are unaspirated. The Spanish consonants /ŋ/, /λ/, /ɣ/, /χ/, /r̃/, and /β/ are absent in English (Perez, 1994).

Some sounds that are grossly similar in English and Spanish are produced differently. For example, /t/ and /d/, which are apical and aspirated in English, are dentalized and unaspirated in Spanish. Compared to English, Spanish has fewer consonants in word-final positions. Only /s/, /n/, /r/, /l/, and /d/ are produced in word-final positions. Therefore, omission of final consonants may be more frequently observed in native Spanish speakers who speak English as their second language.

Spanish and English differ in their consonantal blends. Spanish consonantal clusters are fewer and simpler. The /s/ cluster, common in word-initial positions in English (e.g., *school*), does not occur in Spanish (*escuela* for *school*). While medial consonantal clusters are common in both languages, final clusters are rare in Spanish; both languages contain /l/ and /r/ clusters (Stockwell & Bowen, 1983).

Tables 5.3 and 5.4 provide a summary of some of the major characteristics of Spanish-influenced English.

ACTIVITY

Identify the following: the projected number of Hispanics who will live in the United States by the year 2050, the eight major dialects of Spanish spoken in the United States, the number of consonants that make up the Spanish language, the English consonants that are absent in Spanish, the only consonants in Spanish that are produced in the final position of words.

Table 5.4

MAJOR ARTICULATORY AND PHONOLOGICAL CHARACTERISTICS
OF SPANISH-INFLUENCED ENGLISH

Spanish Articulation Characteristics	Sample English Patterns
Possible dentalization of /t, d, n/ (tip of tongue placed against back of upper central incisors)	
Frequent devoicing of final consonants b/v substitution	dose/doze berry/very
Deaspiration of stops (sound seems to be omitted because said with little air release)	
ch/sh substitution	Chirley/Shirley
/d/ voiced *th*, /z/ voiced *th* (no voiced *th* in Spanish)	dis/this, zat/that
/t/ voiceless *th* (no voiceless *th* in Spanish)	tink/think
Insertion of schwa sound before word-initial consonant clusters	eskate/skate espend/spend
10 different word-ending sounds: *a, e, i, o, u, ɪ, r, n, s, d*	word-ending sounds may be omitted
Silent /h/ in word starting with /h/	'old/hold, 'it/hit
/r/ tapped or trilled (tapped /r/ similar to tap in English word *butter*)	
No /ʤ/ sound (e.g., in *judge*); y sometimes substituted	yulie/julie
Frontal /s/ produced more frontally than in English	Possible frontal lisp sound
ñ pronounced like ny (e.g., *baño* = bahnyo)	
ee/ɪ and ĕ/, ah/ă substitutions due to 5 vowels—*a, e, i, o, u* (ah, ĕ, ee, o, oo)— and few diphthongs	peeg/pig, leetl/little pet/pat, stahn/stan

Note. Adapted from *Multicultural Students With Special Language Needs* (Table 6.2, p. 68), by C. Roseberry-McKibbin, 1995, Oceanside, CA: Academic Communication associates. Copyright 1995 by Academic Communication Associates. Reprinted with permission.

Speech Sound Learning in Latino Children

Researchers on speech sound learning in children of Spanish background have used varied methods and subject populations (Brice & Brice, 2009; B. A. Goldstein, 1995, 2000, 2004; Kohnert, 2007). Some investigators have sampled monolingual Spanish-speaking children, while others have sampled English–Spanish bilingual children with varying degrees of proficiency in each language. A majority of studies have sampled Spanish-speaking children in Mexico and the United States. Data have been reported also on Dominican, Puerto Rican, Bolivian, and Venezuelan children living in the United States (B. A. Goldstein, 2004; B. A. Goldstein, Fabiano, & Washington, 2005; Kayser, 1995). Most studies have used the cross-sectional method of simultaneously sampling children from different age groups.

Studies on typical speech sound learning in Spanish-speaking children include those by Acevedo (1991); De la Fuente (1985); Fabiano-Smith and Goldstein (2010a, 2010b); B. A. Goldstein (1988); B. A. Goldstein, Fabiano, and Washington (2005); B. A. Goldstein and Iglesias (1996); Gonzalez (1981); Jimenez (1987); Linares (1981); and M. Mason, Smith, and Hinshaw (1976). However, only a few investigators have analyzed speech sound production in Spanish-speaking or English–Spanish bilingual children with speech sound disorders (B. A. Goldstein, 1993; Meza, 1983).

The results of several studies of normally developing Spanish- or Spanish–English-speaking children may be summarized as follows (Brice & Brice, 2009; B. A. Goldstein, 1995, 2004; Kayser, 1995). Normally developing infants of Spanish background produce CV syllables containing oral and nasal stops and front vowels. Spanish-speaking children master the basic five vowels by age 18 months. Most Spanish phonemes are mastered by age 4. Dialectal features of the child's community may be evident by age 3. Some phonemes, especially [ð], [χ], [s], [n], [tʃ], [r], and [l], may still be difficult for children at the end of their preschool years. Consonant clusters also may remain difficult. Such phonological patterns as cluster reduction, unstressed syllable deletion, stridency deletion, and tap or trill /r/ deviations may still be evident by the end of preschool. However, such phonological patterns as velar and palatal fronting, prevocalic singleton omission, stopping, and assimilation may no longer be evident in the speech of those children. During the early elementary years, some children may still exhibit errors on the fricatives, affricates, liquids, and consonant clusters (B. A. Goldstein, 1995). Generally, phoneme acquisition in monolingual Spanish-speaking children is similar to that in monolingual English-speaking children (B. A. Goldstein, 2004; B. A. Goldstein et al., 2005).

Phonological patterns and articulatory errors found in Spanish-speaking children are similar to those found in English-speaking children. Vowel errors are few, but they do exist. Errors on /o/ may be the most frequent (B. A. Goldstein & Pollock, 2000). A majority of children with phonological disorders tend to exhibit cluster reduction, unstressed syllable deletion, stopping, liquid simplification, and assimilation. These patterns are similar to those found in children who speak American English. There may be some exceptions, however. For example, Spanish-speaking children may exhibit unstressed syllable deletion longer than English-speaking children mainly because of the generally longer words in Spanish (B. A. Goldstein et al., 2005).

Spanish–English-speaking bilingual children at age 4 may make more consonant and vowel errors in English. They may exhibit a greater number of phonological patterns and for longer duration than monolingual English- or Spanish-speaking children. Intelligibility of English speech in bilingual children also may be lower than that in monolingual English-speaking or Spanish-speaking children (Gildersleeve, Davis, & Stubble, 1996; Gildersleeve-Neumann & Davis, 1998). With increasing age, such differences in bilingual children tend to decrease, however.

B. A. Goldstein and colleagues (2005) evaluated phonological skills in children who were predominantly either English- or Spanish-speaking and compared them with the skills of Spanish–English bilingual children. The results of their study did not reveal significant differences in the phonological skills of 5-year-old children who spoke only one language (Spanish or English) or spoke both languages. The mono- or bilingual status of children was determined by parental report, not by language samples. Additional studies by Fabiano-Smith and

Goldstein (2010a, 2010b) involving 24 typical 3- to 4-year-old children with low socioeconomic status have shown that Spanish–English-speaking bilingual children may attain overall speech sound mastery at a slower rate, although still within the normal limits. Accuracy of both Spanish and English consonant production was somewhat lower for bilingual children than it was for monolingual children speaking either language. Bilingual children performed generally well on sounds that are shared in the two languages. Frequency of occurrence of sounds in Spanish, however, did not correlate well with accuracy of consonant production in that language. Similarly, bilingual children's accuracy of English consonant productions did not correlate well with the frequency of occurrence of English consonants.

Further research is needed to answer the following questions: (1) whether Spanish–English bilingual children have poorer phonological skills than monolingual children, as indicated in the Gildersleeve-Neumann and Davis (1998) study; (2) whether the skills in the two languages are comparable, as indicated in B. A. Goldstein and colleagues' (2005) study; (3) whether any difference that may exist is limited to younger children; (4) whether bilingualism has any negative effect on the rate of speech sound learning or mastery levels of that learning at any given age, as suggested by the Fabiano-Smith and Goldstein (2010a, 2010b) studies; and (5) whether frequency of occurrence of consonants in the two languages are related to speedier or more accurate speech sound learning, as suggested by Paradis and Genesee (1996) but contradicted by Fabiano-Smith and Goldstein (2010a, 2010b). Research also needs a method that is more valid than parental reports to establish the mono- or bilingual status of children.

Assessment of Speech Sound Disorders in Latino Children

Assessment of speech sound skills of bilingual Latino children poses the same challenges clinicians face in providing services to any bilingual client. The standard question is whether to assess the child in Spanish, in English, or in both. To answer this question, the clinician should determine the dominant language for each child. As we noted earlier, parental report is often used; a rough gauge of the number of hours spent speaking the two languages also may be used. Better skills in one of the two languages may be a deciding factor, as may be the number of months or years spent speaking or learning each language. A first-grade child who has been speaking Spanish all along and is just now beginning to learn English will have stronger Spanish than English. It is obvious that the variables that affect language dominance interact with each other to produce the final outcome.

It is likely that a disorder found in one language will be found in the other language, as well. It is probably unusual to see a child with a significant phonological disorder (not just differences) in one language but normal phonological skills in the other. Therefore, unless the child is a monolingual English speaker of Hispanic background, assessment must be completed in both Spanish and English.

To assess a child's Spanish speech and language skills, clinicians should have Spanish fluency or access to a professionally trained interpreter. This interpreter should speak the same dialectal form of Spanish (e.g., Cuban, Mexican) as the child and should have training in interpretation and some background in clinical linguistics. The interpreter should provide the stimuli and administer sound evocation procedures in the same manner as the clinician. He or she should have adequate training in response recording and scoring.

Clinicians may administer standardized Spanish tests of speech sound production. The interpreter who helps the clinician should have adequate training in standardized test administration, response recording, and scoring according to the test manual. Although they may not be suitable to assess children of all ethnocultural backgrounds who speak Spanish, several standardized Spanish tests are now available:

- *Spanish Preschool Articulation Test* (Tsugawa, 2002). Helps assess Spanish phoneme production in children within the age range of 2-6 through 5-5; standard and percentile scores are provided for the different age groups.
- *Preschool Language Scale–5, Spanish Screening Test* (Zimmerman, Steiner, & Evatt-Pond, 2012b). A Spanish screening test that includes an articulation and connected speech screening, among other language measures.
- *Preschool Language Scale, Fifth Edition Spanish* (Zimmerman, Steiner, & Evatt-Pond, 2012a). A Spanish language test that includes items to assess speech sound productions.
- *Assessment of Phonological Processes–Spanish* (Hodson, 1986). Helps identify phonological processes in unintelligible Spanish-speaking children. Identifies priority patterns for intervention.
- *Spanish Articulation Measures, Revised Edition* (SAM; Mattes, 1994). Helps screen or assess Spanish consonant production and phonological patterns in children 3 years and older; includes criterion-referenced probes for speech sound productions in conversational speech, as well as normative information on speech sound learning in Spanish.
- *Spanish Language Assessment Procedure, Third Edition* (Mattes, 1995). A Spanish language test that includes an articulation screening test.
- *Test of Phonological Awareness in Spanish–TPAS* (Riccio, Imhoff, Hasbrouck, & Davis, 2004). Helps assess phonological awareness in children age 4-0 through 10-11 by testing initial and final sound matching in target words, rhyming, and sound deletions.
- *Contextual Probes of Articulation Competence–Spanish* (B. A. Goldstein & Iglesias, 2006). Offers both a quick screen and full assessment test; helps assess frequently occurring phonological patterns; probes the production of all Spanish sounds in a variety of phonetic and phonological contexts and identifies facilitating (correct) contexts.

Many tests are available if the assessment goal is to sample productions of English phonemes, as well. These tests and related procedures are described in Chapter 6. One English test that is also sensitive to certain Spanish patterns of production is the *Fisher-Logemann Test of Articulation Competence* (Fisher & Logemann, 1971). This test samples consonants in the intervocalic positions, in which many Spanish consonants are produced. Therefore, the test may help assess articulation differences in English that are influenced by Spanish (Perez, 1994).

Assessment of articulatory and phonological skills should include a comprehensive speech sample. Clinical decisions should not be based solely on the results of standardized tests, as most of them assess phoneme productions in single, isolated words. Dialectal differences and phoneme productions in connected speech are important to assess. Properly structured speech samples, collected with client- and culture-specific stimuli and considerations, also avoid the biases inherent to standardized tests.

To diagnose speech sound disorders in bilingual children, the assessment data should be analyzed to describe a child's articulatory and phonological skills in Spanish and English. Yavas and Goldstein (1998) suggest that the clinician should describe (1) common and uncommon phonological patterns in the first and second languages, (2) bilingual phonological patterns, (3) interference patterns, and (4) dialectal features.

Research on several language families suggests *common and uncommon phonological patterns across languages* (see Yavas, 1994, 1998, and Yavas & Goldstein, 1998, for a review of studies). For example, such phonological patterns as cluster reduction, final consonant deletion, final consonant devoicing, stopping, velar fronting, palatal fronting, liquid simplification, labial assimilation, velar assimilation, nasal assimilation, and weak syllable deletion are common across many languages, including those belonging to such different families as Germanic (English and Swedish), Romance (Portuguese, Spanish, and Italian), Sino-Tibetan (Cantonese), and Altaic (Turkish). These phonological patterns represent simplified productions of adult models.

Although the patterns just described are common across languages, a particular pattern may not exist in a specific language. For example, children learning a language that does not have consonant clusters (e.g., Turkish) obviously could not exhibit consonant cluster reduction. Another notable fact about patterns across languages is that individual sounds may be differently affected within the same pattern. For example, although liquid simplification or substitution is a common pattern across languages, different sounds may be substituted for the liquids in different languages. In English, /w/ is a typical substitution for /r/. However, /r/ may be replaced by /l/ in Portuguese, /d/ in Spanish, and /h/ in Swedish (Yavas & Goldstein, 1998).

Common patterns found in children who are normally learning different languages also are found in children with speech sound disorders. As in any language, patterns of simplification that persist beyond certain age limits are considered clinically significant. Beyond the common patterns, children who exhibit clinically significant speech sound disorders also exhibit some uncommon patterns. Uncommon patterns are those that are found in the speech of children with a diagnosis of a speech sound disorder but are not found in the speech of normally developing children (Yavas & Goldstein, 1998). Examples of uncommon phonological patterns given by Yavas and Goldstein include unusual cluster reduction (e.g., *ren* for *train*), initial consonant deletion (*ep* for *tape*), liquid nasalization (substitution of /m/ for /l/ in Portuguese), frication of stops (e.g., *van* for *ban*), nasal gliding (e.g., /j/ for /l/), and delabialization (e.g., /s/ for /b/). Of the several unusual patterns, only two—initial consonant deletion and backing—have been documented in all languages studied so far. Unusual cluster deletion is also common across languages, except for Turkish. Liquid nasalization was found only in Portuguese and Swedish; frication of stops is evident in English and Spanish; nasal gliding is documented in Portuguese, Italian, and Swedish; and delabialization is reported only in Swedish (Yavas & Goldstein, 1998). Such generalizations may change when other languages are studied, however.

Identifying *patterns of speech sound production*—another goal of assessment—needs more research. Clinicians cannot make valid clinical judgments based on data separately gathered on English and Spanish speech sound learning. Clinical judgments should be based on dual patterns of learning in bilingual children. We have earlier noted some conflicting data on patterns of speech sound learning in monolingual and bilingual children (Fabiano-Smith & Goldstein, 2010a, 2010b; Gildersleeve, Davis, & Stubble, 1996; Gildersleeve-Neumann & Davis, 1998; B. A. Goldstein et al., 2005). We need more firm evidence to conclude that at all age levels, monolingual and bilingual children learn their speech sound patterns either in the same manner or in a different manner.

It is known that in bilingual speakers the speech sound patterns of one language influence the other. Therefore, *describing patterns of interference* from one language to the other is an important goal of assessment of bilingual children (Yavas & Goldstein, 1998). Weinreich (1953) has described certain patterns of bilingual interference. For instance, a bilingual child may confuse two phonemes in the second language if they are not differentiated in the primary language. A child whose primary language is Spanish may treat the English /d/ and /ð/ as the same because in Spanish, they are not separate phonemes but only allophonic variations. On the other hand, a bilingual child may produce two allophonic variations of the same sound in the second language as two separate sounds because they are separate in the primary language. A child whose primary language is English might produce the Spanish /d/ and /ð/ as separate phonemes because they are separate in English.

Yavas and Goldstein (1998) also suggest that besides segmental interference (interference at the phoneme level), there may be rhythmic interference due to differences in language. Syllable duration errors (syllables that sound too short or too long to a native speaker) and variations in syllable stress patterns (stressing the wrong syllable, failing to stress the right syllable) may be observed because of such differences in the two languages of a bilingual child.

It is common knowledge that learning two languages may result in a dialectal variation of the second language. Thus, description of the dialectal features of a bilingual child is another important goal of assessment (Yavas & Goldstein, 1998). Because no dialectal variation of any language is a disorder (American Speech-Language-Hearing Association, 1983), a diagnosis of a speech sound disorder is not made on the basis of dialectal variations. As noted previously in the context of African American English, a variation is an error only when it is so in the primary language.

In essence, an appropriate assessment of bilingual children's speech sound skills accounts for the features and characteristics of the primary and the secondary language of the child. Persistence of error patterns beyond the expected age range is still the main criterion for diagnosis of a disorder. However, distinguishing error patterns from variations due to interference requires a clear knowledge of the structure and use of the two languages a child speaks.

Treatment of Speech Sound Disorders in Latino Children

Generally, information on speech sound patterns in bilingual children is more extensive than that on treatment. There is no controlled evidence that shows that treatment of bilingual children involves unique principles. Until such evidence is produced, it is appropriate to assume that basic treatment principles, described in Chapter 7, and typically used in treating monolingual children with speech sound disorders, will hold well in treating bilingual children. All children need specification of acceptable and unacceptable responses, manipulation of physical stimuli (e.g., pictures), modeling of correct responses, shaping when necessary, reinforcement for correct production, corrective feedback for incorrect responses, sequencing treatment from simpler to more complex response topographies, parent training in supporting newly acquired skills in naturalistic settings, and so forth (Hegde, 1998, 2008a, 2008b).

Within the broadly applicable treatment procedures, different procedures may be more or less effective with certain children. Selection of stimuli, for example, should be consistent with the child's home environment and culture. Stimuli unfamiliar to the child may be ineffective or inefficient. Certain kinds of reinforcers may be more or less effective with specific children (Hegde, 1998).

Some general guidelines on treating bilingual children include the following from Yavas and Goldstein (1998). First, the clinician should treat phonological patterns exhibited with similar error rates in the two languages. The deviant patterns may have to be treated in both languages, as they are likely to be exhibited in both. In selecting initial treatment targets, the clinician should consider the nature of the two languages. For instance, if a language does not have many final consonants (e.g., Spanish), final consonant deletion would not be an initial treatment target.

Second, the clinician should treat phonological patterns that are exhibited in the two languages with unequal frequency. For instance, final consonant deletion will affect English and Spanish unequally. The deletion problem will be more serious in English than in Spanish. Nonetheless, the problem will affect intelligibility in both languages. Hence, it is appropriate to treat the pattern in both.

Third, the clinician should treat patterns that are evident in only one language. After treating errors that are exhibited in both languages with equal and unequal frequency, the clinician should make a quick assessment to isolate the deviant patterns in one or the other language. The clinician would then target those patterns for treatment. For example, final consonant devoicing is likely to be found in both Spanish–English bilingual children and monolingual English-speaking children. Therefore, final consonant devoicing would be a treatment target for these two groups. However, that pattern is not commonly found in monolingual Spanish-speaking children, for whom it is not a treatment target (Yavas & Goldstein, 1998).

Asian and Pacific Islander Languages

Asians are a significant minority population in the United States. Speech–language pathologists working in public schools are likely to encounter many children of Asian backgrounds who may be in need of clinical services. Unfortunately, treating language and phonological disorders in children of Asian backgrounds poses significant challenges to speech–language pathologists because of the enormous variety of languages and numerous dialects that exist in Asia.

People living in Asian countries and the Pacific Islands are ethnoculturally and linguistically so varied that the terms *Asian* and *Pacific Islander* do not do them justice;

the terms have only helped create some stereotypes. People living in China, the Indian subcontinent, Southeast Asia, and the Pacific Islands are culturally and linguistically different from one another. Even within Southeast Asia, countries are culturally and linguistically varied. For example, Vietnamese and Malaysians and Indonesians and Thai people have contrasting religions, customs, and languages. Many countries have multiple languages and dialectal variations. China alone has more than 80 languages and countless dialectal variations (Cheng, 1991, 1995, 2002). There are more than 20 major languages in India, each having numerous dialects (Shekar & Hegde, 1996). The vast region of Asia is home for many language families including (1) Sino-Tibetan (e.g., Thai, Yao, Mandarin, Cantonese); (2) Indo-Aryan, Indo-European, or Indic (e.g., Hindi, Bengali, Marathi); (3) Dravidian (e.g., Kannada, Tamil, Telugu, Malayalam); (4) Austro-Asiatic (e.g., Khmer, Vietnamese, Hmong); (5) Tibeto-Burman (e.g., Tibetan and Burmese); (6) Malayo-Polynesian or Austronesian (e.g., Chamorro, Ilocano, Tagalog); (7) Papuan (e.g., New Guinean); and (8) Altaic (e.g., Japanese, Korean).

Many Asian-born Americans are bilingual or even multilingual speakers and speak English that is influenced by their native language. They vary from one another in how they speak English because of their diverse native languages. Some general characteristics of Asian American English are summarized in Table 5.5.

It is quite possible that some of the characteristics listed in the table do not apply to all Asian speakers. Therefore, clinicians should not entertain linguistic stereotypes about Asian languages or speakers of Asian background.

Phonological Characteristics of Asian Languages

Because of the wide variety of languages and language families that exist in Asia, it is not possible to describe a single set of phonological patterns of *Asian languages*. One would have to describe many patterns. Only certain major phonological characteristics of Asian languages can be highlighted. A list of such characteristics is included in Table 5.6.

Once again, it should be noted that the phonological characteristics listed in the table may not hold true for all speakers of Asian languages. Because it is not possible to give a detailed description of phonological patterns of hundreds of Asian languages, clinicians who assess Asian children should evaluate their phonological patterns according to those found in the child's first language. Clinicians should also develop local resources, including information on the phonological characteristics of Asian languages spoken in their service area, and consult linguistic experts in regional universities who specialize in those languages.

Clinicians face different challenges in different parts of the United States. For instance, the Hmong are concentrated in a few states, including California and Minnesota. Clinicians who have Hmong in their service area need to develop information on their language. Chinese and Koreans are concentrated in several metropolitan areas, including San Francisco, New York, and Los Angeles. Asian Indians are concentrated in many metropolitan areas, including the San Francisco Bay area, Los Angeles, Chicago, and New York. Clinicians need to develop resources specific to the Asian languages they are expected to face in their service area. What follows is a description of a few specific phonological characteristics of selected Asian languages, as contrasted with those of English.

Table 5.5

MAJOR CHARACTERISTICS OF ENGLISH INFLUENCED BY ASIAN LANGUAGES

Asian Language Characteristics	Sample English Utterances
Omission of plurals	Here are two piece of toast. I got five finger on each hand.
Omission of copula	He going home now. They eating.
Omission of possessive	I have Phuong pencil. I like teacher dress.
Omission of past-tense morpheme	We cook dinner yesterday. Last night she walk home.
Past-tense double marking	He didn't went by himself.
Double negative	They don't have no books.
Subject–verb–object relationship differences/omissions	I messed up it. He like.
Singular present-tense omission or addition	You goes inside. He go to the store.
Misordering of interrogatives	You are going now?
Misuse or omission of prepositions	She is in home. He goes to school 8:00.
Misuse of pronouns	She husband is coming. She said her wife is here.
Omission or overgeneralization of articles	Boy is sick. He went the home.
Incorrect use of comparatives	This book is gooder than that book.
Omission of conjunctions	You I going to the beach.
Omission of, lack of inflection on auxiliary *do*	She not take it. He do not have enough.
Omission of, lack of inflection on forms of *have*	She have no money. We been the store.
Omission of articles	I see little cat.

Note. Adapted from *Multicultural Students With Special Language Needs* (Table 7.1, p. 81), by C. Roseberry-McKibbin, 1995, Oceanside, CA: Academic Communication Associates. Copyright 1995 by Academic Communication Associates. Reprinted with permission.

Chinese Versus English

Cantonese and Mandarin are the two main dialects of Chinese spoken in the United States. The majority of Chinese Americans speak Cantonese (Li & Thompson, 1987). The dialectal variations of Chinese may be mutually unintelligible. Words in both dialects are written logographically: Each word is a graphic symbol, not a combination of letters. Across dialects, words are written similarly although pronounced differently. Thus, even though the spoken forms of dialects are mutually incomprehensible, printed forms are intelligible. Chinese is a tonal language; the same word can have different meanings when spoken with

Table 5.6

MAJOR ARTICULATORY AND PHONOLOGICAL CHARACTERISTICS OF ENGLISH INFLUENCED BY ASIAN LANGUAGES

Asian Articulation Characteristics	Sample English Utterances
Deletion of final consonants in English.	ste/step, li/lid
Reduction of polysyllabic words	effunt/elephant
Wrong syllabic stress patterns	di versity/diversity
Possible devoicing of voiced cognates	beece/bees, pick/pig
r/l substitution	lize/rise, clown/crown
/r/ omission	gull/girl, tone/torn
No voiced or voiceless *th*	dose/those, tin/thin zose/those, sin/thin
Epenthesis (addition of *uh* sound in blends, ends of words)	bulack/black, wooduh/wood
ʃ/tʃ substitution	sheep/cheap, beesh/beach
/æ/ nonexistent in many Asian languages	block/black, shock/shack
b/v substitutions	base/vase, beberly/Beverly
v/w substitutions	vork/work, vall/wall
p/f substitutions	pall/fall, plower/flower

Note. Adapted from *Multicultural Students With Special Language Needs* (Table 7.2, p. 82), by C. Roseberry-McKibbin, 1995, Oceanside, CA: Academic Communication Associates. Copyright 1995 by Academic Communication Associates. Reprinted with permission.

different vocal pitch. Different meanings may be communicated by the same word by saying it with high pitch, low pitch, rising pitch, or rising-then-falling pitch.

The Mandarin and Cantonese dialects of Chinese do not contain consonant clusters. Hence, learning such clusters in English can pose difficulty for a Chinese speaker. Also, unlike English, the two dialects of Chinese have relatively few sounds in word-final positions; Cantonese has seven final consonants, whereas Mandarin has only two. Therefore, Chinese speakers learning English may omit many final English consonants (e.g., *offi* for *office*, *fi* for *fish*; Cheng, 1991).

If a sound is similar in Chinese and English, a Chinese speaker may substitute the Chinese sound for the English sound. For example, a Cantonese speaker may substitute /ʃ/ for /s/, as these two sounds are phonetically similar in Chinese. Chinese speakers also may use a Chinese sound as a substitute for a sound that is present in English but absent in Chinese. For example, neither Mandarin nor Cantonese contains the English /θ/. Therefore, speakers of these two dialects may substitute /s/ for /θ/. Consequently, the speakers may say *sin* for *thin* (Cheng, 1991).

Two other variations found in speakers of Chinese include stress and intonational patterns. Syllable stress tends to be misplaced in speaking English. An intonational pattern that is more appropriate to Chinese may be heard in the English speech of native Chinese speakers.

Clinicians may consult Cheng (1991), Li and Thompson (1987), and Chan and Li (2000) for additional information on Chinese speech sound patterns and language production. Chan and Li (2000) describe Cantonese speech sound patterns and contrast them with English sound patterns.

South Asian Languages Versus English

South Asia includes the countries of the Indian subcontinent. This region is home to several language families, including the Indic languages of the Indo-European (Indic) family and the Dravidian languages. Indic languages are spoken mostly in Pakistan, Bangladesh, and northern parts of India. Indic is a large family of languages and includes Urdu, Hindi, Punjabi, Marathi, Bengali, Gujarathi, Sindhi, Oriya, and Assamese. Most of these languages are derived or heavily influenced by Sanskrit, an ancient Indo-European language of India. Although these languages share many common features, there are significant differences among them. Hindi, being a dominant language of northern India, is the official language of the country (Shekar & Hegde, 1995, 1996).

Dravidian languages are spoken mostly in the four states of south India. Kannada, Tamil, Telugu, and Malayalam are the four major languages of the Dravidian family. There has been significant borrowing among the languages of the Indo-European and Dravidian families, and both families have heavily borrowed from Sanskrit, forming common words between most Indian languages.

The sound systems of the Indic and Dravidian languages share many common features. For example, Hindi, an Indic language, has five short vowels with their long counterparts. Kannada, a Dravidian language, has the same number and variety of vowels. The vowel length is phonemic in both languages. However, Hindi has nasalized vowels, and nasalization of vowels can make a difference in meaning. In Kannada, and other Dravidian languages, nasalized vowels may be heard in some dialects, but they do not make a difference in meaning. Syllabic stress is typically not distinctive in most languages of India (Shekar & Hegde, 1995, 1996).

A distinguishing feature of most languages of India is their aspirated stops. Both the Indic and Dravidian languages have aspirated stops of both the velar (e.g., gh) and bilabial (bh) variety. Another distinguishing feature is their retroflex consonants. For example, the English /d/, /t/, and /l/ have retroflex variations in most languages of India. Yet another feature of the languages of India is the lack of difference between the English /v/ and /w/ in many contexts. In most languages, /v/ is a bilabial fricative (as against the labiodental fricative in English). When /v/ is followed by a back vowel, it is pronounced as a /w/. These are among several features of the languages of India that create difficulties for Asian Indians who speak English as their second language (Shekar & Hegde, 1995, 1996).

Languages of India differ in their tonal characteristics. Asian Indians who speak English as their second language may often exhibit a rhythm that is different from the native English rhythm. Because the languages of India are phonetic (each sound is represented by a letter of the alphabet), there usually is no confusion between printed words and their pronunciation. Therefore, Asian Indians learning English may find the phonetic realization of printed English confusing or difficult. The English of Asian Indians has several other unique characteristics that are described in Shekar and Hegde (1996).

Southeast Asian Languages Versus English

Southeast Asian languages are spoken in Vietnam, Thailand, Laos, Cambodia, and Burma. Like most other parts of Asia, Southeast Asia is rich in linguistic diversity. Different language families are represented in the region. For example, Vietnamese is a member of the Mon-Khmer branch of the Austro-Asiatic family of languages, as is Khmer, the language of Cambodia. Hmong, another language of the region, is a member of the Sino-Tibetan linguistic family. Thai, or Tai, spoken in Thailand, is a member of the Kadai or KamTai language family. All these languages have numerous dialects.

Vietnamese is a phonemic, monosyllabic, tonal language. It has three major dialects (southern, central, and northern), each spoken in a different geographical region (Hwa-Froelich, Hodson, & Edwards, 2002). The influence of Chinese, Malay, and French on Vietnamese has been documented; about one-third of Vietnamese words are Chinese (McWhorter, 2000). Most educated Vietnamese speak a formal and an informal variety of their language. Vietnamese contains 22 consonants and 12 vowels (Hansen Edwards, 2006). The final consonants can be only a voiceless stop (/p/, /t/, and /k/) or a nasal (/n/ and /ŋ/). The majority of words in the language have only one syllable, although speakers speak not in monosyllabic words but in multisyllabic combinations of monosyllabic words (Hwa-Froelich et al., 2002; Thompson, 1965). Although a majority of syllables in Vietnamese are closed, the language does not contain consonantal clusters in word-final positions (Hansen Edwards, 2006). Therefore, Vietnamese speakers speaking English as a second language may correctly produce single-syllable final consonants but not syllable-final consonant clusters. Syllabic stress is not used to signal difference in meaning. Vietnamese speakers may have particular difficulty with the following English phonemes, which are absent in their language: /tʃ/, /θ/, /ð/, /p/, /g/, /dʒ/, /ʒ/, /s/, /v/, /i/, /ɛ/, /æ/, and /ʊ/.

The **Hmong** are originally from southern China but over the centuries have migrated to Southeast Asia, especially to Laos. Because of their work for the United States during the Vietnam War, the Hmong are now a significant minority in certain parts of the United States, predominantly in central California and parts of Minnesota and Wisconsin. There are just over 260,000 Hmong Americans (http://www.hmong.org). Several dialects of Hmong are spoken in Laos, Thailand, Vietnam, and China, but Hmong Americans tend to speak one of two main dialects: White (Hmoob Dawb) or Green (Moob Leeg). A writing system, developed only in the 1950s, is based on the White Hmong. Although Hmong has 56 initial consonants, it has only a single final consonant, /ŋ/. Many consonants have aspirated and unaspirated varieties. The sound comparable to English /r/ is a stop, not a liquid. Its aspirated form may sound like /t/, and its unaspirated form may sound like /d/ (Cheng, 1991, 2002). Consonant clusters are produced only in the initial position of words. English sounds /z/ and /w/ are absent in Hmong. The language also lacks English central vowels that have an /r/ coloring.

Hmong is a tonal language. Meaning is distinguished by eight tones: high, high falling, mid-rising, mid, low, low breathing, short low, and abrupt end. There are 13 vowels in the White dialect and 14 in the Green dialect; none are reduced to the schwa. Six basic vowels, two nasalized vowels, and five diphthongs complete the vowel inventory.

English final consonants and final consonant clusters may pose a particular difficulty for Hmong speakers. They also may pronounce with undue stress the English vowels that are unaccented and often reduced to the schwa (Cheng, 2002). When compared to younger

Hmong children, older Hmong children have better English-language skills than Hmong-language skills, suggesting that their English begins to dominate their native language (Kan & Kohnert, 2005).

Khmer is the language of Cambodia. However, Cambodians also speak French, Thai, Lao, Chinese, and Vietnamese. One aspect that distinguishes Khmer from such other Southeast Asian languages as Laotian and Vietnamese is that it is not a tonal language. As in English, intonational contours vary within and across sentences. Khmer contains mostly disyllabic or monosyllabic words. In disyllabic words, Khmer speakers typically stress the second syllable. The Khmer alphabet is derived from Sanskrit and Pali, the two ancient languages of India. While many classic Khmer words are derived from Sanskrit, most contemporary and technical words are derived from French (Cheng, 1991).

Khmer contains both aspirated and unaspirated consonants. The language contains only two fricatives but contains 50 vowels and diphthongs. Both short and long vowels exist in the language. Khmer has extensive and unusual consonantal clusters. It has 85 initial consonantal clusters but no final clusters. The language contains many initial clusters that do not exist in English. For example, clusters that are in Khmer but absent in English combine the following sounds: *mty, sd,* and *kn* (Cheng, 1991, 2002).

Some Khmer speakers who speak English as their second language tend to exhibit the following substitutions: /k/ for /g/, /v/ for /w/, /f/ for /b/, /tʃ/ for /s/, and /s/ or /t/ for /θ/. Omission of several final consonants, including /r/, /d/, /g/, /s/, /b/, and /z/, also may be noted in Cambodian English speakers (Cheng, 1991, 2002).

Thai is the official language of Thailand, and many scholars consider it a member of the Tai language family (Comrie, 1990; Hudak, 1990; Strecker, 1990). Thai is heavily influenced by the Sanskrit and Pali languages of ancient India.

Thai has 20 segmental consonants including aspirated consonants (e.g., k$^\text{h}$, as in Indic and Dravidian languages of India). All consonants are used in initial positions. Initial consonant clusters include the following: *pr, pl, phr, tr, thr, kr, kl, kw, khr, khl,* and *khw*. Final consonant clusters are not used in Thai (Hudak, 1990). The phonemes /r/ and /l/, though distinguished in Thai, may not be distinguished in fast conversational speech. Thus, some Thai people speaking English as a second language may confuse the two.

Thai has nine vowels. Each may be short or long. It also contains several corresponding diphthongs. The syllabic structures of Thai are associated with distinct tones, as Thai is a tonal language. The tones used in Thai include a low tone, a mid tone, a high tone, a falling tone, and a rising tone (Hudak, 1990). The final syllable in disyllabic and polysyllabic words receives the most prominent stress. Thus, a native Thai speaker may use different stress patterns than the usual ones when speaking English.

East Asian Languages Versus English

The Philippines, Korea, and Japan are among the East Asian countries from which significant numbers of individuals have migrated to the United States. Filipinos, the people of the Philippines, speak at least 75 languages, all belonging to the Malayo-Polynesian group. **Tagalog** is the national language of the Philippines. Ilocano and Visayan are among the other major languages spoken in this country of multiple islands.

Tagalog contains 16 consonants, five vowels, and six diphthongs. It does not contain the following nine English phonemes: /v/, /z/, /θ/, /ð/, /dʒ/, /f/, /ʃ/, /tʃ/, and /ʒ/. A Tagalog native speaker of English may omit some of those sounds. The Tagalog sounds /p/, /b/, /s/, and /t/ are similar to /f/, /v/, /z/, and /ð/ in English. Therefore, a native Tagalog speaker of English may substitute the former set of sounds for the latter.

Korean, the language of Korea, is a member of the Altaic language family, with significant Chinese influence (Ball & Rahilly, 1999; Ladefoged & Maddieson, 1996; Lee, 1999). The Koreans in the two countries (North and South Korea) speak the same language. Korean has several mutually intelligible dialects.

The Korean language has 21 consonants and 10 vowels (Kim, 1990). The language has no consonant clusters in word-initial or word-final positions. Therefore, English consonant clusters may be expected to create problems for a native Korean speaker. Fricatives and affricates occur only in word-initial and -final positions. Consequently, a native Korean speaker may have difficulty with English fricatives in word-final positions. Korean speakers of English tend to omit word-final fricatives. Korean /r/ and /l/ are allophonic variations of the same phoneme; therefore, while speaking English as a second language, Koreans may use one for the other (Cheng, 1991, 2002). Also, /l/ does not occur in initial position in Korean speech; it does occur in writing in the initial position, but in speech it is either deleted or pronounced as /n/. In most cases, /h/ in the word-medial (intervocalic) position is deleted (Kim, 1990).

Korean has no labiodental, interdental, or palatal fricatives. Consequently, some native Korean speakers who use English may exhibit the following substitutions: /b/ for /v/, /p/ for /v/, /s/ for /ʃ/, /t/ for /tʃ/, and /ʤ/ for /ð/.

A distinguishing feature of Korean is the tendency to nasalize a non-nasal stop if it occurs before a nasal sound in a word (Kim, 1990). The stops /k/, /p/, and /t/ are pronounced as /ŋ/, /n/, and /m/, respectively (Kim, 1990). Cheng (1991, 2002) gives the example of native Korean speakers who may say *banman* for *batman* in English. Korean vowels do not contrast in length. Therefore, English vowels that do contrast in length (e.g., /i/ vs. /I/) may be difficult for native Korean speakers.

Syllable stress is not a characteristic of Korean. Intonational variations, therefore, are minimal. Consequently, when native Korean speakers speak English, the speech may sound flat and monotonous. Expressing meaning through rising intonation, as in asking a question, may be difficult for Korean English speakers.

Japanese, spoken by the entire population of Japan, belongs, somewhat controversially, to the Altaic family of languages. Various scholars have suggested that Japanese is a member of the Indo-European, Sino-Tibetan, or Dravidian family. Modern written Japanese uses modified Chinese characters. Even though politically shielded from foreign influence or invasion in all its history, Japanese has a surprising number of foreign words, including numerous words from Chinese and several from Korean, Arabic, and Persian (Shibatani, 1990). Japanese is technically not a tonal language, although accentuation in it involves significant pitch differences.

Japanese has five standard vowels: /a/, /i/, /u/, /e/, and /o/. Some dialects have up to three additional vowels, and others have only three. In contrast to its counterpart in English, the Japanese /u/ is unrounded. Another contrast is that the high vowels /u/ and /i/ are devoiced (not pronounced) when they are surrounded by voiceless consonants. They are not devoiced in initial positions or when they are accented (Shibatani, 1990).

Japanese has 18 consonants, as well as some double consonants (e.g., /kk/ and /pp/). A significant characteristic of Japanese is the palatalization and affrication of dental consonants. For example, /s/ before /i/ is changed to /tʃ/; /z/ before /i/ or /u/ is changed to /dʒ/; /t/ before /i/ is changed to /tʃ/; and /d/ before /i/ is changed to /dʒ/ (Shibatani, 1990). The /n/ is the only word-final phoneme in Japanese.

Native Japanese speakers using English are likely to substitute /r/ for /l/, /s/ for /θ/, /z/ for /ð/, /j/ for /ð/, and /b/ for /v/. Japanese speakers also may add a vowel to words ending in consonants (e.g., *beddu* for *bed* or *milku* for *milk*) (Cheng, 1991).

Arabic Versus English

Arabic is the language of the Arabs. Most Arabs are Muslims, but not all Muslims speak Arabic. For example, Muslims in Pakistan and India do not speak Arabic; they speak an Indo-European language called Urdu. The term *Arab* does not refer to a race, religion, or nationality; it refers to the people of the Arabian Peninsula. Arabs may be of different races (e.g., Negro, Berber, or Semitic) and they live in different countries (M. E. Wilson, 1996).

Arabic is spoken predominantly in countries of the Middle East and North Africa (e.g., Egypt). There are many variations of this language, as it is spoken in Saudi Arabia, Jordan, Iraq, and many smaller Persian Gulf countries in the Arabian Peninsula, as well as Egypt, Sudan, Libya, Algeria, and Morocco in North Africa (W. F. Wilson, 1998).

More than 160 million people worldwide speak Arabic (M. E. Wilson, 1996). It is a member of the Semitic branch of the Afro-Asiatic family of languages, which comprises over 175 languages. Hebrew also is a member of this large language family (Hetzron, 1990). Arabic is a minority language in several countries around the world, including Russia, Iran, and the United States. Variations of classic Arabic are spoken by Muslims living in many countries on all continents (Kaye, 1990; W. F. Wilson, 1998). Arabic is the official language in 20 countries (M. E. Wilson, 1996).

Standard or classic Arabic has 28 consonants, although some sources indicate 32 consonants (Kaye, 1990; M. E. Wilson, 1996). It has several consonants that are absent in English (e.g., emphatic consonants, voiceless and voiced uvular and pharyngeal fricatives). Five emphatic consonants are /t/, /d/, /ð/, /s/, and /q/. The first four have non-emphatic cognates, transcribed without the underscore. Emphatic consonants in Arabic are produced with the root of the tongue retracted toward the back wall of the pharynx. Classic Arabic contains three basic vowels (/a/, /i/, and /u/) and their long versions, for a total of six. Modern variations of Arabic have borrowed or evolved such other vowels as /e/ and /o/. Various dialects of Arabic spoken in different countries have somewhat different consonant and vowel systems.

A few other unique characteristics of the Arabic phonological system are noteworthy. In many Arab dialects, /q/ may be voiced. The /p/ is absent in classic Arabic. However, in modern Arabic speech, /b/ that appears before a voiceless consonant may be devoiced to yield a /p/. In most linguistic contexts, many Arab speakers may simply substitute /p/ for /b/. Another sound absent in classic Arabic is /v/.

Stress is an ill-defined phenomenon in most Arabic dialects. Each of the four syllables in a word, for example, may receive stress in different dialects. Generally, stress is prominent (1) on the first syllable of a CV syllable, (2) on a long syllable in a word containing only one long syllable, and (3) on the long syllable toward the end of a word that contains multiple long syllables. Because of these differences, English stress patterns may pose special problems for native Arabic speakers who speak English.

A noteworthy feature of Arabic is that the written and spoken forms may be significantly different (Amayreh, 2003). Modern standard Arabic, the formal form of the language, is rarely spoken but is used mostly in religious contexts, drama, and literature. At home, on the street, and in shops, people speak mostly a colloquial variety of standard Arabic. Children begin to learn standard Arabic only when they enter school. Another noteworthy feature is that some consonants have variant forms—all accepted. For example, /q/ may be produced as [q], [k], [g], or /ʔ/; /ð/ may be produced as [ð] or [d]; /θ/ may be produced as [θ] or [t], and so forth.

....

ACTIVITY

Identify some phonological differences between English and the following Asian languages: Chinese, South Asian languages, Vietnamese, Hmong, Khmer, Tagalog, Japanese, Arabic.

....

Speech Sound Learning in Children Speaking Asian Languages

It is likely that the speech sound learning of Asian children in their home countries has been studied to various extents. Unfortunately, much of this information is not readily available to the U.S. clinicians. Detailed studies of speech sound learning of children speaking American English and a particular Asian language are not available, either. This is the kind of information most urgently needed for speech–language pathologists who need to assess and treat Asian American children with speech sound disorders.

A study of phonological acquisition in children speaking Cantonese was reported by So and Dodd (1994). The authors also reported data on children with phonological disorders. Generally, Cantonese children acquired their phonemes at a faster rate than English-speaking children. Anterior Cantonese phonemes were acquired sooner than were posterior phonemes. Oral and nasal stops and glides were acquired before fricatives and affricates. These are consistent with data on acquisition of English phonemes. Cantonese children exhibited phonological patterns that were similar to those found in English-speaking children.

So and Dodd (1994) reported that by age 4-0, Cantonese children exhibited phonological patterns relatively infrequently, but the patterns they exhibited were generally similar to those exhibited by children acquiring English phonemes. Children with a phonological delay or disorders tended to exhibit such phonological patterns as cluster reduction, affrication, final consonant deletion, final glide deletion, fronting, backing, and assimilation.

Amayreh and Dyson (1998) reported on the acquisition of Arabic phonemes in children living in Jordan. Note that this was not a report on English–Arabic bilingual children living in the United States. The data showed that, for the most part, the pattern of acquisition of Arabic phonemes was similar to that found for English first-language learning. At early age levels, medial consonants were produced more accurately than were final consonants. Stops (e.g., /b/, /t/, /d/, and /k/), fricatives and affricates (/f/, /h/), and sonorants (/m/, /n/, /l/, and /w/) were acquired the earliest (75% correct in all positions between the ages of 2-0 and 3-10). Other stops (e.g., /t/, /d/, /q/, and /ʔ/) were acquired late (after age 6-4). Acquisition of most other phonemes fell into an intermediate stage (between the ages 4-0 and 6-4). Arabic children acquired /b/, /t/, /d/, /k/, /f/, and /l/ earlier than the ages generally reported for those acquiring the same phonemes in English. On the other hand, five phonemes (/θ/, /ð/, /h/, /r/, and /j/) were acquired later in Arabic than in English (Amayreh & Dyson, 1998). A follow-up study (Amayreh, 2003) demonstrated that even 8-year-olds did not correctly produce some late consonants (e.g., /θ/, /ð/, /z/, /t/, /d/, /s/, /ð/, and /q/). Lack of mastery of these consonants even at age 8 was attributed to lack of input because of their absence in spoken Arabic and their increased difficulty of production (Amayreh, 2003).

Assessment of Speech Sound Disorders in Children of Asian Background

The sheer variety of Asian languages makes it extremely difficult for any clinician, including those of Asian background, to make an appropriate assessment of a bilingual Asian American child's speech production skills. In the absence of data on speech sound learning in many Asian American bilingual children, clinicians can assume that the patterns of development in such children are not radically different from those found in English phonological acquisition. Exceptions reported in the literature should be carefully noted, however. For example, Arabic children's acquisition of certain consonants may be more delayed than usual, although we do not know whether that trend will hold true in Arab American children. Clinicians can make tentative clinical decisions based on their knowledge of phonological acquisition in general and on what is known about the particular child's phonological patterns. Knowledge of parental expectations and educational and social demands made on the child will be helpful in making clinical decisions.

An important factor to take into consideration is the potential interference from the first language in the production of English phonemes. Therefore, a general understanding of the phonemes of the particular Asian language of the child and how they might affect the production of English phonemes would be helpful in assessing a child with a potential speech sound disorder. With the help of an interpreter and any available information on the phonological system of the child's first language, the clinician needs to determine what phonological patterns observed in English are consistent with the child's first language and what patterns are inconsistent and hence deviant. The overall approach to and philosophy of assessing a child with an Asian American background would be the same as those advocated for Spanish-speaking or African American children.

Treatment of Speech Sound Disorders in Children of Asian Background

There is little or no research that contradicts the assumption that evidence-based phonological treatment procedures (described in Chapter 7) may not be effective with children of Asian background. J. Ray (2002) has provided uncontrolled case study data to support the use of standard treatment with Asian American children who have speech sound disorders. Her study reported on a child of Asian Indian background who was exposed to two Indian languages at home and English in the school. In English, the child exhibited final consonant deletion, gliding of liquids, cluster reduction, deaspiration of stops in initial positions, and devoicing of final consonants. In the two Indian languages, the child exhibited the same three patterns—final consonant deletion, gliding of liquids, and cluster reduction. Treatment was offered only in English, and improvement in articulation was evident in all three languages.

Clinicians should experimentally evaluate the effectiveness of various treatment procedures in treating bilingual and multilingual children. Furthermore, in planning treatment, clinicians should consider the child's language and communication style and the influence of the first language on English.

The general guidelines offered for treating Spanish–English bilingual children also are relevant in planning treatment of speech sound disorders in children of Asian background. As suggested by Yavas and Goldstein (1998), deviant patterns evident in both languages, errors that are unevenly distributed in the two languages, and errors that are unique to one of the languages may all be targets of intervention.

Working With Children Who Speak Varied English Dialects: General Guidelines

Children speak a variety of English dialects because of different primary dialects and primary languages. African American children, for example, whose primary dialect is African American English are speaking a dialect of American English. Similarly, children who first learned a language other than English may speak a different dialect of English, learned as a second language.

In the previous sections of this chapter, we summarized assessment and treatment guidelines specific to each ethnocultural group. In this section, we summarize some general guidelines on working with children with varied English dialects because of their different ethnocultural and language backgrounds. In assessing and treating such children, the clinician should adopt as many of the following as are relevant and needed in a particular case:

- understand the characteristics of the child's first language (e.g., Spanish) or primary English dialect (e.g., AAE), including its phonological, morphologic, syntactic, and pragmatic features and how they contrast with those of English

- appreciate the communication style of the child and his or her family

- assess the family resources to obtain and continue treatment services for the child

- procure help, if needed, from government or other agencies that could support clinical services for the child

- appraise the family members' dispositions toward and beliefs regarding speech and language disorders, their causes, and chances of improvement

- obtain available information on the child's phonological development in his or her first language

- study the patterns of interference from the child's first language or English dialect (as in the case of an African American child)

- obtain the services of a competent interpreter who speaks the child's native language, if needed to complete assessment and treatment planning
- train the interpreter in conversational speech sampling, helping with clinical interviews, and test administration
- use standardized tests that have been normed on children from the particular ethnic or linguistic group the child client belongs to
- avoid tests that are known to be culture biased or suspected to be biased against the child's ethnocultural background
- let the conversational speech samples, preferably involving the parents, other family members, or caregivers, be the primary data for analysis of phonological skills
- analyze speech sound disorders in light of the first language or dialect of the child
- determine whether a disorder exists in both the languages or dialects spoken by the child
- make sure that multiple family members understand and agree with the treatment recommendations for the child
- select treatment targets in both the child's languages
- treat the disorder in the primary language as well as the second language or dialect
- assume tentatively that the basic treatment principles (e.g., modeling, shaping, positive reinforcement for correct productions, and corrective feedback for incorrect productions) may hold true for children of varied ethnocultural backgrounds
- expect to modify treatment procedures to suit the individual child (e.g., although the general principle of positive reinforcement may hold, a particular type of reinforcer, such as verbal praise, may be less effective than a token in a given case)
- carefully collect treatment data to sustain or modify the assumptions made in assessing and treating children
- target a dialect not spoken by the child for treatment (e.g., MAE for a child who speaks AAE) only if the family, the child, or both request it
- note that according to the position of the American Speech-Language-Hearing Association, no dialectal variation of a language is a deviation or a disorder
- develop resources on the language and culture of minority children in the service area; have a list of linguistic experts in local or regional universities, bilingual speech–language pathologists in the area, and consultants who might be of help
- identify various Web sites that provide information on different languages and cultures

- watch for new publications in professional journals on language and speech sound learning by minority children
- refer the child to a bilingual speech–language pathologist who speaks the child's language
- be the child's advocate

Summary of the Basic Unit

- Each language is spoken in its own manner. Each variation of a language is a dialect, and no dialect of a language is a basis on which to diagnose a language or speech sound disorder.

- To assess and treat articulation and phonological disorders in children who are bilingual, bidialectal, or both, the clinician needs to know the characteristics of the primary language or dialect.

- A dialectal variety of English that has received much attention is African American English (AAE), or Black English. AAE is not a substandard variety of Mainstream American English; it has its own phonological, syntactic, semantic, and pragmatic rules. The origin of AAE may have been a **pidgin,** a simple form of communication that develops between two verbal communities with no common language. A pidgin develops into a more complex **Creole** when it is passed on to the next generation as the primary means of communication.

- Native Americans speak a variety of languages; many Native American languages are either extinct or on the verge of extinction. Native American languages belong to different language families. Because of this, their phonological systems vary tremendously. Therefore, clinicians need to develop resources for given languages spoken in their service area.

- After English, Spanish is the second-most widely spoken language in the United States. People of Spanish background are classified as Hispanic or Latino, which does not refer to the race of an individual. Hispanics in the United States have origins in different countries, but most are from Mexico. Children who speak a version of Spanish as their primary language and then learn to speak English are likely to show a variety of phonological characteristics of their primary language.

- Asian American children are a linguistically and ethnoculturally diverse group. Children in this group as a whole speak many primary languages that belong to different language families, including the Indo-European and Dravidian (languages of India), Sino-Tibetan (languages of China, Thailand), Austro-Asiatic (languages of Vietnam, the Hmong), Tibeto-Burman (languages of Tibet, Burma), and Altaic (languages of Japan, Korea). Therefore, clinicians should develop resources on the Asian language or languages spoken in their service area.

- The clinician working with children of varied ethnocultural and linguistic backgrounds needs to follow certain guidelines as summarized in the preceding section of this chapter.

Advanced Unit: Theoretical and Clinical Issues

In the Basic Unit of this chapter, we have summarized research on dialectal variations typically found in children belonging to various ethnocultural and linguistic minority groups. In this Advanced Unit, we will take a look at some theoretical and clinical issues that are relevant to bilingualism and bidialectalism. Whether the issues discussed in bilingualism also are relevant for a more complete understanding of African American (AA) children may be debatable. The difference between AA children who speak African American English (AAE) and those who speak English as a second language is obvious: Though it might influence learning of MAE, AAE is itself an English dialect; therefore, AA children are not bilingual. Nonetheless, potentially important technical similarities between AA children and bilingual children cannot be ruled out. A child whose primary language is other than English learns English as a second language. Clinicians deal with two apparent phenomena—acquisition of a secondary dialect of the same language and acquisition of a second language.

Children facing the task of acquiring a different dialect or a different language experience certain common problems. Their primary dialect or language influences the acquisition of their secondary dialect or second language. As our previous discussions in this chapter have made clear, the clinician's concern is to take into account the influence of cultural, ethnic, and personal factors associated with the primary dialect or language that influence the acquisition of the secondary dialect or second language. Although comparative research involving African American and bilingual children is lacking, it is obvious that while acquiring a new English dialect or language, both AA and bilingual children have to contend with differences in speech sound patterns across their primary and secondary dialects, or primary language and second languages. Because these issues are yet to be empirically researched, we address mostly the theoretical issues in bilingual phonology, about which there are plenty of publications. We will point out potential parallels between AA children and children learning English as a second language, however.

Specific Hypotheses and General Theories

Research on the acquisition of a second language or secondary dialect has increased in recent decades. Educational demands placed on bilingual and bidialectal children also have caused increased empirical research. Nonetheless, most hypotheses and theories are concerned mainly with how children acquire their second language.

There are limited hypotheses or general theories of second language acquisition. The hypotheses seek to explain a particular phenomenon and typically consist of a narrow set of observations related to patterns in second language acquisition. General theories, on the other hand, seek to explain second language acquisition in a broader sense. Obviously, the scope of specific hypotheses is narrow, and that of the theories is broad.

Selected Specific Hypotheses Related to Second Language Acquisition

Among the specific hypotheses, we will give a brief description of a selected few. Each hypothesis is designed to answer a specific question.

The first question is **Does second language acquisition result in a single or dual phonological system?** The question is especially relevant to **simultaneous bilingualism**, in which children acquire two languages at a young age and roughly at the same time, typically when the parents speak different languages at home. The question also may be somewhat relevant to **sequential bilingualism**, in which the primary language is well established when the child (or adult) learns a second language. Most researchers, however, have been concerned with the question relative to simultaneous bilingualism.

A single phonological system is described as *undifferentiated*; a dual system is *differentiated*. The question, as expected, has been answered both ways. Some phonologists hypothesize a single phonological system, while others hypothesize a dual system (see Yavas, 1994, 1998, for a review of research and theories). Yavas (1994, 1998) suggests that in the very beginning, the child who is learning to speak two languages nevertheless has only a single phonological system. Around age 2, the two systems may be differentiated.

Whether simultaneous bilingualism results in a single or separate system is a difficult question to answer, because such "phonological systems" are often inferred and not empirically observed. What is empirically observed is appropriate or inappropriate generalizations of the sound production patterns of one language to those of another language. Such generalizations are evident in the observable *phonological repertoires*, not unobservable phonological systems. Once the two languages have been mastered, children will have to exhibit a discriminated phonological repertoire, even if they continue to make a few inappropriate generalizations. Older children and adults also may verbally describe how the sound patterns differ or what rules govern such differences. Regardless of a single or dual phonological system, empirical evidence suggests that children simultaneously learning two languages do so at roughly the same rate (see Patterson, 1999, for a review of studies), which offers a good guideline for making clinical decisions.

The second question is **What kinds of primary language phonological interference are evident in second language learners?** We have summarized in the Basic Unit the kinds of effects the primary language has on the production of the sound patterns of second languages. *Interference*, also called *phonological approximation*, is the phenomenon of speech sounds of a primary language influencing the production of those in a second language (Weinreich, 1953; Yavas, 1998). Phonetic productions from the well-established primary language generalize to the second language. A speech sound that exists in the primary language may be produced as an approximation of a sound that exists only in the second language. Among a variety of interferences, underdifferentiation, overdifferentiation (Weinreich, 1953), substitution, and omission of phonemes are commonly observed.

Underdifferentiation of phonemes is a failure to distinguish two phonemes in the second language if they are not distinguished in the first. For example, in Spanish, /d/ and /ð/ are allophonic variations, not separate phonemes as they are in English. In Spanish, /d/ is produced in word-initial positions after [n], and /ð/ is produced in intervocalic positions. Native Spanish speakers may not distinguish /d/ and /ð/ when they speak English. Another example is a lack of vowel-length contrast in Korean, which means Koreans may fail to differentiate the English /i/ and /I/ in their speech. Behaviorally, underdifferentiation is generalization, albeit inappropriate, in a verbal community.

Overdifferentiation of phonemes is making an unnecessary distinction between allophonic variations of two phonemes as separate phonemes; a native English speaker who speaks Spanish as a second language and treats the Spanish /d/ and /ð/ as separate phonemes illustrates such overdifferentiation. Behaviorally, this is discrimination, although also inappropriate in that verbal community.

Substitution of phonemes also is a phenomenon of generalization from the primary language to the second language because of similar sounds in the two languages. For example, Chinese speakers tend to substitute /ʃ/ for /s/ because the two sounds are similar in Chinese. For another example, because many Spanish consonants are unaspirated, native Spanish speakers who use English may unaspirate aspirated English consonants.

Omission of phonemes illustrates an unusual kind of generalization: A phoneme absent in the primary language is simply omitted in the secondary language, in which that phoneme does exist. Both single phonemes and phonemic clusters are susceptible to this kind of generalization. For instance, native Spanish and Chinese speakers tend to omit final English consonants that do not exist in their native language. Similarly, in consonant clusters, the individual consonant most likely to be omitted is the one that does not exist in the primary language.

Yavas (1998) has provided an excellent summary of various interference patterns found in two or more language learners across a wide variety of languages. His summary includes the following:

- Native Turkish speakers may devoice final English consonants and delete consonants from initial clusters.

- Native Portuguese and Swedish speakers may exhibit weak syllable deletion in English.

- Native Italian, Spanish, and Portuguese speakers may delete final English consonants, as their primary language uses more open syllables; for the same reason, speakers of these languages are less likely to exhibit consonant harmony assimilation, a process that is more commonly seen in speakers whose primary language uses more closed syllables (e.g., English); speakers of these languages also are likely to exhibit prevocalic devoicing and reduced aspiration of aspirated sounds (true for other Romance languages, as well).

- Native speakers of syllable-timed languages may exhibit deviant stress patterns in English; this problem is evident in speakers of such languages as Spanish, Italian, and Turkish.

- Native speakers of Spanish may exhibit fricative stopping (e.g., substitution of /b/ for /v/, as Spanish does not have /v/); Spanish speakers also tend to replace the voiceless fricative /ʃ/ with the affricate /tʃ/.

- Native speakers of Spanish, Portuguese, and Cantonese may confuse high front vowels /i/ and /ɪ/ (e.g., in *peach–pitch* and *leave–live*).

It should be noted, however, that interference from the first language does not explain all variations found in second language production. In fact, only a third of the variations (sometimes described as *errors*) in the second language are thought to be due to interference (Mitchell & Myles, 2004; Richards, 1974). Cross-linguistic research has shown that not all sounds that are absent in the primary language create equal difficulty for the learner of a second language. Some absent sounds are easier to learn than others. Generally, sounds that are extremely rare in human languages are more difficult than those that are fairly common across languages but absent in a given language (Yavas, 1998). For some phonologists, sounds that are common across languages suggest an innate phonological universal. However, as we have seen in Chapter 3, many phonological universals may arise out of anatomic and physiologic constraints on the speech production mechanism (Ohala, 1980). In essence, some or many phonologic phenomena may actually be phonetic, not phonemic.

To determine the source of difficulties in learning a second language, investigators first hypothesized that the second language being learned is a system by itself, with its own internal rules, and they named it *interlanguage*. Unfortunately, a new name for a set of findings does not explain them, especially when the hypothesized causal entity is internalized.

The third question: **Is there a critical age for second language phonological acquisition?** The quality of acquisition of a second language differs across individuals. The range extends from a near-native phonological pattern to a distinct influence of first language on second language production. Some individuals, who have a native-like command of the morphologic, syntactic, and pragmatic aspects of their second language, may still exhibit a distinct and varied phonological pattern. Studies have shown that those who write in a second language as competently as or even more competently than most native speakers of that language may nevertheless retain the influence of their first language in their phonological productions (see Patkowski, 1994, for a review of studies). Obviously, phonological patterns are more difficult to master than are other patterns of a second language.

To explain this difficulty, researchers have suggested that there is a *critical age* beyond which it is much more difficult to acquire the phonological aspect than other aspects of a second language. The critical (also called *sensitive* or *optimal*) age is thought to be between 18 months to 6 years, or even up to the onset of puberty (around 12 to 15 years)—a broad range that gives theorists a wide latitude for being right. However, most data seem to suggest that it is possible to learn a second language with native-like phonological patterns if the learning begins before age 12 or so (see Yavas, 1998, and Patkowski, 1994, for details and critical reviews of studies).

Progressively older persons may still master a second language and speak that language, albeit with a phonological difference, but with no difference in grammatical or writing skills. Although this conclusion is relatively noncontroversial, why it is so has been controversial. Some experts favor a biological explanation of language learning of the kind Lenneberg (1967) initially proposed; accordingly, there are biological limitations to language learning. Others believe that there are too many variables that interact, including many environmental ones, to make a strong case for biological restraints on phonological acquisition. Currently, Lenneberg's biological hypothesis is viewed with skepticism (Brice & Brice, 2009).

An environmental factor that has not received much attention is the manner of exposure to the second language. Naturalistic exposure to the second language, regardless of the age at which the exposure begins, may encourage more native-like phonological skills than formal instruction. Formal instruction by native speakers of a language may encourage more native-like phonological skills than similar instruction by nonnative speakers of the same second language. A second-language–rich environment (Hansen Edwards, 2006) with appropriate reinforcement contingencies may better promote both the learning and the maintenance of a second language than an environment in which it is not regularly produced or reinforced. Age and the manner of second language acquisition may interact to produce certain effects on phonological skills. For instance, the most native-like phonological skills may be acquired if a young child is naturalistically exposed to a second language and also receives instruction from native speakers of that language. Evaluation of the contribution of several such factors to the acquisition of phonological skills in a second language is needed.

....

ACTIVITY

Describe how *age* may affect the phonological acquisition of a second language.

....

Selected General Theories of Second Language Acquisition

Theories of first language acquisition and of second language acquisition both seek to explain language learning, including speech sound learning. As such, the theories include similar concepts and face similar challenges. Theories of second language acquisition face additional challenges: They have to explain not only how a second language is learned, but also whether and how the first and second languages interact and affect the final outcome of second language learning.

Theories of second language acquisition have paralleled those of first language acquisition in many respects. The entire spectrum of conceptual or paradigmatic variations can be found in both sets of theories. Nativist, cognitivist, emergentist, empiricist, interactionist, pragmatist, sociocultural, and sociolinguistic theories, among several others, compete to explain second language acquisition in children and adults (Hansen Edwards & Zampini, 2008; Jordan, 2004; Mitchell & Myles, 2004; Sanz & Leow, 2011). Each viewpoint includes varied subtheories. As a consequence, there are some 60 theories of second language acquisition, though none is comprehensive (Jordan, 2004; M. H. Long, 2000; Mitchell & Myles, 2004) or generally accepted. Consequently, these theories are no more than a *patchwork of insights stitched together* (Jordan, 2004).

Theories disagree on how to explain second language acquisition, as well as on what it is that should be explained. Some divergent theories try to explain the same phenomena (e.g., universal grammar, phonological grammar, phonemic contrasts, or linguistic competence) and thus compete with each other. Others explain different phenomena (e.g., universal grammar, pragmatic communicative skills, or language processing) and thus make little contact with each other. Old theories sometimes acquire new names, suggesting progress where none exists. For example, the Chomskyan nativist theory has been more recently described as a *property theory*, because it is concerned with the nature of the language system to be learned (Mitchell & Miles, 2004). All of this encourages a skeptic view that there are no good theories based on empirical facts, only free speculations. A thorough review of these theories is beyond the scope of this chapter; therefore, we will highlight a few contrasting views.

Chomskyan **nativists** believe that how bilingual children learn their second language is best explained by appealing to the innate Universal Grammar (UG), which contains core syntactic rules that apply to all languages. The UG theory proposes that environmental language input is processed by a "language acquisition device" to arrive at language competence. A similar argument is advanced to explain second language acquisition. Various theorists suggest that second language learners have (1) an indirect access to their second language UG through their first language UG, (2) only partial access to their second language UG, or (3) full access to their second language UG (Jordan, 2004; Mitchell & Myles, 2004). Some critics (e.g., Bates, 2000; Reber, 2011; Sampson, 1997) contend that there is no evidence for the existence of UG, and hence, whatever else that follows from it is invalid. Some *partial* critics say that only grammar is innate, and other aspects of language are not (Butterworth & Harris, 1994); other ambiguous supporters of innate UG theory are not sure what is innate and what is learned (Harley, 2008). In any case, the classic UG-based theories are exclusively concerned with syntax and ignore sociocultural, behavioral, and pragmatic aspects of communication. These theories generally assert that a *collection of utterances* does not reflect the true nature of language (Jordan, 2004; Mitchell & Myles, 2004; Sanz & Leow, 2011); but for speech–language pathologists, utterances—what children say under specified conditions—are indeed data that help in making clinical decisions. Similarly, variations in first or second language production, and the influence of family, social, and cultural factors, are of little concern in any of the UG theories. Again, speech–language pathologists find that such factors are important in understanding a bilingual (or monolingual) child's speech and language skills.

Cognitive theories vary in detail and emphasis, but they generally propose that the key to understanding second language acquisition is an appreciation of how the brain processes information to learn something new. One of the cognitive theories, for example, states that second language acquisition involves the acquisition of a complex cognitive skill (B. McLaughlin & Heredia, 1996). The skill must be practiced to develop fluency in the second language. Underlying, internal, and representational cognitive processes guide second language performance. Information processing is *controlled* in the beginning of second language acquisition, because it depends on short-term memory; eventually, it becomes *automatic* when language sequences are stored in long-term memory. There is a constant and continuous restructuring of internal representations as the second language becomes progressively more automatic (B. McLaughlin & Heredia, 1996). The theory says something that is neither controversial nor explanatory: Initially, second language learning is more deliberate or difficult, and later it becomes more automatic and easier; practice is essential for the skill to improve. That initial information processing is controlled and later is automatic remains an inference based on parallel thinking with little or no explanatory power.

A view that is more empirical than the one previously described is the **interaction hypothesis**. As expected, there are multiple variations of this hypothesis, each subsequently and endlessly modified in some way by others (Mitchell & Miles, 2004). *Interaction* in these hypotheses refers to *communicative* interactions between speakers of native and nonnative languages. Long (1983), who compared the interaction styles of native–native speakers with those of native–nonnative (first and second language) speakers found that the differences lie not so much in grammatical complexity of utterances, but in the use of several conversational tactics. For example, native–nonnative pairs of speakers may more often repeat, check for each other's comprehension, request clarifications, and so forth. Based on this kind of evidence, coupled with other kinds of interactions (e.g., child-directed speech from caretakers, correction of unacceptable speech sound production or syntax), theorists have emphasized the role of conversational interactions as a mechanism of second language learning. An idea inherent to these theories is that the input a child receives should be *comprehensible*, that is, understandable. Comprehensible input is both necessary and sufficient to learn a second language, including its grammar (Krashen, 1985). This view is sometimes described as a separate *input hypothesis* or theory, however. Although the interaction and input hypotheses are more empirical and pragmatic than the nativist–cognitivist pairs of theories, they do not specify the mechanisms of learning. Specifically, it is the contingencies of reinforcement (Hegde, 2010c) that are inherent to interactions between first language and second language speakers that promote second language learning. It is doubtful that a mechanical "language input" is sufficient for learning any language—first or second.

Other theories that emphasize social factors in second language acquisition take a **sociolinguistic** view, sociolinguistics being the study of language in use. Most nativist, cognitive, and purely input-based theories pay little or no attention to speech and language production in social contexts; their main concern is the acquisition of an abstract and formal first or second language grammar, including phonological contrasts. Sociolinguistic theories are more pragmatically oriented; but, again, there are multitudes of theories of this kind. Sociolinguistic theories generally emphasize the observation that language use is highly variable across social situations. This is true of the interlanguage of second language learners whose phonological (as well as other) aspects vary. **Interlanguage** is the second language in the process of being learned; it is a second language whose mastery is in progress but has not been completed yet. It is variable across time and situations, but it is not simply a collection of random errors; the errors the second language learners make are patterned. Interlanguage is an evolving system with its own rules and characteristics (Mitchell & Myles, 2004). It should be noted that although the variability of an interlanguage will decrease, it will not be eliminated even after mastery.

Several linguistic and social causes have been hypothesized to explain variability in interlanguages of second language learners. First, **phoneme markedness** may contribute to variability. Sounds that are the same in the first and second language (called *unmarked* sounds) are mastered more readily because of first language transfer, reducing their variability in production. Sounds that are different (called *marked*) in the two languages are learned with greater difficulty and produced with increased variability because of lack of a first language transfer effect. Second, variability may be due to the gradual **generalization** of specific second language phoneme productions learned in one context or environment, to other contexts and environments over time. During the time when generalization is in progress but not yet complete, correct second language phoneme productions in some situations and incorrect productions in others may contribute to variability. Third, **pidginization** may cause variability. In fact, some linguists believe that second language acquisition and pidgin language formations share similar circumstances: A speaker who needs to communicate with a community that speaks a different language. We have earlier taken note of the possibility that pidgin forms may be one of the origins of African American English. Similarities between pidgin English and the interlanguage of second language learners have been documented (see Romaine, 2003, for details). Schuman (1978) has written that "pidginisation may be a universal first stage in second language acquisition" (p. 110). It may be recalled that such phonological patterns as final consonant deletion and such language features as double negatives characterize both the interlanguage of second language learners and AAE speakers. Although more research is needed to substantiate these and other reasons for interlanguage variability, the ones summarized here seem close to empirical observations.

An additional theory is that of **implicit** and **explicit learning** of languages. *Implicit* learning involves no direct teaching of what is to be learned, whereas *explicit* learning does. Implicit learning is unconscious and effortless, whereas explicit learning is conscious and effortful (Reber, 1993, 2011). Implicit learning leads to tacit knowledge that the person possessing it cannot describe. For instance, children who have mastered certain speech sound production patterns or grammatic structures may not be able to say the rules that presumably apply to such productions. This is because they have learned their language implicitly, from interaction with their caretakers. Parents do not explicitly teach phonological or grammatical rules to children; they just speak to them in natural settings. Children acquire the speech and language patterns they hear in their natural environment. This is probably how the first language is learned, and most likely that is how children learn a second language, as well. Even adults acquiring a second language in a natural environment may, for the most part, learn implicitly. Older children and adults learning a second language in an educational setting, however, are often *instructed* on what to learn; they may be told of certain rules of sound or word combinations. Instructed language learning at any age is explicit. One version of this theory, as applied to language (including phonological) acquisition is described by Ellis (2011). According to Ellis, frequency of use of the particular patterns children hear and the process of generalization are important variables in inducing speaking competence of a second language. Ellis also states that interference from established first language patterns forces greater attention to second language patterns; therefore, both implicit and explicit learning may be involved and may interact in second language acquisition. Implicit learning theories place greater emphasis on the language environment, experience, and language usage and much less emphasis on Chomskyan UG and innateness in acquiring both a first language and a second language (Ellis, 2011).

Multiplicity of theories only suggests that observations are incomplete; new empirical findings lead to new theories. Large-scale theories are sometimes built on the basis of a small set of observational data. Theoretical linguistics, which often eschews empirical and experimental methods, is likely to confound clinicians with more theories, most of them untested, possibly untestable. Many rationalist theories of the nativist and cognitive schools are hard to falsify. Many theories of the same kind coexist because none are rejected; even as competing theories proliferate, none are falsified. What is needed is theoretical restraint until accumulated empirical observations and experimental data can support better theories.

Clinical Research Needs in Bilingual and Bidialectal Phonology

Bilingual and bidialectal phonology has been mostly descriptive, comparative, and theoretical. Research has generally enabled clinicians to understand bilingual and bidialectal children's phonological patterns and make clinical decisions that are consistent with their primary language or dialect characteristics.

Clinicians, however, need to go beyond the descriptive information on dual language characteristics of a bilingual or bidialectal child who might speak African American English and is now learning Mainstream American English. In previous sections, we have addressed the issues related to the assessment and treatment of African American and bilingual children. Generally, tests standardized on mainstream children are inappropriate, and alternative methods of assessment, described earlier, are needed. Any tests used must be standardized on the specific group to which the child belongs and should include test items specific to the language or dialect. As described previously, significant progress is being made in developing alternative assessment procedures for African American children and in developing Spanish speech and language tests.

Similar progress in treatment research is not evident, however. Much of the research continues to be descriptive and theoretical. Therefore, the most urgent need in bilingual and multicultural phonology is controlled treatment research. While recommendations and guidelines on treating bilingual and bidialectal children abound, controlled research on treatment procedures is sparse.

As suggested in the previous section on guidelines on working with bilingual and bidialectal children, clinicians can assume that the basic treatment principles used in remediating disorders of articulation hold well in treating such children, too. Of course, this assumption should be promptly abandoned if controlled treatment research (not just expert opinions or theories) suggests otherwise. Treatment research has generally shown that procedures, not principles, need to be modified to suit individual clients (Hegde, 1998, 2008b). For instance, while one child may react positively to verbal praise for correct productions, another may not. However, the child who does not react positively to verbal praise may react well when tokens are presented for every correct response. Thus, though the effect of a particular reinforcer may vary across children, the principle of positive reinforcement does not.

There is no evidence to suggest that children of different cultural backgrounds are not susceptible to treatment stimuli and response-contingent consequences (e.g., modeling, prompting, positive reinforcement, corrective feedback). Children of different cultural backgrounds may be susceptible to different *kinds* of consequences, as the example in the previous paragraph suggests. There is no compelling reason to assume that bilingual and bidialectal children necessarily require unique treatment procedures. Unless contradicted by experimental data, clinicians can begin using standard treatment procedures and modify them as is found necessary.

The most important consideration in the treatment of bilingual and bidialectal children is the selection of target behaviors. As suggested previously, phonemes that are in error in both languages or dialects and those that are in error in the primary language or dialect should be the treatment targets. Phonemes that are used differently in the secondary language or dialect, due to the influence of the primary language or dialect, should be treated as a matter of *elective* dialectal modification. Except for treatment stimuli that must be child and culture specific, procedures necessary to teach selected target phonemes are unlikely to be different from evidence-based techniques.

Summary of the Advanced Unit

- Bilingual children acquire a different language, whereas bidialectal children (such as AA children) acquire a different dialect of the same language; the two groups face somewhat similar problems

- Some children are **simultaneously bilingual** and others are **successively bilingual.**

- There are **specific hypotheses** and **general theories** of second language acquisition, none widely accepted.

- Hypotheses discussed include the following: (1) Second language acquisition may involve either an undifferentiated single or differentiated dual phonological systems; (2) the primary language may *interfere* with second language acquisition, leading to **under-** or **overdifferentiation, omission,** and **substitution** of phonemes in second language production; (3) there may be a biologically critical age for native-like phonological learning, which may extend up to puberty, although such environmental variables as a second language–rich environment and positive support for learning and maintaining a second language may be even more important.

- Theories of second language acquisition that parallel those of first language acquisition are multiple, contradictory, and partial, with little agreement on what to explain and how; they include (1) the **Chomskyan nativist theories**, which emphasize innate mechanisms of universal grammar acquisition; (2) **cognitive theories**, which emphasize the central neural processing of new information in language learning; (3) **interaction theories**, which emphasize communicative exchanges between speakers of native and nonnative languages; (4) **sociolinguistic theories**, which emphasize language use as well as pidginization (thought to be at least one basis of AAE), as primary mechanisms of second language acquisition; and (5) **implicit learning**, without much awareness or direct instruction, and **explicit learning**, with directed attention and instruction, which may be differentially involved in both first and second language learning.

- There is a great need for developing appropriate client- and primary language–specific assessment tools for evaluating bilingual children.

- In treating bilingual children, clinicians can assume that treatment principles do not change, whereas treatment procedures may need to be modified to suit the individual child. Target phonological behaviors should be selected based on the characteristics of the child's first and second languages.

ASSESSMENT AND DIFFERENTIAL DIAGNOSIS OF SPEECH SOUND DISORDERS

Eloquence is the power to translate a truth into language perfectly intelligible to the person to whom you speak.

—*Ralph Waldo Emerson*

Basic Unit: General Assessment and Diagnostic Procedures for Speech Sound Disorders

A comprehensive and well-structured assessment is essential for the eventual diagnosis of any communication disorder. **Assessment** includes a set of procedures that are used to attain a clear description of the speech sound production skills of a child, with a view to determining whether a speech sound disorder is present. Assessment also includes efforts to understand the specific characteristics of any disorder and contributing factors. Furthermore, it includes an effort to understand the child's family, culture, linguistic background, and communication patterns. The results of such an assessment typically lead to a clinical **diagnosis** of a speech sound disorder (SSD), with a description of its characteristics. A **differential diagnosis** helps determine whether a child has an articulation disorder, a phonological disorder, childhood apraxia of speech, or developmental dysarthria (Strand & McCauley, 2008). In this chapter, we use the term *disorder* to describe impaired speech sound production resulting from a variety of known and unknown causes (please see Chapter 4 for variables related to speech sound disorders).

The assessment and diagnostic process is as exciting as it is challenging. The prudent clinician is careful not to diagnose a disorder when clinical data are merely being collected. In the early stages of assessment, the clinician begins to discern whether a problem does or does not exist; however, it is not until all of the necessary information has been collected, analyzed, and interpreted that an appropriate diagnosis can be made. By following this scientific principle of reserving opinions until the data "speak," the clinician is thus guarded from missing or misdiagnosing a disorder and making inappropriate clinical recommendations.

In this Basic Unit we review the major components of a speech sound assessment that lead to a differential diagnosis. In the Advanced Unit of this chapter, we address specialized assessment issues related to speech sound disorders of neurogenic, structural, and sensory origin, such as *childhood apraxia of speech, developmental dysarthria in cerebral palsy, cleft lip and palate,* and *hearing impairment.*

We limit our discussion of assessment principles and procedures to those that are practical, knowing that clinicians are often limited in time and resources. These limitations are particularly problematic in the public schools, where the majority of children with speech sound disorders are serviced. Assessment procedures must be practical as well as reliable and valid, however, and they should lead to effective treatment.

Overview of Assessment

Although a clinician's specific training, own clinical philosophy, and employer requirements often dictate what is included in an assessment, there are general steps that most if not all clinicians take in assessing speech sound disorders (see Skahan, Watson, and Lof, 2007, for the results of a national survey on assessment practices for speech sound disorders by speech–language pathologists). The clinician may start by reviewing reports written by teachers or related professionals, collecting a written case history, and interviewing the child's parents or caregivers. The clinician then plans out the initial assessment session and selects testing instruments appropriate for the particular child.

The testing area is then prepared so that it ensures the collection of valid data. It is important to eliminate excessive noise, interruptions, and visual distractions. In using standardized norm-referenced tests, the clinician should closely adhere to the recommended administrative procedures to maintain the tests' internal **validity** and **reliability**. A connected speech sample is collected for various types of analyses (to be discussed later). Additional assessments include those of the child's hearing (often tested by a nurse in the school setting), orofacial structures, diadochokinetic syllables rates, level of stimulability, speech rate, and speech intelligibility.

A well-structured speech sound assessment typically yields sufficient information for a clinical diagnosis, which is documented in a written report. The clinician shares the test results, diagnostic impressions, and specific recommendations with the child's parents and other professionals at a closing interview or multidisciplinary educational team meeting, always making sure to communicate the information in a way that is understandable and free of unnecessary technical jargon. Parents are given a copy of all written documents.

Assessment Procedures

What follows is a detailed description of assessment procedures. It contains the major components essential to achieving the goals of assessment. As previously stated, the emphasis in our description is on practical procedures that result in a diagnosis and recommendation for treatment.

Conducting a Speech Sound Screening

A **screening** is a pass-or-fail procedure that can be conducted with a large number of individuals in a relatively short period of time. A *pass* on a screening procedure indicates that no further evaluation is warranted; a *fail* indicates a need for in-depth assessment. Speech sound screenings help identify children who potentially have a speech sound disorder and may require further assessment. Screenings take only a few minutes to complete.

In elementary schools, screenings are typically conducted with children in kindergarten or first grade. Some clinicians also screen children in third grade because mastery of all English sounds is expected by 8 years of age, the age of the typical third grader. Speech–language pathologists may also screen the speech sound production status of referred children to determine if a complete appraisal is warranted. This may save the clinician valuable time since some referrals by related professionals may be well intended but not appropriate.

Screenings are intended to be a quick and easy measure of speech sound productions. They can usually be completed in 10 to 15 minutes. They can be performed with standardized testing instruments or nonstandardized measures designed by the examiner or a group of examiners.

Standardized Screening Instruments

Standardized norm-referenced screening instruments that are commercially available often include normative data and provide a *pass* or *fail* score. Some tests are designed solely as screening instruments, while others are part of full articulation–phonological or language assessment instruments. Speech–language pathologists can choose one of several screening tests. Among these are the *Fluharty Preschool Speech and Language Screening Test–Second Edition* (Fluharty, 2000); *Quick Screen of Phonology* (Bankson & Bernthal, 1990b); and *Speech–Ease Screening Inventory: K-1* (Pigott et al., 1985).

Nonstandardized Screenings

Speech–language pathologists who prefer to use nonstandardized or informal screening instruments may design their own measures. Such screenings may be tailored to a specific population and, thus, may be more suitable than standardized screenings. Screenings may be designed for a particular group's age, ethnocultural background, or bilingualism.

During informal speech sound screenings, the clinician may engage the child in brief conversation or ask specific questions that help evoke spontaneous verbal productions. The clinician notes and records any speech sound errors. (See the companion CD for a nonstandardized screening measure.)

If requests or questions fail to evoke the desired verbal productions from a young child, the examiner may use toys or pictures of objects that have the target sounds in their name. If all else fails, the clinician may ask the child to repeat words that contain the target sounds. It is important to establish adequate rapport with young children to evoke representative verbal productions. Thus, a screening with a young child may take longer to complete than the average 10 or 15 minutes.

Questions designed to evoke speech from older children should conform to the interests of the age group. Older children may be asked to read several sentences containing frequently misarticulated sounds such as the later developing consonants /r/, /s/, /l/, and /θ/. The adolescent student may be asked to read a passage with a representative sample of all the English speech sounds, such as the popular "Grandfather Passage" or "Rainbow Passage." There is an abundance of Internet sites that contain stories the clinician can use during an oral reading screening with older children and adolescents.

The examiner determines the criterion for passing or failing the designed screening measure. Typically, the child's performance is compared to established developmental norms and the phonological system of his or her linguistic community (see Chapter 4 for information on developmental norms and Chapter 5 for ethnocultural considerations). Frequently, the need for a more thorough assessment is obvious to the examiner. However, there are occasions when the child's performance on a screening is not clear-cut. When in doubt, it is wise to refer the child for a more thorough assessment. This will help ensure that a speech sound disorder does not go undiagnosed. This is especially important with very young children, because even a few months can make a significant difference in their articulation and phonological learning.

....

ACTIVITY

Describe the procedures and resources that you could use to conduct a nonstandardized screening.

....

Taking a Case History

A case history offers the needed background information to make a comprehensive assessment. A thorough case history can be gathered by collecting a written case history, reviewing reports written by other professionals, and conducting oral interviews with the child's parents or caregivers. A good case history helps the clinician better understand the child's potential problem. Important factors that may contribute to a speech sound disorder, such as a history of recurrent ear infections, may be revealed in the case history.

The child may also have a history of previous assessments by other specialists, such as a dentist, psychologist, otolaryngologist, neurologist, audiologist, or speech–language pathologist. Requesting all relevant medical and educational records is important in collecting a thorough case history. This information is helpful in thoroughly understanding a speech sound disorder before reaching a diagnosis.

To supplement or clarify the information provided in the written case history and the information obtained from other professionals, it is important to conduct a verbal interview. The verbal interview, also known as an **information-getting interview**, generally takes place prior to or at the initial part of the assessment. It is conducted with the child's parents or caregivers. Generally, the clinician will discuss the child's communicative development and current status; medical, developmental, and social history; and educational history.

Performing an Orofacial Examination

Examination of the orofacial structures is essential in assessing children's speech sound disorders. As reviewed in Chapter 4, research has shown that some speech sound disorders may be directly related to abnormal structure and function of the orofacial complex. For example, children with a severe open bite may also present a frontal lisp, and children with a repaired cleft palate may have **hypernasal** speech and compensatory articulation errors. Therefore, when assessing children with a speech production problem, it is clinically wise to perform a thorough examination of the speech structures. The orofacial examination primarily helps the clinician determine if a speech sound disorder is **organic** or **functional** in nature. An organic disorder is one for which some underlying structural, sensory, or neurological cause or related factor can be identified. The articulation problems associated with cleft palate would be an example of an **organic speech sound disorder. Functional** or **idiopathic speech sound disorders** are not associated with an organic or neurologic impairment.

Tools and Procedures

The clinician needs a light source, such as a small flashlight or penlight, to examine the oral cavity. Use of a glove or finger cot is essential for the health and safety of both the child and the examiner. Applicator sticks and tongue blades can be used to flatten the tongue or to probe certain oral structures. It is preferable to use individually wrapped applicator sticks and tongue depressors for sanitary purposes. Cotton gauze pads can be used to hold on to the child's tongue if necessary. Additional tools used during an orofacial examination are a small mirror and a stopwatch for **diadochokinetic testing** (to be discussed later in this section).

The clinician should try to make the orofacial examination as pleasant as possible for the child. Some clinicians purchase commercial products such as flavored tongue depressors and powder-free examination gloves to help. Many children are much more compliant if testing of their orofacial structures is done in the context of a game. For example, the clinician and the child can pretend to "play doctor." Children often like to take on the role of the doctor, and they will usually be much more inclined to let the clinician examine their mouths after they have had an opportunity to examine the clinician's mouth.

Specific orofacial assessments include the structure and function of the facial muscles, lips, tongue, hard palate, soft palate, and teeth. Any abnormalities in appearance, structure, and function are noted and evaluated. This evaluation helps rule out neurological involvement, including muscle weakness and paralysis; structural deviations, including clefts of the palate and velopharyngeal incompetence; dental abnormalities, including malocclusions, tongue and lip mobility; possible nasal or oropharyngeal obstructions such as enlarged adenoids or tonsils; and so forth. Symmetry of the facial structures and any sign of genetic syndromes also are noted in an orofacial examination.

An important part of the orofacial examination is to measure the **diadochokinetic syllable rates,** also known as the **alternating motion rates (AMRs)** and the **sequential motion rates (SMRs).** These rates refer to the speed and regularity with which a person produces repetitive articulatory movements (Hegde, 2008a). These measurements help assess the functional and structural integrity of the lips, jaw, and tongue through rapid repetitions of syllables. Alternating motion rates are measured through the successive repetition of the same syllable (e.g., /pʌ-pʌ-pʌ/; /tʌ-tʌ-tʌ/; /kʌ-kʌ-kʌ/). Sequential motion rates assess rapid movement from one articulatory posture to another by the repetition of different syllables (e.g., /pʌtəkə-pʌtəkə-pʌtəkə/).

During diadochokinetic testing, the child may be asked to rapidly repeat the selected syllable or syllables. The clinician then counts the *number of syllable repetitions* the child produces within a specific duration, typically 5 seconds. Alternatively, the clinician counts the *number of seconds* it takes the child to make a certain number of repetitions, typically 20 repetitions.

Fletcher (1972, 1978) offers norms for the production of syllable rates by children. His study included a total of 384 children from 6 to 13 years of age. Each of the age groups included 24 boys and 24 girls. The children were asked to repeat /pʌ/, /tʌ/, /kʌ/, and /pʌtəkə/ as rapidly and accurately as possible while the number of seconds required for 20 repetitions was recorded. Fletcher's data should be viewed with caution since the number of children included in the sample was rather small. The following results were obtained:

	Average Number of Seconds								
	20 reps					15 reps		10 reps	
Age	pʌ	tʌ	kʌ	fʌ	lʌ	pʌtə	pʌkə	tʌtə	pʌtəkə
6	4.8	4.9	5.5	5.5	5.2	7.3	7.9	7.8	10.3
7	4.8	4.9	5.3	5.4	5.3	7.6	8.0	8.0	10.0
8	4.2	4.4	4.8	4.9	4.6	6.2	7.1	7.2	8.3
9	4.0	4.1	4.6	4.6	4.5	5.9	6.6	6.6	7.7
10	3.7	3.8	4.3	4.2	4.2	5.5	6.4	6.4	7.1
11	3.6	3.6	4.0	4.0	3.8	4.8	5.8	5.8	6.5
12	3.4	3.5	3.9	3.7	3.7	4.7	5.7	5.5	6.4
13	3.3	3.3	3.7	3.6	3.5	4.2	5.1	5.1	5.7

In general, Fletcher's data show that children's diadochokinetic syllable rates increase with age. Such increase is likely related to a child's gradual neurological and physiologic development and increased speech proficiency. Diadochokinetic rates are most clinically significant in the assessment of neuromotor speech disorders, including **childhood apraxia of speech,** developmental dysarthria, and other speech sound disorders due to poor oral–motor movements. These disorders will be discussed further in the Advanced Unit of this chapter.

Appropriate Referrals

If anything of medical significance is observed during the orofacial examination, the child should be referred to an appropriate specialist. For example, the clinician may refer the child to an orthodontist if a dental malocclusion or bite problem is judged to affect speech sound production. A referral to a pediatrician may be warranted if tonsillitis, or inflammation of the tonsils, is suspected. If hyponasality or hypernasality is observed, a referral to an otolaryngologist is generally appropriate. The implications of the results of the orofacial examination and diadochokinetic testing will be further addressed in the later section "Analyzing and Interpreting the Assessment Information."

Conducting a Hearing Screening

A **diagnostic audiological evaluation** is within the scope of practice of audiologists. Speech–language pathologists may screen a child's hearing, however. The primary purpose of an **audiological screening** is to identify children who may be suspected of having a hearing loss, which may be further evaluated by an audiologist. As addressed in the Basic Unit of Chapter 4, hearing loss is associated with speech sound disorders.

The clinician should gather information about the child's hearing status during the assessment. We believe it is clinically wise to do a hearing screening before administering speech and language tests that require adequate audition on the part of the child. This information helps the clinician anticipate any modifications that will need to be made, such as altering the volume of his or her own voice to a level that facilitates the child's understanding of the tasks presented. Audiological screenings are commonly performed through pure-tone audiometry.

With a pure-tone audiometer, the child's hearing is screened by presenting pure-tone stimuli at 500, 1000, 2000, and 4000 Hz (*hertz*) at a preset intensity level, usually 20 or 25 dB (*decibels*). Although the typical intensity level is 20 or 25 dB, it may be altered to compensate for the level of ambient noise in the testing room. The frequencies tested are most important for the reception of speech stimuli, and the intensity level is usually sufficient to compensate for excessive environmental noise. To avoid missing a mild hearing loss, a more conservative criterion may be used with children by screening their hearing for 500, 1000, 2000, 4000, and 8000 Hz at 15 dB.

A child who fails the audiological screening or of whom a hearing loss is suspected should be referred to an audiologist for a complete evaluation. It is important to inform parents that their child's failure of the hearing screening is not necessarily indicative of a hearing loss. The clinician should stress that a complete audiological evaluation is recommended to rule out the possibility of a hearing loss, which may have important diagnostic and treatment implications.

....

ACTIVITY

Describe what you would do if your orofacial examination revealed a possible nasal obstruction.

....

Administering Standardized Tests

Assessment of speech sound disorders typically involves the use of standardized norm-referenced testing measures, sometimes referred to as *single-word tests*. Many of these tests share similarities; however, each test may also have some unique properties. Therefore, a clinician unfamiliar with a particular test should carefully review the procedures and practice its administration prior to using it for the first time.

Traditional **articulation tests** such as the *Goldman-Fristoe Test of Articulation: Second Edition* (Goldman & Fristoe, 2000) and the *Photo Articulation Test: Third Edition* (Lippke, Dickey, Selmar, & Soder, 1997) provide information about a child's phonetic productions in relation to the types of errors and the word positions in which the errors occur. More specifically, they describe the child's sound system according to substitutions, omissions, distortions, and additions in the initial, medial, and final positions of words. Articulation tests generally sample all English consonants and a selected number of consonant clusters. Although less common, some instruments, such as the *Arizona Articulation Proficiency Scale: Third Edition* (Fudala, 2000), also test vowels and diphthongs. The majority of these tests assess sound production at the word level, but some also assess at the sentence level.

According to the national survey by Skahan, Watson, and Lof (2007) previously discussed, the *Goldman-Fristoe Test of Articulation: Second Edition* is currently the most widely used published articulation test in the assessment of speech sound disorders (51.8% of study participants reported using it), followed by the *Photo Articulation Test: Third Edition* (9.7%) and the *Arizona Articulation Proficiency Scale: Third Edition* (4.9%).

Over the years, several standardized norm-referenced tests have been developed to assess phonological processes (error patterns) in children's speech. Some of these include the *Hodson Assessment of Phonological Patterns: Third Edition* (Hodson, 2004) and the *Khan–Lewis Phonological Analysis: Second Edition* (Khan & Lewis, 2002). These tests are useful in evaluating children who are highly unintelligible and have multiple misarticulations. Unlike traditional articulation tests, **phonological tests** help analyze sound error patterns across words rather than individual phonemes in specific word positions. The assumption behind these tests is that some children may not have problems with the phonetic or motor aspect of speech sound production, but rather demonstrate difficulties with acquisition of the underlying sound system or phonological rules. Therefore, the use of assessment batteries that test for the presence of phonological error patterns may provide a clearer understanding of the child's phonological system. This may, in turn, help in the development of a more efficacious treatment program for the child. In Skahan et al.'s (2007) survey, the *Khan–Lewis Phonological Analysis* is listed as the most frequently used published instrument for the assessment of phonological error patterns.

Some standardized norm-referenced speech sound assessments are comprehensive and provide a means for differentially diagnosing a child's speech sound errors as an articulation or phonological disorder. One such test is the *Diagnostic Evaluation of Articulation and Phonology* (Dodd, Huo, Crosbie, Holm, & Ozanne, 2006), which includes a diagnostic screen, a diagnostic articulation assessment, a diagnostic phonology assessment (with a phonological error pattern analysis), a word inconsistency subtest, and an oral–motor screen. Other specialized tests, such as the *Preschool Motor Speech Evaluation and Intervention* (Earnest, 2001), have been developed to diagnose childhood apraxia of speech and dysarthria.

To meet the needs and requirements of most state and federal funding agencies, several standardized tests provide norm-based guidelines such as **standard scores, percentile rankings,** and **age equivalents,** which help diagnose speech sound disorders and their severity. Many public school districts rely heavily on the use of standard scores and percentile rankings to identify children as eligible or ineligible for specialized services, including speech and language services, under an **Individualized Education Program.** Clinicians should be familiar with basic psychometric measures such as standard scores and percentile rankings to ensure correct interpretation of test results.

The reader is referred to the American Speech-Language-Hearing Association's (ASHA's) online directory of assessment instruments at http://www.asha.org/assessments .aspx for a comprehensive list and general description of articulation and phonological assessments used with children. The directory offers the following information: title, author, publisher, year of publication (most recent revision), age range, administration time, language(s), availability of computerized scoring, and a brief description for each assessment. It also provides contact information for the publishers of the tests and a direct link to their Web sites.

ACTIVITY

Using ASHA's online directory of speech–language pathology assessment instruments, identify and briefly describe at least five different instruments.

Evoking Procedures in Standardized Tests

Most articulation and phonological tests are designed to be relatively quick measures. The child is typically shown a pictorial card and instructed to name a pictured object. Commercially available instruments may allow prompts to evoke the target response if the child is unable to name the picture upon initial visual confrontation. If the child is unable to name the picture with the use of alternative prompts, most standardized tests allow the examiner to model the production for the child to imitate. The use of modeling should be recorded for later analysis.

Whether asking the child to repeat the examiner's production taints the testing results is controversial. Some evidence suggests that evoked (nonimitated) responses are more representative of children's typical responses than are imitative productions (Carter & Buck, 1958; Kresheck & Socolofsky, 1972; Siegel, Winitz, & Conkey, 1963; M. W. Smith & Ainsworth, 1967; K. Snow & Milisen, 1954). However, other research has failed to report a significant difference between picture naming and imitation productions (Paynter & Bumpas, 1977; Templin, 1947). To counteract the possible effects of imitation, some suggest the use of delayed imitation (Hegde, 1998; Newman & Creaghead, 1989). With **delayed imitation,** the clinician casually names the picture and then moves on to the next stimulus word. After a few minutes the picture is presented again in hopes that the child can now name it without the need for **immediate imitation cues.** Despite varying thoughts on the use of imitation, the examiner should model only if the test allows for it. The clinician should take note of any divergence from the standard administrative procedures.

Response Recording in Standardized Tests

As the child produces the target responses, the clinician must record the productions on the recording form or protocol provided by a particular test. The recording method used may vary across examiners, depending on their transcription skills and personal preferences. There are three methods of recording a child's responses: (1) correct/incorrect, (2) type of error, and (3) whole-word phonetic transcription. These are listed according to the method that yields the least to most information. In both the *type of error* and *whole-word* methods of response recording, the clinician typically makes use of the International Phonetic Alphabet (IPA) to identify speech sound errors (please see Chapter 3 for discussion of the IPA and Table 3.1 for the phonetic symbols for the 25 American English consonants, 14 American English vowels, 6 American English diphthongs, and many orthographically written key words). Because the IPA is the most widely used system of transcription in speech–language pathology, it is important that clinicians maintain adequate phonetic transcription skills for accurate recording of errors. The strength of using the IPA to record errors is that it provides a uniform transcription system that can be applied and interpreted by clinicians in the profession. Some limitations on the use of the IPA and phonetic transcription do exist, however, and will be discussed in the upcoming section "Limitations of Phonetic Transcription."

Correct/Incorrect and Type of Error

The simplest method of response recording is to judge each production as either **correct (+)** or **incorrect (–)**. This method does not offer details on the child's productions; it simply identifies the sounds that are produced correctly and incorrectly. It does not identify the types of errors or patterns of misarticulation. This method is most appropriate for speech sound screenings rather than extensive assessments.

In the second, and the more commonly used method of response recording, errors are classified as **omissions, distortions, substitutions,** or **additions** in the initial, medial, and final positions of words. A plus mark or a blank space may suggest correct production of the target sound. Sound **distortions** may be noted by marking a capital D on the recording form, though when used alone, this symbol does not indicate severity of the distortion; therefore, a rating system may be used to suggest severity of misarticulations. Clinicians may use a simple system: 1 for mild distortion, 2 for moderate distortion, and 3 for severe distortion. The clinician can also use **narrow phonetic transcription** to record the type of distortion in addition to the level of distortion.

Sound **substitutions** are identified by phonetically transcribing the sound that was substituted for the target phoneme. For example, if the target sound is /k/ in the word *cup* and the child says [tʌp], then a /t/ is recorded. On forms that provide a space for response recording, it is necessary to transcribe only the sound substituted for the target phoneme. However, when a recording form is not used, a sound substitution is typically written as the following examples illustrate: t/k, p/f, or d/g. The top symbol is the sound produced, while the bottom symbol is the target sound. Care must be taken to avoid the common mistake of reversing the sounds.

Omissions are recorded with a minus sign (–) or a zero (0) in the appropriate space. A minus sign is preferred because it is easy to confuse a zero (0) with the /o/ or the phonetic symbol /θ/. Although less common, some children add sounds to the target words. For example, a child may say "gerin" for *green* or "stopa" for *stop*. **Additions** are best recorded by transcribing the child's entire production.

Most standardized articulation tests document a child's productions according to the *type of error* recording system. As discussed in the next section, this method also has some limitations, although it is more specific than the correct/incorrect system.

Whole-Word Phonetic Transcription

In whole-word phonetic transcription, the examiner phonetically records the child's entire production. Instead of recording the accuracy of a particular sound, this method helps record the accuracy of the entire word production using the IPA symbols. The clinician judges the accuracy of not just the target sound, but all sounds in the word. This method of transcription has many advantages, since some children may produce a target sound correctly but misarticulate another sound within the word. This error would not be depicted if the *correct/incorrect* or *type of error* system was used to judge only a specific target sound.

To illustrate this point, consider that the word *cup* was evoked to judge the production of /k/ in the initial position. If the child said "ku" for *cup*, the production would be marked *correct* if using either the *correct/incorrect* or *type of error* recording system, because the child produced the target sound /k/ correctly. However, if the entire word were considered, an error in production would be identified. Even though the target sound was produced correctly, the non-target /p/ was omitted in the final position. This error would only be recognized if the whole-word phonetic transcription recording system were used. This method of transcription is most appropriate for the identification of phonological error patterns or other patterned misarticulations. From the information it provides, the child's errors can also be identified according to substitutions, distortions, omissions, and additions across word positions. This level of transcription is commonly used in phonological tests and is necessary for deeper phonological analysis, as will be described in upcoming sections.

Limitations of Phonetic Transcription

Although commonly used in transcribing children's speech sound errors, the IPA and the phonetic transcription based on it have significant limitations. The symbols suggest that each phoneme is produced in a discrete manner and that each phoneme has clear boundaries. In actual speech, however, these assumptions do not hold. Phonemes may not be discrete entities, especially in connected speech; allophonic variations are common; phoneme boundaries get blurred in coarticulation (see Chapter 3 for definitions and details). Some productions may not fit the description of any specific phoneme but may sound like something in between two phonemes. In the course of development, for example, children may produce a sound that is intermediate between /s/ and /ʃ/ before the two are produced correctly as distinct phonemes. Such intermediate productions may be described but cannot be transcribed. These problems may get magnified in transcribing impaired speech sound productions.

Instrumental analysis can provide useful information, but it is expensive and impractical for routine clinical work, especially in public schools. Acoustic analysis may show differences when the clinician finds a substitution of /θ/ for /s/, indicating that apparent substitutions have response topographic differences. But it should also be noted that such *covert contrasts* may not be heard by clinicians or other listeners, thus making them immaterial in social communication. Other instrumental analyses of speech may use *cineradiography*, which records moving X-ray pictures of articulatory movement; this exposes young children to radiation and has been used only in a few research studies. *Magnetic resonance imaging* and *ultrasound* recording are other equally expensive research tools to visualize oral movements during articulation. Yet another instrumental device used both in analysis of articulatory movements and as a biofeedback method of treatment is *electropalatography*, described in Chapter 3 (see "Phonetic Versus Phonological Theories" in the Advanced Unit).

Procedures to clinically distinguish various types of inaccurate productions that do not fit the categorical IPA classification have been developed; obviously, these procedures assume that the clinician can hear the differences. Stoel-Gammon (2001) and J. Edwards and Beckman (2008) have suggested that clinicians consider intermediate productions that fall between two clearly demarcated phonemes, indicating whether an intermediate sound is heard more like one or the other sound in question. Such a scoring method would accurately reflect a continuum of error-to-correct productions. Clinicians may devise their own scoring or transcribing methods; our example is as follows:

- [t] for /k/ (unmistakable substitution)
- [t] → /k/ (/t/ for /k/, but more like /k/)
- [t] ← /k/ (/t/ for /k/, but more like /t/)
- [s$_{dist}$] (distorted /s/)

....

ACTIVITY

Identify and describe three methods that could be employed to record sound errors from least information to most information. Describe strengths and weaknesses of using the IPA to record errors.

....

Advantages and Disadvantages of Standardized Tests

Several advantages of standardized norm-referenced articulation and phonological tests make them attractive to use. The first and foremost is the relatively short amount of time it takes for their administration. With a cooperative child, a standardized test can usually be completed in 15 to 25 minutes. For clinicians with a large client caseload, such as school practitioners, time is valuable, and test procedures that are too lengthy are simply not practical.

The second advantage of formal tests is that they provide a representative sample of most, if not all, English consonants and several phonological error patterns, depending on the nature of the test. Most tests evaluate production of sounds in the initial, medial, and final positions of single words. Tests of phonological skills sample a majority of natural phonological patterns. Most clinicians do not have time to collect the many stimulus items that would be needed to obtain a representative sample of sound productions and phonological error patterns if informal measures were used.

The third advantage of norm-referenced tests is that the examiner knows the target word being evoked from the child. This is important with highly unintelligible children, because the occurrence of specific error types or underlying phonological error patterns can be identified only when the target production is known. In conversational speech there is a high probability that unintelligible productions cannot be analyzed for the presence of specific error types or phonological error patterns because the target production cannot be reliably identified.

Despite the many advantages of formal tests, several limitations also need to be considered. Paradoxically, many of the factors that make these tests attractive also contribute to their weaknesses. Probably the biggest disadvantage of most standardized norm-referenced tests is that they assess sound production in single words. Single-word productions may not represent a child's connected speech. Research has repeatedly shown that some children produce more errors in connected speech than in single words (Dubois & Bernthal, 1978; Faircloth & Faircloth, 1970; Healy & Madison, 1987; Johnson, Winney, & Pederson, 1980; Morrison & Shriberg, 1992).

Healy and Madison (1987), in particular, found (1) that connected speech samples revealed a significantly higher number of errors than single-word samples; (2) that connected speech samples revealed a higher number of omissions, substitutions, and distortion errors than single-word samples; and (3) that 35% of all errors in connected speech were produced differently at the single-word level. Andrews and Fey (1986) reported a similar problem for the occurrence of phonological error patterns in single-word versus connected speech samples. They noted a higher incidence of phonological error patterns in connected speech for most of their subjects.

In our own clinical practice we have witnessed young children who do fairly well on standardized single-word articulation or phonological tests but show a significant articulatory or phonological breakdown during conversational speech. This has particular implications for the diagnosis of a disorder, in that potential articulation and phonological disorders may go undiagnosed if formal tests are relied on exclusively.

Limited sampling of sounds and sound contexts in a test is another significant limitation of most standardized tests. Children tested may get one or only a few opportunities to produce a sound. From this limited data, clinicians generalize results to many other untested contexts. Another limitation is an inadequate sampling of vowels. Vowel disorders may be less common than consonant problems, but they do exist and may be missed on certain tests. Finally, standardized tests may be inappropriate for children who speak a dialect not sampled by the test items. See Chapter 5 for details.

Collecting a Connected Speech Sample

Because the production of sounds in single words may not represent a child's articulation and phonological proficiency in connected speech, it is essential to obtain a sample of connected speech during assessment. This will help provide a more valid picture of the child's phonological skills than can be obtained from standardized norm-referenced test results alone (Dubois & Bernthal, 1978; Faircloth & Faircloth, 1970; Johnson et al., 1980; Morrison & Shriberg, 1992; Newman & Creaghead, 1989; Stoel-Gammon & Dunn, 1985). Extended, adequate, and representative speech samples help the clinician (1) find sound omissions, substitutions, distortions, and additions; (2) analyze the phonological error patterns; (3) determine the child's phonetic inventory; (4) explore the syllable and word shapes and any phonotactic constraints; (5) calculate percent intelligibility in known and unknown contexts; (6) evaluate consistency of speech sound errors; and (7) obtain a whole-word measure to determine the child's productions according to their complexity, consistency, and proximity to adult targets.

Strategies to Obtain Extended Speech Samples

Gathering a connected speech sample that is representative of a child's typical productions is not an easy feat. The clinician is usually a stranger to the young child, and more often than not the child may be hesitant to talk. Crying and storming out of the testing room are not the only ways children resist; some children demonstrate their refusal by simply not talking to the examiner. In our experience, the latter can be more common and even more frustrating, especially for inexperienced clinicians. What do you do when a child refuses to talk?

It is important to remember that the sampling process can be very intimidating for a young child who likely has a history of much communicative failure. However, there are things clinicians can do to facilitate a child's interaction (see Text Box 6.1). Many times clinicians make simple mistakes without even realizing it. Following are some suggestions that can help structure the testing process so that a child is more willing to engage in conversation with the clinician (Lowe, 1994; Shriberg & Kent, 2013):

• Interview the parents beforehand to determine the child's interests (e.g., favorite toys, TV shows, friends, foods).

• Create a relaxed, pleasant, and inviting environment. If possible, prepare the testing room with toys and games that the child is familiar with and enjoys.

• Avoid playing 20 Questions as soon as the child enters the testing room. Instead, participate in parallel play with the child and limit your verbal interaction. Establish an opportunity for the child to initiate a conversation. For example, you could place one of the child's favorite toys so that it is visible but out of reach.

• Use toys and objects to evoke connected speech productions as the child warms up to the activity. Use a variety of materials and introduce different topics that will evoke a representative sample of word shapes, phonological processes, and phonemes. Because all English phonemes do not occur with the same level of frequency, you will need to arrange situations that will evoke less frequently occurring sounds.

• Be casual about the presence of the tape recorder, as you are likely to use one. Most children will accommodate to the tape recorder. Children who notice it may ask, "What's that?" We have found that most children will be satisfied by a brief explanation such as, "Oh, I'm recording your voice." Some children enjoy hearing themselves on tape, and hearing their recorded speech actually motivates them to interact more.

• Capitalize on the presence of the child's family members. The child may be more willing to talk with a family member. If possible, record the child speaking with

---

Text Box 6.1. Go ahead and find your inner child

When collecting a sample, try to imagine yourself as a 3-year-old who at such a young age has more than likely experienced significant failure with communication. Your mother or father has promised to take you to a "fun place" but instead carts you to an unfamiliar room where a perfect stranger welcomes you with a smile. In this room there are tongue depressors, flashlights, swab sticks, hand gloves, and various toys. The place looks suspicious; you get the feeling that someone wants something from you. Then this unfamiliar person starts to ask you weird questions like, "Hi, Bobby, how was your trip here?" "Would you like to play with my toys?" "Can you talk to me for a little while?" "Can you tell me about your friends?" Oh, no, suddenly you realize that he or she wants you to talk! Then you do the only thing that seems logical, the only thing that you have control over. You shut down and remain quiet.

In an attempt to avoid this scenario, it is important for the clinician to remember that establishing rapport with the child is of utmost importance for a valid assessment. Although as speech–language pathologists we enjoy the art of conversation, sometimes less is more. Children may open up more quickly if they do not sense any pressure. So, find your inner child, bring out the toys, and enjoy a good game of parallel play until the child lets you know that she is ready to engage. Silliness allowed!

significant others. This will allow you to compare the child's productions across different social situations.

The clinician will usually use toys, objects, books, and pictures to evoke connected speech productions from the child. Again, because some sounds occur with less frequency during spontaneous speech, specific objects that represent those sounds can be used to evoke their production. For example, a toy *fish* may be used to evoke *sh* in the final position.

Some experts recommend collecting at least 80 to 100 words for a representative sample (Ingram, 1981; Shriberg & Kwiatkowski, 1980), while others recommend a minimum of 200 words (Weiss, Gordon, & Lillywhite, 1987). Depending on the child's language abilities and willingness to talk, between 50 and 150 utterances are sufficient to obtain the recommended number of words (Stoel-Gammon & Dunn, 1985). This can usually be accomplished in 20 to 30 minutes, depending on the child's level of interaction. Ultimately, the clinician must decide the number of words and utterances needed for a representative sample of a particular child's speech sound production in connected speech regardless of expert recommendations.

Recording the Sample

An audiotaped or videotaped sample of connected speech will help transcribe the speech and increase the accuracy of later analysis. It is very difficult, if not impossible, to reliably transcribe continuous speech at the time of the assessment. This is especially difficult with highly unintelligible children who have multiple misarticulations. Care must also be taken to ensure a high-quality recording that can be accurately transcribed for individual phoneme productions.

A frustrating situation for a clinician is to gather what appeared to be a great sample only to find out that it is useless because the quality of the recording does not permit a reliable analysis. G. Allen (1984) recommends that noise sources be avoided as much as possible because they frequently affect the quality of the recording. Noisemaker toys can be very attractive to the child but can wreak havoc during later analysis of the information. Soft toys, books, and cloth-covered tabletops that help mute excessive noises should be used, instead.

Another problem for reliable data analysis is the erroneous faith that some clinicians place in their ability to remember what the child said—and in what context during the sample. It is not uncommon for clinicians to find when they listen to or watch their recording that an analysis cannot be made because the target productions or the context of speech cannot be deciphered. A simple way to avoid this situation is to **gloss** or restate the child's attempt into the recording. This will serve as a cue for the clinician during transcription of the sample. When glossing the child's productions, the clinician should do so in a natural conversational style. For example, if a child says, "Ant a," while pointing to a toy car, the clinician can gloss the production by saying, "Joey, did you say you wanted the toy car?" It is not necessary to gloss every production, only those that may be difficult to understand at a later date. When collecting a connected speech sample, the clinician should also make special notations of specific articulatory behaviors such as lingual dentalization, lip rounding, unreleased stops, minor sound distortions, and other facial gestures accompanying speech production.

Transcribing the Sample

After a conversational speech sample has been collected, the clinician must decide the phonetic detail with which it will be analyzed. Some children's productions may require a more thorough analysis than others, depending on their error patterns.

When recording sound substitutions, it is often sufficient to use **broad phonetic transcription.** For example, if the child says, "My gagi buy me a koy [my daddy buy me a toy]," the clinician can record the substitutions as g/d (initial and medial positions) and k/t (initial position). However, some children may use sounds that are not part of the English language, or they may distort certain sounds. Some misarticulations may be due to adaptation or assimilation errors. In such cases, it is more appropriate to use **narrow phonetic transcription** with diacritic markers or non-English sound symbols. Examples of narrow phonetic transcription include the following:

- [d̪ag/dag] (dentalized alveolar stop)
- [z̥u/zu] (devoiced alveolar fricative)
- [βɛri/bɛri] (bilabial fricative for bilabial stop substitution)
- [dɑɣi/dɑgi] (velar fricative for velar stop substitution)

The first two are examples of narrow phonetic transcription through the use of the diacritic marker [̪], indicating dentalization of [d], and [̥], indicating devoicing of [z]. The latter two represent substitutions of non-English sounds for English sounds—[ɣ/g and β/b]. Please refer to Table 3.2 for several diacritic markers and special symbols that can be used for narrow phonetic transcription. Some limitations of using the IPA to record errors were previously discussed in the section "Limitations of Phonetic Transcription." These limitations would also apply to transcription of the child's productions in a conversational speech sample.

....

ACTIVITY

In assessing a shy and highly unintelligible 4-year-old boy accompanied by his mother, what steps and special considerations would you take in collecting a representative speech sample?

....

Advantages and Disadvantages of Connected Speech Samples

A significant advantage of connected speech samples is that they are more representative of the child's typical speech sound skills than single-word tests. Connected speech samples allow for multiple occurrences of various speech sounds, phonological patterns, and syllable shapes, unlike most single-word tests. Furthermore, the child's phonetic inventory, consistency of errors, level of intelligibility, and stimulability can be determined from a connected speech sample. Other variables affecting overall intelligibility, such as rate of speech, restricted jaw movements, loudness, and utterance length, may also come to light during this activity.

Some disadvantages associated with connected speech samples prevent their widespread use in various settings and by all clinicians. A major disadvantage is the time required to collect, transcribe, and analyze a connected speech sample. Many clinicians with a high caseload simply do not have the time to perform such a thorough analysis. Also, some children may be resistant to talking during the testing process despite the clinician's well-structured efforts. Allowing the time to gain rapport with the child or using the child's family in the sampling process can help counteract this problem, but this solution also requires additional time and effort. Furthermore, a connected speech sample gathered from a child who is highly unintelligible is difficult to analyze because the adult model is not always known. Glossing over the child's utterances and structuring the setting so that the target words are known may alleviate this problem to some extent.

Conducting Stimulability Testing

Many clinicians consider stimulability testing a part of assessment. **Stimulability** refers to the child's tendency to make a correct or improved production of a misarticulated sound when given a model or additional stimulation by the examiner. Some standardized articulation tests, such as the *Test of Minimal Articulation Competence* (Secord, 1981), allow for stimulability testing, while others do not. If it is not a part of a standardized test used in assessment, the clinician can easily devise an informal stimulability measure. The Sound Resource Packets on the companion CD provide lists of words and sentences that can be used for stimulability testing of all English consonants and selected consonant clusters.

If multiple sounds are produced in error and time does not permit stimulability testing with all of them, a clinician can limit testing to those sounds that are potential therapy targets in initial treatment sessions. Although most commonly performed in isolation and with syllables, stimulability testing can also be done with words and sentences. The child's individual performance during stimulability testing often dictates the most complex linguistic level that will be examined.

Although there is no standard for what type of stimulation should be provided during stimulability testing, most examiners minimally assess the child's improved production after the clinician's model. For example, the clinician might say, "Joey, listen carefully and say what I say. Say *cow*." The child's correct imitation may be verbally praised. Alternatively, the clinician may enhance visual cues by showing the movements of the articulators in front of a mirror. The clinician also may give tactile cues; with the help of a tongue depressor, he or she can facilitate the tongue placement or movement. Finally, the clinician may combine multiple cues to evoke a correct production. Essentially, stimulability testing is informal, experimental treatment. Its implications have evolved, however, and some aspects are controversial, as we will find out in the upcoming section "Analysis of Related Information."

Performing Contextual Testing

Contextual testing is a special procedure that can help identify a facilitative phonetic context for correct production of a particular phoneme. A **facilitative phonetic context** is a surrounding sound or group of sounds that has a positive influence on the production of a misarticulated phoneme. As reviewed in the Basic Unit of Chapter 3, in connected speech, sounds have an articulatory influence on each other. Sounds misarticulated in some phonetic contexts may be produced correctly in others. Finding sound or syllable sequences in which otherwise misarticulated sounds are produced correctly may help identify initial treatment targets.

The concept of contextual testing is not new. Spriestersbach and Curtis (1951) found that many children who misarticulated /s/ and /r/ produced them correctly in a specific phonetic context (e.g., /s/ in the context of /sp/ and /r/ in the context of /tr/). Supporting that finding, Van Riper and Irwin (1958) also suggested that there are **key words** in which a phoneme can be produced more effectively. They used such words to stabilize the child's production of a target sound in therapy. Since then other researchers have substantiated the finding that sounds influence each other during connected speech (Curtis & Hardy, 1959; Gallagher & Shriner, 1975a, 1975b; Hoffman, Schuckers, & Ratusnik, 1977; Zehel, Shelton, Arndt, Wright, & Elbert, 1972).

McDonald's now classic test, the *Deep Test of Articulation* (McDonald, 1964), is based on the facilitative effects of neighboring speech sounds on a sound produced elsewhere in error. The test examines articulation of speech sounds in multiple phonetic contexts; in this "deep testing," each consonant is tested in approximately 40 to 60 different phonetic contexts in a syllable-arresting (terminating the syllable) or syllable-releasing (initiating the syllable) position. Unfortunately, the *Deep Test of Articulation* is not readily available. However, a more current commercially available nonstandardized phonetic context assessment is the *Secord Contextual Articulation Tests* (S-CAT; Secord & Shine, 1997). The S-CAT is a three-part program that helps clinicians gain contextual information of all consonants, vocalic /r/, some vowels, and 16 different phonological processes. It includes Part 1: "Storytelling Probes of Articulation Competence"; Part 2: "Contextual Probes of Articulation"; and Part 3: "Target Words for Contextual Training." It helps the clinician determine the exact pretreatment status for any phoneme or phonological process, evaluate progress during treatment, and target treatment where it is most needed.

The *Contextual Probes of Articulation Competence–Spanish* (CPAC-S; Goldstein & Iglesias, 2006) is the Spanish equivalent of the "Contextual Probes of Articulation" part of the S-CAT. The CPAC-S helps assess the production of all Spanish consonants in a variety of phonetic and phonological contexts at different production levels (prevocalic/postvocalic words, clusters, and sentences). In addition, it helps identify facilitating (correct) contexts for all tested sounds. Clinicians can use this test and other commercially available or custom-made materials. A now classic motor-based approach that makes use of facilitating phonetic contexts to establish sound production, the **sensory-motor approach** was first introduced by McDonald in 1964. The interested reader is referred to Creaghead, Newman, and Secord (1989) for a thorough review of this approach.

Testing Speech Discrimination

The relation of auditory or speech discrimination skills to speech sound learning and its disorders was reviewed in the Basic and Advanced Units of Chapter 4. Studies have been conducted to determine whether children could discriminate between correct and incorrect productions of sounds they themselves misarticulated. Word pairs reflecting a child's error and the correct production have been used to determine if indeed the child could "perceive" or "discriminate" the difference between the target production and his or her error production. A study by Locke (1980b) revealed that a high percentage of children could discriminate between the correct and incorrect productions of sounds they misarticulated when the examiner presented such productions. Eilers and Oller (1976) reported similar findings. Clinical experience with children who have speech sound disorders would support the notion that children can discriminate their own sound errors when made by the clinician even if they cannot produce the sounds correctly. We have frequently encountered children who attempt to correct the clinician when they are confronted with their own errors. For example, the first author can recall the following conversation with a young client:

Client: "I have a pet **wabbit**."

Clinician: "Oh, really, you have a pet **wabbit**."

Client: "No, I have a pet **waabbit**." (The child was a bit louder and emphasized the target sound although still in error. She also seemed somewhat indignant that I would make such an error.)

Clinician: "That sounds interesting, but I don't know what a **wabbit** is."

Client: "You know. . . . A **wwaabit**—it hops." (The child provided me with a definition of *rabbit* just in case I did not know what the word meant.)

Clinician: "Oh, you mean a pet **rabbit.** I get it."

Client: "Yeah, a pet **wabbit**." (The child seemed relieved that I finally figured out what she was saying.)

In this example, the child clearly auditorily discriminated the correct and incorrect productions of the sound even though she could not articulate it correctly. This child's problem lay with the production of the sound.

On other occasions we have witnessed children who clearly cannot distinguish the difference between the error sound and the target sound. We have found this to be most pronounced in children for whom English is a second language. As reviewed in Chapter 4, the ability to discriminate sound contrasts that are nonnative decreases after the first year of life and continues to deteriorate into adulthood. Children who have difficulty with auditory discrimination of their own error productions and target sounds often make such comments as "I can't tell the difference between what you said first and what you said second." Some children may say, "I can't tell when it's right or when it's wrong."

Research does not suggest that poor auditory discrimination skills cause speech sound disorders. Discrimination may be tested, however, if the clinician suspects that this may be a problem in a particular child. We recommend that such testing be done after the sound production errors have been clearly identified. The clinician can use minimal contrasting pairs to determine whether the child can distinguish between his or her own error productions and the target production. For example, if the child frequently substitutes /i/ for /ɪ/, the clinician could design contrasting word pairs that would assess the discrimination between these two sounds (e.g., *bit-beet, mitt-meat, ship-sheep*).

If poor speech discrimination skills of specific sound contrasts are identified, we strongly recommend against initial auditory discrimination training. As discussed in the Advanced Unit of Chapter 4 and in Chapter 8, studies have documented that speech discrimination training alone does not lead to better production, while production training leads to changes in both production and discrimination (Shelton, Johnson, & Arndt, 1977; G. Williams & McReynolds, 1975). More recent studies that have reported beneficial effects of perceptual (auditory discrimination) training on production have simultaneously offered both production and discrimination training (Rvachew, 1994; Rvachew, Nowak, & Cloutier, 2004), making it difficult to conclude that the latter was necessary. Nonetheless, those who wish to offer auditory discrimination training are referred to Winitz (1989), Rvachew (1994), and Rvachew et al. (2004).

Analyzing and Interpreting the Assessment Information

After the assessment has been completed, the clinician has a wealth of information that must be analyzed. For student clinicians, especially first-time clinicians, this is an overwhelming aspect of assessment and diagnosis. We have often heard our own student clinicians make such comments as "What needs to be done with all of this information?" and "Where do I begin?"

Although they may be somewhat puzzled as to where to go from the assessment data, student clinicians do understand that data collection is only the first step in making a diagnosis and generating specific treatment recommendations. It is only through data analysis and interpretation that the clinician can answer such questions as the following:

- Does a speech sound disorder exist?
- What is the nature of the problem if it does exist?
- What is the severity of the disorder?
- What are the possible compounding or potentially related factors?
- Do the child's errors fit a specific diagnostic label?
- What is the prognosis for improvement?
- Is treatment appropriate?

Analysis of Speech Sound Production

The sound segment information obtained during the assessment can be scored and analyzed through an independent analysis, a relational analysis, or both (Stoel-Gammon & Dunn, 1985). In an **independent analysis,** a child's speech sound productions are described without reference to the adult model. The clinician identifies the sounds that are part of the child's **phonetic inventory,** or those sounds that the child can produce regardless of accuracy in relation to an adult target and that are available for the child to form words (Stokes, Klee, Carson, & Carson, 2005). The clinician can also determine the prosodic (stress) patterns, articulatory features, and syllable structures and word shapes that are within a child's repertoire. Any operating **phonotactic** constraints (word positions in which specific sounds do not occur in the child's speech) also may be determined. The following is an illustrative sample of the type of information that can be gathered from an independent analysis in a fictional child:

- *Phonetic inventory:* limited to *m, n, t, d, k, g, w, j, h,* and all vowels and diphthongs

- *Articulatory features:* produces nasals, stops, glides, vowels; voice and unvoiced sounds; and front and back sounds
- *Syllable structures and word shapes:* limited to CV, VC, and CVCV shapes
- *Phonotactic constraints:* consonants *m, n, g, w, j,* and *h* occurring only in initial position; *t, d,* and *k* occurring only in initial and final positions

In an independent analysis, the clinician simply determines what the child can do, not his or her speech sound errors. Although this type of analysis can be used with all children, it is clinically most useful with very young children, because their productions do not always parallel adult word forms. It can also be used with children who are so unintelligible that the adult target cannot be readily identified.

In the second type of analysis, termed **relational analysis,** the clinician compares (or relates) the child's production to the adult target to identify (1) the types of errors according to substitutions, omissions, distortions, and additions in specific word positions; (2) any absent distinctive features; (3) the evident phonological error patterns or phonological constraints; (4) whole-word acquisition patterns according to correctness, complexity, intelligibility, and variability; and (5) the child's **phonemic inventory** (sounds the child can produce contrastively to make distinctions between words) (Stokes et al., 2005).

To illustrate the application of both types of analysis, let us presume that a child produced the utterance [kʌ]. If the adult target is unknown, the clinician could apply an independent analysis and discover that the child can (1) produce the voiceless velar stop /k/ in word-initial position, (2) produce the vowel /ʌ/, and (3) produce the CV syllable/word shape. No reference is made to the adult target because it is unknown. However, if the target word was known to be *cut* and the child said /kʌ/ instead, the clinician could perform a relational analysis and identify the error as an instance of final consonant deletion (potential error pattern) and possible **positional constraint** of /t/ in postvocalic contexts, in addition to all of the information already derived from the independent analysis.

A combination of an independent and a relational analysis leads to a thorough examination of the assessment data. However, the extent to which the information is examined is highly dependent on a particular child's speech sound skills. Through a relational analysis, the clinician can compare the child's production with the standard adult model and thus perform a sound-by-sound traditional analysis; a manner, place, and voicing analysis (MPV); a distinctive feature analysis; a phonological error pattern analysis; a whole-word measure analysis; and an error frequency and distribution analysis.

Traditional Analysis

Elbert and Gierut (1986) use the term *traditional analysis* to describe one of the earliest methods of analyzing articulation and phonological information. This method of analysis considers two variables:

- the position in which the sounds are misarticulated (initial, medial, or final)
- the type of errors made (omissions, distortions, additions, or substitutions)

This method is most appropriate for children with few articulation errors and relatively good speech intelligibility. The nature of the problem tends to be phonetic (articulatory) rather than phonological.

On occasion, error patterns can be identified in the child's productions even with this simplest of all analyses. For example, the clinician could determine that a child's articulation errors are primarily omissions in the initial position of words, or lateral distortions of all sibilants, or substitution errors that affect all or nearly all alveolar sounds. Most single-word articulation tests help to analyze the assessment information according to error types in initial, medial, and final word positions.

Clinicians continue to make this traditional analysis of assessment data. This analysis may be all that is necessary in understanding the articulatory performance of some children. It is a relatively quick procedure that often yields practical information with children who demonstrate only a few errors. A traditional analysis can also be used with children who have multiple misarticulations, but it may not produce all the information needed for a clear understanding of the extent and nature of the speech sound disorder.

Manner, Place, Voicing Analysis

This type of analysis considers a child's misarticulations in relation to the phonetic features of manner, place, and voicing (MPV). A single-word articulation test that incorporates this type of analysis is the *Fisher-Logemann Test of Articulation Competence* (Fisher & Logemann, 1971).

An MPV analysis can help the clinician derive certain patterns in the sound production errors of some children. Through this type of analysis the clinician may discover that a child frequently substitutes alveolar sounds for palatal and velar sounds, which is a problem with *place of articulation*. A pattern that affects the *manner of production* may be observed in a child who substitutes fricatives for stops or glides for liquids. Multiple substitutions of voiceless for voiced consonants would be described as an error pattern affecting the *voicing feature* of sounds. An MPV analysis may be performed from the information obtained in a single-word articulation test or the connected speech sample. It is not a complicated type of analysis, and it can be done relatively quickly (Elbert & Gierut, 1986).

Clinicians often make the MPV analysis in clinical practice. After identifying particular substitution patterns, the clinician may choose to train one or many **exemplars** of the affected sound class. For example, if velars are frequently substituted by alveolars, the clinician may choose to train one of the velar sounds within the class and then probe for generalized productions to the untrained sounds. Or the clinician may choose to train all velars, /k/, /g/, /ŋ/, simultaneously. This topic will be discussed further in the Basic Unit of Chapter 7.

Linear (Natural) Phonological Error Pattern Analysis

Most clinicians tend to make a **phonological error pattern analysis** in children who display multiple misarticulations and very low speech intelligibility. (See "Linear Phonological Theories" in Chapter 3 for a detailed discussion on the history and theoretical underpinnings of this method of analysis.) In this analysis, the child's speech sound errors are classified according to evident phonological patterns, more historically known as *phonological processes* (see Chapters 1 and 2 for terminological shifts). Phonological patterns have been used to describe sound production errors in children with typical and atypical phonological development. We propose that the term *phonological pattern* be used in reference to typical development and *phonological error pattern* be used in reference to atypical development. This type of analysis is especially useful with highly unintelligible children who have multiple misarticulations.

In the Basic Unit of Chapter 3, we identified the phonological patterns most frequently addressed in the phonology literature according to (1) syllable structure patterns, (2) substitution patterns, and (3) assimilation patterns. Syllable structure patterns include final consonant deletion, syllable deletion, cluster reduction, and epenthesis. Examples of substitution patterns are stopping, velar fronting, liquid gliding, and depalatalization. Assimilation patterns are varied and include labial assimilation, nasal assimilation, prevocalic voicing, and postvocalic devoicing.

Patterns of misarticulation that differ from the more commonly observed phonological patterns have been identified in children with typical as well as impaired phonological skills. These patterns occur infrequently in children with typical phonological skills; thus, they are termed unusual or *idiosyncratic phonological patterns* (Grunwell, 1997a, 1997b; L. B. Leonard, 1985; Stoel-Gammon & Dunn, 1985). Examples of idiosyncratic phonological patterns include the replacement of late developing sounds for early sounds, the use of nasal sounds for /s/ and /z/, click substitutions, and the substitution of stops for glides (Grunwell, 1997a, 1997b; Bankson & Bernthal, 2004; Stoel-Gammon & Dunn, 1985). The reader is referred to Chapter 3 and "Definitions of Other Phonological Processes" on the CD for a review of terms, definitions, and examples of various phonological patterns.

Phonological patterns can be assessed according to their frequency and percentage of occurrence. In **frequency of occurrence,** the clinician simply identifies the number of times a particular phonological pattern occurred in the child's speech sample. In the more specific **percentage of occurrence** analysis, the clinician determines the number of times the child used a particular phonological pattern in relation to the total number of opportunities for occurrence of the pattern. For example, a frequency of occurrence analysis may reveal that a child exhibited velar fronting on five occasions. However, the significance of that information would be enhanced if the percentage of occurrence were also known. Five occurrences of velar fronting would be of greater clinical relevance if the child exhibited this phonological pattern in 5 of 8 total opportunities (63% occurrence) than 5 of 30 total opportunities (17% occurrence). To calculate a percentage of occurrence, the clinician needs to determine the total number of opportunities for the use of a specific phonological pattern in addition to the total number of actual occurrences. The following formula may be used:

$$\frac{\text{Total Number of Occurrences of a Process}}{\text{Total Number of Opportunities for the Process}} \times 100 = \text{Percentage of Occurrence}$$

Most standardized norm-referenced phonological instruments provide the clinician with the total number of opportunities for each phonological pattern tested. The clinician then identifies the actual occurrences by administering the test and recording the child's responses. This predetermined information helps the clinician identify the total percentage of occurrence for each pattern tested. Calculating a percentage of occurrence is a time-consuming task because the clinician needs to ascertain both the number of times the phonological pattern occurred and the total number of opportunities for occurrence of each process under analysis. Because of time restrictions, most clinicians calculate a percentage of occurrence only from the test results rather than from a connected speech sample.

An important clinical issue related to the presence of phonological patterns is the question of when a child's sound productions in fact constitute an error pattern. Although the literature is inundated with various definitions for a variety of phonological patterns, the same is not true for criteria that can clearly identify the presence of a pattern. McReynolds and Elbert (1981a) made the valid point that one occurrence of an omission or substitution error under the definition of a particular phonological process does not signify the presence of a pattern. They also advanced one of the few sets of criteria available to clinicians today for the identification of phonological patterns.

McReynolds and Elbert (1981a) suggest that to qualify as a phonological error pattern, specific errors must have an opportunity to occur in at least four instances, and the error has to occur in at least 20% of the words that could be affected by the pattern. For example, if the child's speech sample contained 10 words with velar consonants, the process of velar fronting would be identified only if the child demonstrated at least two instances of an alveolar-for-velar substitution. One of the problems with McReynolds and Elbert's criterion is that it is rather inclusive. For example, if a child substituted [w] for /r/ in two of eight total /r/ production opportunities, the phonological pattern of liquid gliding would be identified since the 20% criterion would have been met. However, it is questionable whether two instances of a sound substitution constitute a phonological pattern.

A more stringent criterion is offered by Hodson and Paden (1991), who suggest that a phonological pattern have at least a 40% occurrence before it is selected as a treatment target. Phonological patterns that occur in less than 40% of opportunities would be monitored but not addressed in therapy. It should be noted that Hodson and Paden's criterion is intended for the identification of phonological patterns that are in need of remediation rather than the classification of specific phonological patterns. Lowe (2012) suggested that the minimal requirements for qualifying a sound change as a phonological pattern are (1) that the pattern be observed in more than one sound from a given sound class and (2) that the sound change occur at least 40% of the time.

Because of the lack of agreement on criteria for the identification of phonological error patterns in atypical productions, clinicians often rely on their own professional judgment. Over 30 years since Stampe (1979) introduced the concept of phonological processes, quantitative criteria that can be widely used are still elusive. It would be useful to develop a standard definition for individual phonological patterns, so that if a specific quantitative criterion is used, it can be comparable from one source to another.

Another consideration in the identification of phonological patterns is that a single pattern on a specific word is rarely observed in children. Rather, children often produce word forms that reflect the co-occurrence of multiple patterns. For example, a child who produces the word [wat] for *lock* demonstrates the use of liquid gliding and velar fronting on a word. Also, a single production error can be identified as an instance of various patterns. For example, the production of [tut] for *shoot* could potentially be identified as stopping, depalatalization, and alveolar assimilation. The clinician would obviously have to dig deeper and look beyond the production of a single word to identify the patterns that are part of the child's phonological system.

Error Frequency and Distribution Analysis

Gierut and associates originally described a method for analyzing speech samples with a view to find the frequency and distribution of speech sound errors (Gierut, 1985; Gierut, Elbert, & Dinnsen, 1987). Gierut called it the *productive phonological knowledge* approach, and she believed that the error patterns, frequencies, and distributions in a speech sample reflect different degrees of *phonological knowledge* the child may possess. Her approach, however, is clinically useful without the assumption of unverifiable and presumed phonological knowledge the child does or does not possess. Gierut (2008) has acknowledged that her Phonological Knowledge Protocol (PKP) to assess speech sound patterns and errors may be used within different theoretical frameworks, including the nonlinear optimality theory and we think atheoretically as well, as we present it here. The PKP includes 293 words that sample all English consonants in each relevant word position in at least five exemplars. Monosyllabic, disyllabic, and a small number of trisyllabic words are included in the PKP. There is also an Onset Cluster Probe (Gierut, 2008) that may be used to sample two- and three-element initial clusters across a minimum of five different exemplars. Public school clinicians who are under extreme time pressure may find this an impractical analysis, but those who have time to do it may gain a broader as well as in-depth perspective on the child's speech sound production skills.

To make a distributional analysis, a representative speech sample that includes both connected speech and spontaneous single-word utterances is needed. The clinician should sample all target English sounds, sample each sound in at least three word positions (initial, medial, final), sample each sound in each position in more than one word, and sample each word more than one time. The sample should also provide an opportunity for the child to produce minimal pairs (e.g., *core* and *tore*) to assess how the child is using sounds contrastively, as well as morphophonemic alternations (e.g., *play* and *playing*).

Gierut's method is a qualitative rather than quantitative description of error distribution. It differs from the MPV, distinctive feature, and phonological (process) pattern analysis in that it describes (1) the nature of the child's lexical representations of morphemes as adultlike or non-adultlike, (2) the distribution of sounds in some or all word positions and the production of sounds in some or all target words, and (3) the presence of extractable phonological rules. The distribution of correct and incorrect sound productions may be classified according to the following six varieties, although Gierut classified them as six types of phonological knowledge:

1. Sound is always produced correctly in all word positions and for all morphemes (words).

2. Sound is produced correctly for all morphemes and in all positions; however, some optional or obligatory phonological rule may apply.

3. Sound is produced correctly in all positions; however, errors exist in certain morphemes that may have been acquired early and incorrectly (*fossilized forms*).

4. Sound is produced correctly for all morphemes in a specific position but may be produced in error in other positions (*positional constraint*).

5. Sound is produced correctly in a specific word position, but some morphemes may contain errors; sound may be produced correctly for all morphemes in a specific word position but produced in error in other positions (combination of Type 3 and Type 4 errors).

6. Sound is always produced incorrectly in all word positions and for all morphemes.

Gierut infers a hierarchy of phonological knowledge from the variable distribution of speech sound production patterns, including errors. For example, sounds that the child correctly produced in all contexts is thought to reflect *most knowledge* (Type 1), and the sounds that are produced incorrectly in all contexts is said to show *least knowledge* (Type 6 knowledge). Production and error distributions listed in 2 through 5 have intermediate knowledge and are ranked accordingly.

Complex sounds are often considered better initial intervention targets, as they may produce better generalization to untrained sounds. Thus, the clinician can use the differential sound production and error distributions to guide target behavior selection. Gierut's research (2001, 2007) has shown that when more complex sound errors (presumably implying least phonological knowledge) are treated, greater generalization of treated and untreated sounds may be obtained.

Nonlinear Optimality Phonological Analysis

Recall from Chapter 3 that nonlinear approaches are an alternative to linear phonological process-based approaches. Although this approach does not currently hold a strong position in the assessment of speech sound disorders in the clinical setting, it is difficult to predict whether that will continue to be the case or a shift will come in the future. At this time, the traditional manner, place, and voicing and phonological error pattern types of analyses previously discussed are commonly used in clinical practice in speech–language pathology. However, clinicians may wish to stay abreast of this and other developments and critically analyze different perspectives.

As described in greater detail in Chapters 3 and 4, nonlinear optimality theory describes commonly known phonological error patterns in terms of conflicts between faithfulness and markedness constraints. Generally, speech sound errors are analyzed according to markedness constraints (unique properties of a language) versus faithfulness constraints (matching input and output representations). New terms for these patterns have been advanced. Some examples of how nonlinear optimality theory may account for phonological error patterns of linear theory include the following (Barlow, 2001; Barlow & Gierut, 1999); starred items are the markedness constraints, and unstarred items are the faithfulness constraints:

• *Fronting*—The common substitutions are [t/k], [d/g], and [n/ŋ]. These substitutions are explained by the optimality theory constraint *DORSAL, which prevents velar outputs. Consequently, a coronal output (unmarked) emerges instead of a velar output.

• *Stopping*—In this process, stops are substituted for fricatives and affricates. Stops are unmarked; fricatives are marked. Therefore, the OT constraint *FRICATIVES, which prevents fricatives, causes the production of stops instead.

- *Final consonant deletion*—Open syllables (CV) are unmarked (universal), whereas closed syllables (CVC) are marked. Therefore, final consonant deletion is due to the markedness constraint *CODA (no final consonants).

- **MAX*—Consonant deletion (in any word position). *CODA is specific to final consonant deletion.

- **COMPLEX*—Cluster reduction. Clusters are more complex, marked; hence there is a constraint against them. This constraint prevents cluster productions and explains the error pattern of cluster deletions.

- *DEP*—A faithfulness constraint that specifies that input–output segments must match, this prevents any extraneous sound insertion; its violation explains extraneous vowel insertions (e.g., [səwip] for *sweep*).

- *IDENT-FEATURE*—Another faithfulness constraint, it specifies that input features should not be changed in the output. Violation of this constraint explains such error patterns as fronting of velars to alveolars, gliding of liquids, stopping of fricatives, prevocalic voicing, and final obstruent devoicing.

Within a nonlinear framework, understanding and analyzing a child's speech sound productions according to markedness and faithfulness constraints become important for treatment because errors can be re-ranked by demoting markedness constraints below faithfulness constraints. In other words, the universal marked phonological rules of a language are re-ranked (reordered) in treatment so that the faithfulness (input–output) constraints prevail and allow the child to produce phonological patterns similar to adult models. From an atheoretical position, which most clinicians take, the significance of this is that children can be taught sounds and other speech skills that are more difficult than their current skills, something that we have known for years.

Some clinical researchers in speech–language pathology (e.g., Barlow, 2001; Barlow & Gierut, 1999; Bernhardt & Stemberger, 2011; Bernhardt & Stoel-Gammon, 1994) have argued that nonlinear optimality theory offers advantages in the assessment and subsequent treatment of phonological disorders; however, as already stated, clinical application remains extremely limited. This is likely due to poor understanding of nonlinear theory by clinicians not trained in this theoretical framework, or a lack of time needed to complete this very complex and time-consuming method of analysis, or a combination of the two. Unless nonlinear phonological assessments of speech sound production become simpler, more efficient, and easier to use, the nonlinear theory applications in clinical practice will remain limited. As only time can tell, the clinician is encouraged to keep an eye on current developments.

Whole-Word Measure Analysis

Ingram and Ingram (2001) have proposed that clinicians examine the child's *whole-word patterns of acquisition* by measuring whole-word correctness, complexity, intelligibility, and variability. This is a *relational analysis* because it evaluates the child's sound production in whole words (not just individual sounds) in relation to the adult target (Ingram & Ingram, 2001). This is an extension of Bankson and Bernthal's (1990a) and Schmidt, Howard, and

Schmidt's (1983) concept of whole-word accuracy (WWA) in words, although its scope and application is much more comprehensive. Ingram (2000) maintained that although WWA provided valuable information, it was limited because it did not examine words for complexity, intelligibility, and variability in addition to correctness.

Ingram (2000) proposed four distinct but related measures to analyze a child's whole-word production patterns: **proportion of whole-word correctness** (PWC), **phonological mean length of utterance** (PMLU), **proportion of whole-word proximity** (PWP), and **proportion of whole-word variability** (PWV). These measures, which were elaborated on in a subsequent publication (Ingram & Ingram, 2001), can be obtained by transcribing 25 to 50 words selected from a spontaneous language sample that represent a range of common nouns, verbs, prepositions, adjectives, and adverbs used in normal adult conversation; "child words" such as *mommy*, *daddy*, and *tata* are not included in the sample (Ingram & Ingram, 2001). Compound words that are spelled as one word (e.g., *hotdog*, *greenhouse*) are counted as one word, whereas compound words that are written as two words (e.g., *race car*, *teddy bear*) are counted as two separate words. Only one production is counted for each word (except when calculating whole-word variability).

Proportion of whole-word correctness is a rather simple type of analysis that is performed by determining whether the child's word contains any errors. The child's production (transcription) is compared to the adult standard of pronunciation; if a complete match is observed, the word is scored correct; a mismatch is scored as an error. When the number of correct words is determined, the proportion of whole words correct (PWC) is calculated by dividing the number of whole words correct by the total sample size. The following serve as examples of PWC calculation:

- 10 correct words ÷ 50 total sample words = .20 (or 20%) PWC

- 12 correct words ÷ 50 total sample words = .24 (or 24%) PWC

- 15 correct words ÷ 25 total sample words = .60 (or 60%) PWC

Ingram (2002) developed the concept of the **phonological mean length of utterance** (PMLU) as a substitute of sorts for the difficult task of analyzing whole-word *complexity* based on segmental, syllable, and phonotactic properties. Like the traditional mean length of utterance (MLU) for sentences, the PMLU provides a number that increases with an increase in the length of the child's word productions. Note that for PMLU the increase is in the child's word length as opposed to the child's sentence length in traditional MLU. The PMLU focuses on the number of sounds (segments) in the child's word, as well as the number of correct consonants. The following summarizes the procedures that are used to calculate a phonological mean length of utterance:

- At least 25 random words are selected for analysis (rules previously discussed apply).

- Each segment (*consonant and vowel*) in the child's word is counted and given 1 point.

- An additional point is given for each correct *consonant* in relation to the adult target.

- The PMLU is then calculated by adding the total number of points given for the selected sample and dividing by the total number of words. For example, if a child is assigned 65 total points for a 25-word sample, the PMLU would be 2.6 or $(65 \div 25 = 2.6)$.

It is expected that as the child makes progress in learning his or her speech sounds, typically or with treatment, the PMLU would show comparable increases. However, developmental data delineating the average PMLU for specific ages or age groups is currently limited; thus, its diagnostic and treatment application is narrow until large-scale normative studies are completed. That limitation aside, this information can serve as a valuable measure of progress similar to the percent of consonant correct (PCC) measure (to be discussed in the upcoming section "Severity Analysis"); pretreatment measures can help guide goal development and can help document the child's progress after treatment is initiated. For example, if a child's PMLU is 2.0 at the time of assessment, the clinician could develop a related treatment goal of increasing the child's PMLU by targeting word length and consonant correctness. A change in the child's PMLU after treatment is applied could be one of many measures of progress.

The *proportion of whole-word proximity* (PWP) was devised to get an indirect measure of word intelligibility (Ingram, 2000). This measure examines the proximity of a child's word to the adult target—in other words, how closely the child's attempt and the adult target match. It is determined by calculating the maximal PMLU of a target word first and then dividing it into the PMLU of the child's production. For example, the word *banana* has a maximal PMLU of 9 (1 point for each of six segments and 1 additional point for each of three consonants). If the child produces the adult target as [nænə], a PMLU of 6 would be assigned (1 point for each of four segments and 1 additional point for each of two consonants). The target PMLU of 9 is then divided into the child's PMLU of 6, yielding a PWP of .67 for that word. According to Ingram (2000), children tend to display a relatively high PWP from the beginning of phonological acquisition.

The *proportion of whole-word variability* (PWV) is an extension of the more traditional way of looking at production consistency. Consistency has been a factor in the selection of target behaviors for many years (see Chapter 7). In years past it was believed that an inconsistently erred sound would make a good initial intervention target because the child displayed learning readiness; however, recent studies have shown that teaching more complex sounds, misarticulated consistently, may lead to greater phonological change because of the favorable effects of generalization. Thus, consistently erred sounds are now considered better initial targets, especially in phonological intervention programs such as the maximal contrast and complexity approaches (Gierut, 2001, 2007; see also Chapter 8).

In recent years, the need to look at the variability with which the whole word, not just a sound segment, is produced from one attempt to another has been emphasized (Ingram & Ingram, 2001). Whole-word variability is thought to have a connection to speech intelligibility, in that whole words that are produced variably from one attempt to another may not be interpreted as well by the child's listener as those produced in a consistent, predictable manner. The Inconsistency subtest of the *Diagnostic Evaluation of Articulation and Phonology* (Dodd et al., 2006) was specifically designed to look at whole-word production variability.

The core vocabulary intervention approach discussed in Chapter 8 was developed to meet the needs of children whose intelligibility is profoundly affected by variable whole-word productions.

The number of studies on whole-word learning and the clinical implications is currently limited. A small body of research is just beginning to emerge; however, the studies are not comparable and vary from simple case studies to longitudinal studies with children of different language backgrounds (English, Dutch, Finnish, Spanish, and Spanish–English bilinguals) (Bunta, Fabiano-Smith, Goldstein, & Ingram, 2009; Ingram & Ingram, 2001; Saaristo-Helin, 2009; Saaristo-Helin, Savinainen-Makkonen, & Kunnari, 2006; Taelman, Durieux, & Gillis, 2005; Watson & Terrell, 2012). As these measures become better researched and more normative data become available, describing early phonological development at the whole-word level may become more common, and whole-word-level analysis in assessment may provide a way of tracking changes during and following treatment. At this point, these are newer ways of looking at speech sound production; how commonly they will be applied in the clinical setting remains to be seen.

....

ACTIVITY

Briefly describe information derived from each of these speech sound analysis types: traditional analysis, distinctive feature analysis, phonological error pattern analysis, whole-word analysis, error frequency, distribution analysis.

....

Analysis of Related Information

Results of Orofacial Examination and Diadochokinetic Testing

Results of the orofacial examination and diadochokinetic testing help rule out any organic, structural, or neurological variables that may be associated with a speech sound disorder. Such observations as facial paralysis or paresis, abnormal facial movements, drooping of the corner of the mouth, deviation of the corner of the mouth to one side, evidence of repaired cleft of the lip, mouth breathing, inadequate lip seal, inadequate range of motion of the articulators, structural or functional abnormalities of the tongue or soft palate, missing teeth or abnormal teeth alignment, or various other symptoms will help rule out significant organic variables.

Besides structural and functional abnormalities, the clinician evaluates the diadochokinetic rates to evaluate any slowness of articulatory movements. The child's rates may be compared with the available norms previously discussed (Fletcher, 1972).

Medical History Analysis

From the written case history, initial interview, and review of reports written by other professionals, the clinician usually gains a good understanding of the child's current health status and medical history. Occasionally, children bring a history of medical problems and interventions that can affect the diagnosis of speech sound disorders. For example, a child with a history of a repaired cleft lip and palate may manifest unique articulation errors that can be explained by the one-time presence of such structural anomalies. Children with a history of cerebral palsy will have incurred neurological damage that could account for the presence of motor speech sound disorders such as dysarthria. Intellectual disabilities may affect speech sound production skills, especially in children with Down syndrome or Fragile X syndrome. Furthermore, children with a history of recurrent otitis media or fluctuating hearing loss may display sound distortions, substitutions, and omissions typically associated with hearing loss. Not all children's speech sound disorders are associated with structural, functional, or neurological damage. However, when an associated condition is evident or suspected, the clinician should note it in the written diagnostic report and make referrals to other professionals or collect additional data.

Developmental Analysis of Speech Sound Production Skills

In a developmental analysis, the information obtained from standardized tests or a connected speech sample is compared to developmental norms. Such comparison allows the clinician to determine, in part, whether the child's sound errors or error patterns are similar to those typically found in children of the same chronological age or are beyond the average age of mastery. The typical acquisition of speech sound production skills is a relatively lengthy process with significant variations across children. Some children suspected of having an articulation or phonological disorder may simply be producing age-appropriate errors. In such cases, the child's speech sound production skills would be considered typical rather than atypical (of clinical significance).

Speech–language pathologists working in the public school system rely heavily on normative data to make treatment eligibility decisions. Children who appear to be following the normal course of development would not be considered candidates for speech pathology services. This can help the clinician maintain a manageable caseload in a work setting that is well known for serving a remarkably high number of children.

In making a developmental analysis, the strengths and limitations of norms, described in the section "Learning to Produce Individual Sounds and Sound Patterns" in the Basic Unit of Chapter 4, should be considered. The inherent problem of using group data for the evaluation of an individual's performance should always be taken into account. The clinician should treat developmental data as only one of several variables in the diagnosis of speech sound disorders (see Text Box 4.3 for norms and clinical decision making).

Stimulability Analysis

Two widely held beliefs prompt clinicians to routinely assess stimulability for sounds in error. First, it is thought that a child who is stimulable has a better prognosis than one who is not stimulable. Second, it is easier to treat stimulable sounds, and therefore they should be treated before non-stimulable sounds are treated. Unfortunately, there is no strong evidence to support either of these beliefs. Should the clinician offer a more pessimistic prognosis because the child has failed a few attempts at imitating the clinician during assessment? Most children *in treatment* (let alone assessment) need several initial trials before they begin to imitate the clinician's modeled correct productions. Those initial failures probably are not a solid basis on which to offer a pessimistic prognosis for any child. It may prove to be true that stimulable (imitated) sounds are more easily taught than non-stimulable sounds. In their clinical practice, however, most clinicians probably have found it easier to teach initially imitated speech sounds than sounds that are not imitated; the latter need to be shaped.

Although it might be a bit harder to teach non-stimulable sounds, is it worth teaching them first, even if there are stimulable sounds in the child's repertoire that could be taught with greater ease? Evidence suggests that when non-stimulable sounds are taught, positive changes may be noted in both the treated and *untreated* stimulable sounds based on generalization (Klein, Lederer, & Cortese, 1991; Powell, Elbert, & Dinnsen, 1991). Therefore, Gierut (1998) recommends that clinicians treat non-stimulable sounds first. Most clinicians know that sounds that are not stimulable during assessment can be taught; as noted, many sounds are not stimulable even during the first few treatment trials.

Rvachew, Rafaat, and Martin (1999) claim that treatment of stimulable sounds results in a better treatment outcome. In their study, sounds that were not stimulable did not show clinically significant changes when treated with a modified version of the phonological cycles approach (Hodson & Paden, 1983), in which the treatment was offered in small groups and only one phoneme was targeted at a time. The authors selected a second group of children the following school year and offered them the same treatment except that the children received what the authors called "stimulability training" for three individual sessions, each lasting 20 minutes. The stimulability training consisted of "phonetic placement, mirrors, verbal instructions, and auditory-visual models for imitation . . ." (Rvachew et al., 1999, p. 37). This kind of stimulability training progressed from individual sounds to imitation of words and sentences. Children who received such training improved to a greater extent than those in the earlier year who did not receive it. On this basis, the authors concluded that stimulability is related to better treatment outcomes.

It appears that *stimulability assessment* has been stretched to *stimulability treatment* in the Rvachew and colleagues (1999) study. Stimulability treatment is not the same as the traditional concept of stimulability for sounds. While stimulability assessment offers a few modeled trials to see if the child imitates a sound in error, stimulability treatment is simply treatment. Normally, clinicians do not spend 60 minutes assessing stimulability or training stimulability; Rvachew and colleagues spent time training sounds that were not readily imitated. One way of looking at their results is that the modified cycles approach failed in the first year of their study, and when the non-stimulable sounds were individually treated, the outcome improved. Therefore, it may be worthwhile to assess stimulability only if it is further confirmed that it is advantageous to treat non-stimulable sounds first, as Gierut claims. Even then, considering the limited time available for a full agenda of phonological assessment, a thorough understanding of stimulability for target sounds may have to wait until the sounds are base-rated before starting treatment. A base rate is a better measure on which to base clinical decisions. We will describe the base rate (baseline) procedures and analysis in Chapter 7.

Intelligibility Analysis

The conversational speech sample collected during an assessment should be analyzed for the child's speech intelligibility. It is important to assess intelligibility of the child's connected speech, because the primary goal of therapy in most cases is to make the child more understandable.

Clinicians can make a professional judgment of speech intelligibility during conversational interactions with the child. Though they are subjective, experienced clinicians can make reasonably good judgments of speech intelligibility and state their conclusions as a judgment, as, for example: "This examiner judged the child's speech intelligibility to be 50% to 60% during known and unknown contexts."

Clinicians can use various rating systems to describe the degree of intelligibility. Generally a 3- or a 5-point rating scale may be used (Bleile, 1996). On a 3-point scale, 1 would mean *readily intelligible*, and 3 would mean *unintelligible even with careful listening*. The scale can be expanded to 5 or more to include such categories as *mostly intelligible*, *somewhat intelligible*, and so forth.

A more objective analysis should also be performed to supplement the clinician's initial impression of intelligibility. This can be done for both known and unknown conversational contexts. The following steps can be taken in making an objective analysis of the client's speech intelligibility:

1. *Collect a connected speech sample.* Use the sample to assess the child's production of sounds. However, it is important that the clinician select a portion of the sample that was not specifically used for sound production analysis, since the purpose at this point is to assess speech intelligibility.

2. *Transcribe the sample.* Do not make a concerted effort to understand the child as you did during sound production transcription. Rather, listen to the utterance once and transcribe accordingly. This will more closely resemble the natural environment, since the average listener would not have the luxury of recording the child's productions and listening to the sample several times. Write out each word for each utterance. The words may be written orthographically.

3. *Use a symbol that helps depict an unintelligible word.* A dash (—) may be used.

4. *Calculate intelligibility for words.* Divide the total number of intelligible words by the total number of words—for example: 105 **intelligible words** / 250 **total (intelligible + unintelligible) words** = 42% intelligibility for words.

5. *Calculate intelligibility for utterances.* Divide the total number of intelligible utterances by the total number of utterances (an utterance is considered intelligible only if the entire utterance can be understood)—for example: 62 **intelligible utterances** / 200 **total (intelligible + unintelligible) utterances** = 31% intelligibility for utterances.

Please see Chapter 4 for a detailed discussion of speech intelligibility in typical speech sound learning. The clinician may use this information to help guide a speech intelligibility analysis. As a quick review, the following rough guidelines may be used as to the percent of intelligibility that can be expected by certain ages:

- by 19–24 months, 25–50% intelligible
- between 2–3 years, 50–75% intelligible
- between 4–5 years, 75–90% intelligible
- by 5 years of age, 90–100% intelligible, though a few persistent articulation errors may exist

Severity Analysis

Judging the severity of a speech sound disorder is typically a part of the clinical diagnosis. *Severity* refers to the degree of impairment in a particular child, which may range from slight to profound. A severity score may be derived from some tests (e.g., *Test of Minimal Articulation Competence* by Secord, 1981), but not all. When formal testing instruments are not used or those used do not offer a severity analysis, clinicians rely on their own professional judgment for determining the severity of the disorder.

Clinicians consider several variables that may affect the severity of the disorder, including the child's speech intelligibility, the number of sounds in error or the presence and number of phonological error patterns, the consistency of the errors, and the child's age. In general, it can be expected that the higher the number of error sounds or phonological error patterns and the higher the consistency of the errors, the lower the child's speech intelligibility will be. Conversely, the lower the child's speech intelligibility, the more severe the disorder. Although currently there is no standard set of terms, clinicians often use such severity categories as *slight, mild, mild–moderate, moderate, moderate–severe, severe,* and *profound* to suggest the degree of impairment.

In an attempt to provide a more objective measure of severity, Shriberg and Kwiatkowski (1982) developed a metric system that considers the **percentage of consonants correct** (PCC) as an index of degree of impairment. They outlined the following procedures for determining the PCC for a particular child:

1. Collect a speech sample

    - Tape-record a continuous speech sample of at least 50 to 100 words.

    - Determine the meaning of the utterances to ensure accurate transcription. The child's utterances may be glossed to aid later analysis.

    - Identify and exclude any dialectical differences, casual speech pronunciations, or allophonic variations.

2. Consider exclusion criteria

    - Consider only intended consonants in words. Exclude all vowels, including /ɜ/ and /ɚ/. Exclude the addition of a consonant before a vowel, since the intended production is the vowel (e.g., do not score [hon] for *on*).

    - Exclude the second or successive repetition of a consonant. Score only the first production (e.g., in *ba-balloon*, score only the first /b/).

    - Exclude words that are partially or completely unintelligible. Exclude also words whose gloss is questionable. Score only intelligible words or words that can be reliably identified.

    - Exclude target consonants that occur in the third or subsequent repetitions of adjacent words unless articulation of the word changes. For example, count only the consonants in the first two words of the series [kæt], [kæt], [kæt], while the consonants in all three words are counted in the series [kæt], [kæk], [kæt].

3. Determine incorrect consonant productions
   - Score as incorrect the following consonant sound changes: (a) deletions of the target consonant; (b) substitution of another sound for a target consonant, which includes replacement by a glottal stop or cognate; (c) partial voicing of initial target consonants; (d) distortions of a target sound, no matter how subtle; (e) addition of a sound to a correct or incorrect target consonant (e.g., [karks] for *cars*).
   - Count an initial /h/ deletion (e.g., [i] for *he*) and final n/ŋ substitutions (e.g., [rin] for *ring*) as errors only when they occur in stressed syllables. Count them as correct when they are produced in unstressed syllables (e.g., [fidɚ] for *feed her* and [rʌnin] for *running*).
   - Score dialectical differences and casual speech productions based on the consonant the child intended (e.g., [aks] for *ask* is correct in African American English, but [ats] for *ask* is incorrect).
   - Score allophonic variations as correct (e.g., [warɚ] for *water*).

4. Calculate the PCC by using the following formula:

$$\frac{\text{Number of correct consonants}}{\text{Number of correct } plus \text{ incorrect consonants}} = \text{PCC}$$

   - Example:

$$\frac{50 \text{ consonants produced correctly}}{200 \text{ total consonants attempted}} = 25\% \text{ (PCC)}$$

5. Determine the severity level by using the following scale:
   - 85% to 100%   mild
   - 65% to 85%   mild–moderate
   - 50% to 65%   moderate–severe
   - < 50%   severe

According to Lowe (1994), the PCC may be used not only as a severity rating but also as a means of monitoring progress. It is an objective way of determining the severity of a disorder. It may also provide clinicians with a quantitative criterion by which the efficacy of the treatment provided can be evaluated.

Contextual Testing Analysis

Contextual testing is performed to determine if certain phonetic contexts facilitate the correct production of a target phoneme in words. This contextual analysis may be combined with the error distribution analysis discussed previously. It should be emphasized that this type of testing does not help determine the need for treatment. Rather, it helps establish a possible starting point in therapy. By analyzing the results of contextual testing, the clinician notes whether any sound that precedes or follows the target sound helps evoke a correct or improved production. At times patterns of production may be identified that are clinically significant. For example, the clinician may determine that /s/ and /z/ are produced correctly when they precede or follow any alveolar sound. The clinician can promote early success in therapy by taking advantage of such a facilitative context. Stimulus pictures can then be paired so that /s/ and /z/ are preceded by alveolar sounds (e.g., *hat-sun, dad-zoo, moon-soap*, and so forth). Also, through careful analysis of the speech sample, the clinician may identify **key words** for correct production of the target sound. *Key words* can also be used to establish a more consistent production of target sounds at the word level (see Text Box 6.2).

Phonetic Inventory Analysis

A **phonetic inventory analysis** helps the clinician identify the consonants and vowels the child can make without consideration for the contrasting effects of the sound in adult words. The point of interest with this type of analysis is not whether the sound was used in the appropriate linguistic or phonetic context, but whether the child produced the sound according to its articulatory properties. The *Khan–Lewis Phonological Analysis: Second Edition* (Khan & Lewis, 2002) allows for a phonetic inventory analysis.

The child's phonetic inventory can be determined from the information obtained on single-word articulation tests, phonological process or pattern assessments, or a connected speech sample. Stoel-Gammon (1987) indicated that sounds can be considered part of the child's phonetic inventory when they are produced at least two times in words with different base morphemes. Lowe (1994) advanced the following two specific rules for performing a phonetic inventory analysis:

- Sounds that occur at least three times are considered part of the child's productive inventory.
- Sounds that occur one or two times are considered marginal, because such limited occurrence may not be reliable.

A child's phonetic inventory provides clinically relevant information. The clinician may discover that the child's productive phonetic inventory is limited to only a few sounds, reflecting the high number of misarticulations or phonological error patterns in the child's speech. The clinician may also discover a difference in the child's productive phonetic inventory from one word position to another. For example, although a child may produce all stops in the initial position, such sounds may not be part of the child's phonetic inventory

---

Text Box 6.2. The power of a word!

The first author can recall working with a female third-grade student who on standardized assessment demonstrated severe distortion of /r/ and no stimulability. Although contextual testing was not performed with a published instrument such as the S-CAT, analysis of the child's connected speech sample revealed correct production of /r/ in one specific key word—"Dracula." (You never know what the word will be.) That facilitative context was strategically used to establish production of /r/ in additional initial /dr/ word exemplars (e.g., *dragon, drink, drop*) and then to establish production of the singleton consonant /r/. Despite severe distortion of /r/ and poor stimulability on initial testing, the student made quick progress and was dismissed from speech–language services much sooner than expected.

in the final position. Thus, the clinician may choose to teach the production of stops in the final position of words to increase the child's syllable shape repertoire. Furthermore, the phonetic inventory analysis may show that the child's production of sounds is restricted to certain sound classes or types of sounds (e.g., stops and glides). The form "Phonetic Inventory Analysis" found on the companion CD provides a visual representation of the child's productive phonetic inventory and may be used by the clinician to document the child's pretreatment inventory of sounds.

....

ACTIVITY

Describe three ways you could determine a child's speech intelligibility.

....

Making a Differential Diagnosis

Once the various types of analyses have been completed, the clinician typically has enough data to make a differential diagnosis. It is at this point that the clinician decides whether a speech sound disorder exists. If a disorder is present, the clinician now also describes the severity and nature of the disorder. In general, the assessment may lead to one of two general **diagnoses:** (1) normal or typical speech sound production skills or (2) a speech sound disorder.

The clinician may conclude that a child's speech sound productions are typical in the following situations:

- *The errors identified are related to second-language interference, bilingualism, or the use of a particular dialect.* You may recall from Chapter 5 that speech sound production differences are not considered disorders when the child's "errors" are part of a dialectical or linguistic variation. Dialectical or phonological differences may or may not affect a child's speech intelligibility, social interactions, and academic performance.

- *The errors fall within the normal developmental range of mastery for a particular age group.* Typical speech sound learners demonstrate production errors that are not disorders. Speech sound mastery is a gradual process. A 2-year-old child, for example, would be expected to have many more errors than the average 6-year-old. If these two children demonstrated the same errors, the younger child could potentially be diagnosed as having normal speech sound production skills, whereas the older child's productions would likely be considered delayed or disordered. This depends on the errors, of course.

- *The errors are so slight or subtle that they do not have a significant negative effect on listeners.* Some individuals may demonstrate slight or very mild speech sound distortions that may be evident to the trained ear of the speech–language pathologist but not to the average listener. Such errors would probably not affect the child's social or academic life. There are some sound classes that are particularly vulnerable to distortion: sibilants (lisping), liquids (vowelization), and nasals (hyponasality).

In all three cases, the child's or the family's reaction to the speech under consideration is important. If the child or the child's family believes that the speech sound production errors are or may become "handicapping" in the future, the clinician may need to discuss this with the family and possibly reconsider the diagnosis and the treatment recommendations.

Also, children whose speech sound errors are the result of bilingualism or dialectical differences may seek out speech therapy because their social, academic, or future vocational life may be affected by the presence of their dialect. Clinical speech services may be warranted in such a case. However, clinicians in the public school setting need to adhere to state and federal guidelines that may prohibit the provision of speech–language pathology services solely on the basis of dialectical differences or second-language acquisition of English. Children whose errors fall within the normal range of development may or may not be "handicapped" by the presence of certain errors.

If the clinician decides that indeed the child has a speech sound disorder, a description of the disorder is appropriate. For example, the types of errors most commonly observed, any positional or inventory constraints, error distributions, and whole-word production patterns might be described. The clinician can also make reference to the phonological error patterns. In addition, the clinician may specify the type of disorder. Although terminology continues to change over time (see Chapter 1), clinicians may broadly label a child's sound production errors as either an *articulation disorder (impairment)* or a *phonological disorder (impairment)*.

As reviewed in Chapter 1, in clinical practice an **articulation disorder** is evident if the following statements could be made about the child's speech:

- Sound production errors are not typical of the speech of other children the same age.
- Errors are limited to only a few sounds and not necessarily restricted to distortions.
- Errors are not patterned or constrained.
- Errors do not compromise intelligibility to a significant extent, though there may be an occasional misunderstanding.
- Errors are associated with an organic, structural, or neurological origin (whether they are phonetic, phonological, or both).

A **phonological disorder** is evident if these statements could be made about the child's speech:

- Misarticulations are multiple.
- Speech sound production errors are patterned, and from the patterns some rule, constraint, or principle could be extracted.
- Sound productions do not match the adult models.
- Speech is limited in intelligibility.
- Speech is characterized by limited syllable shapes.
- Phonetic inventory is more or less restricted relative to age-level expectations.

Generally, a phonological disorder may be identified from a manner-place-voicing analysis, distinctive feature analysis, phonological process analysis, whole-word analysis, or nonlinear constraint ranking analysis.

Articulation impairment has been subclassified into speech sound disorders with (1) known organic origin (structural and sensory), such as hearing loss, cleft lip or palate, or dental malocclusion; (2) acquired or suspected neurological origin, such as childhood apraxia of speech or developmental dysarthria; and (3) functional origin such as persistent misarticulation of /s/ and /r/ beyond the expected age of development and in the absence of structural or neurological problems. Likewise, phonological impairments have been subdivided into (1) a phonological delay in which error patterns follow mostly a developmental pattern (e.g., final consonant deletion, stopping, and velar fronting) or (2) a phonological disorder in which the child primarily displays idiosyncratic or nondevelopmental error patterns (e.g., backing, initial consonant deletion, child-specific error pattern). We prefer the term *phonological disorder* to describe the presence of developmental, nondevelopmental, or a combination of patterns, as the term *phonological delay* might suggest that the child requires only time, not treatment, to develop phonological skills. Currently, there is no evidence to support that. The use of specific diagnostic terms such as *childhood apraxia of speech*, *developmental dysarthria*, and *tongue thrust* should be reserved for children who demonstrate a sufficient number of the characteristics associated with those speech sound disorders.

An estimate of the severity of the disorder is also important. Speech intelligibility is the most important variable affecting severity judgments. In general, the lower the child's intelligibility, the more severe the speech sound disorder. The clinician may use such categories as *normal, mild, mild–moderate, moderate, moderate–severe, severe,* and *profound* to rate a child's intelligibility.

If any factors are believed to contribute to the speech sound disorder, the clinician should make note of these in the diagnostic report. For example, the child's disorder may result from structural problems associated with cleft palate or malocclusions; suspected neurological problems associated with childhood apraxia of speech or developmental dysarthria; or sensory problems associated with hearing loss.

A diagnostic statement is generally one of the last portions included in a written report. The style and format in which they are written vary from one clinician to another. Diagnostic statements may be written as in the following examples:

- Dee Dee demonstrated a severe functional speech sound disorder as well as severe delay in receptive and expressive language. Her articulation errors primarily consisted of labial and lingual sound distortions. The restriction of tongue and lip movement noted in the orofacial examination may be contributing to misarticulation of these sounds.

- Sammy has a mild speech sound disorder associated with tongue thrust. His specific sound errors included interdentalization of /s/, /z/, /ʃ/, and /ʧ/. His speech intelligibility was not affected by his misarticulations, although they draw negative attention.

- Suzie has a mild speech sound disorder characterized by a lateral lisp of /s/ and /z/. Her speech intelligibility was minimally affected by her articulation errors. No structural problems of the speech mechanism were associated with her articulation errors.

- Frank exhibited a mild–moderate phonological disorder characterized by final consonant deletion, syllable deletion, and velar fronting. His phonological disorder may be related to his history of middle ear infections and moderate conductive hearing loss.

- Christina has a mild articulation disorder characterized by distortions of the /r/ and /l/ phonemes in all word positions. Her voice was also judged to have weak oral resonance due to minimal mandibular and labial movements during speech.

- Bobby exhibited a moderate speech sound disorder characteristic of childhood apraxia of speech (CAS). Error patterns leading to the diagnosis of CAS included the following: sound transposition errors, sound perseveration errors, increased articulation errors with increased word length, and substitution errors primarily affecting fricatives and affricates.

- Edith demonstrated a moderate–severe speech sound disorder characterized by several omission, substitution, and distortion errors.

- John exhibited moderate flaccid developmental dysarthria associated with cerebral palsy and characterized by distortion of stops, fricatives, and affricates. Other characteristics of flaccid dysarthria noted in his speech included hypernasality; a hoarse, breathy vocal quality; and general weakness of the speech musculature.

- Geraldine has a severe phonological disorder characterized by stopping of fricatives and affricates, vowelization of postvocalic /l/ and /r/, and partial reduction of /s/, /l/, and /r/ clusters. Her overall speech intelligibility was clinically judged to be 50% when the conversational context was known. This level of intelligibility is severely delayed for a child Geraldine's age.

- Chad demonstrated age-appropriate articulation skills. Although several errors were noted on the *Goldman-Fristoe Test of Articulation: Second Edition* and a spontaneous speech sample, they were within normal developmental limits for a child of Chad's chronological age. His speech will be reevaluated in 6 months.

Determining the Prognosis for Improvement

A **prognosis** is the estimated course of a disorder under specified conditions. What will happen if treatment is offered or not offered? A prognostic statement is an answer to such a question. Typically, a prognostic statement specifies the expected course of improvement under treatment.

An initial prognosis is based on the *available* information at the time of the assessment. Various **prognostic variables** help in making a professional judgment about a child's anticipated progress. Prognostic variables are factors that can positively or negatively influence the improvement of a child's speech sound production skills. The initial prognosis may change over time.

A well-written prognostic statement has at least three major components: (1) a goal statement, (2) a judgment of success, and (3) the prognostic variables that justify the judgment. The *goal statement* makes reference to what skill(s) the child is expected to achieve. This part should include specifics. For example, the statement "The prognosis is good" is not acceptable, since it does not indicate what the child is expected to learn or achieve. A better statement would be "The prognosis for correct production of /s/ with treatment is excellent."

The above example hinted at the next component of a prognostic statement: the *judgment of success*. This is a clinical judgment that makes reference to how well the child is expected to do in therapy. The terms *poor*, *fair*, *good*, and *excellent* are often used in clinical practice. This judgment, or prediction, is based on the various variables that come to light during the assessment. Prior clinical experience often helps clinicians make such a determination. However, even the most experienced and wisest of clinicians has been proven wrong on occasion. A child who was initially judged to have a poor prognosis might do extremely well in therapy, whereas a child believed to have an excellent prognosis may demonstrate limited progress.

Several variables help decide whether a child has an excellent, good, fair, or poor prognosis for the attainment of a specific goal. Some of these variables are specified in the prognostic statement examples given in the next section. We emphasize, though, that because of the uniqueness of each clinical case, there is no certain set of variables associated with each judgment of success. Ultimately, the clinician must use his or her professional judgment to arrive at a decision. There is very little hard research data to support prognostic statements. Clinicians have the ethical responsibility to provide a child's family with a prognosis for improvement while not guaranteeing the results of treatment (ASHA, 2004).

Clinical experience suggests the following child-centered prognostic variables:

Variable	Underlying Assumption
Severity	The more severe the disorder, the poorer the prognosis and vice versa.
Chronological age	The younger the child at the time of treatment, the better the prognosis.
Motivation	The less motivated the child, the poorer the prognosis for improvement. Motivated clients will likely follow through with assignments, therapy suggestions, and so forth. This variable is most significant with older elementary school children, adolescents, and adults. Young children may be much more motivated by reinforcers manipulated by the clinician.
Inconsistency	Inconsistency in sound production errors may be a positive prognostic variable. Errors that are produced correctly some of the time may be more easily treated.
Associated conditions	Such conditions as a limited attention span; poor cooperation; and neurological, sensory, or developmental deficiencies may slow progress in treatment.
Treatment history	A child with a history of limited progress or poor maintenance of previously learned behaviors may be thought to have a poorer prognosis than a child without such history.
Family support	The stronger the support extended by the child's family, the better the prognosis for improvement. If a child's family takes an active role in therapy, the child may show faster progress and better maintenance than otherwise.

The following are examples of prognostic statements that may be included in diagnostic reports; the style in which they are written varies from one clinician to another. They are provided primarily to illustrate inclusion of a goal statement, judgment of success, and prognostic variables:

- *Example Statement for Excellent Prognosis.* Jamie's prognosis for improved production of /s/ and /z/ with therapy was judged excellent based on the following variables: the mild nature of her articulation disorder, her stimulability for correct production of the erred sounds, her cooperative behavior and good attention span during the assessment, the absence of any structural problems, and the high level of support from her parents.

- *Example Statement for Good Prognosis.* Based on John's age (4 years 2 months), his cooperative behavior, and his stimulability for correct production of some of the erred sounds, his prognosis for improved phonological skills and increased speech intelligibility with treatment this semester was judged to be good.

- *Example Statement for Fair Prognosis.* Jerry was very cooperative during the assessment and has good family support. However, his prognosis for improved articulation skills and increased speech intelligibility with therapy was judged fair at this time because of his age (13 years), the severity of his disorder, and the extent of his hearing loss. His prognosis will be reevaluated according to his performance once treatment has been initiated.

- *Example Statement for Poor Prognosis.* Ron's prognosis for improved articulation skills was judged poor based on the severe nature of his disorder, his uncooperative behavior during the testing process, his short attention span, and a reported history of limited progress and missed treatment sessions. However, in that this clinician has not personally worked with Ron before, his prognosis will be reevaluated throughout the course of treatment.

As the examples make clear, *prognosis* typically means a relatively slow or fast improvement in treatment. A poor prognosis is no basis for denying treatment. There is no ethical or scientific basis for denying treatment to a child whose prognosis is judged poor. A poor prognosis is a warning to the clinician, the client, and the family that they all should expect a long period of sustained hard work ahead.

Making Treatment Recommendations

Regardless of the results of the assessment and the clinical diagnosis, the clinician is obliged to make specific recommendations—to decide whether speech sound treatment is appropriate for a particular child. Not all children tested for a speech sound disorder require clinical intervention. In essence, there are four possible scenarios that can help the clinician decide whether treatment should be recommended or provided:

- *The child has typical speech sound production skills; thus, treatment is not recommended.* The child's errors may be within normal developmental limits; they may be related to linguistic or dialectical differences; or they may be so subtle that the child's social or academic life is not significantly affected. In such cases, treatment should not be recommended unless the child, the family, or both demand it.

- *The child's articulation skills appear to be following the normal course of development; therefore, treatment is not recommended. However, a reassessment after a specified period of time may be warranted.* Some children may be following the normal course of development, and thus treatment is not recommended during the initial evaluation. However, the clinician may recommend that the child's speech sound production skills be reevaluated at a later date to ensure that the child is on the right course of speech sound learning and there is no evidence of a disorder. This type of recommendation is most common for typically learning young children who, the clinician suspects, may simply need time to fully acquire their speech sounds. This recommendation would be inappropriate with older children, since most children can be expected to have adult-like speech sound production skills by 8 or 9 years of age.

- *The child has a speech sound disorder, but immediate treatment is not recommended.* This statement may seem contradictory, but there are occasions when, although a child has a speech sound disorder, the clinician may decide against immediately initiating treatment. An example would be a young child with an unrepaired cleft palate whose articulation errors result from the related structural anomalies. Although a disorder is present, speech–language pathology services may be contraindicated until the cleft is surgically repaired. A clinician may also choose not to recommend treatment if a child's language disorder takes precedence over an articulation disorder. Generally, diagnosis of a disorder leads to treatment; therefore, this recommendation only suggests the postponement of treatment to a more opportune time.

- *The child has a speech sound disorder, and treatment is recommended.* If the clinician decides that the child indeed has a speech sound disorder and treatment is appropriate, other, more specific, recommendations should also be made. For example, the clinician should state how often the child will receive clinical services and how long the sessions will last. Oftentimes, the clinician has little control over these decisions, since his or her place of employment may have set policies.

The clinician also needs to determine which sounds or error patterns will be targeted in therapy. The target behavior selection guidelines are outlined in greater detail in the Basic Unit of Chapter 7. If appropriate, other recommendations may be made to such referring professionals as an otolaryngologist, orthodontist, medical doctor, audiologist, or speech–language pathologist who has a particular specialty.

....

ACTIVITY

Describe some cases in which you would not recommend treatment despite the presence of speech sound errors.

....

Conducting the Final Interview

Assessment ends with a **closing interview,** or in the public schools a **multidisciplinary evaluation team (MET) meeting,** with the child's parents or other caregivers. During the interview, the clinician presents the assessment findings and makes recommendations. It is important to review the information in a clear and concise fashion that is understandable to everyone present. The use of technical jargon should be avoided. Illustrations may be used to facilitate understanding of clinical problems.

Toward the end of the interview, the clinician summarizes the major findings, conclusions, and recommendations. It is important that the clinician ask if the listeners have any questions, thank them for their help and interest, and describe the next steps that will need to be taken according to the recommendations that are being made. It is important that at every point during the closing interview or MET meeting, assessment and diagnostic information be delivered delicately, in a factual yet supportive manner. It is important to remember that you are talking about the listeners' loved one. Families and caregivers often bring with them a lot of emotions that need to be acknowledged and supported.

Writing a Diagnostic Report

Once the assessment has been completed and a diagnosis has been made, the clinician writes a diagnostic report summarizing all of the analyzed information, including all clinical findings, and outlining the treatment recommendations. Because the clinical report becomes an official, and at times legal, document, the clinician should devote sufficient time for its preparation. Also, other professionals often gain some perspective on the clinician's knowledge and competence from the diagnostic report. Reports containing typographic or grammatical errors, poor writing style, and confusing organization and wording may leave a negative impression on the reader.

The exact format, style, length, and degree of detail of clinical reports vary from setting to setting. For example, diagnostic reports written in the university setting are much lengthier and more detailed than those of any other clinical setting. Our own experience in various clinical settings has given us firsthand knowledge of the vast differences in the way diagnostic reports are written. Across settings, diagnostic reports may vary from formatted checklists to one-paragraph reports to six-page reports. The clinician should be flexible and adhere to the regulations of his or her university program or work setting.

Although the length, format, and style of reports vary from one setting to another, the general principles of good writing do not. The reader is referred to Hegde (2010a) for a thorough review of scientific and professional writing in speech–language pathology. Also, diagnostic reports share common features. Regardless of the degree of detail, most reports include the following general categories: identifying information, background information, history, assessment information, diagnostic and prognostic statement, and treatment recommendations. The reader is referred to the file "Sample Diagnostic Reports" on the CD for examples.

Summary of the Basic Unit

- An **assessment** is a series of clinical procedures used to attain a clear description of the speech sound production skills of a child, with a view to determining the presence or absence of a disorder. This determination leads to a clinical **diagnosis.**

- Assessment procedures include reviewing the child's background, planning the assessment session, selecting appropriate testing instruments, making recommendations, and writing a diagnostic report, among others.

- A **speech sound screening** is a quick pass-or-fail procedure that helps determine whether a more thorough assessment is warranted.

- A **case history** is essential to understand the child, the family, and the clinical problem and is obtained by collecting a written case history, reviewing information written by other professionals, and conducting oral interviews with the child and the child's parents.

- An **orofacial examination** helps rule out any underlying structural, sensory, or neurological problems that may be associated with an articulation or phonological disorder. Diadochokinetic testing is typically a part of a thorough orofacial examination.

- An **audiological screening** is a part of the assessment; it helps determine whether the child needs to be referred to an audiologist for a complete evaluation.

- The child's speech productions can be assessed by **standardized articulation tests** and **phonological error pattern tests.** The clinician can record errors using three methods: correct/incorrect, type of error, and whole-word transcription.

- Children's speech sound production skills are also assessed in **conversational speech.** The clinician collects a representative speech sample, which often reveals more errors than single-word productions.

- **Stimulability testing** evaluates whether the child can make a correct or improved production of the error sounds when given a model or additional stimulation (e.g., tactile, visual, auditory, or kinesthetic cues).

- The clinician may perform **contextual testing** to determine whether any facilitative phonetic contexts can evoke correct production of an error sound.

- The clinician conducts **auditory discrimination testing** with children who are suspected of having auditory or speech discrimination problems that may be affecting the articulation of specific sounds.

- Analysis of assessment data may be either independent or relational. In an **independent analysis,** the child's speech productions are described without reference to the adult model. In a **relational analysis,** the clinician compares the child's productions to the adult model and thus determines error types or patterns of production.

- The clinician can perform a **traditional analysis** according to the types of errors in initial, medial, and final word positions. This method of analysis is appropriate with children who exhibit only a few articulation errors.

- A **manner, place, and voicing analysis** may be performed to identify any error patterns in manner of production, place of articulation, or voicing features.

- A **phonological error pattern analysis** may be performed with children who display multiple misarticulations.

- The clinician may also perform an **error frequency and distribution analysis**, a **nonlinear optimality phonological analysis**, and a **whole-word measure analysis.** Additional measures include the **percent consonants correct**, **speech intelligibility**, and **severity of the disorder.**

- The clinician analyzes all relevant information such as that obtained during an orofacial examination, stimulability testing, and contextual testing.

- After analyzing and interpreting all of the relevant data, the clinician makes a clinical **diagnosis,** determines the **prognosis** for improvement, and makes specific **treatment recommendations.**

- The clinician then conducts a **closing interview** with the child's parents and follows up with a written **diagnostic report.**

Advanced Unit: Description and Assessment of Organic and Neurogenic Speech Sound Disorders

In this Advanced Unit, we briefly consider the assessment of speech sound production problems associated with specific clinical conditions, including childhood apraxia of speech, developmental dysarthria in cerebral palsy, cleft palate, and hearing impairment. Unlike speech sound disorders in many children, these clinical conditions are associated with structural, sensory, or neurological variables that affect speech production.

An exhaustive presentation of the special procedures that can be used in the assessment of these disorders is beyond the scope of this chapter. Rather, we would like to introduce the reader to various organic or neurogenic speech sound disorders that will in all likelihood be further addressed in other courses in speech–language pathology. In a simplified outline form, we describe each disorder, the basic information related to its etiology, and assessment objectives and procedures. The reader is referred to the Advanced Unit of Chapter 2 for a review of the anatomy and neuroanatomy of speech production.

Childhood Apraxia of Speech

Apraxia of speech is a motor speech disorder caused by known neurological damage in the dominant language hemisphere. It is most commonly seen in adults and older persons as a result of stroke, traumatic brain injury, tumor removal, surgical trauma, or other sources of brain damage. The disorder is thought to be due to impaired motor planning, programming, and sequential movement for volitional speech production (Yorkston, Beukelman, Strand, & Hakel, 2010). The childhood equivalent of adult apraxia of speech is known as **childhood apraxia of speech (CAS).** Past terms for the disorder include **developmental apraxia of speech** and **developmental verbal dyspraxia,** all emphasizing the idiopathic and developmental nature of the disorder (Forrest, 2003; Hall, 2000; Marquardt, Sussman, & Davis, 2001; Shriberg, Aram, & Kwiatkowski, 1997a, 1997b, 1997c; Shriberg et al., 2005).

The American Speech-Language-Hearing Association (ASHA) has taken the position that CAS is a distinct diagnostic type of childhood speech sound disorder. Controversy about it continues, however, because its etiology is speculative, compared to apraxia of speech in adults, which is diagnosed on the basis of known neuropathology. According to the ASHA (2007) position statement, CAS may occur (1) as a result of known neurological factors such as intrauterine stroke, infections, and traumatic brain injury; (2) as a primary or secondary sign in children with known or unknown complex neurobehavioral variables such as autism, epilepsy, Down syndrome, and Fragile X syndrome; and (3) in the absence of any known neurological factors or lack of association with any neurobehavioral disorder, in which case it would be considered an *idiopathic neurogenic speech sound disorder*.

Despite wider acceptance as a unique diagnostic type of childhood speech sound disorder, *childhood apraxia of speech* continues to be primarily a descriptive label that is most useful in differentiating it from other developmental speech sound disorders, such as articulation disorder, phonological disorder, and developmental dysarthria. Over the years, some "soft" neurological signs—including fine and gross motor coordination problems, gait abnormalities, and difficulties with alternating and repetitive movements—have been reported across study subjects. However, to date studies have not identified a specific neuroanatomical marker or site of lesion that could explain the presence of the disorder (Yorkston et al., 2010).

The best estimate for the current prevalence of childhood apraxia of speech is 0.1–0.2% of the general population, with a greater frequency in males (Flipsen & Gildersleeve-Neumann, 2009). Although the current literature has not advanced a clear list of diagnostic features of CAS that differentiates it from other childhood speech sound disorders, three segmental and suprasegmental features have gained consensus among investigators, including (1) inconsistent errors on consonants and vowels in repeated productions of syllables or words; (2) lengthened and disrupted coarticulatory transitions between sounds and syllables; and (3) inappropriate prosody, especially in the realization of lexical and phrasal stress (ASHA, 2007; Flipsen & Gildersleeve-Neumann, 2009).

Nature of Childhood Apraxia of Speech

The speech characteristics associated with CAS are often inconsistent and contradictory from one source to another. Also, some of the characteristics on which the diagnosis is made are not unique to CAS, as they can also be used to diagnose children with articulation and phonological disorders (Hall, Jordan, & Robin, 2007). Characteristics of CAS described in a variety of sources may be summarized as follows (Hall, 2000; Hall et al., 2007; Lewis, Freebairn, Hansen, Iyengar, & Taylor, 2004; Marquardt et al., 2001; Shriberg et al., 1997a; Velleman & Strand, 1994; Yorkston et al., 2010):

Speech characteristics

- moderate to severe speech intelligibility problems
- greater unintelligibility of connected speech than of single words
- variable speech intelligibility depending on length and complexity of utterances
- variable severity of the disorder from mild to severe

- inconsistent or variable sound errors when the same word is produced on repeated trials; variability of speech problems in the same child across time periods (an important diagnostic indicator)
- unusual articulation errors, errors not usually found in children with functional articulation disorders, or normal articulation, possibly including the following:
    - addition errors (e.g., /gərin/ for *green*; /klæt/ for *cat*; and /kwink/ for *queen*)
    - prolongation errors (e.g., /beːby/ for *baby* and /sːən/ for *sun*)
    - production of sounds that are nonphonemic in English (e.g., glottal plosives and bilabial fricatives)
    - repetition of sounds and syllables
- usual or typical errors of articulation, errors that may also occur in children with functional articulation disorders or in typically learning children, possibly including the following:
    - predominance of omission and substitution errors, although distortion and addition errors also may occur and distortion errors may predominate in some older children
    - more common errors on fricatives, affricates, and consonant clusters
    - possibility of errors on fricatives and affricates continuing longer than in children with functional articulation problems or typical articulation
    - voicing and devoicing errors
    - vowel omissions and misarticulations, primarily distorted vowels and diphthong reduction
- resonance problems, including hyponasality, hypernasality, or nasal emission; likely due to poor motor control of the velopharyngeal mechanism
- problems of **aprosody** (flat prosody) in some children, **dysprosody** (inappropriate variation in frequency and duration) in some children, and the inappropriate use of stress patterns (reduced stress variation and errors on syllabic stress)
- increased frequency of dysfluencies, possibly related to articulatory groping and searching behavior

Sound and syllable sequencing problems

- difficulty producing sounds in correct sequence
- difficulty sequencing sounds in syllables or words, even when the individual phonemes are within the child's phonetic repertoire
- increased difficulty in producing multisyllabic words
- difficulty in sequencing phonemes on diadochokinetic speech tasks
- increase in the number of sequencing errors with an increase in the complexity or length of the utterance
- **metathetic,** or sound reversal, errors (e.g., /mæks/ for *mask* and /ʃɪf/ for *fish*)

Articulatory groping and silent posturing

- silent posturing errors (static articulatory postures without sound production); for example, although the child positions the lips for articulation of /b/, no sound is associated with the gesture—may be more common in older children

- articulatory groping errors, a series of articulatory movements in an attempt to find the correct placement or position for the production of sounds—may be more common in older children

- association of articulatory groping and searching behavior with diadochokinetic tasks

Associated problems

- generally slow progress in therapy

- **"soft" neurological signs,** often presumed from fine and gross motor incoordination

- presence of oral apraxia or difficulty with volitional nonspeech tasks

- slowed **diadochokinetic syllable rates**

- decreased oral awareness **(oral astereognosis)**

- expressive language problems, with relatively better receptive language skills

- associated learning disability in some children

- family history of speech and language problems in some children; perhaps persistence of language difficulties even when speech production improves

These listed symptoms of CAS should be used with caution. They vary to a great extent across children. Features that some consider important (e.g., nonspeech oral movements) may be absent in some children with CAS. Because of such variability, attempts have been made to identify a few essential features that help make a diagnosis of CAS. Some clinicians believe that the three essential features of CAS are (1) struggle, articulatory groping, and trial-and-error in producing speech sounds; (2) difficulty in volitional production of phonemes and sequence of phonemes that the child can otherwise produce; and (3) difficulty executing isolated and sequenced oral movements on command (Murdoch, Porter, Younger, & Ozanne, 1984). We have noted disagreement on oral–motor movements, however. Others believe that inappropriate linguistic stress distinguishes children with CAS (Shriberg et al., 1997c). Although stress problems are often evident to listeners, acoustic measures fail to demonstrate them. A survey of 75 practicing speech–language pathologists, however, has shown that they use up to 50 characteristics, some of them mutually contradictory, to make a diagnosis of CAS (Forrest, 2003). The survey also showed very little agreement among clinicians on the varied characteristics, although the following six characteristics were mentioned often: (1) inconsistent speech sound productions, (2) oral–motor problems, (3) articulatory groping, (4) difficulty imitating modeled sound productions, (5) increased problems with increased utterance length, and (6) difficulty sequencing sounds. Once again, lack of agreement among clinicians on a great variety of features highlights the problem with the diagnostic category CAS. Furthermore, there is some evidence that CAS is overdiagnosed (Davis, Jakielski, & Marquardt, 1998). For these reasons, CAS is still controversial (McCauley & Strand, 2008; Strand, McCauley, Weigand, Stoeckel, & Bass, 2012). Therefore, clinicians should be conservative in diagnosing CAS in children.

ACTIVITY

Describe three segmental and suprasegmental features of CAS that have gained consensus among investigators.

Assessment Objectives for Childhood Apraxia of Speech

There are multiple objectives in the assessment of CAS, including the following:

1. to assess the child's articulation skills and speech intelligibility across varied tasks and situations
2. to assess other communication skills that help develop a child-specific plan of treatment, including the child's auditory comprehension, verbal expression, and reading and writing skills
3. to assess other aspects of communication, including resonance, prosody, and fluency
4. to assess the child's oral–motor skills during speech and nonspeech tasks
5. to determine whether a diagnosis of childhood apraxia of speech is appropriate
6. to describe the nature of the child's speech production problems and make an estimate of severity
7. to distinguish CAS from other speech disorders, such as a functional speech sound disorder
8. to identify potential treatment targets and possible compensatory communication strategies
9. to make a clinical judgment of prognosis
10. to describe the child's strengths and intact skills that may be capitalized on in treatment

Assessment Techniques for the Diagnosis of Childhood Apraxia of Speech

To assess CAS, the clinician can follow some of the general procedures outlined in the Basic Unit of this chapter. Some procedures and activities are more appropriate for diagnosing childhood apraxia of speech in children who are suspected of having this speech disorder. It is recommended that clinicians use the following outline in assessing children suspected of having CAS (S. Haynes, 1985; Lewis et al., 2004; Marquardt et al., 2001):

- Take a developmental history of the child and note problems in sucking, delay in babbling, or slow language development, including limited number of words acquired at successive age levels.

- Assess expressive and receptive language skills; use the standard methods of assessing language production and comprehension.

- Test articulatory proficiency, including simple and complex isolated phonemes, polysyllabic words, and connected speech utterances; administer standardized tests of articulation (e.g., the *Goldman-Fristoe Test of Articulation: Second Edition* [Goldman & Fristoe, 2000]); ~~administer the same items repeatedly~~ (contrary to the standard procedure) ~~to assess inconsistency of productions.~~

- Record a conversational speech sample to analyze articulation errors, groping, and inconsistency of errors on the same sounds.

- Evaluate oral diadochokinetic syllable rates.

- Test for volitional nonspeech movements of the oral muscles, both in isolation and in sequence.

- Assess orosensory perception and oral awareness.

After collecting a thorough case history and screening the child's hearing, the clinician may collect a spontaneous speech sample to assess the child's articulatory performance in connected speech productions. ~~The sample should be tape recorded for later analysis, since it may be difficult to identify all of the symptoms at the time of the assessment.~~ The clinician should pay special attention to any atypical articulation errors and struggling, articulatory groping, and searching behavior that may be suggestive of motor programming problems. Sound prolongations, other forms of dysfluencies, delayed reaction times, silent postures, attempts at self-correction, and articulatory errors should also be noted. The clinician may perform the following tasks for a thorough assessment:

Assess nonimitative speech production skills

- Obtain nonimitative productions of a set of single words that samples all phonemes. Use object- or picture-naming tasks or a standardized articulation test (e.g., the *Goldman-Fristoe Test of Articulation: Second Edition* [Goldman & Fristoe, 2000] or the *Test of Minimal Articulation Competence* [Secord, 1981]) to evoke nonimitative productions. Select stimulus materials that are readily identifiable and appropriate for the child's age to decrease the need for modeling.

Examples

pen	baby
dog	fire
gum	horse
cat	light
mop	nose
table	soap

- Phonetically transcribe the utterances and speech sound errors. Make **whole-word transcriptions** to identify any patterns in production errors or coarticulatory errors (e.g., anticipatory errors, regressive errors, metathetic errors).

- Observe and record any signs of presumed speech motor programming problems (e.g., groping, dysfluencies, false starts, struggling behavior).

- Observe and record speech production problems as the length of the word increases.

Assess imitative speech production skills

- Model individual sounds and syllables and ask the child to imitate.

- Initially, hide your oral movements; if the child cannot imitate, show the normal movements.

- Model a series of shorter and longer words and ask the child to imitate.

  Examples

bat	expensive
hat	attacking
coat	cafeteria
bed	playground
look	computer
fast	principal

- Model a series of shorter and longer sentences and ask the child to imitate.

  Examples

The cat is big.	The cat in the box is black and white.
My mom is nice.	My mother gave me a present for my birthday.
Who wants cake?	I asked everyone, "Who wants chocolate cake?"
I like candy.	My favorite candy is milk chocolate.
I have a toy.	Yesterday, I bought a toy car at the toy store.

Assess the consistency and variability of errors

- Sample speech productions in varied phonetic contexts. Arrange informal tasks or administer formal instruments such as the *Deep Test of Articulation* (McDonald, 1964), the *Secord Contextual Articulation Tests* (S-CAT; Secord & Shine, 1997), or, for Spanish speakers, the *Contextual Probes of Articulation Competence–Spanish* (CPAC-S; Goldstein & Iglesias, 2006).

- Sample speech production in imitative and spontaneous modes. Identify the words the child produces spontaneously and then ask the child to imitate the same words. Note any differences in production.

- Sample production of the same phoneme (in the same word) in multiple trials. Record any articulatory differences in the production of the sound from one trial to another.

Assess diadochokinetic syllable rates, including alternating and sequential motion rates (AMRs and SMRs)

• *Instruct the child*: "Please say [pʌ-pʌ-pʌ] as long and as evenly as you can." Model the response for the client to imitate, "Try doing it like me . . ." (AMR).

• *Instruct the child*: "Please say [tʌ-tʌ-tʌ] as long and as evenly as you can." Model the response for the client to imitate, "Try doing it like me . . ." (AMR).

• *Instruct the child*: "Please say [kʌ-kʌ-kʌ] as long and as evenly as you can." Model the response for the client to imitate, "Try doing it like me . . ." (AMR).

• *Instruct the child*: "Please say [pʌ-tə-kə] as long and as evenly as you can." Model the response for the client to imitate, "Try doing it like me . . ." (SMR). The word *buttercup* may be substituted for [pʌ-tə-kə] with children who have difficulty following through with repetition of [pʌ-tə-kə].

• Record any groping or struggling behaviors observed during this task. Then compare the scores obtained for a particular child with established developmental data for the production of diadochokinetic syllable rates in children (Fletcher, 1972, 1978).

Assess intelligibility of speech

• Assess intelligibility from the conversational speech sample; use the procedures described in the section "Intelligibility Analysis" in the Basic Unit of this chapter.

• Assess intelligibility at different levels (syllables, words, phrases, and sentences).

Assess resonance problems

• Assess hypernasality, hyponasality, and nasal emission by clinical judgment.

• Use a nasal mirror to judge nasal emission in the production of non-nasal sounds.

• Visually inspect the velopharyngeal mechanism as part of the orofacial examination.

• When necessary and feasible, use mechanical instruments to diagnose resonance problems.

Assess prosodic problems

• Clinically evaluate the appropriateness of pitch and loudness variation.

• Clinically evaluate the stress patterns.

Assess fluency and dysfluencies

• Count the frequency of each dysfluency type exhibited in the speech sample.

• Count the frequency of each dysfluency type exhibited in an oral reading sample.

Standardized or formal instruments for the assessment of CAS include the two versions of the *Apraxia Profile* (AP; Hickman, 1997), the *Preschool Profile* and the *School-Age Profile*; the *Kaufman Speech Praxis Test for Children* (KSPT; Kaufman, 1995); the *Oral Speech Mechanism Screening Examination: Third Edition* (OSMSE-3; St. Louis & Ruscello, 2000); the *Screening Test for Developmental Apraxia of Speech: Second Edition* (STDAS-2; Blakeley, 2001); the *Verbal Dyspraxia Profile* (VDP; Jelm, 2001); and the *Verbal Motor Production Assessment for*

Children (VMPAC; Hayden & Square, 1999). See McCauley and Strand (2008) for a review and evaluation of these tests.

Developmental Dysarthria in Cerebral Palsy

Cerebral palsy (CP) is a nonprogressive neuromotor disorder resulting from brain damage in the developing fetus or infant. Because of the early onset of this disorder, it is often described as **congenital**, even if the damage occurs shortly after birth. The brain damage does not worsen as the child gets older, but a child's functional movement and posture disturbance may deteriorate over time (S. H. Long, 1994). Cerebral palsy may be classified in relation to when the brain damage occurs as **prenatal** (before birth), **perinatal** (during birth), or **postnatal** (after birth). It often co-occurs with problems with behavior, sensation, perception, cognition, and communication (Rosenbaum, Paneth, Leviton, Goldstein, & Bax, 2007). The incidence of cerebral palsy is estimated at about 2.0–3.6 in 1,000 live births (Flexer, Gillette, & Wray, 1997; Hegde, 2008a; Hustad, 2010; Mecham, 1996). Most children diagnosed with cerebral palsy grow into adulthood, and it is estimated that 800,000 Americans currently live with this condition (Hustad, 2010).

Etiology and Nature of Cerebral Palsy

There is no single etiology for cerebral palsy, and the actual cause is unknown in about 40% of cases (Hegde, 2008a; Long, 1994; Mecham, 1996). **Prenatal factors** associated with cerebral palsy are multiple and include exposure to radiation, intrauterine infections including HIV, exposure to drugs, exposure to metal toxicity, fetal anoxia or deprivation of oxygen, damage caused by blood infiltration in the nervous system, cerebral hemorrhage, chromosomal abnormalities, placental abruption or premature detachment of the fetus, and brain growth deficiency. Any of these factors may cause injury to the nervous system of the developing fetus.

Complications during the child's delivery have been listed as **perinatal factors**. These include trauma to the child's brain during delivery in a few cases, cerebral hemorrhage during the birthing process, and anoxia. **Postnatal factors** include premature birth, asphyxia, sepsis (blood toxicity or microorganisms in the blood), cerebral hemorrhage, inflammatory diseases of the brain (encephalitis and meningitis), and head trauma.

Because the severity and exact nature of the disorder varies across children, various systems have been used to classify the types of cerebral palsy. A system based on the distribution of limb paralysis uses the following categories:

- **quadriplegia**—paralysis involving the trunk and all four extremities
- **diplegia**—paralysis of the corresponding extremities on both sides of the body
- **paraplegia**—paralysis of the lower trunk and both lower extremities
- **hemiplegia**—paralysis of one side of the body
- **monoplegia**—paralysis of a single extremity

This classification system is limited, in that it does not highlight the type of paralysis associated with the disorder. A classification system based on the neuromuscular characteristics of cerebral palsy, or the damaged neurological system, results in the following categories:

- **spastic**—The most common type, occurring in about 70–80% of children with cerebral palsy (Hustad, 2010), it is related to pyramidal system lesions (upper motor neuron damage) and is characterized by increased muscle tone, an exaggerated stretch reflex, and slow, effortful, jerky, voluntary movements. It accompanies about a third of the other types of cerebral palsy.

- **dyskinetic**—This type results from extrapyramidal damage and occurs in approximately 15% of cases. It is characterized by abnormal patterns of posture or movement, including involuntary, uncontrolled, and recurring movements of the entire body. Dyskinetic CP includes athetoid and dystonic forms. **Athetoid cerebral palsy** is characterized by the presence of slow, writhing involuntary movements when volitional actions are attempted; fluctuating muscle tone, from normal at rest to hypertonic with voluntary movements; and increased involuntary movements with stress or distraction. It may be seen in newborns who have severe **jaundice** or **kernicterus**.

- **ataxic**—This type also is less common, occurring in 5–10% of diagnosed cases. It is caused by damage to the cerebellum or its control circuits. It is characterized primarily by a disturbed equilibrium, resulting in balance and posture problems. It affects the force, rhythm, and accuracy of movement of the entire body, including the trunk, hands, arms, and legs. Ambulating children may show a wide stance and an unsteady gait. Poor control of hand and arm movements may result in overshooting and intention tremor. The child's reflexes and muscle tone may or may not be affected.

- **mixed**—This is a combination of more than one type, the most common being a combination of spastic and athetoid types, resulting from both pyramidal and extrapyramidal lesions. Although the paralysis is mixed, one type usually predominates. The mixed type occurs in about 30% of all cases.

The two classification systems described above are primarily based on the neuromotor symptoms of the disorder. However, cerebral palsy is often associated with many other problems, including speech and language disorders. The motor speech sound disorder associated with cerebral palsy is known as **developmental dysarthria** (Hodge & Wellman, 1999). It can affect one, various, or all parameters of speech production: respiration, phonation, resonance, articulation, and prosody. At least six types of dysarthria have been identified by various researchers: flaccid, spastic, ataxic, hypokinetic, hyperkinetic, and mixed (Caruso & Strand, 1999; Darley, Aronson, & Brown, 1969a, 1969b, 1975; Duffy, 2005; Freed, 2012; Vogel & Cannito, 2001; Yorkston et al., 2010). Major speech characteristics of the different types are given in the following list:

- **flaccid dysarthria**—hypernasality, nasal emission, imprecise articulation (plosives and fricatives are especially affected because of poor intraoral pressure), breathiness, harsh voice, audible inhalation or inspiratory stridor, monopitch, monoloudness, and short phrases

- **spastic dysarthria**—hypernasality, imprecise articulation (consonants and vowels), harsh voice (strained–strangled vocal quality), effortful grunting at the end of vocalizations, excessively low pitch, pitch breaks, monoloudness, reduced stress, excess and equal stress, slow rate of speech, and short phrases

- **ataxic dysarthria**—imprecise articulation, irregular articulatory breakdowns, distorted vowels, prolonged phonemes, prolonged intervals between words or syllables, excess and equal stress, harsh voice (similar to a coarse voice tremor), monopitch, monoloudness, loudness control problems, variable nasality (occasional hypernasality and nasal emission), slow rate of speech, and general "drunken" speech quality

- **hypokinetic dysarthria**—imprecise articulation, repetition of phonemes, repetition of syllables (palilalia) in about 15% of cases, mild hypernasality in about 10–25% of cases, reduced vital respiratory capacity, irregular breathing, faster rate of respiration, hoarse voice, continuously breathy voice, tremulous voice, low pitch, monopitch, monoloudness, reduced stress, inappropriate silent intervals, short rushes of speech, variable and increased rate in segments, and short phrases

- **hyperkinetic dysarthria**—imprecise articulation, distorted vowels, inconsistent articulatory errors, voice tremor, intermittent strained voice, voice arrests, harsh voice, intermittent hypernasality, slow rate, excess loudness variations, prolonged inter-word intervals, inappropriate silent intervals, equal stress, audible inspiration, forced and sudden inspiration and expiration

- **mixed dysarthria**—symptoms depend on the types that are mixed and include the dominant symptoms of the independent types that are mixed (e.g., symptoms of both spastic and ataxic dysarthria)

The degree of neuromotor involvement will determine the degree of communicative impairment (Hegde, 2008a; Mecham, 1996). Children with mild cerebral palsy may not have significant communication problems, while those with severe cerebral palsy may be affected to such an extent that verbal communication is not functional. Approximately 75–85% of children with cerebral palsy show obvious speech problems. Speech intelligibility may be reduced as a result of poor articulation along with decreased loudness control, respiratory inefficiency, poor intraoral air pressure, and hypernasality. Hustad (2010) offers the following divisions, according to the degree of speech and language impairment:

1. no functional speech—severe motor involvement or anarthria

2. limited speech—moderate to severe motor impairment and significantly reduced speech intelligibility that helps meet some but not all communication needs

3. reduced speech intelligibility—mild to moderate speech impairment and reduced speech intelligibility; speech functional for communication and social interaction in known contexts

4. obvious disorder with intelligible speech—mild speech impairment with good speech intelligibility despite obvious dysarthria

5. no detectable speech disorder—speech sound production and intelligibility similar to those of typically learning children of the same age

Specific speech symptoms according to articulatory, resonatory, phonatory, respiratory, and prosodic problems include those listed below (adapted from Hegde, 2008a). Some symptoms listed may seem to contradict each other, highlighting the different types of neuromotor involvement that are associated with cerebral palsy:

Articulatory problems

- generally, more severe articulation problems with athetosis than with spasticity
- generally inefficient or imprecise articulation as a result of affected muscle strength, tone, speed, and range of movement
- slurred speech quality, especially with ataxic cerebral palsy
- significant difficulty with tongue-tip sounds, especially with spastic or rigid cerebral palsy
- articulatory conspicuousness, especially in athetoid cerebral palsy as a result of involuntary movements
- difficulty phonating or prolonging sounds
- predominance of omissions over substitutions or distortions
- greater difficulty with sounds in word-final positions than in other positions
- such phonological processes as cluster reduction, stopping, depalatalization, fronting, and gliding
- less proficient articulation in connected speech than in single words

Resonatory problems

- hypernasality due to velopharyngeal dysfunctions
- nasal emission due to velopharyngeal dysfunctions
- poor oral resonance due to difficulties with controlling intraoral breath pressure

Phonatory problems

- weak voice
- poor volume in some cases
- poor control of loudness, which may result in irregular bursts of loudness
- loss of voice toward the end of sentences and phrases, which may result in a whisper
- high pitch in some cases
- strained vocal quality in some cases due to hyperadduction of the vocal folds
- breathiness in some cases due to hypoadduction of the vocal folds

Respiratory problems

- persistence of rapid breathing rate beyond the first year of infancy (as compared to the normal slowdown of the rate as children mature)

- possibly excessive diaphragmatic activity and reduced activity of the chest and neck muscles
- flattening or flaring of the rib cage
- indented (sucked-in) sternum
- air wastage during speech production, resulting in short phrases or weak productions of final segments of sentences

Prosodic problems

- monotone
- monoloudness
- lack of smooth flow of speech
- general dysprosody as a result of respiratory, phonatory, resonatory, and articulatory problems

Associated problems

- slow and jerky jaw movements
- impaired or discoordinated tongue movements during speech production
- slow diadochokinetic syllable rates

Other problems associated with cerebral palsy, including hearing loss, mental retardation in about 50% of cases, attentional deficit, language disorders, and general learning disorders, may compound the child's speech difficulties. All of these may also affect the diagnosis of an articulation or phonological disorder, the prognosis for improvement, the selection of treatment objectives, and the general course of treatment.

ACTIVITY

Identify the six different types of dysarthria discussed in the chapter and the key speech features for each.

Assessment Objectives for Cerebral Palsy

There are multiple objectives in the assessment of the speech disorders associated with cerebral palsy. Because of the known benefits of early intervention, it is not uncommon for the assessment process to begin before the first birthday of children who are suspected of having cerebral palsy. Specific assessment objectives include the following:

1. to work closely with members of the assessment team, which may include medical specialists, nurses, psychologists, audiologists, educators, social workers, physical therapists, occupational therapists, and other professionals
2. to assess the child's relevant physiological structures during the oral–motor examination:
   - head control with stability of the neck and shoulder girdle (related to later mobility of the oral structure)

- a coordinated pattern of respiration and phonation (related to development of abdominal muscles)

3. to assess the communication deficits typically associated with cerebral palsy

4. to assess the child's strengths and intact skills so that the treatment plan capitalizes on what the child can do

5. to conduct follow-up assessments as needed because the child likely will need long-term care

6. to determine the child's potential for use of an alternative/augmentative communication system if verbal communication is not a feasible option

Assessing Children With Cerebral Palsy

In assessing children with cerebral palsy, the clinician should consider all aspects of child development. Periodic assessment will be needed as the child grows older and skills change (improving up to a point). Repeated assessments will help evaluate any deterioration in skills that may be addressed in rehabilitation. The following observations and assessments may be performed:

Observe and obtain information on neuromotor functions

- Obtain or request reports from the child's physicians or neurologist.
- Take note of the listed neurological symptoms during the assessment.
- Consult with such other specialists as physicians, physical therapists, psychologists, special educators, nurses, and occupational therapists.

Observe and obtain information on motor development

- Use a developmental scale or checklist to assess the child's motor and general behavioral development.
- Obtain systematic information from the parents about the child's motor developmental milestones.
- Consult with other specialists who may have knowledge of the child's motor development.

Obtain information on cognitive development

- Obtain a copy of the child's psychological report.
- Make clinical judgments based on your assessment of the child's speech and language development.

Assess speech disorders and speech intelligibility

- Observe and make note of any pre-speech behaviors such as the influence of abnormal body tone and movements on the speech mechanism; the presence of any structural deviations of the speech mechanism; muscle tone; general feeding, sucking, chewing, biting, and swallowing behaviors; breathing patterns; the presence of early speech behaviors such as cooing and babbling; and so forth.

- Take an extended speech and language sample if the child is verbal. Analyze the information according to any articulation errors, speech intelligibility, and patterns in production.
- Obtain a speech sample that involves the child and the parent or another family member to distinguish any differences in speech production across social situations.
- Administer a formal articulation or phonological assessment test. Assess the errors according to standard procedures and analyze any patterns in the child's misarticulations.
- Make clinical judgments about speech intelligibility for single words and sentences and with or without contextual cues; make a more detailed analysis of articulation skills when intelligibility is reduced.
- Consider any oral structural deviations (e.g., tongue weakness, asymmetries in the tongue and soft palate, abnormalities of the jaw, unusually high palate, malocclusions).
- Consider functional oral–motor problems (e.g., oral apraxia; lateral tongue deviations; sluggish movement of the tongue; uncontrolled movements of the facial muscles; chewing, sucking, and swallowing problems).
- Analyze the speech samples for individual sound errors and for patterns of errors (e.g., final consonant deletion, cluster reduction, fronting).

Assess prosodic problems

- Take note of stress patterns, intonation, rate of speech, and pauses.
- Make clinical judgments about prosody.

Assess voice and respiratory problems

- Make clinical judgments about vocal loudness and pitch and their social adequacy and age and gender appropriateness.
- Judge whether variations in loudness and pitch are smooth and normal or jerky and abnormal.
- Take note of voice quality (e.g., harshness, hoarseness, breathiness, strained–strangled voice).
- Take note of any difficulty in voicing that may be due to vocal folds that are either hyperadducted or hyperabducted.
- Judge the adequacy of breath support for speech.
- Take note of any breathing abnormalities.

Assess resonance problems

- Observe the presence of hypernasality, hyponasality, nasal emission, and reduced oral resonance. A mirror may be used to determine the presence of hypernasality and nasal emission, as discussed under the assessment of dysarthria.
- Consider the resonance data along with information on the child's velopharyngeal functioning.

Assess oromotor dysfunctions

- Complete a detailed orofacial examination.

Assess the need for augmentative and alternative communication

- Assess the child's oral communication potential.

- Assess the verbally limited child's potential for a variety of alternative and augmentative communication devices that might be used. Accomplish this with a team of professionals that includes an occupational therapist and a physical therapist.

Cerebral palsy is a medical diagnosis consistent with a history of damage to the developing brain that occurs before or soon after birth. It is associated with various neuromotor symptoms, behavioral patterns, and communication problems. The speech-language pathologist's primary responsibility is to assess and treat the speech, language, and communication problems of children with cerebral palsy.

Cleft Lip and Palate

A cleft is an opening in a normally closed structure. Various structural malformations affect the tissue, muscles, and bony processes of the upper lip, alveolar process, hard palate, soft palate, and uvula. Such a congenital anomaly results in an opening in the hard palate, the soft palate, or both. Although less common, clefts of the upper lip also occur (Bzoch, 2004; Kummer, 2014; Moller & Glaze, 2009; Peterson-Falzone, Hardin-Jones, & Karnell, 2001). Cleft palate is the most prevalent birth defect in the United States (Moller & Glaze, 2009).

Cleft lip and cleft palate occur during embryonic development. For a variety of reasons, the growth and fusion of the palatal and lip structures are disrupted. Normal closure of the lips generally occurs in the 5th to 6th week of gestation, while the hard and soft palates tend to fuse at about the 8th to 9th week (Golding-Kushner, 1997). Because of their separate embryonic points of fusion, cleft lip and palate do not always coexist. It is not uncommon for a child to have a cleft palate but an intact lip, and vice versa. Cleft lip with or without palatal involvement is thought to have a different etiology than isolated palatal clefts.

The incidence of cleft palate is 1 in 500–1,000 live births (Gorlin & Baylis, 2009; McWilliams, Morris, & Shelton, 1990; Peterson-Falzone et al., 2001). However, incidence rates in the United States have been reported to vary across cultural groups, with the highest incidence in Native American, followed by Japanese, Chinese, non-Hispanic Caucasian, and African American, children. Clefts of the lip and palate affect males twice as often as females, while isolated cleft palate occurs twice as often in females as in males. Overall, nearly half of all the children affected have a cleft of the lip and palate; one quarter show a cleft of the lip only; and another quarter show a cleft of the palate only.

The presence of a cleft palate with or without a cleft lip may be associated with various communication disorders, including speech sound disorders. Less severe clefts that are medically and surgically managed early in life may not affect communication. The more severe the malformation and the more delayed the surgical and medical intervention, the greater the severity of a communication disorder. Communication disorders may be more common in children with clefts that are part of a genetic syndrome.

Etiology and Nature of Cleft Lip and Palate

The origin of clefts is multifactorial. Many genetic, environmental, toxic, and embryonic developmental factors interact to produce clefts. Clefting has been associated with autosomal-dominant genetic syndromes such as Apert syndrome, Stickler syndrome, van der Woude syndrome, Waardenburg syndrome, and Treacher Collins syndrome. Other syndromes associated with cleft lip or palate are Pierre Robin syndrome, Crouzon syndrome, and Shprintzen syndrome. Environmental teratogens (toxins) such as excessive alcohol consumption, illegal drug use, and prescription drug use (e.g., anticonvulsants, thalidomide) during pregnancy have also been associated with cleft lip and palate (Peterson-Falzone et al., 2001).

There are many classification systems used to describe clefts. Each has its limitations, and none is accepted universally (Bzoch, 2004; Hegde, 2008a). A cleft of the lip can be categorized as complete or incomplete depending on its extension. An incomplete cleft of the lip may be only a minor notch or may extend almost to the nostril, while a complete cleft includes all of the lip and continues into the floor of the nostril. A cleft lip can be unilateral (only on one side, which is usually the left) or bilateral (on both sides). As previously indicated, a cleft of the lip can occur with or without a cleft of the palate (Bzoch, 2004; Peterson-Falzone et al., 2001; Hardin-Jones & Karnell, 2001; McWilliams et al., 1990).

A cleft palate can involve the hard and soft palates. The anterior two-thirds of the roof of the mouth make up the hard palate, while the posterior one-third makes up the soft palate. The hard palate has a bony foundation and a muscular overlay. The soft palate is composed only of muscle and mucosa.

Various communication disorders are associated with cleft lip, cleft palate, or both. These may originate from the structural abnormalities associated with clefts. They may also stem from one or a combination of problems that can accompany this disorder (e.g., middle ear infections, hearing loss, intellectual disabilities, and velopharyngeal incompetence). The lists that follow this paragraph provide the characteristics of the speech sound disorders, laryngeal and phonatory disorders, and resonance disorders associated with cleft lip and palate. The severity of these disorders runs along a continuum. Isolated cleft lip rarely results in misarticulations, while bilateral complete clefts of the hard and soft palates lead to the most severe speech problems (Hegde, 2008a).

Speech sound disorders
- greater difficulty with voiced sounds than with unvoiced sounds
- particular difficulty with sounds that require a buildup of **intraoral pressure,** resulting in weak production of fricatives, affricates, and stops (**pressure consonants**), especially in cases of cleft palate
- substitution of nasal sounds for non-nasal sounds, although substitutions may not be genuine; added nasal resonance may be due to **velopharyngeal inadequacy,** leading to a resonance, rather than a speech, sound disorder
- audible or inaudible nasal emission while producing voiceless sounds
- distortion of some vowels
- **compensatory errors,** which are sound substitutions made in an attempt to compensate for inadequate closure of the velopharyngeal mechanism, often by

posterior movement of the tongue to stop the air or to produce friction noise, including the following:

- substitution of glottal stops /ʔ/ for stop consonants
- substitution of laryngeal stops for stop consonants and laryngeal fricatives for fricatives (involving posterior movement of the tongue so as to move the epiglottis toward the pharynx to block the air or to create friction noise)
- substitution of pharyngeal stops (/ʕ̥/ unvoiced, /ʕ/ voiced) for stop consonants and pharyngeal affricates for palatal affricates (involving posterior movement of the tongue to make contact with the pharynx to build up pressure that is suddenly released or to constrict the air to create friction)
- substitution of posterior nasal fricatives for fricatives /Δ/ (accomplished by using the posterior dorsum of the tongue and the soft palate to create friction noise)
- substitution of mid-dorsum palatal stops (/ɟ/ voiced, /ɟ̊/ unvoiced) for /t/, /d/, /k/, and /g/ (involving raising the mid-dorsum of the tongue toward the hard palate to build pressure)
- substitution of mid-dorsum palatal fricatives for fricatives and mid-dorsum palatal affricates for affricates (created by moving the mid-dorsum toward the hard palate to create friction of the built-up pressure)
- production of nasal fricatives for various sounds (also called *nasal snorts*, *nasal rustles*, or *nasal friction*)
- substitution of velar fricatives (/χ/ unvoiced, /ɣ/ voiced) for velar stops /k/ and /g/

• reduced speech intelligibility to varying extents, depending on the number and types of articulation errors

Laryngeal pathologies and phonatory disorders

Most phonatory disorders are due to velopharyngeal inadequacy, which leads to hyperfunction of the voice.

• increased prevalence of voice or phonatory disorders in children with cleft palate

• higher frequency of vocal nodules (possibly due to strain on the vocal folds caused by compensatory articulation)

• hypertrophy and edema (swelling) of the vocal folds

• hoarse voice

• reduced vocal intensity (possibly due to velopharyngeal inadequacy)

• monotonous voice

• strangled vocal quality (possibly due to excessive effort and tension exerted to avoid hypernasality)

Resonance disorders

- hypernasality on vowels and voiced oral consonants (possibly due to inadequate velopharyngeal closure and restricted mouth opening)

- hyponasality

- denasality (near absence of nasal resonance on nasal sounds)

Associated problems

- velopharyngeal incompetence resulting in inadequate closure of the velopharyngeal port

- history of recurrent middle ear infections

- hearing loss (conductive hearing loss, due to recurrent middle ear infections, in approximately 50% of children with cleft palate)

- language disorder (often associated with a cleft that is part of a genetic syndrome)

- initially delayed language development (normal language possible by about age 4)

....

ACTIVITY

Identify and describe some of the speech sound production problems commonly associated with cleft palate.

....

Assessment Objectives for Cleft Lip and Palate

Because clefts of the palate and lips are a congenital anatomic growth disorder, the initial assessment is usually performed soon after the child's birth. Many hospitals have a craniofacial clinic, where children with congenital disorders are assessed by a team of specialists (e.g., pediatrician, nurse, dentist, orthodontist, speech–language pathologist, physician, counselor, audiologist). The surgical repair of cleft lip and palate is done by a team of medical specialists. A speech–language pathologist is a member of the multidisciplinary team identifying and managing the communication problems. Specific objectives for the assessment of speech problems associated with cleft lip and palate include the following:

- to work with other members of the team of professionals

- to determine the communication disorders typically associated with cleft lip and palate

- to make periodic assessments of communication to help plan surgical intervention

- to suggest communication treatment targets if speech problems persist after surgical intervention

- to assess the child's strengths and intact skills

Assessing Children With Cleft Lip and Palate

In the assessment of the communication problems associated with clefts of the lip and palate, the clinician can follow the general procedures outlined throughout the Basic Unit of this chapter. The clinician should collect a comprehensive history and conduct a thorough interview. The collection of a thorough health and developmental history is extremely important because medical and surgical interventions are common in children with cleft lip and palate. Some children may have a history of recurrent otitis media or eustachian tube dysfunction and concomitant hearing loss. The clinician should get clear information on the child's speech and language development.

Assess Connected Speech Production

The actual assessment can start by taking a conversational speech sample, which may be initiated during the interview process. The clinician notes the child's speech characteristics and any other obvious behavioral or structural symptoms. If the child can read, the clinician can also assess connected speech during an oral reading task by asking the child to read passages that are age- and reading-level appropriate. The sample may be audio- or videotaped for later analysis.

Assess the Speech Production Mechanism

Because clefts of the lip and palate are craniofacial structural problems, it is essential to conduct a thorough orofacial examination, using the guidelines given in the Basic Unit of this chapter in the section "Performing an Orofacial Examination." The clinician should pay special attention to unrepaired clefts. If the clefts have been surgically repaired, the clinician can make a judgment about the adequacy of the repair. It is important to note that movements of the soft palate during sustained production of /a/, a typical activity during an orofacial examination, may not always be a valid indicator of soft palate movement in connected speech or the adequacy of velopharyngeal closure. A clinical judgment of hypernasality or hyponasality may be more appropriate to evaluate velopharyngeal closure in connected speech.

Assess Speech Sound Production Errors

Because children with cleft lip and palate often display specific speech sound production difficulties, the clinician may consider and focus on the following:

Assessing possible articulation and phonological problems

- Words and sentences that contain stops, fricatives, and affricates (pressure consonants), which are difficult for children with cleft lip and palate, are especially useful.

- To assess the child's production of all English sounds, administer a norm-referenced standardized articulation or phonological assessment, paying close attention to compensatory substitution errors and any consonants that are typically affected by velopharyngeal insufficiency such as stops, fricatives, and affricates.

- Assess stimulability for an improved production of the error sounds with a combination of auditory, visual, tactile, and kinesthetic cues to facilitate correct production of the sounds that are misarticulated.

- Note any difficulty with the motor production of sounds, along with phonological error patterns that may exist independently of the effects of cleft lip and palate.

Assessing possible phonatory problems

- Note any voice disorder, including a breathy, harsh, hoarse, or excessively soft voice.

- Note vocally abusive behaviors such as excessive coughing, throat clearing, or snorting, as well as the use of compensatory articulatory gestures that may place undue strain on the vocal folds.

- Refer the child for a diagnostic voice evaluation if warranted.

- Assessing possible resonance disorders

- Determine the presence of hypernasality and nasal emission based on the child's connected speech.

- To observe the velopharyngeal mechanism, ask the child to say, "Ah," which also provides an opportunity to note the movement of the soft palate (e.g., its symmetry, tone, range, speed).

- Assess nasal airflow by holding a mirror under the nares as the child prolongs the vowel /i/; because of the absence of nasal resonance on this vowel, the mirror should remain clear during its production unless the child is hypernasal.

The initial assessment and subsequent surgical management of cleft lip and palate are managed by medical specialists. The speech–language pathologist is primarily responsible for assessing and treating the child's speech, language, and communicative problems.

Hearing Impairment

As discussed in Chapter 4, hearing loss is a known variable of impaired speech sound production. **Hearing impairment** or **hearing loss** refers to reduced **hearing acuity**, which can range from mild to profound. Severity of hearing loss is typically categorized as follows:

- **slight hearing loss**—hearing thresholds in the 16–25 dB HL range
- **mild hearing loss**—hearing thresholds in the 26–40 dB HL range
- **moderate hearing loss**—hearing thresholds in the 41–70 dB HL range
- **severe hearing loss**—hearing thresholds in the 71–90 dB HL range
- **profound hearing loss**—hearing thresholds that are 91 dB and higher

A child whose hearing loss falls between 16 and 90 dB HL is **hard of hearing**, as previously described. A child whose hearing threshold is above 90 dB is **deaf**.

Etiology and Nature of Hearing Impairment

The causes of hearing loss are multiple and varied. Most causes are organic, although some individuals may experience **psychogenic** hearing loss. The most common types of hearing loss are conductive, sensorineural, and mixed.

Conductive hearing loss is characterized by the interrupted transmission of sound to the cochlea. The interruption may occur in the outer or middle ear, but the latter is more common. A common cause of hearing loss in children is recurrent *otitis media*, more commonly known as middle ear infections. Other causes of conductive hearing loss include the following:

- otitis externa (inflammation of the external auditory canal, "swimmer's ear")
- collapsed ear canal, most common in elderly females
- osteomas (benign bony tumors of the external auditory canal)
- disarticulation of the auditory ossicular chain (separation of the ossicular bones)
- aural atresia (closed external auditory canal)
- stenosis (narrowing of the external auditory canal)

Sensorineural hearing loss results when the hair cells of the cochlea or the fibers of the acoustic nerve (cranial nerve VIII) are damaged. Specifically, damage to the hair cells constitutes a *sensory loss*, while damage to the acoustic nerve is best described as a *peripheral neural loss*. This type of loss is permanent, because the structures damaged do not regenerate.

Fetal alcohol syndrome, maternal drug addiction, congenital disorders, and low birth weight have been implicated in sensory hearing loss. Isolated *peripheral neural loss* is relatively rare. It may result from a tumor of the cranial nerve (CN) VIII, which is the most common of the cranial tumors. Demyelinization, or damage to the myelin sheath of the acoustic nerve, may also result in this type of hearing loss.

A combination of conductive hearing loss and sensorineural hearing loss is called **mixed hearing loss.** Mixed hearing loss may result from a combination of the causes described for pure conductive and pure sensorineural hearing loss.

The specific communication disorders found in a child with hearing loss depend on (1) the degree of hearing loss; (2) the age at which the loss was incurred; (3) the kind and quality of intervention; (4) the age at which the intervention was initiated; (5) the extent of family support; and (6) the presence of other physical, cognitive, or sensory problems. The speech problems associated with hearing loss may be summarized as follows (adapted from Hegde, 2008a):

Articulation problems
- omission of initial and final consonants and consonant clusters; omission of /s/ across word positions
- substitution of voiced consonants for voiceless consonants, nasal consonants for oral consonants
- distortion of sounds, especially of stops and fricatives

- some vowel substitutions, imprecise production of vowels with increased duration, breathiness before their productions
- addition of sounds, especially an intrusive schwa between consonants in blends (e.g., /bəlu/ for blue)
- inappropriate release of final stops (e.g., /stap^h/ for /stopʔ/)

Voice and resonance problems

These are most pronounced in the deaf.

- high-pitched voice, harshness, hoarseness, breathiness
- nasal emission on voiceless consonants, hypernasality on voiced consonants and vowels, hyponasality on nasal consonants
- lack of normal intonation

Fluency and prosodic disturbances

- generally limited fluency, increased rate of dysfluencies, inappropriate pauses during speech
- slow rate of speech, abnormal flow and rhythm
- abnormal intonation patterns

Associated language and literacy problems

- generally limited vocabulary, poor comprehension of words with multiple meanings and those that are abstract, metaphoric, and proverbial
- slower acquisition of grammatical morphemes, omission of grammatical morphemes, slower acquisition of verb forms
- shorter sentences, fewer varieties of sentence types
- pragmatic language problems, lack of elaborated speech, insufficient background information, and occasional irrelevance of speech
- poor reading comprehension, writing that mirrors the existing verbal language problems

Assessment Objectives

The child may be assessed by a team of specialists, including speech–language pathologists, audiologists (responsible for diagnosing the hearing loss), teachers of deaf and hard of hearing children, regular classroom teacher, social worker, psychologist, and other professionals. The SLP's primary responsibility is to assess the communication disorders that may result from a hearing loss, as follows:

- to assess the child's articulation skills and speech intelligibility across varied tasks and situations
- to assess other aspects of speech, including voice, resonance, and prosody
- to assess other communication skills, including auditory comprehension, verbal expression, and reading and writing skills

- to describe the nature of the child's speech production problems and estimate their severity
- to identify potential treatment targets and possible compensatory communication strategies
- to make a clinical judgment of prognosis
- to describe the child's strengths and intact skills

Assessing Speech Problems Associated With Hearing Impairment

In assessing the communication problems associated with hearing loss, the clinician can follow the general procedures outlined throughout the Basic Unit of this chapter. A comprehensive history should be collected, and a thorough interview should be completed. The child's developmental and medical background is extremely important. It is crucial that the clinician become familiar with the type and degree of hearing loss and inquire about the age of onset of the disorder. Children with congenital or **prelingual** hearing loss may exhibit more severe communication problems than children whose loss is acquired or **postlingual.** The type and extent of prior educational, therapeutic, and medical interventions should be determined.

The clinician may conduct the following specific assessments to gain a thorough understanding of the child's speech sound production skills and areas of difficulty:

Assess auditory perception or speech discrimination problems

- The clinician should consult with the audiologist to determine what information the child can receive from a speech signal presented without visual cues (Elfenbein, 1994).
- The clinician can administer a test such as *Wepman's Auditory Discrimination Test: Second Edition* (Wepman & Reynolds, 1986) to assess discrimination between various kinds of speech and nonspeech stimuli. This test helps to identify children who may have an auditory discrimination impairment and potential difficulty in learning the phonics necessary for reading.
- The child's speech discrimination skills should be considered relative to associated language problems.

Assess the orofacial structures and speech mechanism

- If the child's hearing loss is part of another disorder (e.g., cleft palate, cerebral palsy), the clinician may need to perform a comprehensive orofacial examination.
- If the child's speech problems are a result of the hearing loss only, a less detailed orofacial examination may be sufficient.
- The procedures for conducting an orofacial examination, as outlined in "Performing an Orofacial Examination" in the Basic Unit of this chapter, can be used with deaf and hard of hearing children to rule out any problems with the speech production mechanism.

Assess speech sound production

- Administer a standardized test such as the *Goldman-Fristoe Test of Articulation: Second Edition* (Goldman & Fristoe, 2000) or the *Hodson Assessment of Phonological Patterns* (Hodson, 2004).
- Analyze the error patterns.
- Pay special attention to the typical speech errors of deaf and hard of hearing children.
- Use narrow phonetic transcription to fully capture the extent of the child's errors, because many will be sound distortions.

Assess connected speech production

- The clinician should collect a conversational speech sample to supplement single-word articulation tests.
- Children who are hard of hearing, like hearing children, may demonstrate better articulation skills in single-word tests than in connected speech.
- If the child can read, the clinician can also assess connected speech during an oral reading task.
- The speech sample should be analyzed for articulation and other speech problems. Phonological patterns should be described.
- The child's speech intelligibility should be determined from the conversational speech sample.

Assess voice and resonance problems

- Children who are hard of hearing may exhibit voice or resonance problems that warrant further assessment.
- Clinical judgment may be made regarding voice quality, hyper- and hyponasality, and loudness and pitch and their variations; instrumental assessment may be considered when needed (Hegde, 2008a).

The speech–language pathologist may implement a treatment program for the speech sound and other disorders of communication diagnosed in the child. The clinician and other professionals serving on the team should maintain regular communication with each other.

....

ACTIVITY

Identify the hearing thresholds associated with the degree and severity of hearing loss: slight hearing loss, mild hearing loss, moderate hearing loss, severe hearing loss, profound hearing loss.

....

Summary of the Advanced Unit

- The speech–language pathologist may be involved in the assessment of clients with speech disorders of an organic or neurogenic origin.

- **Childhood apraxia of speech** is a motor speech disorder; in most cases, it is of unknown etiology. Children with apraxia of speech exhibit sound substitutions and distortions, groping articulation, and lack of volitional control of the oral mechanism for speech production.

- **Cerebral palsy** is a nonprogressive neuromotor disorder resulting from brain damage before, during, or shortly after birth. Spastic, athetoid, ataxic, rigid, and mixed are the subtypes. Speech characteristics associated with cerebral palsy are similar to those found in dysarthria.

- **Dysarthria** is a group of motor speech disorders caused by various neurological diseases and associated with muscle weakness, paralysis, or discoordination. Types of dysarthria include spastic, flaccid, hyperkinetic, hypokinetic, ataxic, and mixed. Specific speech characteristics accompany each type. All aspects of speech production can be affected in dysarthria, including articulation, phonation, resonation, respiration, and prosody.

- A **cleft** is a structural malformation affecting the tissues, muscles, and bony processes of the upper lip, alveolar process, hard palate, soft palate, and uvula, caused variously by genetic and environmental factors. A child with cleft palate may exhibit speech sound, resonance, and voice problems.

- **Hearing impairment** or **loss** refers to reduced **hearing acuity** and can range from mild to profound. The terms **hard of hearing** and **deaf** are differentiated by the extent of hearing loss in an individual. The most common types of hearing loss are **conductive, sensorineural,** and **mixed.**

- Children with hearing loss may exhibit problems with articulation, resonance, prosody, and voice.

A COMPREHENSIVE AND EVIDENCE-BASED TREATMENT PROGRAM FOR SPEECH SOUND DISORDERS

It is not sufficient to know what one ought to say, but one must also know how to say it.

—Aristotle

Basic Unit: Treatment Principles and Procedures

This and the next chapter are devoted to treatment of speech sound disorders in children. Clinicians will find a variety of treatment approaches or programs, all recommended by their developers as the one to be used exclusively. In Chapter 8, we describe several such programs, and the clinician may choose one of those programs to treat SSDs. We believe, however, that the clinician needs to do considerably more than follow a single described program. This is because most programs or approaches do not include everything a clinician needs to do to treat children with SSDs. Program authors assume that clinicians know how to perform the required procedures that are not described in their program. They may not give details of base rating, systematic probing, or reinforcer selection, for example. Some programs do not describe the sequence with which treatment proceeds from simpler levels to the conversational level. Most do not specify the types of consequences for a child's correct and incorrect responses. Others, especially the nonlinear phonological approaches, are excessively theoretical for the clinician. No treatment evidence compels the clinician to incorporate those abstract theoretical concepts into treatment; they just inject unnecessary complications into treatment.

Each program developer concentrates on what is unique to his or her approach: cycles, phonemic contrasts, multiple phonemes, stimulability, concurrent teaching, and so forth. Most programs known to the clinicians are different only in the way they characterize the target responses (teaching individual phonemes, eliminating phonological error patterns, demoting or promoting constraint rankings, teaching to a specified criterion or cycling), but they do not differ in the actual teaching of specific phoneme production; all treatment programs require other missing elements like base-rating, reinforcing or providing corrective feedback, treatment sequencing, and so forth. In essence, few treatment programs are comprehensive. The traditional Van Riper approach is more comprehensive than some of the newer approaches, although the newer approaches are better researched.

Not everything in a treatment program is a technically defined treatment variable; these are two different things. A *treatment program* is an overall plan of treatment; *treatment variables* are those technical operations the clinician performs in treatment sessions to teach specific target skills—such as the correct production of selected speech sounds, syllable or word structures, or other speech-related skills. A comprehensive program would include target behavior selection and base rating, for example, but these are not treatment variables. The clinician should probe for generalized production of either individual sounds or sounds within an error pattern, but probes also are not treatment. One can select treatment stimuli based on phonemic contrast or opposition, but this is not treatment. In the multiple phoneme approach, the clinician selects more than one phoneme for teaching, but such selection itself is not treatment—it is simply an overall treatment strategy. *Treatment variables come into play only when the clinician sits down with the child and begins to teach; anything done before that is treatment planning rather than treatment.* Experts describe the treatment variables in their programs with varying degrees of specificity; some may skip this altogether, concentrating on what is unique about their approach: their own ways of conceptualizing the target speech sound production skills.

Therefore, various treatment programs described in the next chapter, though they sound very different from each other, could possibly achieve their goal of teaching speech sound production by performing some of the same technical operations (manipulating treatment variables). These technical operations, more or less explicitly stated in different programs, include the following:

- describing the target behavior (correct production of specific sounds, whole words, syllable or word structure) to the child

- modeling the correct production

- demonstrating how correct production may be achieved (e.g., via phonetic placement)

- asking the child to imitate the clinician's modeled production

- reinforcing the correct production or an approximation of it

- giving corrective feedback for an incorrect production

- fading modeling and evoking progressively more spontaneous sound productions and reinforcing them or giving corrective feedback

A speech sound is taught this way in most if not all the programs described in the next chapter. It does not matter whether a program is called a traditional approach, cycles approach, phonological contrast approach, nonlinear phonological theory approach, stimulability approach, core vocabulary approach, or complexity approach; in each of these apparently different approaches, speech sound productions are taught the same way: by manipulating the specific treatment variables just listed. In the treatment program described in the Basic Unit of this chapter, we have addressed all of the treatment variables typically used in the treatment of speech sound disorders. We have made every effort to describe the treatment variables with sufficient detail to allow clinicians to modify as needed to meet the individual needs of their clients.

Treatment Program Considerations

This Treatment Program Is Appropriate for All Speech Sound Disorders

The program described in this chapter is good for treating children with articulation disorders as well as phonological disorders. In treating speech sound disorders, the primary goal is to teach sounds (what some call *content*) or word structure (what some call *frame*) that are absent in a child's repertoire or to increase the level of correct production for what is present at a low level. This goal holds regardless of whether the errors are classified according to individual sound productions, phonological patterns of linear theory, or phonological constraints of nonlinear theory (see Chapters 3 and 4 for these theories). No single sound error, word structure, constraint, pattern of multiple errors, or inappropriate constraint rankings can be changed without teaching some individual sounds or sound structure that may promote generalized production of other, untreated sounds.

Clinicians may gain the impression that current phonological or linguistically oriented approaches that are researched for their efficacy do not use behavioral teaching methods. But this is an erroneous impression, because in all approaches, whether they are described as linguistic, cognitive, phonological, linear, nonlinear, sensory–motor, cognitive, traditional, minimal pairs, multiple phonemes, contrast, maximal oppositions, multiple oppositions, or phonotactic, the actual teaching of speech sounds in error is indeed accomplished through behavioral treatment procedures that include instructions, modeling, positive reinforcement, corrective feedback, shaping, manual guidance, prompting, fading, and other behavioral techniques. One typical limitation of phonological-linguistic treatment researchers is that they devote much time and space to describe their linguistic concepts while giving only a sketchy impression of how they actually teach sound skills in treatment sessions. That is because linguistics and phonology have no treatment procedures. Rather, they simply suggest some unique ways of analyzing speech sound errors. Linguistic error analysis and treatment data interpretations precede and follow, respectively, behavioral treatment to establish correct production of speech sound skills. Consider, for instance: How does a clinician eliminate an error pattern of final consonant deletion? Only by teaching or increasing production of a few final consonants and then probing for generalized production of other, untreated, final consonants within the error pattern. How does a clinician eliminate velar fronting in which such velar sounds as /k/ and /g/ are replaced with such more frontally produced sounds as /t/ and /d/? Only by teaching the correct production of /k/ and /g/. Further, how does a clinician establish a minimal contrast between the child's atypical production /s/ for the target production /ʃ/? Only by establishing or increasing production of the target /ʃ/ in a set of words that could be paired to contrast with the target /s/; the contrast is established through production training. Those correct productions may be taught only by modeling and reinforcing correct responses, among other procedures.

Clinicians may use phonological theories to analyze assessment results and interpret treatment data, but they should consider the possibility that errors may be organized with adherence to no theory and treatment data may be interpreted with no help from phonological theories. Initially, grouping errors on the basis of phonetic principles, though it may now seem like a throwback to the pre-phonological era, is a good start; in this respect, taking preliminary guidance from natural phonological processes may be good. Identifying patterns by phonetic principles may be more empirical than grouping them according to abstract nonlinear constraints and constraint rankings, because natural phonological patterns are phonetically based—that is, they are based on anatomic and physiologic variables that affect articulation. Only treatment data, however, will tell the clinician whether the error patterns—identified on any basis—are valid. For example, if treating several final consonants results in generalized production of some of them but not the others, those not generalized do not belong to the final consonant deletion pattern. Only those that are generalized belong to the treated speech sound class. Thus, the behavioral treatment and generalization can identify more valid patterns or classes of speech sounds and their errors than phonological theories. This means that posttreatment patterning of speech sound errors will be more valid than theoretically based pretreatment patterning.

This Treatment Program Is Comprehensive and Modifiable

We offer this program because, as noted before, none of the specific or specialized treatment approaches are described in a sufficiently comprehensive way to be applied by clinicians. Nonetheless, all well-researched treatment approaches, including the traditional, linear, and nonlinear phonological approaches, have elements clinicians may find valid, useful, and practical enough to be incorporated into a comprehensive, evidence-based program. For example, from the minimal contrast approach (which evolved from linear theory), the clinician may teach target sound production in a contrasting manner and select picture stimuli (minimal pair word sets) that depict that contrast. Selected contrastive sound productions would still have to be taught with the behavioral treatment procedures, however. In this chapter we offer a comprehensive program that describes fundamental treatment variables. The program described in this chapter may be applied in all clinical settings, across all children, regardless of a diagnosis of articulation disorder or phonological disorder. The clinician may need to effect only minimal modifications in the program to make it suitable for individual children.

We recognize, however, that a clinician may wish to use one of the specific treatment approaches described in the next chapter. If so, the clinician has two choices: First, he or she may apply that procedure wholesale, which we think is unlikely because neither the programs nor their descriptions are comprehensive. Second, the clinician may add missing elements to the selected program (e.g., the maximal contrast approach or the minimal pair intervention approach) and modify it to make it suitable to individual children before implementing it. Although in this chapter we have tried to include all of the components of a comprehensive treatment program, the clinician is free to select and combine treatment elements as he or she pleases. In any case, we do not expect the clinician to use the comprehensive program described in this chapter in addition to a specific program described in the next chapter.

Evidence Base for This Comprehensive Program

The treatment procedures described in this chapter are based on well-researched principles of learning. Their efficacy in establishing and maintaining target skills of various kinds has been demonstrated in numerous experimental studies (Baldwin & Baldwin, 2000; Carr et al., 1994; Hegde, 1998; Kaiser & Gray, 1993; Maag, 1999; Reichle & Wacker, 1993; Scheuermann & Hall, 2008). Behavioral treatment of communicative disorders has been supported by many experimental studies in the past (see Hegde, 1998, for a review of various studies), and it continues to receive support in current treatment research.

Support for using behavioral procedures to establish correct speech sound production comes from many well-controlled single-subject experimental design studies, the first of which were published in the 1970s (Bailey, Timbers, Phillips, & Wolf, 1971; R. D. Baker & Ryan, 1971; Bennett, 1974; Camarata, 1993; Costello & Ferrer, 1976; Costello & Hairston, 1976; Costello & Onstine, 1976; Elbert, Dinnsen, Swartzlander, & Chin, 1990; Elbert & McReynolds, 1975; Elbert, Powell, & Swartzlander, 1991; Fitch, 1973; Gierut, 1989, 1990, 1992, 1998; Gierut & Champion, 2001; Gierut, Morrisette, & Champion, 1999; Gierut, Morrisette, Hughes, & Rowland, 1996; Koegel, Koegel, & Ingham, 1986; Koegel, Koegel, Voy, & Ingham, 1988; McReynolds, 1972; McReynolds & Bennett, 1972; McReynolds & Elbert, 1981b; McReynolds & Engmann, 1975; Murdock, Garcia, & Hardman, 1977; Saben & Ingham, 1991; Tyler, Lewis, & Welch, 2003; A. L. Williams, 2000; A. L. Williams & McReynolds, 1975; among many others). These and other studies have used the behavioral procedures of instruction, modeling, manual guidance (phonetic placement), prompts, positive reinforcement, corrective feedback, and others that promote generalization and maintenance of correct speech sound productions.

Support for the procedures described in this chapter also comes from almost all current phonological treatment efficacy studies. Phonological treatment efficacy studies examine the use of instruction, modeling, positive reinforcement in one form or another, some behavioral criteria to guide movement from imitated productions to spontaneous productions, probing for generalization, and additional treatment if generalization fails; these are the essence of all articulation treatment programs researched in the past several decades, as well as in recent years. The actual treatment procedure with which sound productions are taught in Gierut's (1989, 1990, 1992, 1998) extensive experimental research studies on phonological disorders is entirely behavioral. Others who use explicitly phonological analysis of error patterns also use only the behavioral methods to teach speech sound productions (e.g., see M. Allen, 2012; Stoel-Gammon, Stone-Goldman, & Glaspey, 2002).

Some programs may use terms that suggest nonbehavioral elements of treatment. The popular term *scaffolding*, for example, is positive reinforcement; while the construct of positive reinforcement has a rich history of experimental research supporting the principle that some consequences of behaviors reliably increase those behaviors, there is no such evidential history behind the construction industry–based construct of scaffolding. Similarly, the term *recasting* is simply modeling and corrective feedback. Instead of *reinforcing* or giving *corrective feedback*, some prefer to give just feedback, but reinforcers and corrective feedback are based on replicated experimental research. The difference between an explicitly behavioral and presumably nonbehavioral phonological-linguistic approach is this: Those who take a phonological and linguistic approach analyze and reanalyze, classify and reclassify speech sound errors based on theories; but they teach speech sound productions with the same behavioral methods as those who take a more explicit behavioral view of SSDs. After obtaining their treatment data, clinicians with a phonological-linguistic orientation interpret their data in light of their theory; those with an explicitly behavioral approach eschew such theoretical interpretations as speculative. There is no difference, however, in how the two sets of clinicians or researchers teach the production of individual sounds to children. The emphasis the phonological-linguistic researchers place on linguistic theories in their treatment research papers and books has obscured their actual methods of teaching speech sound productions to children. All phonological-linguistic treatment research on SSDs published in recent years supports the behavioral methods of teaching speech sound productions. If the phonological-linguistic treatment researchers made their treatment descriptions specific and explicit, its essence would be as behavioral as the comprehensive treatment program described in this chapter. It is important to note that behavioral treatment techniques have received the most support in the treatment efficacy research on SSDs and are becoming more explicitly supported in phonological theory circles. For example, Gierut, who adheres to a nonlinear complexity phonological theory approach, states that, in the absence of definitive research data that support the use of one treatment program over another, "it is only safe to say that basic principles of phonological learning may be employed including, for example, the use of modeling, corrective feedback, successive approximation, and branching" (2004, p. 7). We might add that those procedures, including positive reinforcement, are behavioral (operant) learning principles not unique to phonological learning.

Treatment Program Elements

Clinicians develop treatment programs after a valid assessment and diagnosis have been made, as described in the previous chapter. The clinician includes in a treatment program all the steps necessary to begin, implement, and end the program for children under treatment. Accordingly, a comprehensive SSD treatment program minimally includes the following components:

1. selection of child-specific target behaviors (treatment goals and objectives)
2. establishment of pretreatment baseline measures of speech sound production skills
3. selection and preparation of stimulus materials
4. selection and implementation of successful sound-evoking techniques
5. development and implementation of an individualized treatment program
6. implementation of various strategies that help strengthen the child's generalized responses and maintain the target speech production skills
7. involvement of the child's family and significant others in the treatment process
8. completion of a follow-up assessment and provision of booster treatment as necessary
9. use of specific treatment activities that help maximize the child's performance

The goal of this Basic Unit is to offer a practical perspective on the total treatment process. We will begin with the target selection process and end with a discussion of several strategies that can be used to ensure maintenance of the trained sounds or phonological skills. In the Advanced Unit, specific procedures for the treatment of organic and neurogenic speech disorders, such as childhood **apraxia of speech, developmental dysarthria in cerebral palsy, cleft palate,** and **hearing impairment,** will be provided as a general introduction to the remediation of those disorders.

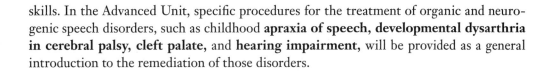

ACTIVITY

Summarize the components of an SSD treatment program, in your own words.

Selecting Potential Target Behaviors

The initial step in offering treatment for any disorder is the selection of functional target behaviors. **Target behavior** is a standard term that refers to any skill or action that is taught to a client, patient, or student (Hegde, 1998; Hegde & Davis, 2005). When speaking of speech sound disorders, target behaviors are the skills taught by the clinician to improve the child's sound production skills, word structures, phonological skills, speech intelligibility, and overall communication effectiveness. In most clinical settings, target behaviors are termed *treatment goals and objectives*.

Short-Term Objectives and Long-Term Goals

The clinician selects target speech sounds and phonological skills for training in light of the child's specific needs. The clinician also selects short-term objectives and long-term goals. *Short-term objectives* are skills that can be trained in a relatively short period of time (e.g., 2 weeks, 1 month, 3 months). They are the steps on the way to achieving the long-term goals. *Long-term goals* are the more broadly defined communicative behaviors that the child needs to learn to improve his or her overall communication skills (e.g., age-appropriate articulation skills, improved phonological skills, improved intelligibility, self-correction skills, and maintenance of skills over time and across situations). Obviously, it takes a longer period of service to reach the long-term goals.

In clinical practice, long-term goals are the speech sound production skills that the child is expected to learn by the end of a specified treatment period (one semester in most university settings and one academic year in most public school settings). Short-term objectives help support the long-term goals. The ultimate long-term goal is always the maintenance of the trained speech sound production skills in the child's natural environments across varied situations with the ultimate goal of attaining normal and effective communication (Kamhi, 2006).

General Considerations

The assessment data will have identified the sounds that are misarticulated, the operational word structure constraints, and the phonological error patterns that are evident in the child's speech. However, because children with speech sound disorders misarticulate many sounds or exhibit several phonological error patterns at the same time, the clinician must select and prioritize the order of treatment for these. Adequate long-term goals and short-term objectives can be established only if the child's individual needs are carefully considered.

Hegde and Davis (2010) identify four guidelines for the selection of potential target behaviors that can be applied across communication disorders, all of which acknowledge the importance of adapting treatment to meet the functional needs of individuals. If speech and language services are to have long-lasting effects, clinicians must teach communication behaviors that are meaningful in the child's life.

The clinician may *select treatment targets that create an immediate and socially significant difference in the child's communicative skills* for social communication, academic achievement, and future occupational performance—such as sounds that are most frequently used in conversation and misarticulated by the child and whose correction will most improve intelligibility in natural environments. The clinician may also *consider selecting the most useful behaviors that may be produced and reinforced at home and in other natural settings* because such behaviors are likely to be sustained over time. *Behaviors that help expand the child's communicative skills,* such as word exemplars that can be easily expanded into phrases and sentences, may also make good intervention targets. Furthermore, it is imperative that the clinician select target behaviors that are *appropriate for the individual child and his or her language and culture.*

A clinician who takes a client-specific approach to therapy can better meet the needs of the child and the entire family unit. Furthermore, the clinician who embraces this treatment philosophy is naturally more sensitive to the child's cultural and linguistic differences. If the individual needs of a particular child are to be met, his or her cultural and linguistic diversity should always be considered (please see Chapter 5 for further information on culture and communication and bidialectal and bilingual phonology).

Criteria for Target Behavior Selection

Many experts have suggested various criteria that may be considered in the selection of individual sounds and errors to be targeted, analyzed according to linear or nonlinear phonological theory (for reviews, see Gierut et al., 1996; Powell, 1991). An analysis of assessment results will have shown the frequency with which the child misarticulates various speech sounds that may or may not be grouped. The next step is to select and prioritize the treatment targets, so that the child's communication needs are met.

Target behavior selection is mostly a matter of sequencing. Clinicians and families generally agree that misarticulated sounds should be corrected. Therefore, all sounds in error are potential targets. But some will be more immediate targets than others. Assuming no positive change occurs in the other problematic sounds or patterns, they, too, will be treatment targets in due course. Therefore, the dilemma of target behavior selection is really not what to teach, but when to teach what, which implies a sequence. What follows is a review of commonly suggested criteria for the selection and sequencing of treatment targets.

Speech Sound Targets Based on Developmental Norms

Traditionally, the most widely used criterion of speech treatment target selection is normative data on speech development. Clinicians are often urged to select "age-appropriate" speech and language skills. In treating a 5-year-old child, for example, target sounds are those mastered by a group of 5-year-old children in the normative sample study. If the child to be treated has not mastered sounds that even younger, normally developing children have mastered, those sounds are especially relevant targets. The treatment of sounds then should be dictated by the earliest to latest normally acquired sounds. The same logic is applied to phonological error patterns.

Within the normative strategy, it is generally considered unwise to select sounds that are mastered at higher age levels than the child's current age. Several reasons have been advanced to justify this view. First, it has always been believed that skills that are typically mastered chronologically earlier are simpler than those acquired later. Simpler skills, of course, are assumed to be easier to teach than more complex skills. Second, the normative sequence of skill acquisition may be clinically inviolable. If all normally developing children in the population acquire speech sounds in a certain sequence, violation of the normal sequence could create problems in treatment, although no one has specified what the problems might be.

Although still popular, particularly in the public schools, the normative criterion of target selection for treatment has several problems (Kamhi, 2006; Lof, 2012). Children learn phonological skills at varying rates; individual differences are important. A child's unique and individual needs may not be met if developmental norms are used exclusively. An important point is that developmental norms are a statistical representation of the average performance of an entire age group. By definition, norms neutralize individual uniqueness and variations (Hegde, 1998). Lowe (1994) states that norms are "useful for determining delays in development or eligibility for a remedial program, but they are probably not the best resource for choosing intervention targets" (p. 176). The use of *norms* is the most uncritically practiced violation of individual uniqueness in clinical and educational disciplines.

Ultimately, whether developmental norms should guide target behavior selection will depend on controlled treatment research, not on arguments that do not seem to settle any issue. Language treatment research has shown that morphologic skills may be taught ahead of developmental norms (Capelli, 1985; DeCesari, 1985). Similarly, some evidence suggests that teaching phoneme productions ahead of developmental norms may indeed be better than teaching in accordance with the norms. In a treatment study, Powell and Elbert (1984) reported that there is no particular reason to teach "developmentally appropriate" sounds; they found that generalized correct productions were more likely when children were taught later-developing, rather than earlier-developing, consonant clusters. Elbert and McReynolds (1975) showed that children who were taught later-developing fricatives in word-final positions exhibited correct generalized productions of those phonemes in untrained words; without additional training, the children also produced earlier-developing sounds. Gierut and colleagues (1996) reported that when children were taught phonemes that were more advanced (later acquired) in relation to their chronological age, positive changes in *untreated* sound classes were evident. No such changes were associated with teaching phonemes that were early acquired. Therefore, we will regard developmental norms as only a broad guideline in selecting target phonemes. If data of the kind cited are replicated, experimental criteria that are clinically more meaningful than the developmental norms will be sustained.

Treatment Targets That Are Readily Taught

Another common recommendation is to select targets that are easier to teach, particularly in the initial stages of treatment. This recommendation suggests that treatment targets should be selected from the child's existing phonological repertoire. In some ways, this is the opposite of the normative criterion that requires the clinician to select what the child should be producing because of his or her age.

Both children who are normally learning the speech sounds of their language and children who have a speech sound disorder produce phonemes at varying accuracy levels. Some sounds may be produced correctly all the time, and some may be produced incorrectly all the time. The remaining sounds may fall in between. A treatment recommendation that stems from this empirical observation is that the sounds that do exist, but not at the expected levels, should be the treatment targets. One specific recommendation is that sounds that have a low base rate of correct production (e.g., between 20% and 40%) should be treated first. Those that are produced at a higher level (e.g., 60% or higher) on base rate trials may not require treatment; if necessary, they may be treated later. Also, treatment of sounds that are not produced at all (0% accuracy) on the base rate trials should wait until those that are produced at a higher (but still not the expected) level are treated.

As we noted in Chapter 6, stimulability is another notion that serves as a treatment target selection criterion. Some sounds produced in error may be produced correctly when modeled or when additional stimuli (e.g., a demonstration of phonetic placement) are added. Accordingly, it is recommended that stimulable sounds should be more immediate targets than those that are not stimulable. A related recommendation suggests that, because sounds produced with visible articulatory movements (simply called *visible sounds*) are easier to teach than those whose movements are more obscure, such sounds as the more visible bilabials should be taught before the less visible velar sounds.

From a phonological error pattern standpoint, the recommendations are to treat (1) error patterns whose frequency is less than 100%, (2) error patterns that occur only in certain phonetic contexts but not in others, and (3) error patterns that affect sounds that the child produces correctly elsewhere (M. L. Edwards, 1983). Such phonological error patterns are also described as *unstable* or *inconsistent*, meaning that on occasion they are not evident in the speech of the child. If affected sounds are produced correctly occasionally or in specific contexts, the phonological error pattern in question is on its way out, and the treatment can hasten its exit.

An opposite recommendation also can be found in the clinical literature. If a phonological error pattern is evident at low frequency, with the possibility that it is being "suppressed" naturally, then perhaps the treatment is not needed. Therefore, Hodson and Paden (1991) recommend that if the frequency of a phonological error pattern is less than 40%, it should not be treated. To be treated, an error pattern should occur with high frequency, more than at least 40%.

The strength of the recommendation that clinicians should first treat sounds with a low frequency base rate, sounds that are stimulable, and phonological error patterns that are inconsistent (have less than 100% occurrence) is that initial treatment sessions may thus produce faster results. The approach seeks to strengthen what is already taking place in the speech of the child. This strength may be neutralized, however, if treating existing skills results in faster improvement only in those skills but does not produce generalized effects (changes in untreated sounds, sound classes, or patterns). This possibility has led to the next recommendation for target selection.

Targets That Produce Extensive Generalization

Generalization is an indirect behavioral effect of treatment. When some skills are taught, other skills that belong to the same response class may show positive changes because of generalization. For instance, when only a few fricatives are taught, the remaining fricatives may be produced without any treatment. Successful production of untaught behaviors as a result of similar behaviors being taught is known as **generalized production.** Generalized productions are a treatment goal because positive changes in untreated sounds save much time and training effort. Therefore, potential for generalization is a consideration in target behavior selection.

Research on the generalized production of untreated phonemes has produced mixed results. It is not uncommon to find in a single study a range from little generalization to considerable generalization to untreated sounds within and across children. Significant individual differences are typical in the results across studies reported. For instance, Powell (1991) reported that the child who was taught the production of the fricative [z] in word-final positions produced untrained voiced fricatives (in the same word-final positions) with only 25% accuracy and unvoiced fricatives with only 31% accuracy. The child also produced (untrained) voiced word-final stops with 33% accuracy but no generalized productions of unvoiced word-final stops. Generalizations to cognate sounds were predicted, but the observed generalizations were neither sufficient nor clinically significant. Saben and Ingham (1991) found that the minimal pairs method applied to two children did not result in generalized production of the phonemes in words that were not taught. Also, the intervention had no effect on untreated phonemes affected by the targeted phonological error patterns.

Treatment research on several specific variables thought to produce differential effects on generalized production also has produced varied and sometimes contradictory effects. For instance, Gierut (1990), in her treatment study of three children, reported that maximal opposition pairs (sounds that contrasted in more than two features; see Chapter 8 for details) were better than minimal opposition pairs (sounds that contrasted in no more than two features) in producing generalization effects. Even so, individual differences dominated the results. Correct generalized production based on maximal opposition training varied from 43% to 86%. One of the three children produced the same generalized productions (86% accuracy) under both the treatment conditions (minimal and maximal oppositions).

Research on whether treatment of more consistently produced errors produces better generalized effects than that of inconsistently produced errors also has yielded somewhat conflicting results (see Tyler et al., 2003, for a review of studies). While some evidence has linked consistency of errors to better generalization (e.g., Forrest, Dinnsen, & Elbert, 1997), other evidence has failed to link the two variables (Powell, Elbert, & Dinnsen, 1991; Shriberg & Kwiatkowski, 1994). However, consistent errors may still be better treatment targets because of the possibility that inconsistent errors—like those that are stimulable—will be spontaneously corrected, as the child is already producing those sounds correctly in some contexts. At least initially, consistently misarticulated sounds and phonological error patterns that occur more frequently (e.g., 40% or more, as suggested by Hodson & Paden, 1991) may be treated; if warranted, treatment may be later extended to inconsistently mis-articulated sounds.

Discussion on generalization effects has recently been concerned with the level of generalized productions to untrained targets when more versus less complex sounds along some linguistic hierarchy, degree of markedness, level or number of distinctions, or extent of phonological knowledge are taught initially. Although results have been mixed, the majority of studies have shown than when more complex targets are taught, greater phonological change through generalized productions to untrained targets is observed (Dinnsen, Chin, & Elbert, 1992; Gierut, 1990, 1991, 1992, 1998, 1999, 2005; Gierut & Champion, 2001; Pagliarian, 2009; Tyler & Figurski, 1994; A. L. Williams, 1991, 2000, 2006a). Primarily because of the work of Gierut and colleagues, it is thought that if greater sound system-wide change is desired, good initial complex targets may be those that are later developing, are more marked, are nonstimulable, are consistently erred, have maximal or multiple distinctions, and are higher along some hierarchy or constraint ranking, among other factors (see Chapter 3). In a treatment study, failed generalization poses methodological and conceptual problems. The methodological problem is the number of treatment exemplars needed to be trained to obtain satisfactory levels of generalized productions. When generalization fails to materialize in a study, one wonders whether treating additional exemplars would have made a difference. For example, was it necessary to train more than one fricative in the previously mentioned Powell (1991) study to obtain greater generalization to other fricatives? The conceptual problem is perhaps more serious. Is it possible that the phonetic or phonological classification of sounds does not reflect empirical response classes? In other words, is it possible that sounds grouped according to phonetic or phonological variables may really not belong to a single class? Or that all fricatives may not be the same? Similarly, stops or affricates or nasals may be linguistically different, but are they really different behaviorally? We do not know. There usually is impressive generalization within empirically valid response classes. However, when there is little or no generalization, we may be dealing with behaviorally separate responses that are grouped according to some rationalist theory with little empirical basis.

Targets That Affect Intelligibility the Most

Selecting treatment targets that make a notable difference in intelligibility in the shortest possible intervention period makes clinical and common sense. Therefore, some clinical researchers suggest that the targets that affect speech intelligibility the most in children should be the initial treatment targets (M. L. Edwards, 1983; M. L. Edwards & Bernhardt, 1973; Hodson & Paden, 1991).

A phonological error pattern that occurs frequently or affects a large number of sounds may significantly reduce a child's intelligibility. Therefore, such error patterns may be better initial targets than the ones that affect fewer sounds. Stopping, for instance, is a good initial target because it affects many sounds. Hodson and Paden (1991) suggest that each phonological error pattern may be rated for its effects on intelligibility. Error patterns that affect intelligibility the most should receive treatment on a priority basis. This recommendation may be interwoven with other recommendations for treatment target selection, however. For instance, consistent errors and errors on a larger number of sounds produce the most negative effects on intelligibility. If consistent errors are the treatment targets, the clinician might address speech intelligibility concurrently.

A related concept that may be considered in selecting treatment targets is *homonymy*, which refers to the use of a single word for multiple words, resulting in significant loss of meaning. For instance, a child who exhibits stopping of fricatives may say [pɪt] for *his*, *fish*, and *sit*, resulting in severely unintelligible speech. Therefore, clinicians may target reduction or elimination of homonymous word forms as the initial target for treatment. A specific phoneme contrast approach designed to eliminate homonymy is the *multiple-oppositions approach*, described in Chapter 8. In this method, the clinician simultaneously teaches all error sounds within a rule or pattern by using multiple-opposition word pairs. A. L. Williams (2000, 2003) gives the example of a child who substitutes [t] for /s/, /k/, /tʃ/, and /tr/ and as a consequence produces the single word *tip* for *sip*, *Kip*, *chip*, and *trip*. Instead of contrasting [t] with each of the error sounds separately, the multiple-oppositions approach, as Williams describes it, will create such treatment word pairs as *tip-sip*, *tip-Kip*, *tip-chip*, and *tip-trip* for simultaneous training. Such pairs contrast the [t] with all of the error sounds at the same time.

Another related recommendation is that any unusual, deviant, or **idiosyncratic** error pattern a child might exhibit should be targeted in treatment, perhaps on a priority basis (M. L. Edwards, 1983). For example, velarization, lateralization, frication of stops, or glottal replacement may make a good initial target, since they call attention to the child's speech to a much greater extent than a more common error pattern, such as cluster reduction. Elimination of unusual error patterns may result in rapid improvement in intelligibility of speech.

Still another related recommendation is that when a child misarticulates multiple sounds, treatment should simultaneously target multiple sounds (Gierut, 2001; Hodson & Paden, 1983). Such a treatment may result in more rapid and more extensive changes in sound productions, thus improving intelligibility.

The variables that affect intelligibility discussed so far are all characteristics of misarticulating children. One other factor that may be directly or indirectly related to intelligibility is a characteristic of the language the children speak, rather than the children themselves. For instance, the same misarticulating sound may be treated in words that occur either more frequently or less frequently. This is more a lexical than a phonological consideration. There is some limited evidence that when treated words are of high frequency in the language, better generalization may be obtained than when treated words are of low frequency (Gierut, Morrisette, & Champion, 1999; Morrisette & Gierut, 2002).

Summary of Guidelines on Target Behavior Selection

Much of the research on target behavior selection summarized in the current and previous chapters may leave the clinician without strong and unambiguous guidelines. This is because research studies themselves have not produced such guidelines. Each guideline has limitations and is threatened by actual or future contradictions. Therefore, the clinician needs to be in constant touch with research studies that continue to support certain guidelines, suggest new guidelines, and contradict well-established guidelines. No matter how well established guidelines are, clinicians should be suspicious of those that are simply expert opinions (without experimental evidence to support them). Furthermore, although a particular guideline may be popular, if it is based on a single study, the clinician should watch for replications that may support or refute a guideline.

In the absence of much replicated evidence, clinicians can tentatively use guidelines based on one or more controlled treatment research study while watching for replications that either confirm or contradict them. Ultimately, treatment research evidence will guide target behavior selection. Currently, some tentative criteria that may be suggested based on research to date are as follows:

1. **If immediate success in initial treatment sessions is more important than generalized effects,** the clinician may select sounds that are easier to teach. These will include stimulable sounds, sounds with higher than zero base rates, visible sounds, sounds that are in any way easier for a given child because of individual differences (e.g., a particular child may find it easier to learn an intuitively complex sound than a simple sound), sound errors that are inconsistent (i.e., produced correctly in some contexts), and phonological error patterns that occur significantly below 100% (i.e., patterns that are on their way out).

2. **If more immediate generalized productions and marked positive effects on speech intelligibility are paramount,** the clinician may select sounds that are complex, sounds that are consistently misarticulated, sounds that are nonexistent in the child's repertoire, phonological error patterns that affect the greatest number of sounds, error patterns that are idiosyncratic, patterns that reduce homonymy, patterns that are exhibited in 100% of opportunities or close to it, words that contain maximal phoneme feature oppositions, and words that contain maximal or multiple-phoneme feature oppositions (see Chapter 8 for maximal and multiple featured oppositions).

3. **Regardless of initial success or generalization considerations,** the clinician should select sounds that are ethnoculturally appropriate for the child, sounds that are in the child's dialect, sounds that are not in the dialect only if the child or the family demands their treatment, sounds in words that are important in view of the child's academic success (e.g., reading assignments, language work in the classroom, literacy considerations), sounds in words that are most frequently used in the child's language, and sounds still produced in error or phonological patterns that are still active regardless of previous guidelines followed.

Regardless of the target behavior selection strategy used, the clinician should assess the effects of just taught speech sounds on untreated sounds that were in error on baselines. For instance, the clinician should probe to find out whether teaching the correct production of one member of a cognate pair (e.g., /s/) results in the generalized production of the other member (e.g., /z/). After having taught a few final consonants to eliminate the final consonant deletion error pattern, the clinician should probe for the production of other, untreated final consonants that were missing on the base rate trials. Obviously, sounds that are produced on the basis of generalization are eliminated as future treatment targets.

A point to be kept in perspective at all times is that all errors may have to be corrected. The clinician who selects visible sounds, sounds that are stimulable, and error patterns that occur with 100% frequency may find at the end of the treatment that sounds that were not visible, sounds that were not stimulable, and error patterns that occurred only at 30% frequency still need to be treated. A clinician may have to go back and treat the errors and phonological error patterns that are still present in the child's phonological system.

A final point to be made about target behavior selection concerns phonological error patterns. When an error pattern is selected for reduction or elimination, the clinician still selects individual sounds to be taught. A phonological error pattern may be eliminated only by teaching certain individual phonemes. If theorists' predictions hold, teaching only a few sounds within a pattern is sufficient to eliminate the entire pattern.

....

ACTIVITY
Determine the best strategy for selecting treatment targets for children with SSD.

....

Deciding on the Number of Sounds to Teach

After selecting the most appropriate initial target sounds, the clinician must determine the number of sounds that will be taught at one time to a child who misarticulates multiple sounds. In the traditional articulation treatment approach (see Chapter 8), no more than two target sounds are trained at any one time. Some clinicians concentrate on a single sound because this can result in more rapid progress. Others think that children may be confused with simultaneous training of multiple targets.

In the not too distant past, simultaneous treatment of multiple phonemes was considered an important development in the profession (Bradley, 1989; McCabe & Bradley, 1973, 1975). It is now commonly believed that such an approach may result in rapid overall progress, improved intelligibility, and treatment efficiency. Within this clinical framework, new sounds may be introduced before the old ones reach mastery criterion, or several sounds may be worked on concurrently. The **multiple-oppositions approach** is a phonological contrast approach that includes as targets multiple errors across a sound class or error pattern (A. L. Williams, 2000, 2003). The stimulability intervention approach (discussed in Chapter 8) also targets multiple nonstimulable sounds for intervention (Miccio & Williams, 2010). Another, experimentally supported view, known as the **concurrent treatment method**, is that two to four sounds may be simultaneously treated at multiple response complexity levels (words, phrases, or sentences) in a randomized sequence (Skelton, 2004; Skelton & Hagopian, 2013; Skelton & Kerber, 2005; Skelton & Price, 2006; Skelton & Resciniti, 2009).

Although the single sound (or few sounds), simultaneous multiple sounds, and concurrent complexity levels training approaches have been found to be effective or result in improvement (Costello & Onstine, 1976; Elbert & McReynolds, 1975, 1978; Hodson & Paden, 1991; McReynolds, 1972; McReynolds & Elbert, 1981b; Skelton, 2004; Weiner, 1981; A. L. Williams, 2000, 2003), the individual clinician must determine what is appropriate for a particular child. While one child's progress may be slow under simultaneous teaching of multiple sounds, another child may show rapid progress under the same method, possibly because of such variables as the child's motivation, intellectual level, language skills, and learning proficiency. The best way is to experiment a little in the initial treatment sessions. It may be better to start with multiple phonemes or complexity levels. If training proves difficult, the clinician can limit the number of target sounds or levels taught in a given segment of treatment.

Establishing Baselines

As stated earlier, the assessment data, though helpful in making a diagnosis, may not be adequate in establishing reliable and valid pretreatment performance levels that will eventually help assess the child's progress under treatment. Assessment tests and conversational speech samples may not adequately sample each phoneme production in sufficient frequency; most single-word tests offer no more than three opportunities to produce a specific phoneme. This is an extremely limited sampling of behaviors. Test results also do not reveal the percentages of pretreatment errors needed to evaluate progress in treatment.

The clinician may counteract this problem by establishing **baselines** of the *potential* treatment targets before starting therapy. Baselines are measured rates of behaviors in the absence of treatment (Hegde, 1998). In essence, baselines provide quantitative pretreatment information that can be used to (1) evaluate the child's progress over time, (2) establish clinician accountability, and (3) modify treatment procedures if the child's rate of improvement is not as expected. In an era of third-party payers and legal vulnerability, it is extremely important that the clinician establish clinical accountability. It is not sufficient to report that a child is "doing very well" or "improving very much." Parents, employers, and third-party payers are increasingly demanding detailed documentation of children's progress. However, it is nearly impossible to reliably measure progress if the child's pretreatment performance is unknown. Therefore, the extra time taken to establish baselines is worthwhile. See the companion CD for a modifiable and printable form titled "Baseline Recording Sheet," which may be used to collect a baseline of potential target behaviors.

Baseline Procedures

There are four steps in establishing baselines of various communicative disorders. These steps may be modified to suit individual needs or for specific disorders (Hegde, 1998).

Specify the Treatment Targets in Measurable Terms

The first step is to specify the treatment targets in clear, specific, measurable terms. Globally stated treatment targets such as "improved articulation" or "decreased stopping of fricatives" are too general and impossible to measure. On the other hand, clearly written target behaviors such as the following can be easily measured:

- production of /s/ in initial-word position at the word level
- reduction or elimination of stopping by teaching /f/, /v/, and /s/ in all word positions
- production of CVC words
- establishment of the contrast between [t] and [s] in initial position of words
- production of the [+ continuant] distinctive feature in CVC words

Target objectives such as these identify the initial intervention targets and specify the **response topography**, or the complexity level of training. Clinicians can compare the child's performance during baseline measures with the selected treatment targets and decide whether they are indeed appropriate. Many of us may often have taught a particular phoneme because a child did not produce it correctly on standardized or formal testing, only to find out through baseline procedures that he or she can already make it with 90% accuracy. What can account for this discrepancy?

The child may have produced the sound incorrectly in a particular phonetic context or in a particular word during articulation testing. However, baseline trials provide multiple opportunities for the production of a single sound in specific word positions across several words. Therefore, baselines are more accurate than the results of articulation testing. If the clinician had not established the baselines, he or she may have erroneously attributed the child's improved performance in the initial treatment phase to the treatment itself.

Prepare the Stimulus Items

The second step in establishing baselines is to prepare the stimulus items and design events, questions, and prompts that will evoke the target responses. It may be noted that the same stimulus materials used during baseline trials will be used in treatment sessions; the type of treatment approach selected (not the precise treatment procedures) will influence stimulus preparation, as noted shortly. To evoke sounds in isolation, modeling may be all that is needed. No particular physical stimuli (such as pictures) are needed. However, physical stimuli will be needed to evoke sounds in words, phrases, and sentences on baseline (as well as treatment) trials. Therefore, the clinician should select the words to be taught and pictures that represent them. If the target phoneme was /s/ in word-initial position, for example, the clinician may select pictorial representations of *soap, soup, sock, sick*, and *sun*. On the other hand, if a contrast approach is used in treatment, the clinician selects pairs of stimuli that depict minimal, multiple, or maximal homonymous or nonhomonymous contrasts (e.g., paired pictures to evoke *sip-ship, Sue-shoe, cap-tap, car-tar*; see "Phonological Contrast Approaches" in Chapter 8 for details). With very young children, the clinician may also use real objects to increase the child's participation. Sometimes, children respond better to items that can be manipulated. However, it is not always possible to use real objects that represent the word containing the target sound. For example, if the target sound was /l/ in the initial position and one of the selected words was *lost*, then an object would not be the best prompt. A picture representing the concept of "lost" or a stimulus question (e.g., "When people can't find their way home, they are...") might be a better option.

There are several commercially available stimulus pictures for speech sound production therapy. However, these are marketed for general clinical or educational use and are not tailored to a specific child; such stimuli may be irrelevant to a child from a diverse ethnocultural community, for example. Often the clinician must compile stimulus pictures from an array of sources to meet a child's individual needs. As the sequence of training is shifted to more complex response levels, these pictures may also be used to evoke production of the target sound in phrases and sentences.

If the clinician plans to use the multiple-oppositions or maximal-oppositions contrast approaches in treatment sessions, the pairs of target words will be child specific. Only after making a thorough analysis of the child's misarticulations can the clinician generate pairs of stimulus words that have either maximal or multiple phonemic contrasts. The clinician then can find pictures to represent the selected target words.

The stimulus items the clinician eventually chooses should be unambiguous and appropriate for a particular child's age, cultural background, and language skill level. If possible, stimulus items from the child's natural environment should be used during baseline trials and later in treatment. This may help in the eventual maintenance of target behaviors in the natural setting (to be discussed further in upcoming sections). At least 20 single or paired stimulus items are needed for each target behavior (Hegde, 1998).

To help clinicians get started, various simple and complex words for treating individual sounds are provided in the Sound Resource Packets on the companion CD.

Prepare a Recording Sheet

The third step in establishing baselines of various communicative disorders is to prepare a recording sheet for the child's responses. A clearly designed yet detailed recording sheet helps the clinician document the child's pretreatment performance. The clinician can design a recording sheet to use routinely. In preparing a recording sheet, it is important to design one that can be used with various treatment targets. As indicated earlier, the companion CD provides a sample "Baseline Recording Sheet" that may be personalized and printed for your clinical use.

Administer the Baseline Trials

In the fourth step, the clinician administers the selected stimulus items in discrete trials. A **discrete trial** is a structured opportunity for the child to produce a given target; in this case, the target is the selected speech sound. Discrete trials are separated from one another by a short time interval, typically a few seconds, so that there is a clear beginning and a definite end to each trial.

Baseline trials can be administered on both evoked and modeled trials (Hegde, 1998). **Evoked trials** do not include modeling; **modeled trials** obviously do. Other stimuli, such as pictures, objects, and questions (e.g., "What is this?") are common to both kinds of trials. The administration of modeled trials can yield useful clinical information. If the child can imitate certain modeled sound productions, the clinician may opt to treat them in the initial phase of the treatment. However, if the child's production of specific target sounds does not improve with modeling, the clinician may either begin with those that are imitated or use such additional stimulus control procedures as **phonetic placement, shaping,** and **sound approximation.** The following steps help administer discrete evoked baseline trials (adapted to illustrate **base rating** of /f/ in the initial position of words):

1. Place a stimulus picture in front of the child or demonstrate the action or event with objects; if using a contrast approach, show a pair of pictures. For example,

   • Show the child a picture of *fish* or *fat* (or a pair of pictures).

   • Lift four fingers to evoke the word *four*.

2. Ask the relevant predetermined question, such as,

   • "What do you see in the picture?" (or "What is this? And what is that?" in case of a stimulus pair)

- "What is swimming in the water?"
- "The boy is not skinny, he's . . ."
- "How many fingers do I have? Let's count them . . . one, two, three . . ."

3. Wait a few seconds for the child to respond. The amount of time needed before presentation of the next stimulus item may vary across children depending on their individual needs.

4. Record the response on the recording sheet. Record a correct response with a plus mark and an incorrect response with a minus. Record a lack of response by "NR" (for "no response").

5. Pull the picture toward you or remove it from the subject's view. It is important to separate the trials and to avoid the possibility of the child continuing to respond to a previous stimulus item after a new stimulus item is presented.

6. Wait 2 to 3 seconds to mark the end of the trial. The number of seconds may vary depending on the child's individual needs.

7. Return to step 1 to initiate the next trial until all trials on the 20 stimulus items (words, phrases, sentences) have been completed.

Modeled baseline trials are conducted in a similar fashion as evoked baseline trials with added modeling of correct sound productions. For instance, after showing the picture of a fish, the clinician asks, "What do you see in this picture?" and immediately models the response, "Bobby, say *fish*." It is important to model immediately after asking the question to avoid a competing response from the child.

Selecting the Initial Level and Sequence of Training

Baselines, in addition to providing reliable pretreatment measures of target sound productions, help identify the level of response complexity that is an adequate starting point for training. For example, the child who produced a sound in words with only 10% accuracy on modeled baseline trials will probably need some initial training at the sound or syllable level. However, if the accuracy score during baseline trials was 50% in evoked word productions, therapy should start at least at the word level.

In the traditional approach to therapy, the starting point for production training has always been isolated sounds or nonsense syllables. Van Riper and Erickson (1996) started training with sounds or nonsense syllables to "avoid the long history of usage that has so strongly reinforced the error. It's easier" (p. 239). Because in recent years the emphasis has been on meaningful differences in words, the most widely recommended starting point for therapy is at least the word level. As stated by Lowe (1994), "It is at the word level that sounds make a difference, and it is at the word level that children can perceive the function of sounds in communication" (p. 180). Selecting functional, high-frequency words for initial treatment may help meet the child's communication needs. It is best to begin treatment at the word level when possible because words are functional in everyday situations.

We have noted earlier that high-frequency words may be useful in treatment and generalization. More frequently used words are familiar to children and meaningful in everyday communication. Other lexical variables that are useful to consider include the phonetic contexts that facilitate correct productions (Lowe, 1994). Such contexts can be made progressively more complex (e.g., longer words in later stages of treatment). Words from the child's classroom curriculum that also help teach the selected sounds may be especially relevant.

Generally, the higher the response complexity level at which the treatment may be started, the more efficient the treatment. For instance, if treatment of target sounds can be started in phrases or simple sentences, the progress may be more rapid than if treatment were started with sounds or syllables. Unfortunately, it is not practical with many children who may fail to respond well when treatment is initiated at a complex level. In our clinical experience, more often than not children need some initial production training at the isolation or simple syllable level for sound establishment. If therapy must be initiated at the sound or syllable level, it should progress to the word level as quickly as possible. If adequate baselines are established, a clinician can easily determine the level of response complexity that is most appropriate for a particular child.

There is very little research on the sequence that should be followed once the sounds in isolation or the sounds in syllables or words are taught. Highly structured treatment procedures generally recommend that the clinician systematically proceed from the simplest (e.g., the sound in isolation) to the most complex level (e.g., conversational speech). The child has to meet the selected mastery criterion at each level to proceed to the next level. It is assumed that simpler skills are easier to teach than more complex skills and that simpler skills help build more complex skills. The different levels of training would normally not be mixed in a single treatment session. That treatment can be successful if using the simple-to-complex sequence is clear (Baker & Ryan, 1971; Van Riper & Emerick, 1984). However, the observation that the traditional sequencing of target skills will result in improvement is no evidence that it is indeed more effective than other, experimental sequences. We noted earlier that addressing complex phonological error patterns, teaching sounds that are consistently omitted, teaching sounds that are nonexistent in a child's repertoire, addressing errors with word pairs that are maximally opposed, and using word pairs that contain phonemes with multiple phonemic oppositions may be more effective than their respective alternatives.

Skelton (2004) performed a study with an experimental single-subject design to evaluate the effectiveness of simultaneously teaching target sounds at simpler as well as more complex levels of speech sound production. In this **concurrent treatment,** he randomly intermixed simple and complex training tasks. The simplest level of training was imitation of the sound in single syllables, and the most complex level was production of the target sound in evoked conversational segments. By randomly mixing 29 levels of response complexity, Skelton avoided the traditional progression of the simple-to-complex sequence of treatment. In each treatment session, he randomly presented exemplars from all levels of complexity. All four 7-year-old children in the study learned their target sound in this random sequence and showed generalized productions, as well. Skelton's results add support to the emerging view that it is not always necessary to follow either the normative sequence of speech sound acquisition or the traditional simple-to-complex treatment sequence. Subsequent studies by Skelton and associates have found that the concurrent treatment method (1) can be successfully used to treat preschoolers, (2) can be successfully adapted to treat multiple sounds in children with a phonological disorder, (3) can lead to greater correct production in training conditions and in generalized productions than the traditional incremental method, (4) can be successfully used in a small group format, and (5) can be successfully adapted to treat children with childhood apraxia of speech (Skelton & Funk, 2004; Skelton & Hagopian, 2013; Skelton & Kerber, 2005; Skelton & Price, 2006; Skelton & Resciniti, 2009; Skelton & Richard, 2013).

ACTIVITY
Identify how you would select the initial treatment targets for children with SSD.

Developing Measurable Objectives

After baselines have been collected and the response level for training has been determined, the clinician must define the target behaviors in measurable or operational terms. The baseline information helps the clinician determine whether the selected target behaviors are indeed appropriate treatment objectives. **Treatment objectives** (also called short-term objectives) can be defined as the skills the clinician plans to teach on the way toward achieving the selected treatment targets or **long-term goals.**

Although long-term goals may be written in somewhat more general terms, short-term objectives must always specify how a certain goal will be achieved. The clinician must address the specific skills targeted, the anticipated outcomes, the predicted level of accuracy, and the situations in which the child will be expected to use the newly acquired skills. Measurable **short-term objectives** help chart the child's progress in treatment. By measuring the response rates before, during, and after treatment, the clinician can collect evidence of improvement, thus justifying treatment.

Measurable objectives also allow external observers to verify the results of the clinical services provided. Many health-care agencies, insurance companies, and other third-party payers not only recommend that such documentation be kept but actually demand it for the continuation of services. Over the years, we have moved toward a health-care and educational era that puts great emphasis on the documentation of progress. No longer are agencies willing to pay for services unless improvement is measured and quantified. Such improvement can only be documented if the goals and objectives of therapy are clearly stated from the inception of treatment.

What exactly constitutes a measurable objective or target behavior? A well-written target behavior specifies the following (Hegde, 1998):

1. the *response topography* or actual skill targeted (e.g., production of /s/)

2. the *quantitative criterion* of performance (e.g., 90% accuracy)

3. the *response mode* (e.g., discrimination versus production training)

4. the *response level* (e.g., in words or sentences)

5. the *response setting* (e.g., in the clinic or in the child's home)

6. the *number of speech samples or sessions* in which the target behavior productions are to be documented (e.g., across three sessions)

The components of a measurable target behavior will vary somewhat depending on the child's skills and treatment needs. The style in which they are written may also need to be suited to a specific clinical setting. The quality of the statement should not suffer by such variations.

Only the observable behaviors (i.e., seen, heard, touched) can be measured. Therefore, the selected skills for training must be those that can be counted, tallied, or identified. Roth and Worthington (2011) advise that in writing behavioral objectives, a clinician needs to use verbs that denote an observable activity.

Examples of observable activities and appropriate verbs include *point, repeat, match, name, tell, ask, count, write, say,* and *lift.* All of these behaviors can be measured. Nonmeasurable activities include *think, believe, discover, feel, appreciate, remember, understand,* and *know.* Although these are certainly action words, their corresponding behaviors cannot be directly observed. We cannot observe a child's thinking, knowledge, feelings, or appreciation. The only way we can assume knowledge, feelings, and the like is through observable behaviors such as a person's performance and crying and laughing. A current popular system of writing goals that has made its way to the educational field, including speech–language pathology, is that of S.M.A.R.T. goals (P. J. Meyer, 2006; O'Neill & Conzemius, 2006). The letters that create the mnemonic come from the five key words that describe the characteristics of well-defined goals, as follows:

- *Specific*—Goals should be specific and clearly defined.
- *Measurable*—Goals should be measurable, observable, and written in tangible terms.
- *Attainable*—Goals should be attainable and consider the underlying skills needed for attainment.
- *Relevant*—Goals should be relevant, realistic, and outcome focused.
- *Time bound*—Goals should be time bound and provide a clear time frame for achievement.

The following lists provide a sampling of measurable short-term objectives for individual sounds, phonological error patterns, contrasts, constraints, complexity, and other behaviors that may contribute to improved speech sound production skills:

Treatment objectives for individual sounds (phonetic approach)
- 90% correct evoked production of /s/ and /z/ in single words across three clinical sessions
- at least 90% correct production of /r/ in conversational speech produced at the clinic, at school, and in the child's home across three speech samples
- production of initial /d/ with 80% accuracy in 10 untrained words during evoked trials in the clinical setting
- spontaneous production of /k/ and /g/ in sentences with 90% accuracy over three consecutive sessions in response to the clinician's questions
- correct production of /s/ in the initial position of words used in two-word phrases evoked on a set of 20 discrete trials at 90% accuracy

Treatment objectives for phonological error patterns and minimal contrasts (linear approach)

- reduction of final consonant deletion by teaching 90% correct production of the following sounds in the word-final position, measured across three clinical sessions: /p/, /k/, /t/, and /m/
- elimination of stopping by teaching 90% correct production of the following fricatives at the conversational level measured in three treatment sessions: /s/, /f/, /θ/, and /ʃ/
- reduction of syllable deletion by training 20 client-specific multisyllabic words in two-word phrases with 90% accuracy observed across three sessions
- eliminate the presence of velar fronting by training 90% correct production of /k/, /g/, and /ŋ/ in conversational speech across three speech samples gathered in the client's home
- establish the contrast between singleton consonants and consonant clusters by training 80% correct production of the following /s/ + stop clusters in the initial position of words: /st/, /sp/, and /sk/
- train 90% correct production of initial /l/ in 10 contrastive minimal word pair sets at the word and sentence levels (e.g., *wet-let, whip-lip, white-light*).

Treatment objectives for phonological constraints, maximal contrasts, and complex targets (nonlinear approach)

- establish 80% correct imitation of the target error sounds /t/ and /ʃ/ in maximal contrast word pairs (e.g., *tie-shy, two-shoe*)
- decrease positional constraints for /p/ by increasing correct production of final /p/ in words and sentences
- establish 90% correct production of the following Type 6 Productive Phonological Knowledge sounds (those with least knowledge) in trained word exemplars: /ʃ/, /l/, and /Θ/
- promote (establish) the dorsal place node by teaching 80% correct production of /k/ and /g/ in initial word position at the word and sentence levels
- increase the production of variable **syllable word shapes** by targeting at least 80% correct production of [CVC], [CCVC], and [CVCC] words in sentences in three consecutive clinical sessions
- establish 90% correct productions of the nonstimulable sounds /s/, /l/, and /k/ in words and assess for generalized production to untrained error sounds

Other possible treatment objectives (mixed approaches)

- eliminate the presence of **homonymous word forms** by training 90% correct production or acceptable approximation of *words affected by homonymy*, in three consecutive sessions
- increase the child's phonetic inventory of sounds by training 90% correct production of the following consonants in a set of 10 untrained words at the sentence level during evoked discrete trials: /t/, /k/, /s/, and /f/

- train a reduced rate of speech to facilitate precise articulatory contacts in conversational speech, the client maintaining a rate of 125 words per minute across three 10-minute conversational speech samples in the home situation

- establish consistent production of 50 functional target words across three separate probe measures

- produce at least 90% accuracy in self-correcting articulation errors of /s/ and /z/ in conversational speech observed across three consecutive treatment sessions

....

ACTIVITY

Identify the treatment goal for a child who does not produce /s/ in any word position.

....

The above objectives are not meant to be all inclusive, and they can certainly be tailored to meet a particular child's needs. The response mode, response level, accuracy criterion, and stimulus conditions should be altered to fit the child's assessment and baseline performance and adjusted according to the child's changing performance once treatment is initiated (see Text Box 7.1). The clinician's own treatment philosophy often dictates whether the target behaviors will be written in terms of individual phonemes; phonological error patterns; or nonlinear markedness, hierarchies, or constraints; or a combination of these. The style in which treatment objectives are written may vary from setting to setting or clinician to clinician, but the essential components of S.M.A.R.T. goals should always be included. We have always emphasized the importance of writing measurable and observable goals that clearly delineate the target behaviors and conditions for achievement.

Text Box 7.1. Children often surprise us

Linda is a bright, outgoing, and extremely verbal third-grade student whose mother referred her for a speech evaluation because of her misarticulation of /r/. On initial assessment Linda showed severe distortion of /r/, /ɚ/, and /ɝ/, no stimulability, and poor self-awareness skills. Her speech intelligibility was significantly affected by the lack of contrast between her intended words and her actual productions, especially in quick, connected speech. Her severe sound distortions drew much attention to her speech. At the initial multidisciplinary information-giving meeting it was agreed that because of Linda's level of distortion, poor stimulability, and limited self-awareness, her S.M.A.R.T. goal for the 1-year Individualized Education Program (IEP) period would be to increase her production of /r/, /ɚ/, and /ɝ/ to 90% accuracy at the sentence level. Everyone involved agreed that this was an achievable goal. To everyone's surprise, but extreme delight, 1 month after services were initiated, Linda achieved her IEP goal of 90% production of her target sounds at the sentence level, and 3 months later she was already working at the conversational speech level inside and outside of the speech room. Linda's self-awareness skills improved quickly once services were initiated and direct attention was drawn to correct versus incorrect productions. Four months into her program, the focus of services shifted to Linda's maintenance of skills through a well-established home practice program. Her treatment program had to be adjusted to address her quicker than anticipated progress. Linda's case illustrates the occasional need to quickly adjust a student's prognosis and treatment plan because actual performance differs from anticipated results.

Planning and Developing a Treatment Program

Before implementing treatment, the clinician should write a treatment plan, the format and style of which will depend on the employment setting. For example, federal and state laws mandate that school clinicians write and implement an *Individualized Educational Program (IEP)* or *Individual Family Service Plan (IFSP)* for children who receive special education services, which include speech and language treatment. The exact format of the IEP or IFSP is usually developed by the *Special Education Local Plan Areas (SELPAs)* in a particular state or district, although the content is generally similar across local areas. In these cases, the clinician has little flexibility as to how the plan of treatment should be written.

Treatment plans, whatever their form, minimally state the **long-term goals** and **short-term objectives** selected to meet the needs of a specific child. The plan may be simple or comprehensive, again depending on the guidelines of the clinician's employment. A comprehensive treatment program has several components:

* *The child's identifying information*—The treatment program provides the child's name, age, address, diagnosis, and so forth. The child's background information, the results of the assessment, and the recommendations for treatment are summarized in a clear and concise manner.

* *The target behaviors selected for training*—The target behaviors (treatment objectives) may be described in measurable terms, so that the daily performance data may be recorded to assess the child's progress.

* *The potential treatment procedures and the tentative sequence of training*—The plan describes the treatment methods that will be used to establish and stabilize correct production of the target sound(s). In addition, the treatment sequence (progression from a sound in isolation to words to phrases to conversational speech), the potential reinforcers to increase the correct production of speech sounds, and corrective feedback to minimize or eliminate speech sound errors and other undesirable behaviors are described.

* *The selected maintenance procedures*—The plan describes the procedures that will be used to promote maintenance of correct speech sound productions. How the clinician will train the family members and caregivers to prompt and reinforce the target responses in nonclinical situations may be described, as well.

* *The dismissal criterion*—A dismissal criterion (e.g., 90% speech sound accuracy in conversation in natural settings) specifies when the treatment may be terminated. However, practical problems may result in dismissal before the mastery criterion is met. Lack of progress despite modifications to the treatment program, lack of parent participation, lack of follow-through with home assignments, poor attendance, inability to arrive at therapy on time, self-dismissal, and so forth may result in treatment termination.

* *Follow-up and booster treatment*—Follow-up consists of periodic evaluation of speech sound productions to ensure their maintenance over time. The initial follow-up session may be scheduled 3 months after the child's dismissal, and subsequent sessions may be held at biannual or annual intervals. If any of the follow-up assessments indicate a decline in the target response rate, booster treatment—treatment offered to bolster the correct response maintenance—may be provided.

We offer details of a treatment program that includes these components in subsequent sections. We emphasize that the treatment plan is a flexible document, which will be modified, in most cases, by the data the treatment sessions generate.

Establishing Correct Productions of Speech Sounds

Children who cannot correctly imitate the target sound in words may need such additional procedures as phonetic placement, sound approximation, modeling, verbal instructions, and prompts. Production training may begin by first establishing the sound in isolation and then progressing to more complex levels. This is the behavioral process known as **shaping.** The final target of speech sound production at the conversational level needs to be broken down into gradual steps to increase the child's likelihood of success.

We first describe the various procedures that help the child either imitate or produce the sounds relatively more spontaneously. The clinician implements these procedures before the child gives a response. We next describe what the clinician does to increase and strengthen the correct speech sound productions.

Phonetic Placement

Phonetic placement techniques have been used from the beginning of articulation treatment (Nemoy & Davis, 1937, 1954; Scripture & Jackson, 1927), and they may be essential if the child cannot produce the target sound correctly. The clinician must then employ special techniques to evoke production of the sound. He or she may directly teach articulatory positions and ways of modifying the airstream. Maintaining voicing for voiced sounds also may be taught.

Most clinicians teach correct articulatory positioning by description and demonstration; placements may be demonstrated in front of a mirror. The clinician may use such simple devices as a tongue blade to manipulate and hold articulators in place. Breath indicators for mouth and nose (the simplest is a tissue or even the hand held under the nose or mouth) may be useful. Spectrographic graphic displays will provide visual feedback. Diagrams and pictures of articulatory positions for different sounds are another method of demonstration. Electropalatography is a research tool that, if available to the clinician, will provide a more dynamic view of the tongue during articulation. Feeling laryngeal vibration helps distinguish voiced versus unvoiced sound productions.

The clinician's physical manipulation of the child's articulators is known as manual guidance (Hegde, 1998), as well as **tactile-kinesthetic cuing** and **tactile-kinesthetic stimulation.** In **manual guidance,** the clinician physically assists the child in the production of the target sound. For example, in teaching the production of /b/, the clinician may shape the child's lips for appropriate seal using his or her fingers. In teaching correct phonetic placement for the production of /l/, the clinician may use the following techniques:

- touch the child's alveolar ridge with a tongue depressor, cotton swab stick, or gloved finger to indicate the place of articulation for the [l]
- touch the child's tongue tip with a cotton swab stick and ask him or her to place the tip of the tongue against the alveolar ridge

- instruct the child to keep the tip of the tongue against the alveolar ridge, or "bumpy spot," and to say [ə], resulting in a distorted [l]
- ask the child to continue saying [ə] and drop the tip of his or her tongue at the same time, resulting in the syllable sequence [lə]
- identify the syllable sequence as the "right" sound and provide the child the selected **reinforcer** (e.g., sticker, chip, etc.)
- continue the sequence until the sound is well established

Please see the companion CD for a description of various facilitative techniques, including phonetic placement procedures, that can be used to establish production of all American English consonants. These techniques are located in the Sound Resource Packets designed for each of the English consonants.

Successive Approximation (Sound Shaping)

Successive approximation, or sound shaping, is a technique that capitalizes on a sound that the child can already make to help him or her learn a new sound (Bleile, 1996; Hegde, 1998; Secord, 1989; Secord, Boyce, Donohue, Fox, & Shine, 2007). The sound used to facilitate the production of the target can be either a speech sound or another type of sound (e.g., growling noises, "car" noises for the production of /ɚ/) that the child can make without difficulty. Sound approximation is needed because of the complexity of sounds and the ineffectiveness of just asking the child to "say [p]" to evoke its production. Speech sound productions need to be broken down into initially simple and progressively more complex response components that will eventually lead to the final target.

Successive approximation guides the child through a series of graded steps, each progressively closer to the target sound. The clinician first targets a related sound or an initial response in the child's repertoire that could be related to the final target sound. The clinician then arranges instructional steps that help the child move from the initial response (a sound that the child can produce) to the terminal response (the target sound). For example, if the child cannot produce [b] but can produce [p], the latter would be a likely starting point, since these sounds share the same place of articulation and manner of production. It would not make good clinical sense to attempt to shape [b] from [k], since the sounds do not share any articulatory features.

Shriberg (1975, p. 104) provides an example of a sound-shaping procedure that can be used with a child who misarticulates /ɚ/. In the following example, the clinician is helping the child shape [ɚ] from [l]:

1. "Stick your tongue out" (model provided).
2. "Stick your tongue out and touch the tip of your finger" (model provided).
3. "Put your finger on the bumpy place right behind your top teeth" (model provided).
4. "Now put the tip of your tongue lightly on that bumpy place" (model provided).
5. "Now put your tongue tip there again, and say [l]" (model provided).

6. "Say [l] each time I hold up my finger" (clinician holds up finger).

7. "Now say [l] for as long as I hold my finger up, like this" (model provided for 5 seconds). "Ready? Go."

8. "Say a long [l], but this time as you're saying it, drag the tip of your tongue slowly back along the roof of your mouth—so far back that you have to drop it." (Instructions accompanied with hand gestures of moving fingertips back slowly, palm up.)

Sound approximation also includes other techniques. For instance, Shriberg's evocation procedure for /ɚ/ includes phonetic placement, modeling, detailed verbal instructions, and physical prompting.

Modeling

Modeling is a component in all treatment programs, regardless of their theoretical orientation. It is used in the treatment of all communication disorders. In modeling, the clinician produces (or models) the target response the child is expected to produce. The child is then encouraged to repeat the target sound modeled by the clinician. The child's response to the clinician's model is called **imitation** (Hegde, 1998).

Modeling is successful if the child can imitate the selected target response with some level of accuracy; if the child cannot imitate the sound, the shaping technique is needed. Modeling may be used at all levels of response complexity, including the sound in isolation, syllables, words, and sentences.

Training should begin at the most complex response level at which the child can imitate the target sound. The goal is to shape the response from the simple level to the ultimate goal of sound production in conversational speech. When modeling, the clinician asks the child to watch his or her mouth closely and to listen very carefully as the sound is produced. The child is then asked to repeat the target sound. Clinicians may also highlight the sound by *vocal emphasis* (Hegde, 1998).

In **vocal emphasis**, the clinician may model the target sound (or the sound in a word) and increase its vocal intensity or duration. Sounds that can be prolonged (such as fricatives) may be modeled with increased duration. For example, if the target were /s/ in syllables, the clinician would highlight /s/ by modeling it more loudly and prolonging its production (e.g., "Johnny, say [sssssssi]").

In the establishment phase of sound production, modeling is frequently used in conjunction with phonetic placement and successive approximation. For example, in phonetic placement, the child may be asked to imitate the placement of the tip of the tongue against the alveolar ridge. More detailed information on how modeling should be implemented and eventually faded may be found in Hegde (1998) and Hegde and Davis (2010).

Verbal Instructions and Prompts

Instructions are verbal stimuli that help facilitate a person's actions (Hegde, 1998). In treatment, instructions are almost always given on how to produce a sound; they are given neither about the phonological rules the child is supposed to follow nor about the mental representations or cognitive processes that presumably underlie sound productions.

When modeling alone is insufficient to get an imitated response, detailed verbal instructions preceding the model may increase the probability of a child's correct imitation. Clinicians commonly offer descriptions such as the following: "See the back part of my tongue? I'm going to make it go up really high, like this. Then the back part of my tongue is going to touch the top part of my mouth way in the back. Can you see? Now I'm going to make our sound like this: /kakaka/. Okay, now I want you to try to make the sound. Go ahead. Remember to use the back part of your tongue."

To further increase the likelihood of a correct response, the clinician may use prompts. **Prompts** are similar to hints or cues that help draw responses from reluctant persons. Verbal instructions and prompts are invariably used in conjunction with other facilitative techniques, including phonetic placement, successive approximation, and modeling.

Prompts can be verbal or nonverbal (Hegde, 1998). **Vocal emphasis** is a **verbal prompt** that is frequently used in articulation therapy; it was previously described under "Modeling." In vocal emphasis the clinician highlights the target response by vocalizing it more loudly or by prolonging its production (e.g., "Bobby, say [zzzzzzu]"). Some verbal prompts do not contain any part of the expected response but can still serve to facilitate correct production of the target sound. Examples of these include the following: "Remember, your tongue needs to stay inside your mouth when you make your sound" and "Before you start, I want you to think about where your tongue should be." Such prompts as "Don't forget the sound at the end of words" may help eliminate final consonant deletions.

Nonverbal, or **physical, prompts,** also known as visual cues or visual stimulation, are often used in speech sound treatment. They are similar to physical signs and gestures that may help the child visualize correct production of the target sound. For example, if training appropriate articulatory placement for [l], the clinician may demonstrate tongue-tip contact against the alveolar ridge by doing the following:

1. placing the right hand under the left hand

2. identifying the left hand as the alveolar ridge and the right hand as the tongue

3. lifting the fingertips of the right hand to make broad contact with the bottom front portion of the left hand

Physical prompts should not be confused with manual guidance (Hegde, 1998). In manual guidance, the clinician physically manipulates the child's articulators directly. When providing physical prompts, however, the clinician merely demonstrates the production of the sound; there is no physical contact with the child. Physical prompts may be especially useful when working with children who have sensory aversions such as a strong gag reflex that prevents the clinician from using direct manual guidance or phonetic placement procedures.

These various procedures, which are implemented before the child either imitates the clinician or produces a response that is evoked (not imitated), are followed by steps the clinician takes to increase and strengthen the correct responses. Positive reinforcement of various sorts is inherent to all treatment sessions. Also inherent are procedures that help reduce the error responses (corrective feedback). All clinicians are familiar with reinforcement and corrective feedback, because they will have used them in treating not only speech sound disorders, but all disorders of communication. Therefore, we provide only a brief overview of these procedures as a quick reminder.

Paired Stimuli

The pairing of picture stimuli to facilitate the correct production of a target sound in words was first promoted as an approach to treatment of speech sound disorders in the 1970s by Weston and Irwin (1971), which led to the subsequent publication of the *Paired Stimuli Kit* (Irwin & Weston, 1975). Although Irwin and Weston's training kit is no longer commercially available, the essence of their approach can still help strengthen the production of a target sound in words, thus bypassing the need to establish target sound production in isolation and syllables. This method requires the identification of one or more **key words**, words in which an error sound is produced correctly because of coarticulatory effects.

If key words do not exist in a child's speech sample, the clinician can create some by teaching them. After key words have been identified or taught, the clinician can then select at least 10 training words that can be paired with the key word and create a training picture board with the key word in the center and the training words arranged around it (see Figure 7.1). The clinician then asks the child to produce the key word followed by each target stimulus word in an alternating fashion to create a training string. So if the key word were *fan*, the clinician would instruct the child to produce the selected stimulus words on the training board (e.g., fan-*five*, fan-*fist*, fan-*fox*, fan-*foot*, fan-*fire*, fan-*fib*, fan-*four*, fan-*fight*, fan-*find*, and fan-*foil*). The child is reinforced for correct productions and given corrective feedback for incorrect productions of the target sound in selected stimulus words. When the predetermined production criterion is reached, training can progress to programmed sentences (e.g., Clinician: "Does the fan have five blades?" Child: "Yes, the fan has five blades"). In this example, *fan* is the key word, and *five* is one of the training words. Irwin and Weston's (1975) original program is much more detailed and has specific steps that need to be followed from a single word to sentences to conversation. We present their program here primarily as a facilitating technique that can be used to capitalize on the effect of coarticulation to strengthen the production of a sound that is known to be produced in at least one key word rather than a comprehensive treatment program.

Positive Reinforcement

A positive reinforcer is any event that follows a behavioral response and thus increases the response's frequency. For example, if the accuracy of a child's target sound increases when the child is given a sticker after each correct response, a sticker would be considered a positive reinforcer. The child who is praised for correct production of a particular speech sound will more often produce the sound correctly; in that case, verbal praise serves as a positive reinforcer. Clinicians who are sophisticated about the various nuances of reinforcement usually are more effective than those who have a simplistic idea of "reward" and "feedback." Because something is called a reinforcer only after it is known to increase the frequency of a behavior, the clinician needs to precisely measure the frequency of speech sound productions in all sessions. This requirement not only helps determine whether the response consequence selected is working, but also helps determine whether the treatment

Training Word 9	Training Word 10	Training Word 1
Training Word 8		Training Word 2
Training Word 7	KEY WORD	Training Word 3
Training Word 6	Client: _____ Phoneme: / / Position: Initial Final Training Word 5	Training Word 4

Figure 7.1. Paired-stimuli training sheet sample (without pictures).

is working. Clinicians should follow a few guidelines in selecting and administering positive reinforcers for correct speech sound productions:

• **Select primary reinforcers only when needed.** Primary reinforcers are consequences that do not rely on past learning because their effects are biologically mediated. Food and drink, examples of primary reinforcers, have their effects without past learning. Food is among the most frequently used primary reinforcer in articulation and phonological therapy. Raisins, candy, M&Ms, cereal, crackers, and other food items have been used by clinicians to increase children's correct productions of the target sounds. Food items may be especially useful with very young children and those with intellectual disabilities who may not initially respond well to verbal praise. Children with autism also respond well to primary reinforcers. Although they are powerful, they also are unnatural, however; they help establish the correct production of speech sounds, but they do not promote generalized productions. Also, in order for a reinforcer to be effective, the child needs to come to therapy sessions having had no recent access to the reinforcer (to have been temporarily deprived of it). For example, if the child had been given juice to drink on the way to the clinic, juice might not be an effective reinforcer because the child might be satiated. Therefore, the clinician should always pair verbal praise with primary reinforcers; once the speech sound production is established at the word level (e.g., 90% accuracy in 10 consecutive trials), the clinician should fade the primary reinforcers and maintain only the verbal praise. Healthy choices and parental permission are other important considerations in using primary reinforcers. Parents themselves may be requested to supply primary reinforcers they approve.

- **Prefer social (secondary) reinforcers. Verbal praise**, the most commonly used positive reinforcer, is a good example of social reinforcers whose effects are due to past learning experiences. Other practical secondary reinforcers include attention, eye contact, smiles, tokens, and informative feedback on performance. These different forms of social reinforcements are typically combined to reinforce correct speech sound productions. For example, while paying attention to the child and maintaining eye contact, with a smile on her face, the clinician may praise the child by saying, "Excellent job! You got it right!" If a token system is used, the clinician may give a token along with all those social reinforcers. **Tokens** and **stickers** are especially useful to teach correct sound productions. The clinician may award a token or a sticker for each correct response, and the child may later exchange them for a gift selected at the beginning of the session. There is plenty of behavioral research on the effectiveness of tokens; in speech–language pathology, tokens are known to reinforce speech sound productions, fluency, and other target skills (Hegde, 1998). Informative feedback, yet another form of social reinforcement, may be just a verbal statement that informs the child of his or her progress in therapy—for example, "Eddie, you got 4 out of 10 /s/ sounds correct yesterday, but today you got 6 out of 10 correct. That is fantastic!" Tokens may be faded as the teaching moves from word and phrase levels to conversational speech. At these more complex levels of teaching, periodic verbal praise (on an intermittent schedule) will be adequate to maintain the target speech sound productions.

- **Begin with continuous reinforcement and shift gradually to intermittent reinforcement.** In the initial stages of therapy, every correct response should be reinforced (**continuous reinforcement schedule**). Although there are no hard and fast rules, it is recommended that the clinician reinforce continuously until each sound is trained at the word level with about 80% accuracy. After meeting this criterion, the clinician may use an intermittent reinforcement schedule. For instance, the clinician may reinforce every other correct response (**fixed ratio 2 [FR2]**) until the child gives 90% correct responses or better. When the teaching is shifted to phrase level, continuous reinforcement may be needed again until the correct response rate increases to 80% or so, at which time an intermittent schedule may be reintroduced. When the sound is taught or strengthened in conversational speech, the clinician may reinforce on a larger **variable ratio schedule. A variable ratio 4 (VR4)** means that roughly on average, four responses are required to earn a reinforcer. The third or fourth or fifth response may be the one reinforced, but four responses would be average. This is a more informal and natural way of socially reinforcing correct speech sound productions.

- **Use reinforcers effectively.** A few general guidelines, followed diligently, will increase the effectiveness of reinforcers: (1) measure correct (and incorrect) sound productions in all sessions to make sure that the reinforcer is effective and correct responses are increasing; (2) reinforce promptly and immediately after a correct response; (3) be unambiguous and clear in your verbal praise (e.g., don't say, "I think you made your sound okay, so here is the token"; instead say, "You made your sound perfectly—here is the token"); (4) show that you are happy with the child's correct responses; be pleasant and show positive emotions as you praise the child or give out a token; and (5) avoid monotony in verbal praise; use different terms and phrases.

Corrective Feedback

The clinician can use corrective feedback to inform a child of an error made while attempting to produce the target sound. When used properly, and always in conjunction with positive reinforcement for correct speech sound productions, corrective feedback helps improve treatment efficiency by reducing speech sound errors on treatment trials. In addition to speech sound errors that need to be reduced, children in therapy may exhibit various extraneous behaviors that need to be reduced. For example, behaviors such as wiggling in the chair, leaving the chair, crawling under the table, crying and whining, and interrupting therapy in other ways (e.g., by asking frequently, "Are we done yet?") need to be reduced so the treatment may be efficient. A few effective procedures are available to reduce speech sound errors as well as behaviors that interfere with treatment:

- **Give corrective verbal feedback for all incorrect speech sound productions.** **Verbal corrective feedback** helps reduce inadequate, inappropriate, and unacceptable speech sound productions. Such statements as "No, let's try it again," "That was not right," or "You forgot to turn your voice on" uttered immediately after a wrong response, are helpful to the child in identifying his or her own wrong responses. This kind of verbal feedback may also explain what went wrong. For example, if a child said *thop* for *soap*, the clinician might say, "Johnny, you stuck your tongue out too much that time. Remember when you make 's' words, your tongue stays inside your mouth."

- **Give mechanical feedback.** Mechanical feedback can be provided through digital technology. Clinicians can use commercial computer software programs and Web-based applications for articulation and phonological therapy. These programs often provide children with immediate feedback about the accuracy of their responses and can help document their progress. Children may be especially responsive to digital feedback of their speech sound accuracy. However, digital technology should never be implemented without the clinician's close monitoring and direction.

- **Withdraw positive reinforcers for incorrect or interfering responses.** An effective way of removing positive reinforcers that may be maintaining undesirable responses is **token withdrawal**, also called **response cost**. Tokens awarded for correct speech sound productions may be withdrawn when incorrect responses are given. While withdrawing the token, the clinician must give corrective verbal feedback. For example, the clinician might say, "Oh! That was not what you wanted to say! I am taking a token back." The same token may be promptly given for the next correct response. The clinician should make sure that she gives more tokens than she takes away.

 • **Use corrective feedback effectively.** In each session, positive reinforcers (verbal praise, tokens) should exceed the quantity of corrective feedback. The child should come to, and leave, the treatment sessions happily. Excessive corrective feedback is often a sign that (1) the treatment task may be too difficult for the child, (2) the reinforcers may not be working, (3) more modeling or prompts may be needed, and (4) maybe a different speech sound should be targeted. If the treatment task is too difficult, perhaps a shaping procedure, which begins with a simpler response related to the final target, may help. Sometimes errors may be reduced (along with corrective feedback) by more frequent modeling and effective prompts. In some cases, the selected (presumed) reinforcer may have to be abandoned in favor of another, more effective one. In all cases, if the errors persist, the clinician should critically examine all aspects of treatment, *including his or her own skill level in the implementation of treatment.*

....

ACTIVITY

Describe *positive reinforcement* and *corrective feedback* in technical terms.

....

Structuring the Treatment Sessions

To be effective, treatment sessions should be a flexible arrangement. Initially, a treatment session is more structured because discrete trials (Hegde, 1998) are the most effective to establish speech sound productions in words. Each **discrete trial** is a distinct opportunity for the child to produce the target sound mostly in words, although a few initial trials may involve isolated sound productions or certain articulatory gestures (e.g., "Put the tip of your tongue here"). As the child becomes more proficient in sound productions, the treatment sessions become progressively less structured, more flexible, more naturalistic, ending in sessions in which relatively spontaneous conversational speech is the vehicle to strengthen the speech sound productions. Such naturalistic sessions are essential to promote generalization of learned speech sound productions to the natural environment.

Although some clinicians may prefer to use play as the main vehicle to teach speech sound productions, play activities often distract from the multiple, rapidly presented treatment trials that are most effective in establishing speech sounds. Play activities may be used as reinforcers, however, in which case, therapy is both fun for the child and effective. For instance, clinicians can give tokens for correct responses, and when the child accumulates a certain number, a 2-minute play activity may be allowed. The treatment process should never be play for the sake of play.

The clinician may learn how best to structure the session by observing the child response patterns in the initial session or two. While some children respond very well to loosely structured sessions from the beginning, others require sessions that are highly structured. The structure should fit the child, not the other way around.

Sound-in-Isolation Level

At the sound-in-isolation level, discrete treatment trials may be conducted as follows. Treatment trials are similar to the modeled base rate trials described earlier. The only difference is that treatment trials include reinforcement and corrective feedback, and base rate trials exclude them. It may be noted that not all sounds can be produced in isolation without an intrusive vowel (e.g., [ə]). The following steps can be individualized to meet the needs of a particular child.

1. The clinician presents multiple **antecedent stimuli** that help evoke the target sound, such as:
    *   verbal instructions on how to produce the sound
    *   a picture that helps evoke the word with the target sound in it
    *   phonetic placement cues
    *   visual and verbal prompts
    *   modeling
    *   combination of facilitative techniques
2. The child is instructed to produce the sound after a specific technique or a variety of facilitative techniques have been provided. A question is asked (e.g., "Danny, what is this?").
3. The clinician immediately models the correct response after asking a prompting question, whose prompt may be in the form of emphasis (e.g., "Danny, say fish").
4. The clinician consequates the child's production in one of the following ways:
    *   A reinforcer (verbal praise, token) is given if the response was acceptable.
    *   Corrective feedback is provided if the response was unacceptable.
5. The clinician records the accuracy of the response on a prepared data collection sheet using a plus or minus sign or NR for correct, incorrect, and no response, respectively.
6. The clinician begins another trial after a few seconds.

Sound-in-Syllable Level

Discrete trials at the syllable level are conducted in a similar fashion as the sound-in-isolation level. The syllable is the simplest response level for sounds that cannot be produced in isolation. Voiced stop plosives, for example, are impossible to make without an intrusive vowel.

After the sound is made with some consistency at the syllable level, the clinician may use a visual stimulus to evoke its production. The clinician can use a **vowel diagram,** in which the letter representing the target sound is paired with various pure vowels (e.g., *ba, be, bi, bo, boo*). This can be successful with students who know or have been taught the sound–letter association. This response-evoking method will provide the clinician an alternative to direct modeling.

At the sound-in-isolation and sound-in-syllable levels it is important to provide many rapidly evoked trials to establish the accurate motor production of the sound. Otherwise, when the treatment moves to a higher level of response complexity (words and phrases), the target sound production may be lost. Also, near perfect production of the sound at the isolation and syllable levels may be emphasized, so that articulatory precision of the sound is not lost in coarticulated speech. Although movement through the various levels of response complexity should be as rapid as possible, it is imperative that the clinician not move on to higher levels of production before correct production is solidly established at the preceding level. The first author has worked with many children who have been moved on to speech sound practice at the conversational level when obvious distortion of the target sound was still present. This is especially problematic with /r/ and all sibilants, as they are particularly vulnerable to distortion in coarticulated speech. Although it may seem tedious to do such intense practice at the isolation and syllable levels at the initial stages of treatment, it is worthwhile in the end, because correct production of sounds can then be sustained in coarticulated speech at increasingly complex levels over time.

Sound-in-Word, -Phrase, and -Sentence Levels

At the word, phrase, and sentence levels, discrete trials are conducted in a similar fashion. The primary difference is the length of the required response. At the word level, the stimulus items are most often pictures, objects, and events depicting a word that contains the target sound. At the phrase and sentence levels, the same stimuli can be used, but the child is now instructed to put the word in a phrase or a sentence. This may be difficult for young children who have not been asked to construct a sentence before. They may not know exactly what to do when instructed to create a sentence with the target word. Therefore, some initial training is usually necessary to facilitate this task. The clinician may need to provide extensive modeling in sentence production, so that eventually a child can create his or her own sentences without the need for modeling. The use of **carrier phrases** (e.g., "I see a . . ." and "I want a . . .") may simplify the task when the initial transition is made from words to sentences. With children who have oral reading skills, the clinician may use written sentences to facilitate production of the target sound at this level. To conduct a discrete trial at the word level, the clinician may do the following:

1. Place the stimulus picture or object in front of the child, or demonstrate the action or event that represents the sound in a word—for example:
    -   show the child a picture of a *rat* or *rain*
    -   swiftly move your legs and arms to represent the action *run*.
2. Ask a relevant predetermined question—for example:
    -   "What do you see in the picture?"
    -   "What is the name of this animal?"
    -   "What is falling from the sky?"

- "What am I pretending to do?"

3. Immediately after asking the predetermined question, model the correct response, assuming that modeling is needed—for example:

   - "Johnny, say *rat*."
   - "Johnny, say *rain*."
   - "Johnny, say *run*."

4. After providing a model, wait a few seconds for the child to respond. The amount of time needed before presentation of the next stimulus item may vary across children; some children require a longer response time

5. Consequate the child's production, either by providing a reinforcer if the response was acceptable or by providing corrective feedback if it was incorrect—for example:

   - "Johnny, you said your /r/ perfectly in the word *run*. Good job."
   - "Johnny, that /r/ came out just wonderfully."
   - "Johnny, that was a perfect /r/. Keep up the good work."
   - "Uh-oh, Johnny, that time your tongue was too flat, and your /r/ sounded like an /a/. We need to try that again."
   - "Johnny, stop. Your /r/ sounds like an /a/ in that word."

6. Record the response on a prepared data collection sheet using a plus or minus sign for correct or incorrect or NR for no response.

7. Remove the stimulus by pulling it away from the child's view and wait for 2 to 3 seconds before presenting the next trial. This is necessary to decrease the possibility of the child continuing to respond to a previous stimulus item and to measure responses discretely on each trial.

8. Return to step 1 to initiate the next trial until all trials are completed.

Discrete trials should not be equated with "boring" treatment activities. Discrete trials are temporally defined opportunities for the occurrence of a response. They are usually incorporated into highly structured tabletop activities; however, they can also be easily infused into structured play activities. For example, to play a *Fishing for Sounds* game, the clinician can paper clip the picture cards used to evoke the sound onto the paper fish. The fish now serve as the stimulus items. In using the discrete trial procedure, the clinician may continue as follows:

1. Place five fish on the ground (the stimulus pictures are attached with paper clips). Then instruct the child to "Go Fish" with a pole containing a magnet on the end of the fishing line. Hint: You may need to guide the child's "fishing expedition" to make this a time-efficient activity. The child may have a difficult time connecting the magnet with the paper clip on his or her own.

2. Ask a relevant question after the child catches a fish (e.g., "Johnny, what do you see on the fish?").

3. Immediately model the correct response, assuming that modeling is needed (e.g., "Johnny, say *cat*").

4. Wait a few seconds for the child to respond.

5. Consequate the child's production, either by providing a reinforcer if the response was acceptable or by providing corrective feedback if it was incorrect.

6. Record the response on a prepared data collection sheet.

7. Put the stimulus item aside and instruct the client to "Go Fish" for another card if the previous response was correct.

8. Instruct the child to try again if the sound production was incorrect or unacceptable and grant the child permission to "Go Fish" for another card only after the sound has been produced correctly.

As can be seen, these trials can still be categorized as discrete because they are temporally separated; however, they are not necessarily stiff or unexciting. The clinician should always think of making play contingent on correct productions. Play is not incorporated into therapy for the sake of play. All activities and treatment trials must be productive.

Speech Sounds in Conversation

At the conversational level, the discrete trial procedure is no longer clinically efficient because natural conversation does not occur in discrete opportunities. Often a conversation is a dialogue; at times it is a monologue. Frequently, there is conversational overlap between the listener and the speaker.

Instead of discrete trials, the clinician may use **open-ended questions** to evoke free-flowing speech from the child. A myriad of activities can be used to ensure that the child has an opportunity to produce the sound in more natural communicative interactions. In conversational speech, unlike discrete trials, the clinician does not have control over the number of times the sound is produced. Rather, the clinician's responsibility shifts to listening for natural occurrences of the target sound and delivering intermittent verbal praise. The clinician may say, "That was a good /s/!" Or "I've noticed that for the last 3 minutes all of your /s/ sounds have been made perfectly. Keep up the good work." At the conversational level, the clinician should continue to provide corrective feedback for inappropriate responses the child may give, possibly because of a lack of self-monitoring. The training of self-monitoring skills becomes crucial at this level (and is discussed further in the upcoming section "Implementing a Maintenance Program").

Using Specific Treatment Activities

Clinicians working with children frequently use fun and exciting treatment activities in hopes that this will increase the child's interest and cooperation in therapy. The activities are presented in a game format so that the children feel like they are playing rather than working. The children's cooperation can indeed be increased if the activities are fun for them. However, the primary goal of therapy is not to keep the child entertained but to improve the production of the target sounds.

Fun and exciting treatment activities must be structured to maximize the child's sound production learning. The target sounds will not improve if the child spends most of the time cutting and pasting or playing in the absence of sound production training. Therefore, clinicians should select treatment activities that will not only increase the child's participation in therapy, but also allow many opportunities for production practice. Furthermore, clinical activities should be planned and organized before the session, so that the treatment time is not devoted to deciding what to do next. Treatment activities should not take more than a few seconds to introduce and initiate.

Creative clinicians devise varied activities that interest the child and afford opportunities to practice speech sound production. The game format of Go Fish was previously described in the context of teaching sounds at the word, phrase, or sentence level. The clinician could also structure a *Let's Give It a Smile* game while teaching sounds. On a sheet of paper, the clinician draws 10 round faces with eyes and nose but no mouth. Each time the child correctly produces a sound a certain number of times (e.g., 10 correct responses), he or she is allowed to draw a smile on the face. In another game format—*Let's Paste Spots on the Dalmatian*—the clinician draws a picture of a Dalmatian dog without any spots on a sheet of paper. Contingent on a certain number of correct productions, the child is allowed to paste a cutout of a spot on the Dalmatian. The game continues in such fashion until several spots are placed on the Dalmatian.

See the companion CD for a variety of specific treatment activities, found in the file "Sample Treatment Activities," that are fun for the child and packed with opportunities to practice speech sound productions.

Moving Through the Initial and Subsequent Treatment Sequence

Soon after treatment is initiated, the clinician will have to make some important clinical decisions. As the child begins to produce the target speech sounds more consistently, the clinician will have to decide when to stop modeling, when a particular exemplar (e.g., the /s/ in *soap*) is tentatively trained, when to pick up another sound for teaching, when to move from the word level to the phrase level, and so forth.

As therapy progresses, the need for special stimuli such as visual prompts, verbal instructions, and modeling will diminish. Although highly necessary in the initial stages of treatment, the use of these stimuli should eventually be faded, because they are not part of the child's natural environment.

Treatment is begun at the most complex level the child can handle. That might be at the isolated sound or syllable level, or it may be at the word or even the phrase level. The treatment then moves progressively into the next higher level, terminating in conversational speech in and outside the clinic.

Essentially, a **target response,** also called an *exemplar,* is any word that contains the target phoneme; it is taught to establish the broader **target behavior,** which is the production of the target sound in varied contexts in conversational speech (Hegde & Davis, 2005). For instance, a correct production of the word *soup* is an exemplar of the target behavior of /s/ production in varied contexts. Teaching usually begins with an exemplar, and soon the clinician may make the following decisions to move the child through different levels of teaching:

- *Discontinue modeling*—The clinician may be more or less stringent about this: either 5 or 10 correctly imitated responses may be a guideline to discontinue modeling.

- *Initiate evoked trials*—Modeling is omitted on an evoked trial. When the child gives 10 (or so) consecutively correct evoked responses (e.g., the word *soup* when shown a picture of soup and asked what *it* is), the clinician may consider this exemplar tentatively trained.

- *Teach additional exemplars*—When one exemplar meets the tentative training criterion, another exemplar may be selected for teaching. Some four to six exemplars may be taught before taking the next step. Research has shown that generalization is a highly individualistic matter. Elbert, Powell, and Swartzlander (1991) report that in articulation treatment, 59% of 19 children studied exhibited generalized production with only 3 exemplars trained. About 21% of the children needed training on 5 exemplars, and 10 exemplars were needed in the case of 14% of the children. Even 10-exemplar training did not result in generalized production in 7% of the children. In behavioral research, about 7 to 10 exemplars are sufficient to produce generalization in most cases (Hegde, 1998; Hegde & Maul, 2006), but individual differences are dominant.

- *Probe for generalized production of the phoneme*—When the child's correct response rate is 90% or better on four to six exemplars, the clinician conducts a probe to see if the child produces the same phoneme in untrained words. The generalized production of a phoneme informs the clinician that the target behavior (a particular sound production, e.g., /s/) has been taught. This probing is done at each level of response complexity—words, phrases, sentences, and conversational speech. To conduct a probe, the clinician evokes untrained words, phrases, or sentences containing the target sound. Generally, if the child produces the trained sound with 90% accuracy in untrained contexts, the target behavior may be considered mastered. If not, treatment may be extended to additional exemplars. Details on generalization and probe procedures are given in a later section titled "Probing for Generalized Responses."

- *Vary the levels of training*—Typically, clinicians move linearly, from the most simple level of teaching a sound (e.g., in a syllable or word) to the most complex (sentences and conversational speech). As noted in an earlier section, target sounds may be taught simultaneously at different levels of response complexity. Skelton's (2004) original and subsequent research (Skelton & Funk, 2004; Skelton & Hagopian, 2013; Skelton & Kerber, 2005; Skelton & Price, 2006; Skelton & Resciniti, 2009; Skelton & Richard, 2013) has shown that a target sound may be simultaneously taught in word, phrase, and sentence levels, all selected levels randomly presented to the child. This might increase treatment efficiency as well as the potential for generalized productions.

Data Collection

Throughout the entire treatment sequence, the clinician should collect data on the child's performance in therapy. This is necessary to establish the clinician's accountability, to document positive changes in the child's skills under treatment, and to evaluate overall progress from the inception of treatment. Parents, clients, third-party payers, government agencies, and insurance companies invest valuable resources for the provision of therapeutic services. They have the ethical and legal right to know if their time and money are being well spent.

Nearly all employment settings require daily documentation of the child's performance in treatment. It is important that the clinician devise or adapt recording forms that allow for such documentation (see the companion CD for several sample recording forms that can be modified and personalized for clinical use). In speech sound production therapy the clinician can judge the child's production of the target sound as correct or incorrect and determine an accuracy percentage. In this manner, the clinician can determine whether the child's skills are improving. The clinician should follow the documentation guidelines dictated by his or her employment agency.

We have found that documentation of the child's performance during every treatment session can easily be incorporated into the treatment of articulation and phonological disorders when the *treatment targets* or *target objectives* are clearly identified. When the clinician is certain about what he or she is teaching and what the child is expected to do, charting is an easy task. When the clinician fails to specify what will be taught, documentation will be difficult or impossible. Incidentally, we have frequently found that documenting the accuracy of responses in front of the child, especially in the case of upper elementary and adolescent children, can be highly reinforcing to them. In our own clinical practice we have often heard children make such comments as "I don't want any more minuses," "How many pluses did I get today?" and "Tomorrow I'm gonna get them all right."

Probing for Generalized Responses

Generalization is an intermediate target of clinical intervention. It refers to "either a temporary production of a recently learned response in different contexts and situations, or the production of new (untrained) responses based on recent or remote learning" (Hegde, 1998, p. 179). For example, after training the production of /f/ at the word level in the clinical setting, the child may show generalized responses of the sound in words produced at home or school (untrained context or situation). Or the child may demonstrate a new, untrained production of /v/ after establishing the production of /f/. In either case, the generalized response occurs in the absence of current and systematic reinforcement.

If the behaviors that initially appeared as generalized responses continue to be produced in the absence of reinforcement, they will begin to decrease and eventually disappear. For this reason, Hegde (1998) describes generalization as a temporary phenomenon that should not be the final goal of treatment. If these behaviors are to be maintained over time, the clinician, family members, teachers, and others cannot simply ignore them and assume that they will continue. Special procedures must be implemented that will guarantee their maintenance over time. These will be addressed under our discussion of response maintenance procedures in "Implementing a Maintenance Program" later in this chapter.

Several types of generalization have been described in the literature. We address those that are most relevant to articulation and phonological disorders in the following list:

• *Generalization to untrained stimulus items*—Also described as **physical stimulus generalization** (Hegde, 1998), this is the production of trained speech sounds in the context of untrained stimuli (new words, phrases, sentences) because of stimulus similarity. This type of generalized responding has been documented when a child who has learned to say *soup* as a response to the picture of a bowl of soup used in treatment goes home and says *soup* when presented with a different bowl of soup. Physical stimulus generalization has been documented in the treatment of speech sound disorders (Arndt, Elbert, & Shelton, 1971; Elbert & McReynolds, 1975, 1978; Elbert et al., 1991; Gierut, 2008; Hoffman, 1983; McReynolds, 1972; McReynolds & Elbert, 1981b; Mowrer, 1971; Powell & Elbert, 1984; Shelton, Elbert, & Arndt, 1967; Skelton, 2004; Skelton & Funk, 2004).

- *Generalization across word positions*—This type of generalized responding refers to the transfer of the production of a sound taught in one position to other untreated word positions. According to Elbert and Gierut's (1986) review of the literature, studies have not conclusively demonstrated that teaching a sound in a particular word position facilitates more generalization than teaching a sound in any other position. Therefore, they conclude that teaching sounds in any position can facilitate generalized responses in untrained word positions.

- *Generalization across response topographies*—The production of the trained sound in response topographies (e.g., syllables, words, phrases, sentences) that were not directly trained exemplifies generalized productions across response (linguistic) units (Elbert & Gierut, 1986). This type of generalization is illustrated by the child who produces /p/ in phrases and sentences despite having been taught its production only in single words. Generalized responding across linguistic units has been documented in the treatment of speech sound disorders (Elbert, Dinnsen, Swartzlander, & Chin, 1990; McReynolds, 1972; Powell & McReynolds, 1969; Skelton, 2004; Skelton & Funk, 2004; Skelton & Kerber, 2005). Generalization at a different level of response complexity speeds up training.

- *Generalization within sound classes*—A **sound class** is a group (or class) of sounds that share certain characteristics or features. For example, /s, z, f, v, ʃ, ʒ, θ, ð/ are categorized under the fricatives sound class because they all share the phonetic feature of frication. As noted in Chapter 2, sounds are classified in several ways. These include (1) cognate sound pairs; (2) manner, place, and voice features; (3) distinctive features; and (4) phonological processes. Studies have reported generalization within sound classes (see Elbert & Geirut, 1986), as well as failure to generalize within sound classes (Saben & Ingham, 1991; A. L. Williams, 1991) This type of generalization has been reported for sound classes as related to (1) *manner, place, and voice features* (McNutt, 1994; Shelton et al., 1967; A. L. Williams, 2000); (2) *feature distinctions* (Costello & Onstine, 1976; McReynolds & Bennett, 1972; Tyler & Figurski, 1994); and (3) *phonological error patterns* (Elbert & McReynolds, 1978; McReynolds & Elbert, 1981b; Powell & Elbert, 1984; Skelton & Kerber, 2005; Weiner, 1981). Generalization within sound classes or error patterns cannot be taken for granted; it must be measured. When there is no generalization to untrained sounds within a class or pattern, the clinician has to teach them.

- *Generalization across sound classes*—This more complex form of generalization implies that sounds that are seemingly unrelated according to their many phonetic features (e.g., manner, place, voicing) could actually affect each other when treated (Gierut, 1985; Weiner, 1981). Gierut (1985) found that teaching production of the voiceless fricative /s/ resulted in accurate production of the voiced /l/. Gierut (1989) found that teaching maximally opposed known sounds resulted in the learning of 16 word-initial untreated consonants. Weiner (1981) reported improved production of final fricative consonants after teaching final stop consonants. He also found that when stopping of fricatives was eliminated, fronting of stops was also eliminated. Tyler and Figurski (1994) found that when they taught production of /l/, a more complex phonetic distinction, to a child of 2 years 8 months with a pretreatment phonetic inventory of nine sounds limited to nasals, stops, and glides, the child's phonetic inventory increased to 21 sounds. Besides adding the trained sound /l/ and three untrained sounds within the existing sound classes, the child added seven sounds in untrained sound classes including fricatives /f, v, s, z, ð/ and affricates /ʧ, ʤ/. Although this type of generalization may initially seem unlikely, it may happen because phonetically unrelated sounds may still form a response class. That is, the phonetic classification of sounds may be faulty. If phonetically unrelated sounds show the generalization effect, then those unrelated sounds are indeed related empirically. Generalization occurs only among empirically related or clustered responses (in other words, response classes). Plenty of treatment research in language has demonstrated that linguistic structural categories are mostly problematic because they are theoretical, not empirically real (Hegde, 1998; Hegde & Maul, 2006). It is likely that phonological and phonetic categories also are not entirely empirical.

- *Generalization across situations*—This refers to generalized productions of clinically established speech sounds in situations in which teaching has not taken place. In this case, there may be a physical setting generalization (to new situations) or an audience generalization (to new conversational partners) (Hegde, 1998). Physical setting generalization of clinically taught speech sound productions has been documented to such untrained environments such as the child's home, classroom, or playground (Bankson & Byrne, 1972; Carrier, 1970; Costello & Bosler, 1976; Olswang & Bain, 1985; Skelton, 2004; Skelton & Resciniti, 2009). Researchers have also reported generalized responding of the target sound to untrained audiences such as teachers and peers (Conley, 1966; Engel, Brandriet, Erickson, Gronhoud, & Gunderson, 1966).

Assessing Generalized Responses

A **probe** is a procedure to assess generalized speech sound productions. After a certain number of target responses (words) have been trained to a selected criterion (e.g., 90% accuracy), the clinician can assess for generalized responses to untrained words, untrained phonemes, untrained positions, and levels of response complexity. For example, the clinician can teach the correct production of the target sound /f/ in a certain number of words (e.g., *fat, four, five, farm, fix,* and *fight*). After these words have been trained to the criterion, the clinician can *probe* for generalized productions to the following:

- untrained words: *fun, feet, fox, fan, phone*

- untrained phonemes (cognate pair): *vine, vest, vote, valentine, vegetable*

- untrained word position: *leaf, half, life, safe, beef*

- untrained response complexity (sentences): *The boy is fat; I am four years old; The farm is big; I like to fix things; I fight with my brother*

Probes can be conducted through discrete trials or a conversational speech sample, depending on the response complexity level at which the sound was taught just prior to probing (Hegde, 1998). **Discrete trial probes** are conducted similarly to baseline trials. The clinician selects stimulus items that have not received prior training (see the examples in the preceding bulleted list), presents them to the child, and records the child's response. However, there is no modeling, positive reinforcement for correct responses, or corrective feedback for incorrect responses on any of the probe trials, unlike the baseline trials. The clinician simply shows the picture, asks the predetermined question, and records the client's response. The child is reinforced for adequate participation (e.g., sitting quietly, responding nicely) but not for correct productions. The clinician then calculates the percentage of correct probe response rates, which is a measure of generalized productions. If the probe response rate is less than the desired level (e.g., 90% correct), the clinician offers additional treatment.

See the companion CD for a modifiable and printable "Probe Recording Sheet" for clinical use.

During a **conversational probe,** the clinician collects one or several conversational speech samples and analyzes them for generalized responding of the trained target sounds. No reinforcing or corrective contingencies are provided during collection of the conversational speech sample. At that point, the clinician assesses the child's production of the target sound in untrained words, situations, response complexity levels, and so forth in the absence of any special prompting.

ACTIVITY

Describe at least three types of generalization that should be targeted in treatment.

Implementing a Maintenance Program

As stated earlier, the ultimate goal of treatment is the correct production of speech sounds in the child's natural environment and the *maintenance* of those skills over time and across situations. The clinician may take certain steps to ensure maintenance of acceptable speech sound production skills. These steps should be well thought out and implemented, not just at the end of the treatment program but from the beginning. Maintenance is a consideration from the beginning of treatment because the kinds of target speech sounds selected and how they are taught might influence maintenance.

In planning for maintenance, the clinician should consider (1) the kinds of sounds to teach, (2) the types of treatment stimuli to be used, and (3) the types and methods of reinforcement and corrective feedback to be given. A summary of these considerations follows:

• *Select child-specific and functional speech sounds with a potential for generalization*—For instance, treating sounds that occur most frequently or sounds that help eliminate a phonological error pattern that affects a large number of sounds may be more effective than treating sounds that occur less frequently or patterns that affect fewer sounds. Treatment targets that help improve intelligibility may help sustain correct productions because they are likely to be reinforced in everyday situations. See the earlier section "Selecting Potential Target Behaviors" for more information.

- *Select treatment stimuli from the child's environment*—If the treatment stimuli are the same as or similar to what the child encounters at home, the correct production of speech sounds is more likely to generalize and be maintained in natural settings. The clinician may give a list of words with target sounds in them to parents of the child and request them to bring treatment stimuli (e.g., pictures, objects, or the child's toys) to the sessions. In the school setting, the clinician may consult with the child's teacher to incorporate into treatment pictures, storybooks, art projects, spelling words, and language materials the teacher uses.

- *Select common verbal antecedents*—Use simple, common, everyday words, phrases, and questions to evoke the target speech sounds. These are the **verbal antecedents** of target productions. The child is likely to encounter the same verbal antecedents at the classroom and home, so the target speech sound productions are likely to be maintained. Examples include the following: (1) for the target of /b/, the clinician says, "Tell me what you're playing with," and the client responds, "My *ball*"; (2) for the target of /k/, the clinician says, "What are you eating?" and the client responds, "Cookies"; (3) for the target of /ʤ/, the clinician says, "What is the title of the book you're reading?" and the client responds, "*Jack and the Beanstalk*."

- *Teach multiple exemplars*—Both generalization and maintenance may fail because the clinician has taught few exemplars of each target speech sound. Increasing the number of exemplars taught is usually an effective method of enhancing initial generalization and subsequent maintenance.

- *Teach complex response topographies*—Terminating treatment at a low level of response complexity is another reason correct speech sound productions may not be maintained. The final phases of treatment should always include the most complex level of treatment: conversational speech, with typical and varied sentence structures and lengths, in which the correct production of target sounds are socially and informally reinforced.

- *Use naturally occurring reinforcers*—If the child responds well to verbal praise, there is no need to introduce any other kind of reinforcer. If used, primary reinforcers (food and drink) or tokens may be faded to maintain target speech sounds on verbal praise.

- *Delay reinforcement*—In the latter part of treatment, now and then the clinician may wait for a few extra seconds to praise the child. Delayed reinforcement is common in everyday situations; thus, the child is likely to sustain correct speech production in those situations because of the similarity between the teaching and natural settings.

- *Use an intermittent reinforcement schedule*—In the latter stages of treatment, the clinician should reinforce every third, fourth, or fifth correct response, rather than every correct response. At the level of conversational speech, reinforcement should be entirely natural; smiles, agreement, attention, and so forth will be constant, but explicit reinforcement for correct speech sound production will occur only occasionally.

- *Invite different people to take part in the treatment sessions*—The clinician can invite colleagues, teacherzs, peers, and others into the treatment sessions in which conversational speech is targeted. These individuals may ask questions, request a personal narration, and just be present when the child talks. The child will then be more likely to produce the targeted speech sounds in the presence of people other than the clinician.

- *Move treatment out of the treatment room*—One reason children fail to generalize and then maintain target speech sound productions is that they are taught in a highly discriminated situation. The clinician should take the child out for a walk while maintaining typical conversation with the child. Correct sound productions may thus be informally and verbally reinforced. The greater the variety of situations in which the target skills are reinforced, the higher the probability that they will be maintained.

- *Teach self-monitoring skills*—Self-monitoring (self-control or self-correcting) is a skill that can be taught by asking the child to evaluate his or her own mistakes immediately following their occurrence. During this time the clinician could withhold corrective feedback and instead ask the child to chart his or her own correct and incorrect productions. The clinician could also videotape a sample of the child's speech, ask the child to evaluate correct and incorrect speech productions, ask the child to stop talking (without a prompt from the clinician) as soon as a sound is produced incorrectly, and so forth. Effectiveness of self-monitoring skills has been evaluated in several studies, with positive results (Koegel, Koegel, & Ingham, 1986; Koegel, Koegel, Voy, & Ingham, 1988; Shriberg & Kwiatkowski, 1990).

- *Teach contingency priming*—Caregivers, teachers, and others not paying positive attention to correct speech sound production is another reason children fail to maintain target speech skills. Teaching children in therapy to prompt others to reinforce their own newly acquired behaviors is called **contingency priming.** The child primes others to pay attention and reinforce. For example, the child might be taught to say, "Mom, did you notice I have been saying my s sounds correctly?" Or "Dad, can you please listen to me when I say some words with k sound in them?" Or "Hey, Jim, what do you think of my r sounds?" Most likely, the child will receive some positive attention from then on. This strategy should be combined with the next.

- *Work with parents and significant others*—Training parents in administering treatment sessions at home and then teaching them to informally reinforce their child's correct speech sound production is one of the most effective ways of promoting maintenance. The parents may initially observe the sessions and then subsequently administer a few trials along with the clinician; the clinician can take this opportunity to train them to verbally praise the child in a natural manner. The child's teachers and siblings may be similarly trained. All who receive this type of training should be able to help by recognizing the target skills the child is supposed to learn and maintain, learning subtle and natural ways of reinforcing them in naturalistic contexts, offering more or less subtle prompts when needed (e.g., showing a particular tongue tip movement to the child or telling the child, "Remember what the speech teacher has told you"), not reinforcing incorrect responses even if they do not wish to provide corrective feedback, and so forth. Current best practice and legislation such as the Individuals with Disabilities Education Act mandate family involvement in the assessment and treatment of communication impairments, including speech sound disorders, and other disabilities. Therefore, it is imperative that the parents' role in treatment be clearly communicated from the outset.

Dismissal, Follow-up, and Booster Therapy

In practice, many children may be dismissed from treatment before their target skills are stabilized in natural settings. Many children in therapy may not even reach the skill maintenance phase. Some children are dismissed after a certain period of therapy. For example, if clinical services are funded by a third-party payer, the clinician has to discontinue therapy when an allotted number of sessions have been completed. The clinician may also dismiss a child from therapy because a neurological, structural, or other organic variable limits the child's progress, which may have reached a plateau.

Children may sometimes be dismissed because of poor motivation to improve. It is the child's responsibility to follow through with assignments, to monitor his or her productions, and to practice correct sound productions as often as possible. In spite of the clinician's best efforts, dismissal may be unavoidable if a lack of motivation continues to interfere with the child's progress. Before dismissing a child, the clinician must seriously evaluate whether everything possible has been done to motivate the child, the teacher, and the family members; whether the selected treatment procedure is known to be effective; and whether all needed treatment modifications to suit the child have been made. If the clinician is satisfied that the treatment followed the best practice, he or she must be willing to dismiss the child.

Although following up with children who have been successful in meeting treatment objectives is more rewarding, following up with children who were dismissed prematurely is an ethically responsible thing to do. Perhaps the child and the family would be willing to work harder the next time. In all cases, a **follow-up assessment** is a quick procedure that helps the clinician determine a child's status. The clinician can record a conversational speech sample or administer a standardized test to reassess speech sound production and the presence of phonological error patterns. If the clinician finds that the child's skills have diminished or regressed after having been dismissed from services, a short period of intervention, called **booster treatment**, may be warranted (Hegde, 1998). After reestablishing the desired skills, the child is dismissed again with another schedule set up for follow-up.

Summary of the Basic Unit

- The comprehensive treatment program described in this chapter is evidence based, includes steps missing from many programs, and is appropriate for treating articulation disorders as well as phonological disorders. Phonological analysis is all about target behaviors, not about treatment procedures.

- It is only by teaching individual sounds that even a phonological disorder can be eliminated. All currently popular phonological approaches use behavioral methods to teach speech sounds.

- Treatment begins with the selection of functional, useful, and ethnoculturally appropriate **target behaviors,** which are typically outlined as **short-term objectives** and **long-term goals.**

- Considerations in selecting target behaviors include improved intelligibility, rapid generalization, improved academic success, low or high base rates of errors, phonological processes that affect a large number of sounds, more frequently occurring sounds, and so forth.

- Either several phonemes or just one or two phonemes may be targeted in a given session; the child's response rate shows a preference for one or the other approach.

- Before starting therapy the clinician identifies the potential treatment target, prepares stimulus items to evoke its production, prepares a recording sheet to document the client's performance, and administers **baseline discrete trials.**

- Treatment should begin at the highest response level possible, although many children may first need a few trials at the isolated sound level.

- The clinician should develop measurable objectives, a quantitative mastery criterion, the response mode, the response level, the response setting, and the methods by which progress will be measured.

- Treatment programs may be written in a simple, comprehensive, or specific format (i.e., **Individualized Education Program, Individualized Family Service Plan**).

- **Phonetic placement, successive approximation, modeling,** and **verbal instructions** and **prompts** help establish the motoric production of speech sounds.

- **Positive reinforcers, primary reinforcers, social reinforcers,** or **conditioned generalized reinforcers** help increase and strengthen correct sound productions. To begin with, reinforcers are delivered on a continuous schedule and faded to an intermittent schedule.

- **Time-outs, response cost, verbal corrective feedback, nonverbal corrective feedback,** and **mechanical feedback** will help reduce **interfering** or **inappropriate behaviors.**

- Initial treatment sessions are highly structured and become progressively more flexible.

- Speech sounds may be **taught initially in discrete trials** but eventually in more spontaneous **conversational interactions.**

- **Generalization may be probed** in untrained response modes, untrained words, untrained settings, and in relation to untrained audiences.

- Various **maintenance procedures** help ensure that the target speech sound productions last.

- **Dismissal may be determined,** a **follow-up schedule** may be established, and **booster therapy** can be provided as needed.

Advanced Unit: Treatment of Organic and Neurogenic Speech Sound Disorders

The basic treatment principles and procedures described in the Basic Unit of this chapter are known to be effective in the treatment of a variety of communication disorders. In this Advanced Unit, we will address a few other procedures and general considerations that may be added to the basic procedures in treating the speech difficulties associated with specific disorders: childhood apraxia of speech, developmental dysarthria in cerebral palsy, cleft palate, and hearing impairment. We previously addressed the characteristics and etiologies of these disorders in the Advanced Unit of Chapter 6. In essence, speech sound production problems found in individuals who have one of these disorders are associated with neurological, physiological, or sensory limitations, and the clinician needs to consider additional variables in treating children with these disorders. The information addressed in this Advanced Unit is meant to be an introduction to the treatment of these organic and neurogenic speech disorders. It is likely that students will have specific courses that focus on the assessment and treatment of these disorders at both the undergraduate and graduate levels.

Childhood Apraxia of Speech

As reviewed in Chapter 6, apraxia of speech is a motor programming disorder of neurogenic origin. Its etiology is better understood in adults. The primary etiology for the neurological damage leading to apraxia of speech (AOS) is a left hemisphere stroke in the frontal lobe, although several other causes have been identified. The onset of the disorder in adults is acute rather than progressive. The severity of apraxia of speech can range from mild to profound, depending on the extent of damage, which often results in varied speech characteristics from one client to another.

Childhood apraxia of speech (CAS) shares common features with apraxia of speech in adults. To date, the neuropathology for CAS has not been documented (see Chapter 6). Many clinicians reserve the label of childhood apraxia of speech for children with a severe speech sound disorder who display many characteristics typically associated with apraxia of speech in adults. Childhood apraxia of speech is primarily a sensory–motor disorder affecting the articulatory and prosodic parameters of speech production. The child with CAS exhibits particular difficulty with fine, rapid, and voluntary movements necessary to produce speech that may be directly influenced by context (Strand & Skinder, 1999; Yorkston et al., 2010). Nonspeech movements may or may not be impaired. Although varied, and at times conflicting, descriptions of CAS have been advanced, the American Speech-Language-Hearing Association (2007) lists the following characteristics as those that have gained consensus: (1) inconsistent errors on consonants and vowels in repeated production syllables and words; (2) lengthened and disrupted coarticulatory transitions between sounds and syllables; and (3) inappropriate prosody, particularly in word or phrase stress patterns.

Treatment procedures for CAS have been drawn from a variety of sources, including adult apraxia treatment and treatment of articulation and phonological disorders in children. Such treatment procedures have been modified to suit the needs of children diagnosed with CAS. A few specific programs also are available (Hayden & Square, 1994; Helfrich-Miller,

1994; Square, 1999; Strand & Skinder, 1999; Strand & Debertine, 2000; Strand & Stoeckel, 2006; Velleman & Strand, 1994; Yorkston et al., 2010). Treatment efficacy data on CAS have recently begun to emerge (Edeal & Gildersleeve-Neumann, 2011; Iuzzini & Forrest, 2010; Knock, Ballard, Robin, & Schmidt, 2000; Mass & Farinella, 2012; Mass et al., 2008; Skelton & Hagopian, 2013; Strand & Debertine, 2000; Strand & Stoeckel, 2006). In general, the treatment for CAS, as for its adult counterpart, tends to follow a sequential organization progressing from simple to complex speech tasks. After specifying the vowels and consonants targeted for remediation, clinicians usually begin treatment at a complexity level judged appropriate for the child. For some children, that level may be syllables, while for others it may be words or sentences. A couple of recent studies (Edeal & Gildersleeve-Neumann, 2011; Skelton & Hagopian, 2013) have experimentally evaluated the efficacy of using a concurrent treatment method in which target sounds are randomly and simultaneously trained at different task levels. Both studies revealed positive results for the use of a random versus blocked practice format. These studies are preliminary and have not yet been replicated, so results should be viewed with caution until further data are advanced.

Most experts, in spite of some differences in approach (ASHA, 2007; Hall, Jordan, & Robin, 2007; Lof, 2009; Square, 1999; Strand & Skinder, 1999; Velleman & Strand, 1994; Yorkston et al., 2010), agree that in treating children with CAS, the following guidelines should be followed:

1. The primary focus of treatment should be the movement patterns and sequence of sounds instead of drill on individual sound productions.

2. Treatment may be started with vowel errors if they are dominant. Generally, treatment may progress from CV or VC to CVC to CCVC syllable shapes to words of varying lengths, then phrases, sentences, and conversational speech.

3. Initial treatment targets may include the earliest developing and most visible sounds. Stimulable sounds also may be preferred.

4. Initial treatment trials may include highly contrasted and easily distinguishable consonants (e.g., /p/, /t/, /k/, /s/) and vowels /o/, /a/, /i/, and /æ/.

5. Sounds that occur more frequently are better targets than are those that occur less frequently. An exception to this rule is the sounds in the child's name and the names of family members.

6. Sounds may be treated in an order of increasing phonetic difficulty: vowels, plosives, nasals, laterals, fricatives, and affricates. Voiceless sounds may be treated before voiced sounds.

7. Sounds may be first trained in the word-initial position.

8. Auditory discrimination training is not important, as sequenced production of speech is the main difficulty.

9. Treatment with frequent short breaks may be beneficial, because fatigue is typically a problem in CAS.

10. Treatment with sound and syllable sequences should be done in the context of meaningful single words; a core vocabulary should be selected for initial treatment.

11. Repeated trials of the same movement patterns are essential.

12. Initial success in treatment is important because a child with CAS may have experienced repeated failure in treatment.

13. Five to seven utterances may be targeted at a time for the child to practice.

14. Each target word or phrase should be practiced a few times (several trials in sequence) before switching to another target.

15. Prompt and effective positive reinforcement and corrective feedback are essential.

16. Slower movement of the articulators is essential to stabilize movement patterns; any modeling provided, as well as the child's imitation, should be produced at a slower rate.

17. Varied carrier phrases (e.g., "I like the . . ." or "I see the . . .") may be helpful in making repeated trials more meaningful.

18. Automatic speech tasks (counting and reciting) may be trained before spontaneous speech.

19. Nonspeech oral–motor exercises should be avoided.

20. The number of responses per session should be maximized to promote more automatic production of speech targets.

Specific Treatment Approaches

Treatment techniques designed for adults with apraxia of speech have been used with children with CAS. Similarly, some procedures initially developed for CAS have been used with adults. Generally, modeling, shaping (described in the Basic Unit), immediate positive reinforcement, and corrective feedback offered in carefully sequenced and repeatedly practiced treatment sessions are expected to yield good results. As with apraxia of speech in adults, the clinician can use auditory, visual, and tactile cues with children to facilitate correct production of the target sounds, words, or phrases. Children with CAS often benefit from a multimodality approach, especially when new sounds are introduced. What follows is a brief overview of selected specific techniques.

A tactile, kinesthetic, and visual cuing system originally developed for the treatment of CAS is called Prompts for Restructuring Oral Muscular Phonetic Targets **(PROMPT;** Chumpelik, 1984; Hayden & Square, 1994). The technique uses specific cues to facilitate the production of speech. It was subsequently applied to adults with apraxia of speech (Square, Chumpelik, & Adams, 1985; Yorkston et al., 2010). This program uses touch, pressure, kinesthetic, and **proprioceptive** cues to facilitate speech production. The approach trains finger placements on the child's face and neck to prompt the place of articulation and manner of production (features) for the articulatory target. The finger placements also provide information about the degree of jaw movement needed and appropriate duration of the syllable or segment. The prompts may be initially used in isolation to facilitate the production of individual sounds but may eventually be chained to facilitate articulatory movements between sounds, to create words in meaningful utterances rather than nonsense syllables (Yorkston et al., 2010). Duffy (2005) indicates that this program is probably most appropriate for children with chronic, severe apraxia of speech whose spontaneous verbal output is very limited and for whom other approaches have failed. Clinicians require specialized training to use the prompts in the PROMPT program. Another tactile cuing method includes the **touch-cue method**, which uses tactile cues to the face and neck along with auditory and visual cues and in three major stages progresses from nonsense syllables to spontaneous speech (Bashir, Grahamjones, & Bostwick, 1984). The **adapted cuing technique** (ACT; Klick, 1985) uses hand motions to prompt the articulatory movements and manner of production of the target productions.

Integral stimulation has been used with both adults and children who have apraxia of speech. This technique integrates an auditory and visual model with the prompt "Watch me and listen to me." The child is expected to imitate the modeled movement in a repetitive fashion. Tactile cues that provide additional information may also be used by the clinician to prompt a response. In addition, the child can be trained to self-cue. The Eight-Step Continuum (Rosenbek, Lemme, Ahern, Harris, & Wertz, 1973) is an example of a structured program that targets meaningful utterances and trains their use in a hierarchical fashion beginning with tactile cues and ending with role-playing activities.

Another comprehensive cuing program is the Dynamic Temporal and Tactile Cueing for Speech Motor Learning (DTTC; Strand & Stoekel, 2006). This program shapes the movement gestures for speech production and the effective use of those gestures in the context of speech. It was derived from the Eight-Step Continuum, but in DTTC, the time between the clinician's stimulus and the child's response constantly changes instead of following a hierarchical sequence of training. Also, in this program there is a constant back-and-forth adding and fading of cues until the child says the target utterance with normal rate and prosody in spontaneous productions (Yorkston et al., 2010).

In a technique called **progressive assimilation,** the clinician attempts to reestablish production of the target sounds from sounds that are not affected or from other nonspeech gestures. This method is similar to the **successive approximation** or **shaping** method described in the Basic Unit of this chapter. For example, the child may be asked to lightly bite his lower lip with his upper teeth and then exhale, which may yield /f/. The child may be asked to tightly pucker his lips and then say /ə/ to derive the production of /u/. The voiceless palatal /ʃ/ may be shaped when the child is asked to protrude his or her lips while making /s/. This method is appropriate for patients with severe childhood apraxia of speech, because they often need to learn or relearn to produce single sounds and syllables (Rosenbek, 1985). The **phonetic placement techniques**, including physically guiding the articulators to specific positions and locations, described in the Basic Unit of this chapter, have also been recommended for children with CAS.

Contrastive stress drills may be used to promote articulatory proficiency and natural prosody in children with apraxia of speech. This approach is especially suited to teach appropriate stresses and rhythms of spoken language. Also used in the treatment of clients with dysarthria, the method uses different phrases and sentences to train stress placement on different words. In articulation training, the clinician constructs phrases and sentences with a single target sound in them (e.g., "My name is Bob" for /b/; "Terry is her name" for /t/). The clinician then asks a series of questions structured so that the child responds with the target phrase while placing extra stress on the target word or sound (e.g., the clinician asks, "Is her name Mary?" and child responds, "No, her name is *Terry*"). The child is likely to stress the target word and thus improve the articulatory proficiency of the target sound. The child is reinforced for the precision of the target sound. A similar procedure is used to train appropriate stress and rhythm in words:

- The clinician creates a series of phrases and sentences (e.g., "Terry likes steak").

- The clinician then asks a question that will force stress on different words in the target phrases or sentences (e.g., "Does Mary like steak?" may evoke "No, *Terry* likes steak"; "Does Terry like pork chops?" may evoke "No, Terry likes *steak*").

- The clinician reinforces the use of appropriate stress on varying words.

With children who have severe childhood apraxia of speech, nonverbal communication systems may be used to facilitate functional communication (see Text Box 7.2). The child may be taught sign language, meaningful gestures, or an augmentative communication system such as the Picture Exchange Communication System (PECS), a communication system in which the child exchanges pictures to communicate (Yorkston et al., 2010); clinicians require special training in the use of PECS. Electronic communication devices may also be used with appropriate candidates. The success of nonverbal communication systems is highly dependent on the child's intellectual abilities and receptive language skills. See ASHA (2007), Caruso and Strand (1999), Hall and colleagues (2007), Velleman and Strand (1994), Vogel and Cannito (2001), and Yorkston and colleagues (2010) for detailed presentations on the characteristics, assessment, and treatment of apraxia of speech in adults and children.

....

ACTIVITY

Identify and briefly describe specific treatment programs and/or general approaches that could be used to treat childhood apraxia of speech.

....

Developmental Dysarthria in Cerebral Palsy

Dysarthria is a group of motor speech disorders resulting from neurological damage that can affect all speech parameters: articulation, resonance, phonation, respiration, and prosody. At least six types of dysarthrias have been identified, including flaccid dysarthria, spastic dysarthria, hypokinetic dysarthria, hyperkinetic dysarthria, ataxic dysarthria, and mixed dysarthria. The etiology of the neurological damage leading to each type of dysarthria is varied, including stroke, progressive neurological disorders, metabolic disorders, inherited disorders, and so forth. We discussed several of these in the Advanced Unit of Chapter 6. Similar to apraxia of speech, various forms of dysarthria are typically noted in adults. Among children who show dysarthric speech are those who have cerebral palsy, traumatic brain injury, tumors, and strokes, with cerebral palsy (CP) being the most common.

You may recall from Chapter 6 that CP is a congenital disorder resulting from brain damage before, during, or soon after birth. Thus, it is generally considered a childhood neurological disorder. As described in Chapter 6, cerebral palsy has been classified into

---

Text Box 7.2. Our role includes being a strong child advocate

As speech–language pathologists, we understand that one of our most important roles is to help children gain valuable communication skills that will improve their social and academic lives. As we work with children with speech sound disorders, our ultimate goal is to facilitate improved production of sounds and phonological skills through direct training to promote greater speech intelligibility and over-all communication effectiveness. As important as those responsibilities are, at times our role expands from speech and language clinician to child advocate. A case in point is that of a Spanish-speaking student whom we will call Javier. Javier was a nonverbal, bright-eyed, and cheerful kindergarten student with profound childhood apraxia of speech who communicated primarily through grunts, pointing, and facial expressions and by guiding the adults in his life to his wants and needs. At the recommendation of his preschool multidisciplinary school team, Javier was placed in a cross-categorical, self-contained classroom with students with mixed disabilities, including severe cognitive impairments, classical autism, and behavioral challenges. His early intervention team based this decision on the belief that the general education classroom would be too difficult for Javier because he was nonverbal. Initially, he adjusted well to his new classroom environment and participated well in his speech and language sessions. He benefited from a highly structured, hierarchical apraxia of speech program to establish early-developing sounds in CV, VC, CVC, and CVCV syllable contexts. Typical of children with profound apraxia of speech, he made steady but very slow progress, and his communication skills continued to be quite limited. However, in working with him, the first author of this book quickly realized that his recep-tive language skills were strong and that cognitively he appeared to be a typically developing child. He showed frustration with his inability to communicate verbally but tried to compensate through nonverbal means. A few months into the school year, Javier's behaviors began to change, as he started to imitate many of the negative behaviors of the students in his cross-categorical classroom. Although his speech and language services continued to improve his speech sound production skills, the first author began to advocate for a different educational placement for Javier, as it had become apparent that his current educational placement was not the least restrictive and most positive environment for him. She involved the school psychologist, who confirmed that Javier's nonverbal intelligence skills were in the average range; consulted with the school district's alternative and augmentative communication (AAC) special-ist, who determined that Javier was an excellent candidate for an electronic communication device; and involved the educational team at his home public school to determine the types of supports he could receive at his neighborhood school. After much (not always easy) advocacy, Javier was placed in the general education kindergarten classroom at his neighborhood school, with a one-to-one aide to assist with the transition, an electronic communication device, and ongoing speech and language services. Although he did not continue on the first author's caseload because of his change of placement, her ongoing consultation with his new team revealed that he was thriving in his new school, making friends, and learning academic concepts with the help of a well-established support system. Yes, one of our most important jobs is improving a child's communication skills, but just as important is advocating for our students' social, emotional, academic, and personal well-being.

---

several types according to the physical manifestations of the disorder (e.g., athetoid, spas-tic, ataxic, mixed). Children with cerebral palsy often have accompanying speech disorders, which can affect all parameters of speech production, including articulation. Based on his-torical data, it is estimated that approximately 70% of individuals with CP have a speech sound disorder (Yorkston et al., 2010). The speech disorder observed in children with CP is usually termed **developmental** or **childhood dysarthria.**

The treatment of children with cerebral palsy is multidisciplinary because of the varied physical, communicative, emotional, intellectual, and social problems that may accompany the disorder. A speech–language pathologist is a member of a team that typically includes a nurse, medical doctor, physical therapist, occupational therapist, audiologist, social worker, and psychologist. The speech–language pathologist should always work closely with the team of specialists involved in the child's medical or rehabilitative care. Clinicians should also work closely with the child's parents and thoroughly explain their role in the treatment process.

Therapy for children with cerebral palsy usually begins in infancy. At this point, the speech–language pathologist's role is primarily to facilitate adequate pre-speech motor movements and adequate motor functioning for swallowing and feeding. Air, Wood, and Neils (1989) emphasize the importance of parent education in communication and language stimulation. Currently, there is limited data on the effectiveness of speech treatment for children with CP (Pennington, Goldbart, & Marshall, 2004, 2005; Pennington, Smallman, & Farrier, 2006; Yorkston et al., 2010). Thus, treatment of dysarthria in children with CP tends to follow approaches similar to those used with individuals with nondegenerative etiologies.

Assuming that the child with cerebral palsy has sufficient sensory–motor functions to support verbal communication, the clinician may or may not need to treat the child's speech sound production skills. Some children acquire fairly normal articulation, while others may require special intervention (Mecham, 1996). In the treatment of speech sound disorders in children with cerebral palsy, clinicians often follow the procedures used with functional articulation disorders with suitable modifications.

The child's skills should be thoroughly assessed, and any sound errors or error patterns should be analyzed. Clinicians may also need to assess the use of any compensatory articulatory postures of the child or the presence of abnormal reflexes (e.g., tongue thrust). Furthermore, the presence of a concomitant neuromotor programming disorder such as apraxia of speech should be ruled out.

Treatment of children with cerebral palsy involves the following considerations:

• Before beginning treatment, the parents and other family members should be counseled about the child's limitations and what the treatment entails; a realistic prognosis may be made to the parents to encourage realistic expectations; the family members' responsibilities in helping the child at home should be emphasized.

• With children who may have a speech and language delay, a home-based early language stimulation program may be necessary.

• If a home speech and language treatment does not produce the desired effects, formal language treatment may be necessary; periodic assessment is needed to make this determination (S. H. Long, 1994).

• Some clinicians recommend methods to control interfering movements of the hand, neck, jaw, and other body parts. The clinician may consider using such devices as a chin strap that controls extraneous movements of the lower jaw or such simple techniques as holding steady an arm that is susceptible to unnecessary movements.

• A child's articulation problems may be limited to a few sounds, or they may be extensive. Generally, the errors are due to muscle weakness. Phonological processes may be evident in some cases.

- Direct treatment targets include bilabial, linguavelar, lingua-alveolar, linguadental, articulatory contacts needed for various speech sound productions. Auditory, tactile, and visual cues will probably be needed to facilitate these movements initially. Other phonetic placement cues, shaping procedures, physical manipulation of the articulators, and modeling should be used as much as needed. These will be gradually faded.

- Increasing the speed of the child's articulatory movements once they have been established becomes the next goal of therapy. Air and colleagues (1989) indicate that this can be done by serial production of voiced and voiceless and nasal and non-nasal sounds. The clinician selects syllable combinations that contain sounds that the child can produce (e.g., /na/, /da/, /ka/, and /ga/). The child then practices repetitive productions of the chosen syllables in two-, three-, and four-syllable sets to increase the speed of the articulatory movements (e.g., /na-ta/, /na-da/, /na-na/, /na-ka/, and /na-ga/). This is done in succession from two-syllable sets to three-syllable sets to four-syllable sets. Eventually, two-word combinations can be introduced.

- If the assessment reveals specific errors (i.e., substitutions, omissions, distortions) or error patterns (i.e., phonological processes), the clinician can use the many procedures described throughout the Basic Unit of this chapter to treat those errors or error patterns.

- Some clients may need to be trained to use compensatory articulatory movements. For example, the tongue blade may be used instead of the tongue tip when the tongue is markedly weak. Also, linguadental contact for nasals may be used when the lips are too weak to achieve an adequate seal.

- Children with cerebral palsy may have an accompanying voice problem. Because of breathing abnormalities (due to poor muscle control), vocal intensity may vary too much. Overabduction or underabduction of the vocal folds may be noticed. These and any other voice problems need to be treated.

- Children with cerebral palsy may need some training in sustaining airflow for speech production. Sustained airflow may be shaped by reinforcing the child in producing progressively longer strings of syllables, words, phrases, and sentences while maintaining normal vocal intensity (loudness).

- Treatment of children with cerebral palsy should target prosodic features, including an acceptable speech rate, rhythm, stress patterns, and pitch variations. Behavioral treatment techniques such as modeling, shaping, positive reinforcement, and corrective feedback will be helpful. If the speech rate needs to be reduced, such techniques as finger tapping and such devices as a pacing board, metronome, and delayed auditory feedback (DAF) may be used. A reduced rate of speech tends to improve speech intelligibility.

- Speech intelligibility may be improved with a slower rate and more natural prosody. If necessary, exaggerated articulation of consonants may be taught, particularly in the medial and final positions, to improve speech intelligibility. An increased open mouth posture to promote better oral projection of sounds also may improve intelligibility.

- With some children, integration of language treatment with speech treatment to minimize the effects of dysarthria may be essential.

- With many children, it may be necessary to target social communication skills (e.g., such pragmatic language skills as eye contact, clarifying the topic of discussion at the outset, appropriate facial expressions, conversational repair strategies) to enhance communicative effectiveness.

• Treatment of literacy skills may be integrated with speech training. The clinician should work closely with the child's classroom teacher, special education specialist if involved, and other school professionals (e.g., psychologists) to design an integrated family service plan.

• In some children, speech does not become a functional mode of communication. Speech may be so severely impaired that the child's intelligibility is significantly compromised. For these children, alternative or augmentative modes of communication (AAC) are most appropriate to facilitate functional communication. Examples of AAC systems include gestural communication, simple communication boards containing words and pictures, and sophisticated electronic or computer devices.

• Associated undesirable or interfering behaviors (e.g., inattention, uncooperative behaviors) should be addressed through behavior management procedures.

• Training family members and others in promoting and maintaining clinically established communicative skills is a significant part of treatment.

As with childhood apraxia of speech, treatment activities designed for dysarthria in children are highly structured and repetitive; speech trials for continued practice play an important role in the treatment of dysarthric speakers. Proper head, trunk, and body positioning are crucial for articulation training. It is difficult to address improved articulatory proficiency if the child is slumped forward in a wheelchair, for example.

As with other speech sound disorders, the clinician determines the phonetic error patterns in a particular child. The behavioral methods discussed in the Basic Unit of this chapter can be used to treat the speech production difficulties in dysarthric speakers. The child is provided instructions and demonstrations to facilitate appropriate placement of the articulators. Phonetic placement and shaping procedures are used as needed. The clinician models the target productions, and the child is expected to imitate. Prompt reinforcement and corrective feedback will help strengthen all skills targeted in treatment. Family involvement at every stage of treatment will assist with the use of trained skills in extra-clinical environments.

....

ACTIVITY

Determine a recommendation for a 4-year-old boy with cerebral palsy who is 20% intelligible to family, friends, and teachers despite early speech intervention efforts.

....

Cleft Palate

Because cleft lip and palate is a congenital disorder (present at birth), intervention for children with this disorder can begin in infancy (Moller & Glaze, 2009). As discussed in the Advanced Unit of Chapter 6, clefting results from the lack of fusion of the upper lip, the hard palate, the soft palate, and/or the uvula early in the embryonic stages of human development. An opening in the palatal regions connects the nasal and oral cavities and can have a significant effect on speech production.

In the United States, surgical management of cleft lip and palate is common practice, and it begins early in infancy; unfortunately, this is not the case in countries where people do not always have access to adequate medical care. Medical specialists use varied surgical methods to fuse cleft lip and palate in infants. The technical aspects of such surgeries are beyond the scope of this chapter. Cleft lip is repaired very early in infancy, at about 3 months of age. It is desirable that the infant be at least 10 weeks old and weigh 10 pounds prior to the initial surgery (Buckley & Landis, 2009; Bzoch, 2004; Golding-Kushner, 1997; Kummer, 2014; Peterson-Falzone et al., 2001). Cosmetic revisions of the nose and lip are done at later ages. Surgical repair of the palate is typically done between 12 and 18 months of age. The primary reason for repair of a cleft palate is to separate the oral cavity from the nasal cavity, which will have a significant positive effect on speech production and swallowing. Surgical repair of cleft palate when the child is between 12 and 18 months of age results in better speech and language development and less maladaptive behaviors (e.g., compensatory articulation errors). Golding-Kushner (1997) indicates that if surgery is delayed until after 2 years of age, children experience a higher risk for severe maladaptive compensatory articulation disorders that can be difficult to treat.

In approximately 15% to 20% of cases, hypernasality due to **velopharyngeal insufficiency** occurs even after surgical closure of a cleft palate (Buckley & Landis, 2009; Golding-Kushner, 1997). In these cases, further surgical intervention may be required in the form of **pharyngeal flap surgery.** This is a secondary surgical procedure in which a muscular flap is cut from the posterior pharyngeal wall, raised, and attached to the velum. The flap is open on either side to allow for nasal breathing, nasal drainage, and production of nasal speech sounds. A pharyngeal flap helps close the velopharyngeal port during the production of non-nasal consonants and thus reduces hypernasality. Construction of a flap that is too wide increases the risk of airway obstruction, snoring, and hyponasality. Another procedure that may be used is **dynamic sphincteroplasty**, in which muscle flaps from the posterior tonsillar pillars are brought together with a short posterior pharyngeal wall flap to reduce the size of the central port during speech production (Buckley & Landis, 2009).

The child with cleft lip and palate often requires several other surgical, medical, or both kinds of interventions. Repair of a **fistula,** which is an opening that remains or appears after surgery, may be needed. An unrepaired fistula can have negative effects on both speech production and eating, depending on its size and location along the palate. The child may also need consistent dental care to promote an adequate oral hygiene program that will help prevent the premature loss of teeth. Also, because orthodontic problems are common in children with cleft lip and palate, orthodontic care may be crucial. Orthodontic problems include malocclusion, cross-bite, rotated or jumbled teeth, and extra teeth. These may or may not affect articulation, depending on the severity of the problem and level of orthodontic care. A prosthodontist, a dentist or orthodontist with a specialty in the construction of artificial teeth and prosthetic oral devices, may also be involved in the client's care. Some children may need the construction of artificial teeth if their permanent teeth are missing or may require other devices, such as a **speech bulb.** This device is designed to eliminate hypernasality in children with velopharyngeal insufficiency. It contains a palatal retainer and pharyngeal extension that terminates in a bulb, usually made of acrylic. The speech bulb serves the same purpose as the pharyngeal flap, in that it helps with velopharyngeal closure by reducing the amount of space in the pharyngeal area. For more detailed information on the medical intervention of children with cleft palate, see Bzoch (2004), Golding-Kushner (1997), Kummer (2014), McWilliams et al. (1990), and Peterson-Falzone et al. (2001).

Speech–language pathologists who work in children's hospitals are often involved in the treatment of children with cleft lip and palate in the neonatal intensive care unit or critical care unit if the child requires further hospitalization after birth. Clinical services at this point include parent education and counseling, and addressing the infant's feeding problems. The speech–language pathologist consults and collaborates with other specialists (e.g., nurses; occupational therapists; audiologists; and medical doctors, including plastic surgeons).

Many children's hospitals have craniofacial clinics, in which a team of specialists frequently assesses the child's needs after she or he is released from the hospital. The child is followed up every 6 to 12 months in the early years to ensure that his or her surgical, dental, cosmetic, communication, and educational needs are adequately met. The frequency with which the child is assessed diminishes as he or she grows older and the rehabilitative needs lessen. The speech–language pathologist is an integral member of the craniofacial team.

Early surgical repair of cleft lip and palate does not guarantee normal speech production skills in all children. Therefore, any child with cleft lip and palate is considered to be at high risk for speech and language disorders. Assuming that problems with phonation, articulation, and respiration occur despite all preventative efforts, the clinician needs to offer direct treatment.

In the treatment of speech sound disorders in children with cleft lip or palate, the clinician can use the general principles for the treatment of functional articulation or phonological disorders. After an assessment, the clinician identifies the specific sound errors or error patterns and decides on the most relevant treatment target for a particular child. The general behavioral treatment principles discussed in the Basic Unit of this chapter can be successfully used to meet the articulation needs of children with cleft palate speech. The clinician should consider the following suggestions, which may be unique to children with repaired clefts (Bzoch, 2004; Hegde, 2008b; Kummer, 2014; Moller & Glaze, 2009; Peterson-Falzone et al., 2001; Scherer, 1999):

- The clinician should educate the parents about the speech mechanism and the possible reason for persisting articulation errors despite surgical repair of the cleft.

- The clinician should consider an early language intervention program to stimulate language skills; improved language skills may have a beneficial effect on speech sound learning.

- The clinician should train the parents to withhold reinforcement for undesirable compensatory behaviors when the need for them has been eliminated by medical management.

- The clinician should target sounds or error patterns that contribute most to reduced intelligibility.

- The clinician should teach more visible sounds before less visible sounds, except for the linguadentals.

- The clinician should begin treatment with vowels and semivowels and move on to nasals, glides, and aspirate consonants.

- The clinician should teach fricatives before stops.

- The clinician should teach accurate production of consonants that are produced with weak articulatory force, as this is a unique problem of children with cleft palate. The force with which consonants are produced may be increased by reinforcing louder production. The clinician may let the child feel the force of the airflow by placing his or her hand in front of the mouth (first the clinician's mouth and then his or her own mouth) as plosives are modeled and imitated.

- The clinician should avoid or postpone training on /k/ and /g/ if the child's velopharyngeal functioning is inadequate.

- The clinician should teach lingua-palatal sounds, lingua-alveolars, and lingua-dentals, in that order.

- The clinician should structure therapy so that it progresses from syllables to words, phrases, and sentences.

- The clinician should use visual, auditory, and tactile cues as needed. Phonetic placement, successive approximation, and modeling should be used frequently initially and faded gradually.

- The clinician should avoid nonspeech oral–motor exercises (i.e., blowing, sucking) to strengthen the velum or tongue, as there is no evidence that such exercises are beneficial.

- The clinician should teach the child to direct the breath stream orally. Visual and tactile feedback can be provided to increase the client's success. The child can be instructed to feel the flow of air on the back of the hand or to see it when a tissue is placed in front of his or her mouth.

- The clinician should teach the child to articulate with less effort and facial grimacing.

- The clinician should train compensatory articulatory productions if structural distortions are present that prevent normal articulation (e.g., if a stiff and short upper lip prevents adequate seal for bilabials, the child may be taught to make an upper teeth–lower lip contact, instead).

Managing resonance problems (especially hypernasality) is a unique aspect of treating children with cleft palate, as such problems are not uncommon in them. Behavioral interventions are inappropriate for resonance problems that are a result of **velopharyngeal incompetence** (structural or physiologic inability to achieve velopharyngeal closure). If the child does not have the ability to achieve velopharyngeal closure, the clinician's efforts to decrease hypernasality will be unsuccessful. In such cases, the child may need medical intervention through a pharyngeal flap procedure or prosthetic device (e.g., speech bulb) before speech therapy can be initiated. Air and colleagues (1989) indicate that a trial period of behavioral speech therapy may be provided in cases where specialists are uncertain whether the child can achieve velopharyngeal closure. A trial period of 3 months is often sufficient to determine whether the resonance problem will need medical intervention.

For children who can achieve velopharyngeal closure, it is important to take steps to reduce hypernasality. Oral resonance may be achieved by occluding the child's nares while he or she makes the target production (i.e., oral sound, word with only oral sounds). Initially, the nares may be occluded during the entire production. As therapy progresses, the clinician may need to occlude the nares only as the child begins the production and then suddenly release as the child is instructed to continue the production. Eventually, the clinician may need to touch the child's nares only lightly to prompt adequate oral resonance. In addition, enhanced loudness or sudden bursts of loudness may facilitate improved oral resonance, since more articulatory effort is needed as the intensity of speech increases. Increased mouth opening may also promote improved oral resonance.

Because there is a high incidence of vocal nodules in children with cleft palate, often due to compensatory efforts or vocal hyperfunction, the clinician should treat problems of phonation in addition to articulation and resonance. The clinician should clearly identify the abusive vocal behaviors (e.g., yelling, screaming, throat clearing, coughing) and provide systematic voice therapy. Because of our emphasis on speech sound disorders, the treatment of vocally abusive behaviors is beyond the scope of this chapter. The reader may consult Boone and McFarlane (2000), Bzoch (2004), Kummer (2014), McWilliams et al. (1990), and Peterson-Falzone et al. (2001) for more information.

ACTIVITY

Describe how you would establish correct production of /ʃ/ in a 7-year-old girl with cleft palate using some of the treatment procedures described in the Basic Unit of this chapter.

Hearing Impairment

As described in Chapter 6, *hearing impairment* refers to a reduced hearing acuity in children and adults. The degree of loss can range from mild to profound. The terms *hard of hearing* and *deaf* are often differentiated. Deaf individuals have a profound hearing loss of at least 90 dB HL. The degree of loss in hard of hearing individuals can range from mild to severe (less than 90 dB HL). People who are hard of hearing typically have some residual hearing that can be maximized through amplification devices such as a hearing aid. The articulatory proficiency of individuals with decreased hearing acuity often varies according to the degree of loss.

The treatment of communication disorders associated with hearing impairment is multifaceted. Articulation difficulties are often only one of the problems associated with hearing loss and deafness; language disorders, learning disabilities, and reading difficulties may accompany a hearing loss. Treatment is provided by a team of professionals, including medical specialists, nurses, audiologists, regular education teachers, special education teachers, interpreters, vocational counselors, and so forth. As a member of such a team, a speech–language pathologist must consult and collaborate with other specialists. Audiologists can provide invaluable information about the type and extent of hearing loss and the amount of residual hearing that exists. It is the audiologist who fits the child with a hearing aid, but all specialists involved in the child's care must be familiar with the intricacies of the amplification device (e.g., how it is turned on and off, how the battery is replaced, how to turn the volume up or down).

Although various aspects of communication can be affected in deaf and hard of hearing individuals, we will offer only a brief overview of the treatment of articulation skills. To reduce the effects of hearing loss on speech and language acquisition, the clinician should start a language stimulation program at an early age. Parent counseling on the effects of hearing loss and the special needs of deaf or hard of hearing children is essential. Parent training in providing language stimulation opportunities is crucial during the infancy and preschool years that are critical for oral language learning.

Formal speech training should be started as early as possible. The younger the child is, the better the prognosis will be for improved articulation skills and natural-sounding speech. The child's family should be involved in treatment from the very beginning to facilitate the use of trained behaviors in the home environment. The family can be specifically trained to conduct therapy sessions at home that parallel the clinician's treatment targets, objectives, and activities.

Even with amplification, the use of visual, tactile, and kinesthetic cues is important in teaching speech sound production in hard of hearing and deaf individuals. Some clinicians use the Ling system for speech training (Ling & Ling, 1978). In this program, sounds are taught through audition first, with the addition of visual and tactile cues as necessary. The clinician may include speech perception or auditory training activities to supplement articulation and phonological training if the client has some residual hearing or functional audition. This may help clarify "auditory confusions" or contrasts between sounds and words (Paterson, 1994).

The general principles and procedures described in the Basic Unit of this chapter are appropriate to meet the articulation and phonological needs of deaf and hard of hearing children. However, the clinician may need to rely more heavily on visual, tactile, and kinesthetic cues to facilitate correct production of sounds in isolation, syllables, and words. The clinician should pay special attention to stops, fricatives, and affricates, since these are especially difficult for children with hearing loss. Omission of consonants in the initial and final positions—a significant problem associated with hearing loss—deserves special attention in treatment. Treatment of /s/ is another particularly important target.

Teaching voiced and voiceless sound distinctions will be especially important in treating children with hearing loss. Paterson (1994) offers a specific treatment for voiceless fricatives (which are often replaced by voiced sounds) that underscores the need for a multimodality treatment approach (e.g., audition, vision, touch, and orosensory modalities). Treatment of fricatives progresses from simple to complex tasks. The child's productions are gradually shaped to match or approximate the target fricatives (see Paterson, 1994, for the details of this approach).

Vowel disorders may be noteworthy in many speakers with hearing loss. Generally increased vowel duration and imprecise or distorted vowels should be addressed in treatment.

Improved voice quality, reduced hypernasality, and a more natural-sounding speech rhythm are other goals of speech treatment. Some children with hearing impairment may need training in social communication skills, as well.

The clinician should be systematic in the use of antecedent stimuli, the selection of target responses, and the provision of feedback. The effectiveness of articulation treatment with deaf and hard of hearing children should be constantly reevaluated to ensure that speech is an appropriate and realistic communication choice.

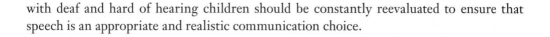

ACTIVITY

Describe how articulation treatment might be similar and different for a child with a functional articulation disorder and one with a moderate hearing loss.

Summary of the Advanced Unit

- Treatment for childhood apraxia of speech is primarily behavioral. It is hierarchical, systematic, and repetitive. Repeated treatment trials (drills) are essential. Several specific treatment approaches include **PROMPT, the touch-cue method, ACT, integral stimulation, DDTC, progressive assimilation, phonetic placement,** and **contrastive stress drills.**

- Treatment of dysarthria includes medical, prosthetic, and behavioral interventions. The clinician systematically targets all aspects of speech production, including articulation, prosody, and voice. Treatment trials are repetitive.

- **Cerebral palsy,** a congenital neurological disorder, is often classified into various types according to the physical manifestations of the disorder. Treatment for children with cerebral palsy typically begins in infancy. Therapy is multidisciplinary, and the speech–language pathologist is only one of several professionals involved in the client's care. Articulation therapy targets accurate articulatory movements for speech and increasing the speed of such movements in gradually more complex syllable units. **Augmentative or alternative modes of communication** are appropriate for children with cerebral palsy who do not acquire functional speech.

- Children with **cleft lip and palate** require surgical intervention to repair the clefts. Primary surgeries of the palate are done between 12 and 14 months of age. Secondary surgical intervention may be needed in some patients for improved **velopharyngeal competence,** closure of **fistulas,** or cosmetic purposes. Traditional methods of therapy can be used to treat the articulation and phonological problems of children with cleft palate.

- **Hearing impairments** can range from mild to profound and may yield varying communication disorders across children with hearing loss or deafness. The intervention for deaf and hard of hearing children is multidisciplinary. Traditional treatment approaches, supplemented by visual, tactile, and kinesthetic cues, can be used with hard of hearing children.

SPECIFIC SPEECH SOUND
TREATMENT APPROACHES

Nothing is more useful to man than to speak correctly.

—Phaedrus, Fables

In Chapter 7 we offered a comprehensive treatment program that can be used with a variety of speech sound disorders, one that takes advantage of various approaches, some of which are described in this chapter; recent treatment efficacy research; and the current best evidence. We made a distinction between a *treatment program* and *treatment variables.* Treatment programs include all steps in treatment, whereas treatment variables are technical operations designed to teach the correct production of sounds (e.g., stimuli, models, prompts, phonetic placement, positive reinforcement, and corrective feedback). These technical operations are common to the comprehensive treatment program described in Chapter 7 and to the specific programs described in this chapter. We suggested that the clinician could make exclusive use of that comprehensive treatment program because it includes elements from these specific programs and describes all steps necessary to teach correct speech sound production to children. The clinician also may use one of the approaches described in this chapter, but none of these includes all the necessary treatment steps or procedures. The clinician would have to add the missing steps, which is what we have done in creating the comprehensive approach described in Chapter 7.

In this chapter, we describe some of the treatment approaches the clinician may consider in treating speech sound disorders in individual children. Our discussion of different approaches is not meant to be all inclusive, as that is beyond the scope of this textbook. Instead, our goal is to offer an introduction to some of the varied treatment programs currently available, some of which (e.g., the traditional approach) have existed for many years, and some of which (e.g., the concurrent treatment approach) are more recent. Readers who desire more detailed information on a specific treatment program are advised to consult published research studies, articles, or other sources expressly devoted to that approach.

We share these different approaches with the full understanding that they may leave the clinician, especially the student clinician, with an incomplete program or perhaps one that has received only partial research support. As indicated in Chapter 7, some researchers omit certain steps involved in treating speech sound disorders on the assumption that most clinicians know them. Specifically, many recently published treatment efficacy studies necessarily exclude such steps as operationally specifying treatment targets, base rating the target behaviors, sequencing treatment, measuring improvement under routine treatment, administering treatment trials, systematically providing feedback to the child, probing for generalized productions, and implementing a maintenance program. Some who do offer such program details use technical terms that they presume the clinician already understands and thus omit exhaustive definitions or explanations. When the researcher or author indicates that a baseline should be collected before starting treatment, for example, the likely supposition is that the clinician knows what a baseline is and how to obtain one. Similarly, if the clinician is advised to probe for generalized productions, the author presumes that the clinician understands the principles of generalization and the procedures involved in conducting a probe. The clinician lacking such knowledge may garner only a partial understanding of a specific program, limiting his or her ability to apply it effectively or as designed. The preceding chapter was explicitly written for that purpose: to provide the clinician with such technical information. If the reader's plan is to read this chapter before Chapter 7, we highly recommend reconsidering that sequence. We believe that clinicians will be able to maximize their understanding of the programs presented in this chapter if they first understand essential treatment program components and treatment variables, so that if some of those details are omitted, the clinician's knowledge can help fill the gap.

How Different Are the Varied Treatment Approaches?

Over the past several decades, researchers and clinicians have proposed various specific treatment programs or approaches to help meet the needs of children with speech sound disorders. Some programs are based on years of empirical research, others have evolved primarily from uncontrolled clinical data (case studies), and still others are based on clinical experience or expert advocacy. Some, such as the traditional approach, gain immense popularity and enjoy wide professional application for years. Others, such as the distinctive features approach, quickly become popular, like a fad, and soon get abandoned, perhaps because of complicated theoretical underpinnings that limit their clinical implementation. Others might enjoy great application but limited empirical validity, prompting experts to warn against their use, as in the case of nonspeech oral–motor exercises. In any case, as approaches come into being, are questioned, and slowly or quickly die off or become established, clinicians often wonder about the difference between the varied approaches.

On the surface and by their titles, most treatment programs sound unique. Clinicians, however, may enjoy knowing that when carefully examined, many of them share several features. They all advocate the selection of particular target behaviors, make use of certain antecedent stimuli (e.g., pictures, objects, written words), expect a response from the child, and provide consequences according to the child's responses (e.g., verbal praise, tokens, play time, verbal corrective feedback). Most of them make use of behavioral learning principles that have been around for years (please see Chapter 7).

What then are the valid differences between the major approaches? The differences are not so much in treatment, technically defined, as in certain other aspects of the programs. The technical definition of *treatment* is the application of variables that change behaviors; treatment is what the clinician does, not what the child does. To change speech sound behaviors, the clinician uses behavioral treatment procedures. Most effective treatment approaches, programs, and plans, therefore, do not differ in treatment procedures. They differ in their analysis of speech sound production errors before and after treatment.

Analysis of errors and sound production patterns before and after treatment is not the essence of the manipulation of variables that induces behavior change. In other words, such an analysis, though important in treatment planning, is not treatment itself. While traditional methods did not pay attention to how multiple errors formed patterns or revealed constraints, phonological approaches were keen on finding such patterns in errors. Such patterns found before treatment help organize treatment targets into classes (e.g., consonants that are deleted in the final position of words, a single phoneme that is substituted for multiple phonemes, sounds that occur only in a specific word position, sounds that are selected based on hierarchical constraints or rankings). When treatment is offered for some sounds in a class or a rule set, the clinician can see whether the other, untreated sounds in the class or rule set change.

In some respects, certain treatment programs differ in *what* they teach, not *how* they teach. For instance, those that target auditory discrimination—also variously known as *ear training, sound discrimination training, auditory bombardment,* and *sound perception training*—target a different class of skills than those that target sound production. Still, differences in target behaviors do not necessarily create differences in treatment procedures. Sound discrimination training, too, is accomplished only through behavioral treatment procedures. The only difference is that in discrimination training, the child's response is nonverbal, whereas in sound production training, the child's response is verbal.

Other differences among treatment approaches are not as crucial in a technical description of treatment, although they are important in how treatment sessions are organized. In some approaches, multiple phonemes may be simultaneously targeted, whereas in other approaches only one or a few phonemes may be targeted. In some approaches, pairs of words that differ in only one physiologic or acoustic property may be targeted (e.g., the minimal pairs intervention approach), whereas in other approaches (maximal or multiple opposition approaches) more than one or even multiple feature differences may be targeted. Some approaches may recommend training a sound or sounds to a specified high-accuracy criterion before moving through the treatment sequence, while others merely stimulate the sounds, with no accuracy criterion required before proceeding to the next step of treatment. Traditionally, most treatments have moved from simple to complex levels of training, whereas a newer approach (the concurrent treatment approach) simultaneously targets different levels of complexity. These program distinctions may make a difference in treatment outcome; hence, they are important to consider in treatment planning. Nonetheless, such distinctions are not differences in technical treatment variables.

In their narrative review of evidenced-based practice for children with speech sound disorders, Baker and McLeod (2011) identified 42 different approaches, with varying quantities and levels of evidence. After their extensive review, they concluded that the evidence "suggested that it is better for children who have a phonological impairment to receive intervention than no intervention at all . . . [but] at the moment, there are few studies that show that one intervention approach is unequivocally superior to another with a particular client group" (p. 115). They recommend increased publications of rigorous and well-designed comparative studies to help clinicians make well-informed, evidence-based decisions. Gierut (2004) recommends that in the absence of definitive research that supports the use of one treatment program over another, the clinician can only safely make use of basic principles of learning such as shaping, modeling, and corrective feedback. It is important to keep in perspective such technical treatment variables (also discussed in Chapter 7) as one reads about the approaches described in this chapter.

....

ACTIVITY

Describe the primary difference between the varied treatment approaches and describe some similarities.

....

What Is Included and Why

That we could not include a description of 42 different approaches or programs in this chapter is obvious. Instead, we include treatment programs that meet one or more of the following criteria: (1) they have withstood the test of time in the sense that they are still in use; (2) they can be adapted to different age groups with modifications, different settings, or different service delivery models; (3) they do not necessitate specialized training for specific program components (e.g., special hand or picture cuing systems); (4) they do not require the use of commercial computer-based learning systems; (5) they do not require the use of special feedback instruments or devices (such as electropalatography) that are unavailable to the average clinician; (6) they are not so deeply rooted in complicated theoretical understandings that only those who comprehend or adhere to that theory can apply it clinically; (7) they are currently popular and thus merit discussion; and (8) they are currently controversial, and the controversy needs to be addressed. We have omitted some programs that were included in the previous editions of our textbook because their use is now limited (e.g., the distinctive features approach), they recommend a specific published component that is no longer readily available (e.g., the sensory–motor approach *Programmed Conditioning for Articulation* [Baker & Ryan, 1971]), their essence may be easily integrated into a comprehensive program as a sound establishment or cuing technique (e.g., paired-stimuli approach), or they are now thought to be part of a more standard treatment philosophy (e.g., the multiple phonemes approach).

With those considerations, we have included the following treatment programs or approaches: the traditional approach, concurrent treatment approach, cycles approach, contrast approaches, complexity approach, stimulability approach, core vocabulary approach, and naturalistic speech intervention approach. We have also addressed controversies surrounding language-based intervention treatment approaches and nonspeech oral–motor exercises. Additionally, we have devoted an entire chapter (Chapter 9) to phonological awareness as related to the treatment of speech sound disorders.

We do not assume that this will meet everyone's expectations. We recognize that class instructors will bring their own training and theoretical philosophies into their teaching and will choose to discuss all of the programs we have presented, only address some, or supplement what we have offered with other approaches. There is much flexibility for each scenario.

In describing the varied programs, we have done our best to stay true to the authors' use of terms, program components, and treatment procedure details when available. In most cases, we reserve critical observations for the summary and evaluation section that follows each program; in some cases, we offer criticism as we briefly summarize procedures that need not be described in detail. We do not advocate the use of one approach over another. As the different programs are studied, it will become apparent that often they contradict each other. For example, some recommend the selection of stimulable sounds as initial targets, while others recommend nonstimulable sounds. Some recommend training sounds to a high criterion, while others specify a service time criterion. Some recommend only one or two targets or complexity levels at one time, while others recommend multiple targets and complexity levels simultaneously. We advise the reader not to let this become too confusing and simply recognize that different program authors or developers have different ways of implementing a treatment program based on their research, clinical experience, or theoretical philosophy. We also remind the reader that often a comprehensive treatment program includes aspects of separate approaches and that the behavioral treatment variables discussed in Chapter 7 draw the most useful elements from many approaches (see Text Box 8.1).

Traditional Approach

The **traditional approach** to articulation therapy, often called the motor-based approach, has gained its name primarily by the length of its existence. The foundation of this well-established approach was laid in the 1920s by several pioneers in speech–language pathology (Scripture & Jackson, 1927; Stinchfield & Young, 1938; Van Riper, 1939). Although many researchers and professionals helped guide the development of somewhat varied traditional approaches, we will concentrate on the most dominant traditional approach, which has been used for many years. Charles Van Riper is primarily credited for its development, popularity, and longevity.

The hallmark of the traditional approach is its progression from sensory–perceptual training to maintenance of the newly acquired speech sound. It is composed of five major phases: (1) sensory–perceptual, or ear, training; (2) production training for sound establishment; (3) production training for sound stabilization; (4) transfer and carry-over training; and (5) maintenance of the learned behaviors across time. Van Riper and Erickson (1996) depict this progression as a staircase of precise steps that the child must surmount on the way to correct sound production.

Although the word *traditional* may connote something that is old, outdated, and not useful, this is not so for the traditional approach to articulation therapy. Many clinicians continue to use elements of this approach. In his conceptualization of establishment, stabilization, and transfer (generalization) of correct production, Van Riper set the stage for refinements and modifications while giving a framework that still is valid: The general sequence he recommended is used with only minor modifications. Some aspects of the traditional approach are now controversial (e.g., sensory–perceptual training) and some missing elements are now considered important (e.g., a pattern analysis of multiple misarticulations, a complexity model for target selection, concurrent treatment at multiple complexity levels).

The following sections outline the traditional approach, beginning with sensory–perceptual training and progressing to the ultimate goal of maintenance of the target sound (see Secord, 1989, for an excellent overview of this approach).

Text Box 8.1. How to evaluate whether a treatment approach is working

To ascertain whether any of the treatment programs discussed in this chapter is working with an individual child, a clinician must follow fundamental clinical steps and procedures. First and foremost, the clinician must thoughtfully consider the selection of child-specific target behaviors, which can vary from a single sound to multiple sounds, to a set of sounds, to an entire class of sounds. The clinician must then define the targets in observable and measurable terms and establish pretreatment baselines. Although at one time the collection of a baseline was considered optional, this step is now required for all goals included in a child's Individualized Education Program.

The clinician then applies the treatment procedures as outlined by the program authors and experts, with as much detail as has been provided. If there are steps that are not included in a particular program, the clinician must fill the gaps with well-established procedures. For example, if the details on sound establishment, modeling, reinforcement, or corrective feedback are not given, the clinician must determine what is appropriate for a particular child. The clinician must then maintain clear progress data that document a child's performance across treatment sessions. If the data identify a steady level of progress, a treatment program may be considered effective. If the collected data demonstrate little to no progress, adjustments will need to be made or a new approach implemented. It is important to remember that a treatment program in and of itself is not effective unless the data show that it is, regardless of expert advocacy. So keep those data sheets handy and be ready to be flexible.

Sensory–Perceptual Training (Ear Training)

In the traditional approach, sensory–perceptual training, also called **auditory discrimination training**, as well as **ear training**, is the first goal of therapy. At this stage a standard for the target sound is identified and defined. The child is not taught to produce the target sound; rather the emphasis is on teaching auditory discrimination between the correct and incorrect forms of target sounds, so that the child can make comparisons.

The essence of **sensory–perceptual training** is that through auditory stimulation practice the child will become aware of his or her own sound errors. This awareness is thought to provide a foundation for production training. The training consists of the following phases: identification, isolation, stimulation, and discrimination. The complexity of the skills trained increases as the child progresses from one phase to another. Research has not clearly shown that it is necessary to teach auditory discrimination training before moving on to speech sound production training. There is no strong evidence that teaching auditory discrimination between speech sounds that are in error will result in their correct production. Furthermore, there is no strong evidence that speech sound discrimination, once established, reduces the production training effort. It is inappropriate to justify speech sound discrimination training on the basis of studies that include both discrimination and production training (Rvachew, 1994; Rvachew, 2007; Rvachew & Brosseau-Lapré, 2010; Rvachew, Nowak, & Cloutier, 2003). Researchers will have to show that pure discrimination training results in correct production of speech sounds in error. In fact, an experimental study by A. L. Williams and McReynolds (1975) has shown that discrimination training produces better discrimination but no change in production. Production training, on the other hand, produces changes in both production and discrimination. A child who learns to produce speech sounds correctly will also discriminate those sounds from other, similar sounds. These results suggest that it is more efficient to teach production because it affects both production and discrimination. Clinicians who wish to offer speech sound discrimination training may find procedural details in Secord (1989) and Van Riper and Erickson (1993).

Production Training: Sound Establishment

After the child has learned to describe the most important acoustic features of the target sound and make judgments about the accuracy of sound productions, the second stage of treatment is initiated. In the production training stage, the goal is to evoke and establish a new sound pattern that will replace the child's error pattern.

The sound-evoking techniques include (1) imitation–auditory stimulation, (2) phonetic placement, (3) contextual cues, (4) motor–kinesthetic cues, and (5) sound approximation (Secord, 1989). Many of these methods were reviewed in the Basic Unit of Chapter 7. Several sound-evoking techniques for establishing individual consonants are provided in the various Sound Resource Packets included on the companion CD for this book.

The clinician uses any combination of sound establishment techniques to replace the error production with correct production. Establishing the correct sounds, especially those of /r/ and /s/, can be difficult. However, this stage can also be fun and exciting. Getting a child to produce a sound that was incorrectly produced in the past can be very rewarding for the clinician. Also, the clinician's creativity can flourish at this stage of articulation therapy.

Production Training: Sound Stabilization

After the target sound has been established, the clinician shifts attention to stabilizing the child's production of the sound at various levels of response complexity. If he or she is following the traditional approach as originally outlined, stabilization training is initiated at the simplest level of production—isolation—and progresses to the most complex level—conversation.

In his discussion of the traditional approach, Secord (1989) outlined the progression of therapy as follows: isolation, nonsense syllables, words, phrases, sentences, and conversation. However, he emphasized that not all clinicians begin at the isolation level. Some believe that the syllable level is the most appropriate place to begin, because in natural speech, sounds do not occur in isolation—for example, if one tries to produce /b/ in isolation, it quickly becomes evident that it cannot be produced without an intrusive /ə/. These clinicians insist that the syllable is the basic element of speech.

Others advocate the word level as the entry point of stabilization training. Proponents of this view argue that words are more meaningful, since by definition phonemes are units that signal changes in meaning. We have addressed this topic in the section "Selecting the Initial Level and Sequence of Training" in the Basic Unit of Chapter 7.

It is generally believed that training should begin at the response complexity level that is appropriate for the individual child. If a child can produce the phoneme in isolation and syllables, it may be clinically efficient to begin training at the word level. In other words, the goal of training is to stabilize the child's production of the target sound at the lowest level at which the child has difficulty and gradually progress to more complex linguistic levels. In the traditional approach, stabilization at one level is considered a prerequisite for entry to the next level. This maximizes the child's chances for success as treatment progresses from one level to the next. This approach is not necessarily the most efficient, as the concurrent treatment, described in the upcoming section "Concurrent Treatment Approach," demonstrates.

Stage 1: Isolation

The goal at isolation is to develop a stronger and more consistent correct production of the target sound through various practice activities. Some of the visual cues used in the establishment phase are also used at this stage. Secord (1989, p. 142) outlined some common tasks that are typically used for sound stabilization at the isolation level:

- practicing prolongation of the target sound
- varying the number of productions emitted at any one time
- varying the intensity with which the sound is produced
- whispering the new sound
- starting and stopping production in response to the clinician's signal
- simultaneously saying and writing the new sound
- responding to large and small letters that represent the target by using loud or soft sounds, depending on the size of the letter cues
- playing "speech games" in which the child responds by producing the target sound a certain number of times when it is his or her turn
- playing with a deck of cards with different numbers used to indicate to the child the number of times to produce the sound
- switching from one sound to another and then back to the target, so that the target sound is produced immediately after the client has repositioned the articulators

Stage 2: Nonsense Syllables

The goal at this point is to help the child develop a stronger and more consistently correct production of the target sound in a variety of nonsense syllable contexts. The target sound may be practiced in a variety of syllable shape contexts and word positions, as the following examples (adapted from Secord, 1989, p. 143) illustrate:

Syllable	Shape	Word Position
/bu/	CV	initial (prevocalic)
/ub/	VC	final (postvocalic)
/ubu/	VCV	medial (intervocalic)
/bum/	CVC	initial (prevocalic)
/mub/	CVC	final (postvocalic)

The vowel can be replaced by any of the stressed vowels to create more nonsense syllables, and the target can be practiced in clusters. Training can shift from nonsense syllables to nonsense words by giving familiar objects funny or silly names.

Stage 3: Words

Stabilization training shifts to true words when the child easily and consistently produces the target sound in nonsense syllables. The target sound is practiced in words using a series of substages, moving from simple monosyllable to complex, multisyllable exemplars. The substages may include the following (adapted from Secord, 1989, p. 145, Table 5.2):

Substage	# of Syllables	Examples for /f/ or /p/
Initial (prevocalic) words	1	*pot, pig, pen*
Final (postvocalic) words	1	*up, mop, lap*
Medial (intervocalic) words	2	*open, upon, epic*
Initial clusters	1	*play, plate, plump*
Final clusters	1	*apple, zipper, opal*
Medial clusters	2	*applause, apply, oppress*
All word positions	1–2	any appropriate word
All word positions	any	*application, prime, stop*
All word positions, multiple targets	any	*paper, popping, proper*

The goal is to teach the child to produce the target sound in a variety of contexts, from simple to very complex words. Word training begins with the use of a core group, typically consisting of meaningful words such as the child's name, family names, social words, and academic curriculum words. When the child produces the target sound consistently in the core group, the clinician expands the group to a larger set of training words.

Stage 4: Phrases

At this stage, training shifts from single words to two- to four-word phrases. This serves as an in-between stage from words to sentences. Carrier phrases such as "I see a…" may be used.

Carrier phrases are simple because only a single word is changed as the target words are practiced in sequence (e.g., "I see the *boat*"; "I see the *bear*"; "I see the *balloon*"; "I see the *baby*"; "I see the *basket*"). Some clinicians skip the phrase stage altogether and begin the sentence level with short, simple sentences.

Stage 5: Sentences

Whether the clinician skips the phrase level or not, the next stage in stabilization training is sentences. The goal is to stabilize production of the target sound in sentences of varying length and complexity. Secord (1989) recommends the following substages of sentence-level stabilization training (examples are for /b/):

- simple, short sentences with one instance of the target sound ("My dog is *big*"; "I want the *ball*"; "My name is *Brenda*")

- sentences of various lengths with one instance of the target sound ("Yesterday I *bought* a doll at the store"; "Why did you *bring* your dog here?"; "My mommy made *bean* soup for dinner")

- simple, short sentences with two or more instances of the target sound ("My *baby* sister likes *bubbles*"; "She *bought* a *blue* dress"; "Daddy made a *big bench*")

- sentences of various lengths with two or more instances of the target sound ("My daddy made a *big bench* for the *backyard*"; "She *broke* Mom's *brown* lamp"; "I like to play with *bubbles*, and I like to play dodge*ball*")

The clinician can use several techniques (Van Riper & Emerick, 1984) to help establish production of sentences: slow-motion speech, echo speech or shadowing, unison speaking, a corrective set, and role playing. In **slow-motion speech** the clinician and the child say the target sentence at the same time using a very slow rate of speech. In **shadowing,** or echo speech, the clinician says the target sentence and then gives the child a signal to indicate that it is his or her turn. The child repeats the sentence as quickly and automatically as possible. In **unison speech,** hand tapping or other signals of rhythm are employed in sentence production. The child follows the clinician's physical movements and prosody as he or she repeats the sentence in unison with the clinician. The **corrective set** capitalizes on an activity that most children enjoy: correcting the clinician. In this activity the clinician purposely misarticulates the target sound and asks the child to correct it. On occasions, children who cannot produce a sentence correctly when instructed to do so are able to model it appropriately when "teaching" the clinician. Finally, **role playing** can be used with children who cannot produce the target sound in a normal training context. The child is instructed to take on a dramatic theatrical role to facilitate correct production of the target sentences.

Stage 6: Conversation

The conversation level is the last stage of production stabilization training before therapy progresses to the transfer and carry-over phase. When the child produces the target sound consistently in sentences of varying length and complexity, the clinician typically shifts production training to conversation tasks. Conversation practice in the treatment room lays the foundation for training in various extra-clinical settings such as home, playground, and classroom.

Production training at this level usually progresses from structured tasks (planned conversation) to unstructured tasks (everyday conversational speech). In structured conversation tasks, the clinician controls the treatment activities so that only words containing the target sound are practiced. For example, the child may be asked to tell a story about several pictured objects that contain the target sound. Another example is to use a city map in which all of the locations and street names contain the target sound (Secord, 1989). Published materials such as "sound posters" are also available. The posters contain a variety of pictured objects, all containing a specific target sound in their names.

Once the child can successfully produce the target sound in structured conversation tasks, the clinician shifts the focus of therapy to natural conversation where no restrictions are placed on the child. Open-ended questions such as "Tell me about your friends at school" and "Tell me about your last birthday party" help evoke conversation.

Transfer and Carryover

One of the most important aspects of articulation training is the child's production of newly acquired skills in extra-clinical situations. It is not uncommon for children who are 100% accurate in the clinical setting to revert to old speech patterns at home, on the playground, in the classroom, and in other natural environments. Because children do not live in the clinic environment or interact only with the clinician, it is necessary to extend treatment to more natural settings and to other people who regularly interact with the child.

The term **transfer** means the same as *generalization*, and the two terms are often used interchangeably. Both refer to the production of clinically established behaviors in various nonclinical settings. In the traditional approach, transfer is differentiated from **carryover**, in that the latter is defined as the production of a newly acquired sound in conversation (Secord, 1989). In the Basic Unit of Chapter 7, in the section "Implementing a Maintenance Program," we addressed several clinical procedures to establish and help maintain generalized productions of target sounds in conversation, evoked in varied settings.

Speech Assignments
The clinician can provide the child with speech assignments that can be completed at home, at school, and in other settings. The speech assignments are prepared so that they meet the particular child's individual needs. The assignments should be practical; they should not be too difficult for the child and the parents to complete independently at home.

Self and Peer Monitoring
The clinician can instruct the child or a significant other (e.g., sibling, classmate, friend) to monitor the child's speech and document any errors. When using classmates or friends as peer evaluators, the clinician should always ensure that school regulations are being followed and that the peer's newfound role does not create emotional conflicts.

Practice in Other Situations
The clinician can design treatment activities so that the child has an opportunity to practice the target sound in various natural-speaking situations. The clinician should ensure that the child has the foundational skills to be successful in more complicated speaking situations.

Proprioceptive Awareness Exercises
The traditional approach emphasizes the need for the child to have adequate proprioceptive skills to monitor his or her own speech productions. The child not only should be able to hear his or her speech productions, but also must be able to "feel" them. Various exercises can be used to enhance the child's proprioceptive awareness, including (1) speaking with earplugs, (2) speaking while wearing earphones that supply a masking noise, (3) whispering, and (4) speaking in pantomime.

Varying the Audience and Setting
The clinician can vary the child's audience to promote production of the target sound with people other than the speech–language pathologist. Speaking situations with the classroom teacher, parents, and other professionals can be arranged outside the clinical setting.

Maintenance

The ultimate goal in articulation therapy is maintenance of the newly learned skills in various natural environments across time. It is important not only that the child transfer and carry over the skills learned in the clinical setting to extra-clinical situations, but also that he or she maintain these skills over time. To promote maintenance of the newly acquired skills, the clinician may arrange follow-up sessions with the child. The child may be seen progressively less frequently—once a month initially for a few months, then once every three months, once every 6 months, and so forth—until he or she is ready for final dismissal from therapy.

....

ACTIVITY

Identify and briefly describe the five major phases of the traditional approach training hierarchy.

....

Summary and Evaluation of the Traditional Approach

Van Riper's 1939 publication is usually cited as the source of the traditional approach, to which others have contributed. The approach has **five phases:** (1) sensory–perceptual training, which includes identification, isolation, auditory stimulation, and discrimination; (2) production training—sound establishment, which includes such procedures as phonetic placement and sound approximation; (3) production training—sound stabilization, which includes training in isolation, nonsense syllables, words, phrases, sentences, and conversation; (4) transfer and carry-over training, which includes various speech assignments carried over in varied settings; and (5) the maintenance program, which includes decreasing frequency of treatment sessions and follow-up.

The traditional approach enjoyed widespread practice until the more explicitly behavioral approaches—and later the pattern-based and contrast approaches—became more popular in the treatment of speech sound disorders. The traditional approach is designed essentially to teach individual sound productions; the approach does not take into consideration potential patterns in errors or target selection factors. This sounds like a limitation now, but until the phonological pattern and complexity approaches in target selection became known and more common practice, it could not have been judged a limitation. Given the state of knowledge when it was developed, the traditional approach was comprehensive; and its basic framework of treatment, which includes skill establishment, stabilization of sound productions in conversational speech, and generalization and maintenance of skills (including self-monitoring and situational variations), has stood the test of time. Most clinicians today agree that these are essential elements of any treatment program. In fact, some of its components, such as generalization, are now considered key to some well-researched programs (see "Phonological Contrast Approaches" and "Complexity Approach" later in this chapter).

The main limitation of the traditional approach is that it includes a variety of specific steps and procedures, some of which may be unnecessary and not clinically efficient. We noted earlier that speech sound discrimination training may be unnecessary and direct production training will save treatment time and effort. Because there has been no systematic experimental evaluation of the total approach as a comprehensive program and of the different elements of the program, it is difficult to judge which components are effective and which ones are not. Possibly ineffective procedures include perceptual training, proprioceptive awareness exercises, unison speech, and shadowing.

One can judge that the overall procedure, even if it includes some questionable elements, is probably effective in teaching speech sound productions, with or without patterns, because even in the current pattern-based approaches, individual sound teaching is the main treatment component. Such judgments are no substitute for treatment efficacy data, however. What is not often explicitly stated in descriptions of the traditional method is that it includes modeling, systematic positive reinforcement for correct productions, and corrective feedback for incorrect productions—all known to be effective in teaching speech sound productions or any other skills, and part of the currently effective phonological treatment procedures. Repeated practice of speech sound productions, varied phonetic and linguistic contexts for such practice, extensive efforts to extend the skills to conversational speech produced in varied naturalistic environments, and teaching self-monitoring skills also can be expected to contribute to the efficacy of teaching speech sound productions. In essence, the traditional approach does contain elements that are now known to be effective.

Concurrent Treatment Approach

As briefly described in Chapter 7, a recent speech sound disorders intervention program that challenges the assumption that treatment should progress through a simple-to-complex task hierarchy has been developed by Skelton and his associates (Skelton, 2004; Skelton & Funk, 2004; Skelton & Hagopian, 2013; Skelton & Kerber, 2005; Skelton & Price, 2006; Skelton & Resciniti, 2009; Skelton & Richard, 2013). Skelton's series of studies have all used single-subject experimental designs and have ruled out extraneous variables and established treatment effects (Hegde, 2003). The treatment method used in the studies is explicitly behavioral in using shaping, modeling leading to imitation, evoked trials with no modeling, positive reinforcement, token reinforcement with backup reinforcers, and corrective feedback. Skelton (2004) evaluated the efficacy of randomized variable practice tasks, known as **concurrent treatment,** in teaching /s/ to four 7-year-old children in a controlled research environment. He used the multiple-baseline-across-subjects experimental design to establish the treatment effects (Hegde, 2003). The participants progressed from a baseline level of 0% to 2% accuracy of the target sound and then to establishment of the sound in CV and VC syllables in block trials. At that point, variable or concurrent practice, in which simple and complex training tasks were randomly intermixed, was initiated. The simplest level of training was imitation of the sound in single syllables, and the most complex level was production of the target sound in evoked trials of conversational segments. By randomly mixing 29 levels of response complexity, Skelton avoided the traditional progression of the simple-to-complex sequence of treatment. By the end of the first randomized concurrent teaching session, the participant had achieved 70% to 100% correct production. All the children reached 80% correct production for all practice tasks within four to six sessions. Generalized productions in untrained tasks were also observed.

A subsequent study by Skelton and Funk (2004) with three preschool-age, rather than school-age, children produced similar results. Targeting one specific sound and applying the concurrent treatment method described in Skelton's (2004) study, the participants increased correct production from 0% to 2% during baseline testing to 47% to 56% in the first teaching session and 80% correct production within the first five sessions. The three participants finished the program with greater than 80% correct productions in evoked (nonimitative) sentences. Probes revealed generalized productions of the target speech sounds to untrained words, phrases, sentences, and brief stories using stimuli not used during experimental treatment conditions.

Although the Skelton (2004) and Skelton and Funk (2004) studies showed that the concurrent treatment approach could successfully be used to train production of single sounds, Skelton and Kerber (2005) sought to experimentally evaluate the approach's efficacy in teaching multiple sounds to four children diagnosed with a phonological disorder. The authors used the multiple-baselines-across-subjects design (Hegde, 2003). In this study, the clinician taught four sounds to each student, simultaneously using an adaptation of the concurrent treatment method. The four participants showed a substantial increase in the percent of correct productions once treatment procedures were implemented for four target consonant clusters or fricatives. The participants progressed from 25% to 56% accuracy in target sound production in the first session and reached the 80% production criterion within seven treatment sessions. Probes for generalized productions showed over 90% correct productions of untaught sounds in single words and over 85% correct production of untaught sounds in story-telling tasks.

Skelton and Price (2006) then completed a comparative study of the concurrent treatment method and the traditional (incremental) teaching sequence in an alternating experimental treatment design (Hegde, 2003). The study included two participants, both of whom showed multiple sound errors before treatment. Two target speech sounds were selected for each participant. Results showed that both treatment participants showed an increase in correct production of their target sounds in both treatment conditions; however, results showed that concurrent treatment produced a higher percent of correct productions during teaching conditions and on generalization probes.

Most recently, Skelton and Richard (2013) experimentally evaluated the efficacy of using the concurrent treatment approach in small groups of up to four participants in a public school setting, the most common service delivery model. The study used the randomized pretest–posttest control group design (Hegde, 2003). The experimental treatment group received concurrent treatment, while the control group received treatment (if needed) only after the study ended. After implementation of the concurrent treatment method, Skelton and Richard found a statistically significant treatment effect; the participants in the experimental group acquired their target speech sounds within 40 30-minute sessions held in small groups. The conclusion was that the concurrent treatment method could be successfully implemented by school-based speech–language pathologists not only with individual students, but also in small groups—which could help ensure delivery of an efficient, as well as efficacious, treatment program. Using a multiple-baseline-across-subjects design (Hegde, 2003), Skelton and Hagopian (2013) further found that the concurrent treatment method could be used to treat multiple sound productions in children with childhood apraxia of speech.

As previously indicated, Skelton's (2004) study used 29 levels of response complexity that were randomly intermixed in a single session. This is in contrast to more traditional programs that sequence the progression of treatment in incremental steps from easy to difficult tasks (e.g., isolated sounds, syllables, words, phrases, carrier sentences, sentences, oral reading, conversation) when a specified training criterion is reached (e.g., 90% correct production). Treatment does not progress from one level to the next until the criterion is reached, because the child is considered not yet ready for the more difficult task. Skelton designed his program to include 29 exemplar (target) types, starting with imitative trials of single syllables and progressively ending with evoked trials of conversational segments (see Skelton, 2004, for full details on exemplar types).

The following general procedures can be extrapolated from Skelton's original and subsequent studies:

1. Target sound or sounds are selected for training.

2. Orientation training is conducted to teach the child the expected response length and mode.

3. Baselines are established to obtain pretreatment measures.

4. Production of the target sound or sounds is established in isolation and then in CV and VC syllables to a training criterion of 8 out of 10 consecutive trials. This helps establish the articulatory context of the sound before treatment tasks are randomized and taught concurrently. These are considered pretreatment teaching trials.

5. Concurrent treatment procedures are initiated after the criterion is reached for the pretreatment teaching trials, as described in #4. A random order in which the target exemplars are presented is generated at the beginning of each session.

6. All 29 exemplar types are taught in the randomized order established by presenting them at least once, with the exception of conversation segments (which are presented four times to balance with other evoked response lengths). Each randomized presentation of all target exemplars, including conversation segments, is considered one pass. As many passes of the randomized exemplar targets as time permits are completed.

7. Each exemplar type is trained to a specific criterion (e.g., four of five consecutive passes for all exemplar types except conversation). Conversation exemplar types may be considered mastered when the target sound reaches 80% correct production within four of five conversation segments.

8. A token system may be used to reinforce correct target sound productions. Tokens may be accumulated for a backup reinforcer. Reinforcement may progress from continuous to a high fixed ratio.

9. Probes are conducted to evaluate generalized productions to untaught exemplars, higher response levels such as natural conversation, and across settings.

The varied studies under different experimental conditions have offered support for the use of the concurrent approach in the treatment of speech sound disorders. It is expected that this newer approach will continue to be evaluated and developed through subsequent studies.

Summary and Evaluation of the Concurrent Treatment Approach

The concurrent approach, developed by Skelton and his associates, challenges the notion that target sounds need to be taught along a traditional hierarchy of simple to more complex tasks (i.e., isolation, syllable, word, phrase, sentence, and conversation). In a series of well-controlled experimental studies, Skelton demonstrated that children can make positive changes on trained targets when treatment tasks are randomly and concurrently trained. Results also showed generalized productions to untrained task stimuli, task response topographies, and settings. Using the concurrent treatment method, children are initially taught to produce the target sound in isolation and syllables to a criterion of 8 of 10 consecutive block trials. Once the sound is established in isolation and CV and VC syllables, training progresses to the random trial presentation of various treatment target types (e.g., imitative trials of single syllables-initial, imitative trials of single words-final, imitative trials of single words-initial, imitative trial of single words-cluster, evoked trials of phrases-initial, imitative trials of sentences-intervocalic). Probes for generalized production to untrained tasks, in natural conversations, and in extra-clinical environments may be obtained.

Subsequent studies have shown that concurrent training can be used effectively with (1) articulation disorders in which a single sound is treated, (2) phonological disorders in which up to four sounds within an error pattern are simultaneously treated, (3) a small group of children with varied target sounds, and (4) childhood apraxia of speech with multiple target sounds. In a comparative study between the traditional hierarchy approach and the concurrent treatment approach, the authors found that while both programs were effective, the concurrent treatment approach produced a higher percent of correct productions during teaching conditions and on generalization probes, indicating greater transfer of learning.

The strength of the concurrent method is that it has been studied under well-controlled experimental conditions that have resulted in positive treatment outcomes. Studies clearly describe the treatment methods. Furthermore, results have been replicated with varied disorders, age groups, and treatment settings. The effects of generalization to untrained tasks have been documented. It is anticipated that ongoing research studies investigating the efficacy of this treatment approach will continue to be well controlled and empirically valid. Areas requiring further investigation might include determining if all response types are necessary to produce positive results. For example, is it necessary to include imitative trials in single syllables, or can treatment progress from the establishment of the sound to the word level and still obtain positive results? Also, is it necessary to train a sound in all positions of distribution, or can training in one position be sufficient to promote generalized productions to untrained positions? Perhaps the efficiency of the treatment program may be increased if a sound is trained in one position and the clinician then evaluates generalized effects to other positions. If generalization to other positions is not observed, other positions of distribution need to be directly trained. However, if generalization to other positions is noted, additional training would not be needed. Furthermore, additional comparative studies between this approach and other treatment approaches are necessary. Replication studies on the use of this treatment approach in a group setting, the most common service delivery model, yielding similar results may add to the program's current strengths.

....

ACTIVITY

Describe how the concurrent approach differs from the traditional approach.

....

Cycles Approach

Hodson and Paden (1983, 1991) advanced a speech sound production treatment approach now commonly known as the **cycles approach.** It was originally designed for severely unintelligible children who exhibited several phonological error patterns and an intelligibility percentage of less than 20% (Prezas & Hodson, 2010). The cycles approach, which has evolved over the last 30 years, targets for instruction certain phonological patterns that are lacking in the child's repertoire. Its theoretical framework is multifaceted, as individual components have been influenced by different phonological theories, including natural (linear) phonology, developmental phonology, and gestural phonology. The reader may consult Prezas and Hodson (2010), Hodson (1989), or Hodson and Paden (1991) for extensive details on the cycles remediation approach to speech sound disorder therapy.

The general procedures included in the cycles approach are as follows (Hodson, 1989; Hodson & Paden, 1983, 1991; Prezas & Hodson, 2010):

1. *Stimulation*—With the use of auditory, tactile, and visual stimulation cues, the child is made aware of the auditory, tactile, and visual characteristics of the target sound.

2. *Production training*—Also called kinesthetic stimulation, production training is offered to evoke sound productions that are incompatible with the occurrence of the phonological error pattern selected for remediation, so that the operation of the error pattern is reduced in the child's speech. The goal is 100% accuracy for all target productions (Prezas & Hodson, 2010), but that does not serve as the criterion for moving from one cycle to another.

3. *Semantic awareness contrasts*—Training with minimal pairs is conducted to increase the child's awareness of the semantic contrast between his or her typical (erred) production and the target production. (The details of the minimal pair intervention approach are described in the upcoming section "Phonological Contrast Approaches.")

The remediation program is planned around cycles, thus the name *cycles approach*. Hodson and Paden (1991) defined a **cycle** as a "period of time during which all phonological patterns in need of remediation are facilitated in succession" (p. 41). They also define it as the "time period required for the child to successively focus for 2 to 6 hr on each of his or her basic deficient patterns" (Hodson & Paden, 1991, p. 96). *Patterns* refers to the specific phonological error patterns or phonological skills targeted for reduction (e.g., final consonant deletion, syllable deletion, stopping, velar fronting). Hodson (1989) emphasized that treatment cycles can range from 5–6 weeks to 15–16 weeks, depending on the number of error patterns and the number of *stimulable* phonemes (error sounds the child can make with modeling or assistance) within each pattern.

Prezas and Hodson (2010) indicate that stimulable sounds are central to the cycles approach and suggest that targeting nonstimulable sounds can be counterproductive because practice of an error sound can reinforce its inaccurate kinesthetic image. Also greater gains, at least in the initial stages of treatment, can be expected on stimulable than nonstimulable sounds when targeted directly (Rvachew & Nowak, 2001). Nonstimulable sounds then are stimulated during therapy sessions but not targeted directly until the child can show stimu-lability. Hodson and Paden (1983, 1991) offer a detailed and elaborate treatment program. The following sections highlight their remediation approach, which can be used with indi-vidual children or modified to a group format.

Identification and Selection of Target Patterns and Phonemes

The first step is to assess the phonological performance to identify the patterns affecting the child's speech intelligibility. Standardized phonological assessment tools and conversa-tional speech samples described in Chapter 6 may be used. A percentage of occurrence for several phonological error patterns will lead to the next step.

The next step is to select target error patterns and specific phonemes. Improved speech intelligibility is the main concern in selection. Therefore, the clinician should ar-range a hierarchy of phonological patterns that the child demonstrated at least 40% of the time during phonological assessment. The phonological error pattern that is the most stimulable is considered the optimal remediation target, so that the child can achieve im-mediate success. Remediation then shifts to the next most stimulable error pattern until all priority patterns are stimulated during one cycle.

Hodson (1989) and Hodson and Paden (1991) identify the following **potential opti-mal primary target patterns** or **phonemes** for beginning cycles, with some recent slight modification (Hodson, 2007):

- *early developing phonological patterns*—word-initial and word-final singletons (stops, nasals, glides), utterances containing two or three syllables (emphasis on appropriate number of syllables rather than accuracy of specific consonants), CVC and VCV word structures
- *posterior and anterior contrasts*—velar stops (/k/ and /g/; however, word-final /k/ before word-initial /k/ or /g/), alveolar stops (/t/ and /d/), glottal fricative (/h/)
- */s/ clusters*—word-initial /s/ clusters (/sp/, /st/, /sm/, /sn/, /sk/) and word-final /s/ clusters (/ts/, /ps/, /ks/)
- *liquids*—/l/ and /r/ phonemes, velar-liquid clusters (/kl/, /gl/, /kr/, /gr/), alveolar-liquid clusters (/tr/, /dr/, /sl/), labial-liquid clusters (/pl/, /bl/, /fl/, /pr/, /br/, /fr/), and postvocalic /ɚ/

Hodson and Paden (1991) also designate some **potential optimal secondary tar-get patterns** and advanced target patterns. These are not targeted until specific criteria have been met, including (1) appropriate syllableness, (2) production of single consonants, (3) some emergence of /s/ clusters and velars, and (4) productions of practice words for /l/ and /r/ without inserting the glide (Prezas & Hodson, 2010). Current recommendations for secondary patterns are (1) palatals (glide /j/, sibilants, and /r/), (2) all other consonant clusters and sequences (e.g., /j/ clusters, three-consonant clusters), (3) other singleton stri-dents (e.g., /f/, /s/, and /z/), and (4) any remaining vowels or diphthongs or prevocalic voic-ing or devoicing difficulties. **Advanced target patterns,** appropriate for upper elementary school–age children, include **multisyllabic words** and **complex consonant sequences.**

Prezas and Hodson (2010) emphasize that patterns that are not yet correctly produced by typically developing children, particularly preschoolers, are inappropriate as primary targets for unintelligible children. These patterns include voiced final obstruents, final /ŋ/, unstressed weak syllables, postvocalic /l/, and voiced and voiceless /th/. Prezas and Hodson further recommend that baseline measures of the treatment targets be obtained to allow for documentation of change following intervention. The authors recommend that treatment progress from individual sessions to group sessions when the child's speech sound disorder progresses from severe/profound to mild/moderate severity levels.

Structure of Remediation Cycles

As noted, the remediation process is organized around cycles. Target patterns are facilitated via stimulation (auditory, tactile, visual), production training of phonemes, and the use of minimal pairs at the appropriate stage of therapy. Hodson (1989) offered the following suggestions for treating target patterns during cycles:

1. Each phoneme exemplar within a target pattern should be trained for approximately 60 minutes per cycle before shifting to the next phoneme in that pattern and then on to other phonological patterns. Intervention can be programmed into a single 60-minute session, two 30-minute sessions, or three 20-minute sessions each week.

2. Ideally, stimulation should be provided for two or more target phonemes within a pattern (in successive weeks) before changing to the next target pattern. In essence, each deficient phonological pattern is stimulated for 2 hours or more within each cycle.

3. Only **one** phonological pattern should be targeted during any one session, so that the child can concentrate on it. Also, patterns should not be intermingled initially in the target words.

4. A cycle is complete when all target phonological patterns have been taught. Patterns are recycled as needed until they emerge (are observed) in conversation.

5. After one cycle has been completed, a second cycle is initiated that will again cover those patterns that have not yet emerged or are in need of further instruction.

6. At least three to six cycles of phonological remediation, involving 30 to 40 hours of instruction (40 to 60 minutes per week) are usually required for a child to become intelligible.

Instructional Sequence for Remediation Sessions

Within the framework of cycles, individual sessions follow a specific instructional sequence. Although developed in a university phonology program, the program can be adapted for use in schools, clinics, and hospitals. The sequence consists of the following:

1. *Review of previous session*—At the beginning of each session, the prior week's production practice word cards are reviewed, unless a new pattern is initiated during the cycle. If the target patterns are changed, the previous session's cards are set aside for a later cycle.

2. *Auditory bombardment*—Auditory bombardment is provided through slight amplification, usually with an auditory trainer, for about 2 minutes. The child, who is wearing headphones, simply listens while the clinician slowly reads approximately 12 words containing the target sound. The clinician may demonstrate the child's error and contrast it with the target. The list of words is repeated twice if the client remains attentive. At no point during this activity is the child allowed to repeat the target words. At the end of the auditory bombardment activity, the child is allowed to repeat one or two words into the microphone from a different list containing possible production practice words.

3. *Target word cards*—The child draws, colors, or pastes pictures of three to five target words on large index cards. The name of the picture is written on each card by the child's speech–language pathologist or parent. The picture cards are controlled for their phonetic environment to ensure that they are not too phonetically complex for the child to produce.

4. *Production practice*—The child participates in game-based production practice activities that include auditory, tactile, and visual stimulation at the word level. Shifting experiential-play activities every 5–7 minutes helps to maintain a child's interest in repetition of the target words. Usually, the child is instructed to produce five words per target sound in a single session. The child also produces the target words in conversation. A variety of games are used in each session. These activities are the heart of an instructional session.

5. *Stimulability probing*—Prior to ending the session, the target phoneme for a specific pattern to be addressed during the next session is selected based on the child's performance on stimulability testing. Modeling, slight amplification, and cuing may be provided during such testing.

6. *Auditory bombardment (repeated)*—Slightly amplified auditory bombardment, with no opportunity to produce words, is repeated using the 12-item word list from the beginning of the session.

7. *Home program*—Parents or significant others are asked to read the 12-item word list used in the auditory bombardment task once a day until the next therapy session. The child is also instructed to review the target word list by naming the picture cards for a week at least once daily. The time devoted to this activity each day may be as little as 2 minutes. Involvement of the parents or significant others in the home is viewed as an extremely important component of the program for carryover of the learned skills.

Selection of Production Practice Words

To avoid failure, practice words that will maximize the child's performance, especially in the early stages of treatment, should be selected. For example, if the remediation target is elimination of final consonant deletion, it is wise to initially select practice words that are CVC in structure versus more complex, multisyllable words such as *telephone*. As treatment progresses and the child's skills improve, the practice words may increase in complexity. Hodson (1989) suggests the following in selecting practice words:

- Select words versus nonsense syllables for production practice.
- Use monosyllabic words with facilitative phonetic contexts during the initial cycles.
- Avoid words containing phonemes produced at the same place of articulation as the substitute phoneme during early cycles. For example, *cat, can, kiss, kite, goat,* and *gun* would be inappropriate practice words for remediation of velar fronting.
- Use words for which actual objects can be incorporated, especially for preschool children.
- Select production practice words that are appropriate for each child's vocabulary level.

Remediation Activities

Hodson and Paden (1991) recommend the use of experiential-play activities and minimal contrasting pairs as part of the remediation sessions. **Experiential-play activities** are structured so that they are reinforcing for the child. Examples of such activities are the *Flashlight Game* (finding picture cards with a flashlight and naming each card), *fishing, bowling,* and *tic-tac-toe.*

Minimal contrasting pairs (details of which will be discussed in the upcoming section "Phonological Contrast Approaches") can be incorporated into therapy. Minimal pairs may help the child recognize the semantic difference between the target word production and his or her typical production.

....

ACTIVITY

Identify some of the *optimal primary target patterns* or *phonemes* for beginning cycles in the cycles intervention approach.

....

Modified Cycles Approach

For purposes of their study, Tyler, Edwards, and Saxman (1987) developed an altered version of the cycles approach, aptly called the *modified cycles procedure.* Using a single-subject AB study design, they sought to evaluate the effectiveness of two phonological approaches: the perception-production minimal pairs and cycles procedures. In this modified version of the original cycles approach, a cycle is defined as 3 weeks of intervention. One pattern is the single focus of training during that 3-week cycle. Two target sound exemplars are chosen for each pattern. Services are provided in twice-weekly sessions, with one target sound being the focus of one of the two therapy sessions in the week. At the beginning and end of every session the clinician provides auditory bombardment by reading a list of 25 words containing the target sound. Contrary to the original cycles approach, in the modified cycles approach the list is read without amplification.

The emphasis of each session is on numerous correct productions of the target sound in 5–10 carefully selected words. Auditory and visual cues are used as needed, but once the child is able to readily imitate the target, they are strategically faded to allow for spontaneous productions. The child's parents are given the list of words containing the target sound, along with pictures representing the words, for daily home practice at the appropriate level. A different target sound is the focus of the second session, unless the child achieves 20% accuracy or less, in which case a second session is spent on the same sound.

At the end of week 1, the next pattern is introduced and worked on for a week in the same fashion previously described. This is repeated until all three patterns have been targeted, at which point the cycle is considered complete. The cycle is then repeated using the same training sound and the same stimulus words, unless a probe administered at the end of the first 3-week cycle indicates that the target sound is produced with less than 50% accuracy, in which case the target sounds (or patterns) are changed for the new cycle. If probe measures indicate that the target sound is produced with greater than 50% accuracy, training shifts to the carrier phrase or sentence level for those sounds. Probes are also conducted to assess generalized productions of untrained sounds within the pattern.

Other modified versions of the cycles approach include those used by Almost and Rosenbaum (1998) in a randomized controlled trial study, Rvachew et al. (1999) in a within-subjects pre- and post-study design, and Culatta, Setzer, and Horn (2005) in an uncontrolled case study. It should be noted that although these studies made use of a modified cycles approach in their research studies, the versions differed from each other, and none examined the independent effectiveness of the approach.

Summary and Evaluation of the Cycles Approach

Hodson and Paden's (1983) cycles approach is a pattern-based program for children with severely unintelligible speech due to several phonological error patterns. The procedure consists of sound awareness **stimulation** through auditory, tactile, and visual cues; **production training**; and **semantic awareness** contrast training. The remediation program is planned around cycles—a period of time during which all phonological patterns in need of remediation are facilitated in succession.

Treatment cycles range from 5–6 weeks to 15–16 weeks, depending on the child's number of deficient patterns and the number of stimulable phonemes within each pattern. **Primary** potential target patterns include (1) early developing phonological patterns, (2) posterior/anterior contrasts, (3) /s/ clusters, and (4) liquids. **Secondary** patterns include voicing contrasts, vowel contrasts, singleton stridents, other consonant clusters, and other residual context-related processes. Each **remediation session** includes a review period, auditory bombardment, color-and-paste activity with target word cards, production practice, stimulability probing, a second period of auditory bombardment, and home activities.

The cycles approach may be one of the most widely used pattern-based treatment procedures. No systematic controlled evaluation of this approach as a total program has been published. The method has not been experimentally compared against other procedures known to be effective (e.g., the minimal pairs, maximal contrasts, complexity approach, or other behavioral treatment programs). Some studies (Rvachew et al., 1999; Tyler et al., 2002) that were not explicitly designed to test the effectiveness of using a cycles approach nonetheless report success with the method (although their cycles format varied from the original cycles approach). A study by Tyler et al. (1987) that was specifically designed to test the effectiveness of a cycles approach obtained positive results; however, the program was significantly modified from its original version in format, so efficacy implications are limited (see the section just above on the modified cycles approach). Other researchers have made use of a modified cycles approach in their study but without controlling the independent effects of the approach (Almost & Rosenbaum, 1998; Culatta et al., 2005; Rvachew et al., 1999). Well-controlled experimental studies are needed to establish the approach's independent effects and relative effects when compared with those of other methods. It would also be interesting to perform a well-controlled study comparing the efficacy and efficiency of a modified cycles approach and the more classical cycles approach.

The cycles approach consists of several elements whose independent effectiveness remains unknown. The method combines both auditory bombardment and production practice, but it is not clear what separate and independent effect the auditory bombardment has on phonological learning. Whether the experiential-play activities have any effects of their own is also not clear. Whether the selection of stimulable and less complex targets is the best approach to intervention needs to be evaluated in light of current generalization research. Kamhi (2006) indicated that research is needed to investigate efficiency aspects of this multiple-component and comprehensive program.

Phonological Contrast Approaches

In the treatment of speech sound disorders, the **contrast approaches** have gained wide acceptance and clinical implementation. These approaches are most frequently used in remediating phonological error patterns, but they may be integrated into any treatment where enhanced phonemic contrasts would improve speech intelligibility. The goal of contrast therapies is to increase the effectiveness of a child's communication by establishing the lost phonemic contrasts in his or her speech.

Phonological contrast approaches are theoretically based on the linguistic phoneme feature analysis. We pointed out in Chapter 3 that phonemes are defined as the basic units of meaning in language. The advent of the distinctive feature theory, also described in Chapter 3, suggested that a phoneme is a collection of distinct and separately analyzable features, and phonemes help contrast meaning mainly because of differences in features that characterize speech sounds. In selecting treatment targets, the contrast approaches pay special attention to distinctly different features (feature contrasts). Distinctive phoneme features do not play a significant role in treatment target selection in most other approaches. Although the notion of features is involved in phonological pattern analysis, as well as the nonlinear phonological constraint analysis, the target sounds are not explicitly grouped according to contrasting distinctive features. Contrasting sound features are the main criterion of target selection in contrast approaches. The oldest of the contrasting approaches, the minimal pair intervention approach, is most closely aligned to the theory of linear (natural) phonology, while more current methods such as the maximal contrast and interrelated complexity approaches are more greatly influenced by nonlinear phonological theories. The reader may refer to Chapters 3 and 4 for a review of phonological theories and their clinical applications.

The contrast approaches to treatment do not imply new treatment procedures, as defined and discussed in Chapter 7. Treatment procedures are still behavioral (e.g., use of stimuli, modeling, corrective feedback, successive approximation). The approaches suggest that treatment targets may be fine-tuned to promote better generalization of training effects to untrained phonemes—an important advancement in treatment research. In essence, contrast approaches do not offer any new answers to the question of *how* to teach phonemes (which is technically a *treatment* question) but do offer novel answers to the question of *what* to teach children with speech sound disorders. Of course, the question of what to teach can make a difference in treatment outcomes; therefore, it is an important question and has guided the development of newer approaches such as maximal contrasts and complexity.

There are at least three ways in which phoneme contrasts have been used in target behavior selection: *minimal contrasts*, *maximal contrasts*, and *multiple contrasts*. Phonemic contrasts are also described as *oppositions* in linguistic theories. Therefore, *contrasts* and *oppositions* mean roughly the same (Barlow & Gierut, 2002; A. L. Williams, 2000). One can characterize the three variations as *minimal opposition*, *maximal opposition*, and *multiple opposition* tactics of target behavior selection in the treatment of speech sound disorders. In phonological contrast therapies, two or more target sounds with contrasting features are taught primarily in words (but also in phrases and sentences as needed) with the help of behavioral treatment techniques. All three approaches use *minimal pair word sets*, which have been defined as sets of words that differ by only one phoneme (Barlow & Gierut, 2002), as treatment stimuli to evoke sound production. The kinds and the number of contrasts selected for intervention is what makes the difference between the minimal, maximal, and multiple contrast approaches. The type of contrasts used in the minimal and multiple oppositions approaches have also been called *homonymous*, as the primary aim is to reduce the level of homonymy in the child's speech. Those used in the maximal contrast approach are referred to as *nonhomonymous* because reducing the homonymy that results between the child's error productions and target productions is not the main goal.

Minimal Contrast (Minimal Pair Intervention Method)

In the **minimal contrast method,** the phoneme contrast is limited to one or just a few features; thus, the contrast is *minimal*. For example, the first sounds in the word pair *bat-pat* differ minimally; only the *voicing* feature distinguishes (or contrasts) the initial phoneme in the two words. The difference in meaning is signaled by that feature alone. The first sounds in the minimal pair *tea-key* differ in place of articulation; the first sounds in the minimal pair *toe-so* differ in the manner of production. Other examples of minimal contrasting pairs include *thick-sick*, *bend-mend*, and *pig-big*. Because the phonemes are contrasted in pairs of words and classically word pair distinctions have been minimal, the minimal contrast approach is traditionally and more commonly known as the **minimal pair intervention method.**

The use of minimal pair training is currently more common than the maximal or multiple oppositions mainly because the former is the older (Ferrier & Davis, 1973; Weiner, 1981); the latter two are relatively new (Gierut, 1989, 1990a; A. L. Williams, 2000), although the trend is beginning to change in light of more current research. Several case studies as well as treatment efficacy studies with single-subject experimental designs have produced data supporting the effectiveness of the minimal pair intervention method (Elbert & Gierut, 1986; Gierut, 1989, 1990; McReynolds & Bennett, 1972; Weiner, 1981). The minimal pair intervention approach has included treatment goals within the framework of developmental phonological processes (patterns), nondevelopmental or unusual phonological processes (patterns), distinctive features, and sounds consistently in error or absent from phonetic or phonemic inventories (E. Baker, 2010).

This intervention has been applied in a variety of clinical settings, including university, school, child care, home, and hospital sites. Most research studies have been conducted using an individual intervention model, but this approach has also been used in a group format. Service delivery models have varied in the number and length of weekly sessions. The minimal pair approach has been used as a primary method of intervention and as a component of such other intervention programs as Hodson's cycles approach (discussed earlier). Although originally used with children with moderate to severe phonological disabilities displaying at least six phonological processes (patterns) (Blache, Parsons, & Humphreys, 1981), it is now considered most appropriate for children with mild to moderate phonological impairments (A. L. Williams, 2000), who display only a few consistent sound errors or error patterns. Current research has shown that children with a moderate to severe phonological impairment displaying multiple and inconsistent error patterns may be better served by a multiple oppositions or maximal oppositions approach (Baker, 2010).

The general procedures of the minimal pair intervention can be extended to maximal contrast training with some modifications. The inclusion of perceptual training has varied across studies, with some omitting it completely, and others introducing perception training first, followed by speech production training.

Although a variety of minimal word pairs can be formed randomly, the classic version of this approach requires the use of word pairs that contrast the child's typical (error) production and the target production, or word pairs produced as homonyms by the child. For example, if the child fronts velar consonants, substitutions such as *tea* for *key* and *date* for *gate* may result. The clinician would then select pictures that represent the minimal word pair as stimulus items (e.g., pictures illustrating *tea* and *key*). The child's typical production does not always result in a meaningful word, however. For example, a child who fronts velar consonants may produce [tau] for *cow*, and obviously [tau] does not have meaning in the English language. Because minimal contrast training is linguistic in nature, it is important to use productions that are semantically meaningful. In such cases, the clinician can use his or her creativity and grant such nonsense words meaning (e.g., the child may be told that [tau] is the name of a fictitious animal, which may be drawn as a stimulus). It is recommended that the clinician select 5 to 10 word pairs representing the target contrasts.

Perceptual Training

Once the minimal word pairs (target words and cognate pairs) have been selected for treatment, the clinician has the choice of either including or excluding perceptual or auditory discrimination training of the sound contrasts. In perceptual training, the clinician begins by selecting the word pairs that represent the target contrast. The clinician then places both pictures in the word pair in front of the child and asks him or her to "point to the _____." For example, if the target contrast is open syllables versus closed syllables with a child who deletes final consonants, word pairs such as *bee-beat*, *see-seat*, and *bow-boat* could be used. The clinician tells the child, "I want you to show me the *bow*. Point to the bow. Perfect. Now I want you to show me the *boat*. Point to the *boat*, please. That was great." Perceptual training may continue until the child achieves the predetermined criterion.

To date, there is no compelling evidence to support perceptual training. As noted under the section on the traditional approach earlier in this chapter, there is experimental evidence that production training is usually sufficient (G. Williams & McReynolds, 1975). Furthermore, the child who says *see* for *seat* (final consonant deletion) rarely confuses the act of *seeing* as an object to sit on. Most single-subject experimental studies on minimal or maximal pair treatment have excluded perceptual training and yet have produced good results (e.g., Gierut, 1989, 1990, 1991, 1992). We believe that production training is a priority, to increase the efficiency of services. If the clinician is still concerned with auditory discrimination, he or she can probe for it after production training and, if necessary, train it then.

Minimal Pairs Production Training

In production training using meaningful minimal pair interactions, the child is required to verbally produce the selected minimal pairs. The word pairs are selected for remediation of the child's error patterns. In the previous example of deletion of final consonants, the clinician may select word pairs such as *bow-boat*, *bee-beet*, *toe-toad*, *pie-pine*, and so forth. The same approach can be used with a child who substitutes one sound for another as in [t/k]. Word pairs such as *tea-key*, *tar-car*, and *ten-Ken* may be appropriate in this case. The clinician then obtains pictures that illustrate the words in the selected pairs. Typically, 5 to 10 word pairs containing the target sound and depicting the contrast are recommended.

The training sequence may be structured as follows:

1. The clinician places the word pairs in front of the child, models both the target and the contrast words, and asks the child to imitate them.

2. The clinician provides several opportunities for production of the target and contrast words during imitative trials.

3. The clinician reinforces the child for correct production of the target and contrast words.

4. The clinician then asks the child to spontaneously name the pictures. At this point the clinician instructs the child, "Say the name of the picture that you want and point to it at the same time." If the child is not sure, the clinician can model the action by saying, "Let us pretend that you want the picture of *beet*. Point to *beet* and say the word. I will then give you the picture." Such introductory trials may be conducted not to train perception but just to familiarize the child with the required action. The clinician gives the child the picture he or she names. For example, if the child says *bee* but points to *beet*, the clinician hands the picture of *bee*, which creates semantic confusion and need to repair communication. The child may say, "No, not that one." The clinician provides the child with appropriate corrective feedback such as, "Oh, you meant to say *beet*, but it came out *bee*. If you want *beet*, you should say *beet*, not *bee*. To say *beet*, you need to put the *t* sound at the end. Try it

again: *beet, beet, beet.*" If the child says *beet* correctly, the clinician hands over the picture of *beet* and, if necessary, a tangible reinforcer such as a token. The child is also given meaning-based feedback such as, "Here you go, you wanted the picture of *beet*, and you said *beet*. I understood you clearly this time."

Note that in this type of minimal pair teaching, the child is saying both words—the correct target word (*beet*) and the incorrect word (*bee*) with phoneme omission in this case. In some cases, it may be necessary to spend some time on teaching the production of the target sound in a more traditional manner (e.g., phonetic placement or manual guidance of the articulators, as described in the Basic Unit of Chapter 7) before implementing the minimal pair method. In an attempt to avoid this, it is now recommended that the child be stimulable or show at least 40% correct imitative production of the target sound exemplar(s) before initiating minimal pair training on a specific target (Tyler, 2005). After teaching a few exemplar pairs to a specific criterion, the clinician can probe to see if other untrained phonemes in the class are being correctly produced on the basis of generalization. For example, after training a few target consonants in the final position of words, the clinician could probe for generalization to untrained final consonants in untrained words.

Treatment sessions would typically consist of approximately 20 trials of each of the target minimal word pairs (with or without the minimal pair picture stimuli). Production practice activities may be incorporated into different games, each lasting about 10 minutes. The games are designed to allow the child multiple opportunities to say the target words within a *semantically meaningful* context. During production training, the clinician makes use of contrasting picture stimuli (target words and cognate pairs), modeling, articulation instruction (e.g., placement cues) when needed, verbal praise for correct productions, and instructional corrective feedback for incorrect productions. The clinician may obtain picture stimuli from an array of commercially available published resources, as well as many free Internet sources.

The child's progress is continually monitored not only for generalization of the trained features to untrained words containing those features, but also for the production of those features in conversational speech. If the target features do not generalize to untrained linguistic levels, the clinician should work on additional exemplars (treatment words) or progress to direct training at higher levels such as phrases and sentences.

Maximal Contrast (Maximal Opposition)

In the **maximal contrast** method (also known as maximal opposition), the word pairs selected for phonological treatment have multiple feature contrasts, or maximal opposition between contrasted phonemes. While contrasts in minimal pairs may involve place, manner, or voicing features, contrasts in maximal pairs may involve all three, in addition to other distinctive features. For instance, the word pair *chop-mop* contains maximal opposition because the two initial phonemes differ on several features including [sonorant], [nasal], [voice], [anterior], [coronal], [high], and [strident]. Other examples of word pairs with maximal contrasts include *chain-lane, can-fan, gear-shear, see-bee,* and *thumb-gum*. As in minimal pairs, maximal opposition also contrasts two sounds using minimal pair word sets, but the *features* on which the sounds contrast are many, as against one or two.

As mentioned earlier, in the classic implementation of minimal pair intervention, one word is the target (correct) and the other word is the comparison (child's incorrect production). In maximal opposition, the child's errors are not used for comparison. Instead, a sound the child correctly produces that is maximally different from the error (target) sound is used for comparison with the target word (H. Goldstein & Gierut, 1998; Barlow & Gierut, 2002). As A. L. Williams (2003) illustrates the approach, suppose a child substitutes /t/ for /ʃ/ and says *top* for *shop*, *tip* for *ship*, *two* for *shoe*, and *tack* for *shack*. In the minimal pair intervention approach, the child's error and the correct productions form a pair to be used in treatment (e.g., *top-shop*, *tip-ship*). On the other hand, in the maximal opposition treatment, /t/ would not be contrasted with the target /ʃ/. Instead, an entirely different sound within the child's repertoire, one that is maximally opposed to the target /ʃ/, would be contrasted with it. A. L. Williams (2003) gives the hypothetical examples of /m/ as a potential contrasting sound. The resulting maximal opposition pairs might be *me-she*, *Mack-shack*, *my-shy*, and *mall-shawl* to teach the correct production of /ʃ/ to eliminate the /t/ substitutions.

Once the maximal opposition pairs are formed, treatment proceeds as described under the minimal pair intervention model. In essence, the difference between the minimal and maximal pairs is in the contrasting pairs, not in the treatment procedures per se. Out of the extensive amount of research that has been done on the maximal contrast approach over several years, an interconnected but slightly diverse program has emerged. Research on this diverse program has demonstrated that the selection of complex target behaviors (the *what* of intervention) leads to wider phonological generalization. This program, commonly referred to as the complexity approach to intervention, will be discussed in an upcoming section of this chapter. As the reader reviews that program, it is important to consider it in light of the varied contrast approaches discussed in this section.

Multiple Contrasts (Multiple Opposition)

In the **multiple contrast method,** also called the **multiple opposition method,** selection of target sounds for treatment is similar to the minimal pair approach but differs from it by creating minimal contrasting pairs for all or most of the errors simultaneously (A. L. Williams, 2000, 2003, 2006b, 2010). The method is especially useful for children who substitute a single sound for multiple sounds, resulting in extensive *phoneme collapse* and consequent *homonymy* (production of the same word for a different word). As A. L. Williams (2003) illustrates, suppose a child substitutes /t/ for /s/, /k/, /tʃ/, and /tr/, considered a rule set. Consequently, the child would produce a single word in place of multiple words, such as *tip* for *sip*, *Kip*, *chip*, and *trip*, displaying widespread homonymy. The major goal of the multiple contrast method is reduction of the homonymy that results from multiple and inconsistent errors on the same sound. In the minimal pair intervention approach, the clinician selects one sound to be contrasted at any one time in treatment. For instance, for a child who fronts the velar /k/ by substituting it with /t/, the clinician may select /t/ and /k/ for contrast and create such minimal pairs as *tight-kite*, *tan-can*, and *two-coo* to teach discriminated productions. If there is no generalized correct production of other target sounds, the clinician may create additional minimal pairs, for /d/ and /k/. Thus, in each instance, only one sound contrast is treated.

In the multiple opposition approach, on the other hand, minimal pair word sets would be created to contrast all error sounds simultaneously. According to A. L. Williams (2003), multiple opposition pairs would include exemplars for the child's entire rule set, instead of just one or two exemplars from the set. Thus, to continue with Williams's example of the child who substituted /t/ for /s/, /k/, /tʃ/, and /tr/, a multiple opposition training set would include four minimal pairs, each involving one of four error sounds (i.e., a /t/ and /s/ pair, a /t/ and /k/ pair, a /t/ and /tʃ/ pair, and a /t/ and /tr/ pair), and all four pairs would be treated simultaneously. Multiple sets, each set including all four contrasts, would be used in training, as in the following example:

- set 1: *tin-sin, tin-Kin, tin-chin, tin-trin*
- set 2: *tease-sees, tease-keys, tease-cheese, tease-trees*
- set 3: *two-Sue, two-coo, two-chew, two-true*

All four target sounds, /s/, /k/, /tʃ/, and /tr/, are contrasted in each set.

Sometimes the phoneme collapse ratio is low, meaning that the child's production is substituted for only a few sounds. Multiple contrasting pairs could then be formed for the child's production and all of the target (error) sounds, similar to the minimal pairs intervention approach. When the phoneme collapse ratio is high, however, from a practical clinical standpoint multiple, contrasting pairs could be formed for only some of the error sounds. The clinician would have to decide which sounds would make the best initial intervention targets. In such a case, A. L. Williams (2000) recommends (1) choosing target (error) sounds that would create a maximal contrast or greater distinction from the child's production, with the goal of creating greater phonological change (as in the maximal contrasts approach) and (2) selecting sounds that could expand the child's repertoire of sounds and features. Williams (2000) gives an example of a child with a high-phoneme collapse in which /t/ is substituted for initial /k/, /tʃ/, /s/, /ʃ/, /st/, /sk/, /tr/, /kr/, and /kt/ (voiceless nonlabial obstruents and clusters). Based on the guidelines of creating contrasts with maximal distinctions while also selecting sounds that could add to the child's repertoire of sounds and features, the target sounds for the multiple opposition approach could then include /k/, /tʃ/, /s/, and /tr/, which are sounds that are in maximal contrast to the child's production and expand the child's repertoire. Multiple minimal word pair sets could then be formed for /t/ and /k/, /t/ and /tʃ/, /t/ and /s/, and /t/ and /tr/.

Once the multiple word set targets are formed, the treatment procedures used in multiple oppositions would not be much different from those in the other contrast approaches. The same behavioral treatment method is used to teach correct production of the target phonemes. A. L. Williams (2000, 2010) outlines the following four specific phases of treatment, which have been applied to both the minimal and multiple contrast approaches (see A. L. Williams, 2010, for more specific details):

- *Phase 1: Familiarization and production of the contrasts*—The clinician helps the child become familiar with the rule (error pattern), the target sounds, and the pictured stimuli and vocabulary through immediate and direct models and recasts produced with increased stress and intonation of the target sound (vocal emphasis). The clinician uses closed response sets.

- *Phase 2: Production of the contrasts (focused practice) + interactive play (naturalistic activities)*—The clinician allows for intense imitative productions through phonetic practice in naturalistic play activities. The training criterion for moving from imitative to spontaneous production is 70% accuracy across two consecutive training sets, which means 20–50 responses for multiple sets, depending on the number of contrasts being trained. Treatment progresses to spontaneous productions when the child reaches the training criterion at the imitative level. The production criterion in spontaneous productions is 90% accuracy across two consecutive training sets. If the spontaneous production criterion is not reached, the clinician may add new picture cards and continue to train at this level. If the child reaches 90% accuracy in an untrained words probe (narrow generalization), a conversational sample may be obtained to check for generalization to conversational speech (broad generalization), which serves as the final criterion for termination of services for a specific target. The criterion for discontinuation or treatment on a specific target is based on Fey's (1986) criterion of 50% accuracy in spontaneous connected speech. If the training criterion is met, but the conversational criterion is not, treatment progresses to phase 3. The clinician continues to offer immediate corrective feedback through modeling and recasts with increased stress and intonation in salient positions. Toward the end of phase 2, the feedback is delayed. Closed response sets continue to be used.

- *Phase 3: Production of contrasts with communicative contexts*—The clinician arranges spontaneous productions of the contrast sets in more complex linguistic contexts such as phrases and sentences, with the goal of "programming" or promoting generalization. The conversational probe criterion described in phase 3 would remain the same. Feedback is delayed, as opposed to immediate, using semantic confusion and wrong clinician models to encourage self-monitoring. Open-ended responses are evoked.

- *Phase 4: Conversational recasts*—Target training sets are practiced in conversational speech, and feedback is provided through natural recasts, as opposed to programmed feedback, until the conversation probe criterion is met for the specific target (see the section "Naturalistic Speech Intervention Approach" later in this chapter for an explanation of natural recasts).

Like all the other contrast approaches, the multiple oppositions approach is data driven and recommends careful monitoring of the child's performance in therapy, as well as generalized productions outside of training. A baseline of the child's production for each of the targets is obtained before treatment is applied. "Narrow" generalization to untrained words is probed every third session by using 10 untrained words containing the target in the position of training. A "broad" measure of generalization in conversational speech is obtained when the 90% criterion is reached in narrow generalization progress.

Other Ways of Forming Word Pairs

A variation of the minimal pair formation is to pair two target phonemes, both absent in the child's speech. In forming such word pairs, it may be more efficient to select two error sounds that are maximally different (maximally opposed). For instance, for a child who produced /t/ for /ʃ/, minimal pairs would contrast those two sounds; maximally opposed dual-error contrast pairs would include words with /ʃ/, the error sound, and perhaps /r/, another error sound but maximally different from /ʃ/. This is commonly known as the **empty set.**

Gierut (1992, 2001) also suggests that phonemic contrasts may involve *major* or *nonmajor class distinctions*. Manner, place, and voice distinctions are considered nonmajor distinctions (contrasts), whereas the distinctive features [syllabic], [consonantal], and [sonoric] are major class distinctions. In essence, the distinctions between consonants versus vowels; glides versus consonants; and obstruents that include stops, fricatives, and affricates versus sonorants that include nasals, liquids, glides, and vowels are considered major class distinctions. A clinician can pair words whose phonemes contrast on such major class distinctions. Distinctions found in languages in general are considered major.

These alternative forms of minimal pairs can be even more effective than the conventional method (Gierut, 1989, 1990, 1991, 1992; Gierut & Neumann, 1991), but they have somewhat different effects on generalized productions. Generally, contrasting two new phonemes that differ maximally and are absent in the child's speech may produce better generalization than the conventional minimal pair training (Barlow & Gierut, 2002). The reader is referred to Table 8.1 for a quick comparison of the varied contrast approaches.

....

ACTIVITY

Identify and briefly describe each of the three major contrast approaches.

....

Summary and Evaluation of the Phonological Contrast Approaches

The contrast approach involves pairs of words that help teach the child discriminated learning of correct productions of incorrectly produced or omitted sounds. In the **minimal pair intervention approach (minimal contrast),** the target and the comparison sounds differ by a single feature. A single sound contrast is taught at any one time. In **maximal opposition,** the target and comparison sounds differ by multiple features. Word pair sets are constructed by contrasting a target sound with a sound the child produces correctly. Again, a single sound contrast is taught at any one time. In **multiple opposition,** a training set includes contrasts for all or most of the errors, and the entire set that illustrates a rule is taught simultaneously. Other ways of forming word pair sets are by including two sounds that are both absent in the child's speech (**empty set**) and including sounds that differ by major class distinctions.

The contrast approaches are probably the most systematically investigated treatment methods for speech sound disorders. Most studies have used the single-subject experimental design and have systematically assessed generalized productions. The different kinds of word pairs that may result in different extents of generalization have been an experimental concern. Gierut and her associates have been mainly responsible for a series of treatment and generalization efficacy studies with significant positive outcomes (see Barlow and Gierut, 2002, for an overview of several studies).

As researched in recent years by Gierut and her associates, the contrast approaches help vary the target behaviors in such a way as to produce the greatest possible amount of generalization. These approaches do not contain new treatment techniques; they are almost always strictly behavioral. From the multiple contrasts approach, a different but deeply interrelated approach, the complexity approach, has emerged.

Table 8.1

DISTINCTIONS BETWEEN FOUR MAJOR PHONOLOGICAL CONTRAST APPROACHES

Contrast Approach	Leading Expert	Types of Minimal Pair Word Sets Used	Number of Target Sounds	Level of Feature Distinctions	SSD Severity Level	Current Recommended Stimulability Level for Target Sound(s)
Minimal pairs intervention	Weiner and Blache	Minimal word pairs that contrast the child's error (typical) production and the target sound	1 new sound	Usually minimal but can be maximal (error sound vs. minimally opposed target sound)	Mild to moderate	Stimulable; at least 40% imitative production
Maximal oppositions (contrasts)	Gierut	Minimal word pairs that maximally contrast an existing correct sound and the target sound	1 new sound	Maximal (correct sound vs. maximally opposed target sound)	Moderate to severe	Nonstimulable
Multiple oppositions (contrasts)	Williams	Minimal word pairs that contrast the child's error (typical) production and multiple target sounds	Multiple: up to 4 collapsed sounds in a rule set	Minimal or maximal; maximal is preferred (error sound vs. multiple maximally opposed target sounds)	Moderate to severe	Stimulable or nonstimulable
Empty set	Gierut	2 maximally opposed error sounds paired as targets in word pair sets	2 new sounds	Maximal (target sound vs. target sounds that are maximally opposed)	Moderate to severe	Nonstimulable

Complexity Approach

The complexity approach to intervention focuses on *what* is targeted rather than *how* it is targeted (Gierut, 2005). It is a speech production–oriented approach that has garnered much empirical support and repeatedly demonstrated that more complex linguistic input promotes greater generalization to, or changes in, untreated but related targets. This approach was originally developed to meet the needs of children with a moderate to severe functional phonological impairment, although its use has been extended to a range of speech sound disorders. It is considered most appropriate for children who have problems with phonological content (individual sounds) rather than phonological frame (syllable or word structure and shape). The reader is referred to E. Baker and Williams (2010) for a detailed review of the complexity approach, including its theoretical and empirical basis.

As noted, this approach evolved from the contrast intervention methods already described, primarily the maximal contrasts approach, and is founded on years of experimental research. The most notable shift has been from the selection of treatment targets according to feature distinctions such as manner, place, and voice in nonhomonymous maximal contrasts to the selection of complex targets that are trained in a noncontrasting intervention format (E. Baker & Williams, 2010). In essence, the original maximal contrast approach considers maximal contrasts for target selection and teaches those distinctions in contrasting word pair sets; however, the primary goal of the complexity approach is not to teach sounds in contrasting words pair sets, but to select complex target behaviors that could lead to wider phonological change based on generalization.

Complexity of speech sound targets may be determined in different ways. One way is to use the implied hierarchies, which suggest that clusters, fricatives, and affricates are more complex than other speech sound classes. Relative markedness of speech sounds is yet another factor (see Chapter 6 for details). Features that are most marked are less frequently observed across languages and, therefore, are more complex than features that are less marked or unmarked; the unmarked are commonly observed and are the simplest. Another important variable of complexity, especially in Gierut's research, is productive phonological "knowledge." Readers may recall from Chapter 6 that *productive phonological knowledge* (PPK) is inferred from patterns of speech sound production. For instance, the highest level of phonological knowledge is presumed when the child produces all speech sounds consistently. The lowest level of knowledge is presumed when the sounds are incorrectly produced consistently (Gierut et al., 1987). Complexity varies between these two extremes, as does the PPK.

Speech sound complexity also may vary according to the degree of sonority. Speech sounds may be ranked by the amount of sound, or sonority, they hold on a numerical hierarchy ranging from 0 (*most sonorous*) to 7 (*least sonorous*) (Steriade, 1990). Using the sonority rating scale, English sounds are ranked as follows from most to least sonority: vowels = 0, glides = 1, liquids = 2, nasals = 3, voiced fricatives = 4, voiceless fricatives = 5, voiced stops = 6, and finally the voiceless stops = 7. Two-element clusters, with the exception of /s + stop/ clusters, are assigned a sonority score by calculating the difference between the sonority of the individual segments. The child's speech productions can then be analyzed according to their sonority, and sounds that show the lowest level of sonority can be selected as initial complex word targets.

Yet another method of determining speech sound complexity is stimulability. As mentioned in Chapter 6, *stimulability* refers to a child's enhanced production of an error sound when specific elicitation methods (e.g., modeling) are employed. According to Powell (2003), a sound is considered stimulable if it is produced in isolation or in CV, VCV, or VC syllables with at least 20% accuracy following visual and auditory cues (direct modeling). It is believed that a child who demonstrates stimulability for a specific speech sound is showing some level of phonological knowledge. Following the complexity model, sounds with the lowest degree of stimulability, or the lowest level of phonological knowledge, would be considered the most complex and would make good initial intervention targets. When they are taught, other errors may be produced on the basis of generalization (Powell et al., 1991; Rvachew & Nowak, 2001).

Other factors that can guide the clinician's selection of complex intervention targets include the following:

- later developing sounds (more marked, more complex)

- consistently erred sounds (more complex)

- two maximally distinct sounds (two error sounds formed as a contrastive empty set) rather than one sound in a maximal opposition contrast (one error sound and one correct sound used to form maximal contrastive pairs)

Most of the research conducted on complexity-based intervention has been done with individual children in a university clinic setting. A sequential strategy has been used, meaning that one or two carefully selected consonants or clusters are targeted for a specified period of time until the predetermined performance criterion has been met. Sessions are structured so that there is opportunity for massed production practice to increase learning and stabilizing of accurate sound production. Clinicians use the assessment information to select complex treatment targets that can be established using a *nonhomonymous contrasting format* such as maximal oppositions and the empty set, reviewed previously in our discussion of contrasting methods. Or the clinician can use the somewhat newer and less researched *noncontrasting treatment format* (described in an upcoming section), which appears to be the next advancement within the complexity approach.

Gierut (1992, 2008) indicates that when using the *nonhomonymous maximal contrast approach* or the *empty set* to treat complex targets, the clinician needs to select eight nonsense word (NSW) pairs according to the child's individual needs and abilities. The phonetic composition of the selected words is consistent with the phonotactics of the English language (or that of another target language). Contrasting phonemes within the words are presented in the word-initial position. The NSW pairs are assigned meaning by naming characters, objects, and actions in stories. Intervention progresses from imitation to spontaneous productions. During the imitation phase the child is instructed to repeat the clinician's model of each word, and the clinician provides feedback regarding accuracy. Corrective models are provided as needed. When the child reaches 75% accuracy over two consecutive sessions in modeled trials, or when seven sessions have been completed, treatment shifts to the spontaneous production phase. During this phase the child is instructed to produce the same target words independently without a model; this continues until the child reaches

90% accuracy over three consecutive sessions. Treatment activities during the sessions may include sorting, matching, informal story telling, and disambiguation of word pairs.

The *noncontrasting treatment format* has been used experimentally to treat the production of consonant clusters with created nonsense words (Gierut, 1999; Gierut & Champion, 2001). Research data are currently limited, as this is a newer way of structuring treatment within the complexity approach. Up to 16 NSWs containing word-initial consonant clusters are selected as treatment stimuli (exemplars). The words follow phonotactic constraints of the target language and are balanced for canonical structure, phonetic environment, and syntactic category and may include a variety of word shapes. The nonsense words selected for training are assigned meaning through stories. Picture stimuli are displayed on flash cards for production practice. As described in the nonhomonymous contrast approach, treatment is divided into an imitation phase followed by a spontaneous phase using the same accuracy criteria. The primary difference is that the nonhomonymous contrasting approach (maximal, empty set) uses contrasting word pair stimuli, whereas the noncontrasting method does not; sounds and words for training are selected with complexity and generalization factors in mind. The benefits of using nonsense words over real words, which has been an integral procedure component of much of the intervention research done by Gierut and her colleagues, remains to be well understood, and studies are currently limited to retrospective examinations (Gierut, Morrisette, & Ziemer, 2010).

Generally, the complexity approach requires the use of picture stimuli to evoke target productions and makes use of drill-play types of activities during treatment sessions. Gierut (2004) recommends using principles of phonological (sound) learning such as modeling, corrective feedback, successive approximation, and branching to establish complex target sound production. The clinician can create the needed picture stimuli by accessing published picture cards, Internet clip art, or other commercially available sources such as A. L. Williams's (2006a) program *SCIP: Sound Contrasts in Phonology—Evidence-Based Treatment Program*. This computer-based resource contains 100 different nonsense word illustrations that are specifically designed for maximal oppositions, the empty set, and consonant clusters and are ideal when using a nonhomonymous contrast format.

Consistent with the research and clinical approach of Gierut and her associates, the complexity approach emphasizes the need for continual evaluation of the effectiveness of treatment through generalization probes (see Gierut, 2008, for details). A predetermined probe schedule is recommended. The schedule can be *fixed* (such as every third session) or *variable* (such as sessions 1, 2, and 6), with an average probe administration every third session (E. Baker & Williams, 2010). The probe stimuli should be designed so that both within- and across-class generalizations are examined, along with generalizations across word positions and from single words to conversational speech. The effects of intervention on the child's speech intelligibility should also be monitored.

....

ACTIVITY

Identify some of the factors considered in the selection of complex sound and word targets in the complexity intervention approach.

....

Summary and Evaluation of the Complexity Approach

The complexity treatment approach makes a counterintuitive recommendation that more complex sounds be taught before less complex ones. It is a speech production–oriented approach that has received much empirical support and repeatedly demonstrated that teaching more complex response topographies promotes greater generalization to untreated but related targets. This approach has evolved from the contrast intervention methods, primarily the maximal contrasts method, and is founded on years of experimental research. Whereas the original maximal contrast approach considers maximal oppositions for target selection and training essential, the complexity approach eschews teaching sounds in contrasting word pairs, in favor of selecting complex target behaviors that could lead to wider phonological change. The clinician determines the complexity level of speech sounds by considering a child's productive phonological knowledge, sounds that are later developing, sounds that are not stimulable, sounds that are consistently produced in error, sounds that are marked, and so forth. The clinician then teaches the selected targets using either a non-homonymous word contrast format or a noncontrasting training approach. The clinician probes for generalized production, expecting that the selection of complex targets will lead to widespread phonological changes (e.g., generalized productions to untrained sounds).

As previously indicated, the complexity approach enjoys great empirical validity due to many well-controlled research studies evaluating its effectiveness, which is the program's strong suit. However, efficiency studies on the use of this approach in a variety of clinical settings, including public schools and with diverse clinical populations, are currently lacking. As with the contrast approaches, this approach does not offer any new treatment variables, but rather offers a different way of selecting treatment targets based on theoretical understandings and hierarchical implications, or the *what* versus the *how* of treatment. Determining how this method of selecting target behaviors can be effectively integrated into other treatment programs, such as the concurrent treatment approach or cycles approach, could increase its clinical application. Also, many complexity studies have focused on generalized production of trained sounds to untrained sounds but have not examined generalized production of trained sounds to higher response topographies such as conversational speech. It is expected that with additional experimental studies, the complexity approach will continue to evolve.

The complexity approach may be stripped of all the speculative linguistic theories and still be used effectively. Most of the theoretical inferences, including markedness and productive phonological knowledge, are unnecessary to take advantage of teaching more complex speech sounds. Better generalization across sounds or sound classes alone will justify targeting more complex speech sounds for teaching.

Stimulability Intervention Approach

The measure of *stimulability*, which refers to a child's improved production of sounds in error with additional stimulation such as modeling, has a long history in the assessment and treatment of speech sound disorders. In the past, the information gathered from stimulability testing primarily served as a prognostic indicator of general intervention outcomes. This was based on the results of early studies (e.g., Carter & Buck, 1958) that showed that children with strong stimulability skills were likely to have better initial intervention gains than children with poorer stimulability. Studies also showed that, even without intervention, children with high stimulability tended to perform better than children with low stimulability, which served as a predictor of spontaneous learning of error sounds.

In time, stimulability came to be seen as a sound specific measure and not just one of general ability because it was observed that a child could be stimulable for one sound and not for another. Therefore, its clinical use expanded, and it became an indicator of sound-specific prognosis and learning readiness. It was thought that production of a stimulable sound could be more easily mastered. This served as a basis for target behavior selection; stimulable sounds were believed to make good initial intervention targets because they could be more readily remediated, leading to early success and less child frustration in therapy. However, research over the past 20 years (as described in the sections on contrast and complexity approaches earlier in this chapter) has strongly challenged the assumption that stimulable sounds make better intervention targets. There is now empirical evidence showing that treatment of nonstimulable sounds leads to wider phonological change, or, from a behavioral perspective, greater generalization to untreated sounds (please see Chapters 6 and 7 for more details on stimulability). Concerns about the time involved in instruction, the perceived difficulty in teaching a nonstimulable sound, and potential child frustration have been advanced as reasons speech–language pathologists have not widely embraced the treatment of nonstimulable sounds.

In response to these concerns, while taking into account current research on complexity and generalization, Miccio and Elbert (1996) and Miccio (2005, 2009) developed a program that focuses on "enhancing" *stimulability* of nonstimulable (complex) sounds, rather than targeting their full *acquisition* (mastery). In their view, this could help alleviate the concerns expressed by some clinicians regarding the time required, difficulty, and potential frustration of the child when treating nonstimulable sounds. Their program is rooted in research that has shown that (1) stimulable sounds are likely to be acquired even without intervention, (2) nonstimulable sounds are not likely to change without intervention and thus should hold high priority, (3) therapy outcomes could be enhanced by treating nonstimulable sounds because of potential generalization to untreated sounds or higher linguistic environments, and (4) generalized production in the absence of direct intervention is greater on stimulable than on nonstimulable sounds.

Miccio and Elbert's (1996) **stimulability intervention program** was designed to be used with young children between the ages of 2 and 4 with a moderate to severe functional speech sound disorder and severely restricted phonetic inventory. Following Stoel-Gammon's (1987) criteria, Miccio and Elbert consider a sound to be part of a child's phonetic inventory when it occurs in a given position in at least two different words. Children considered to be good candidates for this approach show poor stimulability for most if not all of the sounds absent from their phonetic inventory, significant homonymy, and severely reduced speech intelligibility.

The primary goal of stimulability intervention is to increase the stimulability of all nonstimulable error sounds. Data evaluating it as a comprehensive treatment program are currently limited to a few case studies. Miccio and Williams (2010) state that despite current limited research, "the available evidence indicates that the stimulability intervention approach is a promising intervention with probable efficacy for increasing a child's correct imitative production of sounds that are missing from the phonetic inventory across a wide range of manner, place, and voice characteristics" (p. 189). However, only experimental research can validate Miccio and Williams's assessment.

Although stimulability testing can be performed in a variety of ways because there is no recommended or universal method of assessment (see Chapter 6), the stimulability intervention program uses a modification of Carter and Buck's (1958) *Nonsense Syllable Test*. The child's stimulability is initially base rated (a pretreatment baseline is established) and then probed after treatment is initiated. Production of each target sound (error sound) is modeled first in isolation and then in its positions of distribution across three different vowel (syllable) contexts (e.g., /ɪ/, /æ/, /ɑ/). For example, if the target (error) sound were /k/, stimulability would be determined for the following contexts: /k/ (isolation) and /kɪ/, /ɪkɪ/, /ɪk/; /kæ/, /ækæ/, /æk/; and /kɑ/, /ɑkɑ/, /ɑk/. Sounds such as /k/ that occur in initial, medial, and final positions would have a total of 10 opportunities. Sounds that do not occur in all positions (initial, medial, and final) such as /ŋ/, /w/, /h/, and /j/ would have fewer total opportunities. After conducting the stimulability baseline and probe, the clinician then determines a percentage of correct production for each target sound by dividing correct production by the total number of opportunities. Continuing with our example of /k/, if a child produced it correctly four times, the percentage of correct production would be 40%. This stimulability intervention program considers a sound stimulable when it is produced correctly at least 20% of the time under stimulability testing conditions. Stimulability treatment is production oriented and focuses on establishing correct production of the nonstimulable error sounds. A nonstimulable sound is considered stimulable when the child produces it with at least 20% accuracy on probe stimulability trials, as described. Although this approach has been used primarily in individual treatment sessions, it could also be used in small groups with the appropriate supports. Miccio (2009) describes stimulability intervention as a short-term, 12-week program typically delivered in twice-weekly sessions lasting 45–50 minutes. Nonstimulable sounds are the primary targets, but this program also trains stimulable error sounds so that early success is promoted. The goal is to decrease potential child frustration while working on more difficult (complex) nonstimulable sounds.

The following is a summary of the technical operations and treatment procedures that have been described as part of the stimulability intervention approach (Miccio, 2005; Miccio & Elbert, 1996; Miccio & Williams, 2010):

- The child's phonetic inventory is determined, and a stimulability baseline is established.

- All error consonants (stimulable and nonstimulable) are addressed within each session.

- Sounds are taught either in isolation or in CV contexts.

- Picture cards (drawings) of alliterative characters (people and animals) and hand motions are used to evoke sound production.

- Initially, the alliterative card for each sound is shown and the body or hand motion is made while the clinician models the target speech sound and provides encouragement; the child is not required to produce the target in unison with the clinician.

- Interesting, play-based, and developmentally appropriate activities are used for production practice.
- Play activities allow the child opportunities to imitate the target consonants; the child and the clinician take turns, so that the clinician continually models correct production of the target sound.
- If the child produces the sound incorrectly, the clinician offers corrective feedback through clarification and verbal recasts, a natural model not requiring imitation on the part of the child.
- Verbal praise is used to reinforce correct sound production; small prizes are given for task completion.
- Two to three play-based activities are used per session to maintain joint attention and interest.
- Specific instructions to "listen and watch" and phonetic placement cues are used to shape a more precise imitated production of the target sound when the child becomes more receptive.
- Stimulability probes are conducted to determine whether the number of stimulable sounds has increased and to evaluate their generalization to real words.
- Progress is monitored by administration of a "real word" probe to measure generalization to real words and across syllable positions.
- No response-contingent reinforcement is provided during baseline or probe trials.

The length of the stimulability program is based not on the production of target sounds to a specified criterion, but rather on the delivery of services for no more than 12 weeks. The program's intent has never been to directly train correct production of sounds (stimulable or nonstimulable) to a mastery criterion at any linguistic level. In fact, the program never moves beyond the syllable level and never states that production in isolation or in syllables should reach mastery criterion. The target sounds simply progress from being nonstimulable (less than 20% correct production in stimulability baseline or probe) to stimulable (20% or greater correct production in stimulability probe). Real-word probes are included as a way of measuring generalization, but words are never worked on directly. Sttimulability intervention is recommended as a primer program to prepare children for a more conventional intervention approach (e.g., contrasts intervention).

....

ACTIVITY

Identify how stimulability for error sounds is determined under the stimulability intervention approach and when a speech sound is considered stimulable.

....

Summary and Evaluation of the Stimulability Intervention Approach

The stimulability approach originally developed by Miccio and Elbert in 1996 seeks to enhance the stimulability of sounds in very young children with severely restricted phonetic inventories. It is designed to be a short-term intervention program for children with a moderate to severe functional speech sound disorder, with the goal of increasing the child's phonetic inventory in preparation for another treatment approach (e.g., the contrastive approach, traditional approach). There is no direct teaching of correct production of sounds (stimulable or nonstimulable) to a mastery criterion. In fact, the program never moves beyond the syllable level and never emphasizes that production in isolation or in syllables should reach mastery criterion. A sound simply progresses from being nonstimulable to being stimulable (20% or greater correct production in stimulability probes). The program is based on research findings that (1) stimulable sounds are likely to be acquired even without intervention, (2) nonstimulable sounds are not likely to change without intervention and thus should hold high priority, (3) therapy outcomes could be enhanced by treating nonstimulable sounds because of potential generalization to untreated sounds or higher linguistic environments, and (4) generalized production in the absence of direct intervention is greater on stimulable than nonstimulable sounds.

Experimental studies evaluating the effectiveness of the stimulability intervention are lacking. Evidence is limited to three case studies (Miccio, 2009; Miccio & Elbert, 1996; Powell, 1996). It is debatable whether a 12-week stimulability program is a short-term program; that is almost an entire semester's worth of therapy. If children are frustrated when nonstimulable sounds are targeted in a regular treatment program, why would they not be similarly frustrated in a stimulability treatment program, despite the inclusion of stimulable sounds? An important question is whether sounds trained to the "stimulability" criterion continue to improve in the absence of training conditions. Most likely, the children would still need therapy. Possibly, it is more efficient to begin a regular treatment program than a treatment priming program. These are all empirical questions that require experimental manipulation of variables.

Core Vocabulary (Consistency) Approach

The idea that some children display inconsistent production of the same word was previously discussed in Chapter 6 in the section titled "Whole-Word Measure Analysis." Ingram and Ingram (2001) suggested that some children may demonstrate variability in their production of the same word and proposed the proportion of whole-word variability (PWV) measure as a method of analyzing a child's consistency in production. They also discussed the profound negative effects of word production variability on speech intelligibility and described some potential intervention goals, but to date they have failed to advance any supporting clinical research.

Core vocabulary intervention is a relatively newer approach developed by Dodd and her associates, which in a sense has carried on where Ingram and Ingram left off. According to its developers, it is designed to meet the needs of the approximately 10% of children with functional speech sound disorders characterized by inconsistent errors on the same lexical items (words) in the absence of childhood apraxia of speech (Broomfield & Dodd, 2005; Holm, Crosbie, & Dodd, 2005, 2007). The speech production problem for these children is theorized to be at the level of phonological assembly, which is described as an impaired ability to phonologically plan (not motorically program) the sequence of phonemes that make up a word despite average neuromotor abilities (Dodd, Holm, Crosbie, & McIntosh, 2010).

This approach has been used with children as young as 2 years of age, preschool children, and school-age children. It has been used with a bilingual child in a case study (Holm & Dodd, 1999) and with children diagnosed with Down syndrome in an uncontrolled parent–child interaction training program (Dodd, McCormack, & Woodyatt, 1994).

Inconsistent SSD is identified by assessing a child's multiple productions of the same words in the same phonetic context. The Inconsistency subtest of the *Diagnostic Evaluation of Articulation and Phonology* (DEAP; Dodd et al., 2006) may be used for this purpose. The child is asked to name 25 pictures on three separate trials within one session. Each trial is separated from the next by another activity. A word produced identically regardless of accuracy receives a score of 0, while a word produced differently on at least one of the trials receives a score of 1. The child's total score for all words is converted to a percentage, and a score of 40% meets the diagnostic criterion for inconsistent SSD. Dodd et al. (2010) indicate that the 40% criterion is justified by consistency of production data in children with typical sound production and children with speech sound disorders, as found in Holm, Crosbie, and Dodd (2007) and McCormack and Dodd (1998). Improvement in speech intelligibility is expected with consistency in whole-word production because the child's communication partner is better able to predict the child's target production or communicative intent.

As indicated earlier, core vocabulary intervention is recommended for children at least 2 years of age and is offered in individual, twice-weekly, 30-minute sessions for about 8 weeks, with the ultimate goal of increasing the child's speech intelligibility. A set of 70 core vocabulary words, thus the name of the approach, is selected for intervention with the help of the child's parents and teacher (if applicable). Target words are not selected according to word shape or sound segments. Rather, functional words that the child frequently uses, such as names, places, function words, foods, and preferred toys or things, are selected for consistency training.

The long-term, 8-week goal is for the child to produce at least 70 pragmatically powerful vocabulary words consistently, meaning that each word is produced the same way each time. One of the two major short-term goals is for the child to achieve the best production possible for each target word. The objective is for the child to produce the target words correctly, but if it is not possible, "developmental" errors are accepted (Dodd et al., 2010). The second of the two short-term goals is for the child to consistently use the established best production, whether it is an exact match to the adult target or one that contains errors. In the first of the two weekly sessions, up to 10 target words are randomly selected from the set of 70 words that were chosen with the help of the child's parents and teacher. The clinician elicits and establishes the best production of the 10 target words by initially "drilling" sound by sound and then practicing the obtained best production in games. The child's best production of the first syllable is established by the provision of models and specific feedback. After the best production of the first and second syllables has been established in turn, the two syllables are combined to form the word. If the child produces a word in error, the clinician imitates the child's error production and explicitly explains that the word differed and how it differed. Sounds in words may be linked to letters for additional visual feedback. Most children with inconsistent SSD are able to imitate all sounds, but when a correct production is not evoked with cues and models, the best production may contain "developmental" errors (e.g., [tuti] for *cookie*, [kaut] for *couch*). These procedures are applied to all target words. At the end of the first session the child's parents and teacher are instructed to target the words directly in the child's home and school environment until the second clinical session.

In the second session, the words are practiced some more so that their production can be monitored, and the child is given appropriate feedback when the best production is not made. Games are used to evoke a high number of repetitions for each target core vocabulary word. Picture naming games can be followed by games requiring the target in a carrier phrase and then games that focus on story generation to include one, two, or three of the target words. Games are structured for rapid and multiple opportunities for production of the target words. Toward the end of the second session each week, the child is asked to produce the set of target words that have been the focus of therapy for that week, three times each. Words that the child can now say consistently are removed from the list of words to be learned. Words that continue to be produced inconsistently remain on the original list and are readdressed in another week. This is considered a test procedure. Words that are mastered can be displayed on a wall chart. This is similar to the initial assessment data procedures in administration of the Inconsistency subtest of the DEAP.

Since this intervention approach relies heavily on the provision of feedback by the child's parents and teacher in extra-clinical environments, it is important that they are trained to recognize the child's best target production and to offer appropriate feedback. Probes are conducted every 14 days to monitor generalization of consistent whole-word production to untreated words (in sets of 10). Consistency of production, as well as an increase in the child's percentage of consonants correct (PCC), which is described procedurally in the Basic Unit of Chapter 6, is expected to be achieved within the 16 half-hour sessions. The authors propose that once the child's phonological system becomes "stabilized" (words are produced consistently), another treatment program, such as minimal contrasts, can be applied to address continued speech sound production errors.

....

ACTIVITY

Describe how inconsistent speech sound disorder is differentiated from childhood apraxia of speech.

....

Summary and Evaluation of the Core Vocabulary (Consistency) Approach

The core vocabulary approach, developed by Dodd and her associates, is an intervention method that establishes consistent word production in children with moderate to severe functional speech sound disorders. These children may produce inconsistent pronunciation of the same lexical items from one attempt to another in the absence of childhood apraxia of speech. Variable productions of the same word may affect how understandable the child is, because listeners, including family members, may not be able to accurately predict the communicative target or intent. This program is recommended for children at least 2 years of age and is offered in individual, twice-weekly, 30-minute sessions for about 8 weeks, with the ultimate goal of increasing the child's speech intelligibility. Target words are not selected according to word shape or sound segments. Instead, commonly selected training words are those the child frequently uses for names, places, function words, foods, and preferred toys or other things. Daily practice facilitated by parents or caregivers at home is an essential part of the program. Words are trained in sets of 10 each week until the best approximation or correct production is consistently established.

The strength of the core vocabulary approach is its emphasis on increasing the child's immediate communicative success by improving production of misarticulated words that are part of the child's existing lexicon. In essence, the words that the child already produces are made more understandable to the child's immediate listeners, such as parents and teachers. Its emphasis on the whole word rather than individual segments is socially relevant. Involvement of the child's family and other communication partners such as teachers is also a valuable component of this program. A primary weakness at this time is that the effectiveness of the core vocabulary approach has been advanced primarily through case studies (Dodd & Bradford, 2000; Dodd & Iacono, 1989; McIntosh & Dodd, 2008), and experimental studies are currently limited to just a few (Broomfield & Dodd, 2005; Crosbie, Holm, & Dodd, 2005). The individual components of the program have not been experimentally evaluated. For example, is the involvement of parents and teachers an essential component for positive treatment outcomes? By implication, if a clinician suspected that a child would not receive such extra-clinical support, would this approach not be useful, beneficial, or recommended? As with the stimulability approach, this program is intended to be a primer for more traditional intervention methods (e.g., cycles, contrast). Because this program is intended for children with moderate to severe speech sound disorders, it is likely the children will still need therapy after 8 weeks of core vocabulary intervention. It may be more efficient to begin a regular empirically validated treatment program, instead of a treatment priming program followed by another program.

Naturalistic Speech Intervention Approach

Like the core vocabulary approach previously discussed, the naturalistic intervention for speech intelligibility and speech accuracy approach (here referred to as the naturalistic speech intervention approach for ease in discussion) seeks to improve a child's overall speech intelligibility and whole-word accuracy. The specific methods used in the two programs differ, however. This approach, developed by Camarata (1993, 1995, 1996, 2002), has a social language framework and is intended for children with a severe speech sound disorder whose speech intelligibility may be profoundly compromised and whose *immediate* communication needs may not be met by intervention methods that focus on individual sound accuracy.

For purposes of his intervention program, Camarata (2010) defines *intelligibility* as the degree to which a listener understands what the speaker says when the target is uncertain and *speech accuracy* as the correctness with which an individual phoneme or speech sound is made. This program is thought to be most appropriate for children who have a severe speech sound disorder and may not be ready for or compliant with a more traditional service delivery model of sitting, listening, and producing on demand (e.g., preschoolers, children with developmental disabilities such as Down syndrome, and children with autism spectrum disorder). It is intended to be a two-tiered approach, which initially seeks to improve overall speech intelligibility so that intended messages are better understood by the child's listeners and then focuses on improving the accuracy of individual speech sound errors. Some children with developmental disabilities, however, such as those with Down syndrome and cerebral palsy, may never achieve typical sound production, and thus improving their overall speech intelligibility through compensatory speech productions and target approximations may prove to be a more socially relevant focus of intervention. For those who do show potential for greater sound accuracy, sound-specific goals can be developed.

Before initiating treatment, the clinician follows the standard assessment procedures discussed in Chapter 6 and obtains sufficient information on the child's sound production accuracy, error patterns, whole-word production patterns, speech intelligibility, stimulability, oral–motor skills, and much more from which to make clinical decisions. Since this program focuses on increasing the child's speech intelligibility, it is imperative that the clinician determine the method that will be used to judge pretreatment and posttreatment levels of speech intelligibility to determine the child's progress and the effectiveness of treatment.

This approach is considered child-led, so the clinician is mostly responsible for manipulating the environment so that the child naturally attempts to communicate. For quieter children, the clinician may need to select toys and activities that are of high interest to evoke communicative attempts. The communicative interactions may be between child and clinician, child and parent, child and teacher, and child and peer. Treatment sessions focusing on speech intelligibility may take place in the clinic, home, or school environment—in fact, in any setting where spontaneous communication attempts occur, such as the school cafeteria, playground, and park. However, accuracy training of specific target sounds are more suited to traditional one-to-one interaction in a clinical setting between the child and the clinician or between the child and the parent with the clinician acting as facilitator. Services have been typically delivered in two to three weekly, 30–60-minute sessions.

In the initial phase of treatment, the goal is on increasing the child's functional rather than ideal speech intelligibility by indirectly establishing closer approximations of the whole-word structure of the adult target. What is important at this point is not the ideal production of the sounds within the word, but rather sound and word approximations that could potentially be better understood by the child's listener. Naturalistic activities that may facilitate child initiations include watching videos, playing games, looking at picture stimuli cards, reading books, playing with objects, and spontaneous conversation.

The foundation of this approach is on the provision of natural feedback through recasts. *Natural recasts* refer to corrective feedback that is given to the child in a naturalistic fashion without requiring the child to imitate the adult's model. They are designed to provide a corrective model to the child without interrupting communicative interactions. More specific to speech sound disorders, a *speech recast* is an "adult utterance that immediately follows a child utterance, gives a neutral or positive evaluation of the meaning of the child's utterance, and is an exact or reduced imitation of the word(s) that the child attempted to say, only using adult pronunciation of the attempted words (Yoder, Camarata, & Gardner, 2005, p. 35). Yoder et al. give an example of a child who says, "This a wion [lion]," and a possible clinician recast of "Yes, a lion." Novel word order, word endings, and vocabulary are not added to the child's utterance in a speech recast (Camarata, 1996). This distinguishes the speech recast from language recasts in which new grammatical information and vocabulary may be provided.

Conversational interactions in which natural recasts are used may proceed as follows: The clinician presents a game activity. The child makes a comment about the game that is difficult to understand—for example, [a em] for "want game." The clinician then provides a natural recast by saying, "Want game? Here you go." The conversational interactions continue, with the clinician offering corrective recasts when appropriate. Exaggerated cues through vocal emphasis of the targets are not provided. If naturalistic intervention procedures are applied to speech (sound) accuracy in which certain sounds are targeted, the clinician can provide word-level phonological recasts focusing on the target sound in an attempt to indirectly improve production. This can be done for individual sounds or sounds representing a phonological pattern (e.g., /t/ and /d/ for velar fronting). Words containing the target sounds are introduced into naturalistic interactions (e.g., board games, Go Fish). The minimal pair intervention concept could also be used by including words that the child produces in a homophonous fashion. Furthermore, words that represent target phonemic contrasts could be introduced into naturalistic interactions. Camarata (1993) provides an example of a child who says, [hi ə wop], and the clinician recast of "Yes, a rope." At the speech accuracy level when specific sounds are targeted, the clinician preselects materials so that a large number are available for inclusion in the training activities. Speech accuracy training can be provided for one or more targets. As the child's overall speech intelligibility improves and begins to display "readiness," more direct ways of improving speech sound accuracy can be employed, using treatment techniques such as phonetic placement, shaping, modeling, corrective feedback, and reinforcement.

The clinician needs to monitor positive effects to speech intelligibility and sound accuracy training by obtaining pretreatment (baseline) information of overall speech intelligibility and any specific target sounds or patterns. Because this approach seeks to increase overall intelligibility, it is imperative that the clinician not vary the measures used to judge or calculate speech intelligibility from pre- to posttreatment measures, because this would cloud the effects of treatment.

....

ACTIVITY

Provide an example of a natural recast that could be provided to a child who says [ai wa aʔi] for "I want cookie."

....

Summary and Evaluation of the Naturalistic Speech Intervention Approach

The naturalistic speech intervention approach was developed by Stephen Camarata to meet the needs of highly unintelligible children with moderate to severe speech sound disorders who may not display readiness for a more traditional intervention approach in which one or more sounds are trained to a mastery criterion using a discrete trial format. The naturalistic approach is designed to be implemented in two phases. The first phase focuses on increasing the child's speech intelligibility for whole words through recasts and acceptable approximations. The second phase focuses on increasing the child's speech accuracy of selected sounds through recasts initially followed by a more traditional articulation or phonological approach (e.g., the contrast approach) when the child shows increased maturity and readiness. It is most appropriate for preschool-aged children or children with developmental delays.

At the core of the naturalistic intervention approach is the provision of feedback through **natural recasts**, or corrective feedback that is delivered in a naturalistic fashion and does not require the child to imitate the adult model. Its developers emphasize that this helps avoid interrupting natural communicative interactions between the child and the listener. More specific to speech sound disorders, a **speech recast** is adult feedback that immediately follows a child utterance and gives a neutral or positive evaluation of the meaning of the child's utterance. It provides an exact or reduced imitation of the word(s) that the child attempts to say, only using adult pronunciation of the intended words. Recasts can be provided by a speech–language pathologist, trained parents, teachers, and others involved in the child's life.

The naturalistic approach seeks to increase speech intelligibility in highly unintelligible children who have experienced a great extent of communicative failure. By targeting the child's overall intelligibility through the establishment of word approximations rather than accurate production of individual sounds to a specified criterion, the child's overall communication may be improved. The empirical basis for this approach lies primarily in research studies that have been conducted on the acquisition of morphological skills through natural recasts of the targets (Camarata, Nelson, & Camarata, 1994; Yoder et al., 2005). However, experimental studies focusing on the use of a naturalistic speech intervention approach through recast models and feedback to improve speech intelligibility and speech accuracy are currently limited (Camarata, 1995; Yoder et al., 2005). Studies that examine the comparative effectiveness of natural and speech recasts and established behavioral methods such as positive reinforcement and direct corrective feedback are necessary. Also, standard methods of assessing speech intelligibility for pre- and posttreatment measures are currently lacking and are needed to evaluate progress. Additionally, the point at which a child is considered ready for a more conventional articulation or phonological approach for improved speech sound accuracy is currently unclear and needs to be determined. Comparative experimental studies are needed to determine whether starting with a primer that progresses to a more conventional program is more or less effective than, or equally as effective as, simply starting with a conventional program.

Language-Based Treatment Approaches for Phonological Disorders

We will briefly describe an approach to phonological treatment that has so far produced inconsistent research data. It is well known that in many children language and phonological disorders coexist. In addition to pragmatic communication deficiencies, language disorders may include limited vocabulary, limited syntactic structures, and missing morphologic features (e.g., the regular and irregular plurals, possessives, articles, the present progressive, pronouns, prepositions). Some researchers have investigated whether it is possible to induce phonological change in children by treating their language disorders. Such language treatment need not have phonological targets, practice for sound productions, or explicit reinforcement or corrective feedback for sound productions. Language treatment may use a variety of methods, including naturalistic interactions in which the child's unclear statements are clarified, story telling and retelling, clinician's imitation of child's language structures, prompts, sentence completion tasks, restatements of child's productions, expansion of child's telegraphic productions, and so forth (Fey et al., 1994; Norris & Hoffman, 1990; Tyler, 2002; Tyler & Sandoval, 1994; Tyler et al., 2002). If the intent of a language treatment study is to document the changes in phonological skills as an indirect effect of such a treatment, the researcher needs to show that explicit teaching of such morphological skills as the plural /s/, /z/, and /ɪz/ (e.g., in *cups*, *bags*, and *oranges*, respectively); the past tense /d/, /t/, and /ɪd/ (e.g., in *bored*, *walked*, and *painted*, respectively); and other language targets that may inadvertently treat phonological skills is not included.

Studies have not produced convincing data to show that it is indeed better to target language skills to induce phonological skills than it is to treat the phonological skills directly. A few studies have shown that language treatment may have a beneficial effect on phonological skills with no explicit training (Hoffman, Norris, & Monjure, 1990; Matheney & Panagos, 1978; Tyler et al., 2002; Wilcox & Morris, 1995). Some of these studies had a small number of subjects. The Hoffman and colleagues (1990) study had only two subjects, whose language problems were mild or near normal.

Other studies, some that included fairly large numbers of children, have produced conflicting results. When they treated only the language disorders in 25 children with moderate to severe language and phonological disorders, Fey and colleagues (1994) failed to demonstrate significant effects on phonological skills in a controlled group design study. In an uncontrolled case study, Tyler and Sandoval (1994) found that in 6 children, language treatment alone had no significant effect on phonological skills. However, Tyler and colleagues (2002), who used an experimental group design, found that 10 children who received language intervention first showed improvement in language and phonological skills; they then received phonological treatment. Another group of 10 children who received phonological treatment first showed improvement only in phonological skills; their morphological skills improved only after following the language treatment. The authors concluded that language treatment can affect both morphological and phonological skills, whereas phonological treatment affects only what is treated. Their results contain certain puzzling elements, warranting a cautious interpretation. First, after 24 weeks of treatment, changes were higher in phonological skills than in language skills, even in the group that received language treatment first. Could the language treatment somehow be more tuned to phonological skills than to language skills themselves? Second, the standard deviations for the means were extremely large, in some cases higher than the mean, suggesting great individual differences within the group. Third, regardless of statistical significance, the amount of improvement did not exceed 35% for phonological skills and 20% for morphological skills. In essence, both the treatment effects, despite their statistical significance, were clinically weak. It is not clear from evidence accrued so far that it is more efficacious to indirectly treat phonological skills by a more exclusive language treatment. Additional research is needed to justify an exclusive language treatment to remediate phonological disorders in children. However, in routine treatment of children who have language and phonological disorders, both kinds of skills may be simultaneously targeted. Various morphological features that are intertwined with articulatory productions may be treated to improve both sets of skills (e.g., the plural and the possessive /s/ and /z/, the past tense /d/ and /t/). In selecting words and phrases for language treatment, the clinician may consider the child's articulation targets (e.g., if /s/ is an articulation target, socially significant words starting with /s/ may be the language targets, as well).

A language- or literacy-based approach that has received considerable attention in recent years is the metaphonological or phonological awareness approach. The correlation between phonological awareness problems, literacy problems, language problems, and severe speech sound disorders, particularly those considered more phonological in nature, has been well established. By virtue of this correlation, it has been argued by proponents of a language- or literacy-based approach that the effective treatment of severe speech sound disorders should include phonological awareness training, or at least some elements of it. However, this notion has not been empirically substantiated. To address these important issues, we have written an entire new chapter. The reader is referred to Chapter 9 for discussion of phonological awareness as it relates to speech sound disorders.

....

ACTIVITY

A 5-year-old boy on your caseload misarticulates /s/ in all positions and also omits the regular plural marker in words. Identify some possible target word exemplars that could be used to simultaneously teach both skills.

....

Nonspeech Oral–Motor Exercises: An Update

We will finally address the question of nonspeech oral–motor exercises (NSOME), special exercises designed to improve the strength and control of the speech articulators, in treating speech sound disorders. The value of these exercises continues to be hotly debated, perhaps as an outgrowth of the call for evidence-based practice in the field of speech–language pathology. Except for perceptual training of speech discrimination, the treatment approaches described so far in this chapter directly teach speech sound production skills.

Similar to the argument that perceptual training is a precursor to production training in articulation treatment is the argument of some experts that before production treatment or in conjunction with it, children need to be offered NSOME that do not include any sound production attempts. The precise reasons for this recommendation remain unclear (Clark, 2010). Despite the fact that a majority of children treated for speech sound disorders do not have clinical symptoms of neuromotor deficits, the assumption is that because speech is a motor act, exercises designed to improve nonspeech motor strength and control should be important in speech treatment (Hall et al., 2007; Marshalla, 1996; P. G. Meyer, 2000).

It is important to note that the controversial aspect of NSOME is its application in the treatment of functional speech sound disorders in children who evidence no motor control problems. There is also controversy when it is applied to the treatment of children with evident sensorimotor control problems, such as apraxia of speech and dysarthria; however, that controversy and debate may be for slightly different reasons. Any level of controversy stems from the central concern that NSOME do not involve speech production, and that valuable time and resources may be better spent in teaching speech sound production skills directly.

Before proceeding it is important to define NSOME, to avoid confusion of terms. Lof (2009) and Lof and Watson (2008) define NSOME as any treatment technique that does not require the child to produce a speech sound but is used to indirectly "influence" the development of speaking abilities. They may be considered an array of methods and procedures that theoretically influence tongue, lip, and jaw strength and increase their tone, range of motion, control, and resting postures (Lof, 2009; Ruscello, 2008b). They may also include procedures that provide sensory stimulation to the lips, jaw, tongue, soft palate, larynx, and respiratory muscles with the goal of influencing the physiologic foundation of the speech mechanism to improve its function for speech production (McCauley, Strand, Lof, Schooling, & Frymark, 2009; Lof, 2009). To date, many of these methods and procedures lack experimental data to support the stated or implied claim that NSOME influence the production of speech and facilitate more efficient treatment of speech sound disorders. Despite the lack of research supporting their use, it has been indicated that in both Canada and the United States, 85% of speech–language pathologists use NSOME in their treatment of speech sound disorders, and 71% of SLPs make use of them in the United Kingdom (Hodge, Salonka, & Kollias, 2005; Joffe & Pring, 2008; Lof, 2009; Lof & Watson, 2008).

A variety of NSOME have been recommended for children with speech sound disorders. These include various exercises of the tongue (e.g., brushing parts of the tongue to increase oral awareness; elevating the tongue tip while holding the jaw stable; protruding the tongue without lip or jaw movements; moving the tongue sideways; touching the tip of the nose with the tongue; touching the chin with the tongue tip) and lips (e.g., puckering, smiling, mouth opening and closing, sucking actions). Lof (2009) specifies that the most frequently used exercises include (listed in rank order of use): blowing, tongue push-ups, pucker-smile, tongue wags, big smile, tongue-to-nose-to-chin, cheek puffing, blowing kisses, and tongue curling. The presumed benefits of these exercises were improvement in tongue elevation, awareness of the articulators, tongue strength, lip strength, lateral movements of the tongue, stabilization of the jaw, protrusion of the lip and tongue, control of drooling, velopharyngeal competence, and sucking ability (Lof, 2009).

NSOME should be differentiated from the oral–motor movements that have been used throughout the history of our profession to facilitate the production of speech sounds through shaping, phonetic placement cues, physical manipulation of the articulators, and so forth (discussed in the Basic Unit of Chapter 7). The key difference is that the latter have a direct connection to specific sounds targeted for intervention, whereas NSOME target improvement in the strength, tone, range of motion, control, and resting posture of the articulators with the hope that such improvement will transfer to sound production. A boy who is asked to stick out his tongue and hold for 10 seconds a Cheerio placed on its tip, with the goal of strengthening the tongue, is being given a nonspeech oral–motor exercise, while another who has his alveolar ridge rubbed with a Q-tip and is then asked to place his tongue tip against the "tickle spot" and say /ə/, with the goal of evoking /l/, is being provided direct stimulation of the articulators for target sound production. In both scenarios the ultimate goal may be the correct production of /l/, but in the first, strengthening of the tongue may or may not transfer to correct production of /l/; even more important, the presumed higher tongue strength may be unnecessary to produce the target speech sound. In the latter scenario the movements taught are specifically designed to evoke correct production of the sound. To further illustrate, a girl who is asked to suck a milkshake through a straw or blow into a specific horn for lip strengthening is being given a non-speech oral–motor task, while another, whose lips are first physically shaped into a rounded position, is asked to "blow" air at a Kleenex placed in front of her for visual feedback, to stimulate the production of /p/, is being encouraged to perform an oral–motor movement directly involved in speech production.

Several comprehensive reviews of studies on NSOME have concluded that there is no evidence that such exercises help improve speech production (Forrest, 2002; Lass & Pannbacker, 2008; Lof, 2009; McCauley et al., 2009; Ruscello, 2008b). Lof (2009) lists several reasons for questioning the clinical use of nonspeech oral–motor exercises: (1) there is no clear-cut evidence that teaching a part of the articulatory gesture will transfer to the entire gesture; (2) the articulatory strength required for production of sounds is actually low; (3) "improvements" in articulatory strength are highly subjective because they are difficult, if not impossible, to measure without special instruments (see Text Box 8.2); (4) there is not much relevancy between many of the oral–motor movements taught (e.g., tongue to nose, puffing cheeks) and the actual speech gestures desired; (5) although identical structures are used for speech and nonspeech activities (e.g., feeding, sucking, swallowing, breathing), their functions are independent and are mediated by different parts of the brain; and (6) warm-up exercises are not required for tasks that do not maximally tax the system, such as speaking, which uses only a minimum (10–20%) of the muscular strength available.

That nonspeech oral–motor exercises should be avoided with children who have functional articulation or phonological disorders seems obvious in light of current research. But what about their use with children who have organic or neuromotor-based speech sound disorders, such as childhood apraxia of speech, dysarthria, and cleft lip or palate? Can this be justified, and does it fall under the parameters of best practice? Experts now concur that children with childhood apraxia of speech have adequate oral structural movements for nonspeech activities. Furthermore, their difficulty in producing volitional movements involved in speech production cannot be attributed to muscle weakness. Therefore, there is no need to offer muscle strengthening exercises or other exercises that focus on nonspeech activities. As already discussed in the Advanced Unit of Chapter 7, the target of intervention with children who have childhood apraxia of speech should be improved planning, sequencing, and coordination of muscle movements for speech, because it is a disorder of coordination and not one of a muscular strength deficit (ASHA, 2007).

Duffy (2005) suggests that nonspeech oral–motor strengthening exercises may be appropriate for a small number of patients with acquired dysarthria, though their use even with that population is increasingly controversial (Hustad, 2010; Hustad & Weismer, 2007; Lof, 2009; Ruscello, 2008b; Weismer, 2006). Duffy's (2005) suggestion may also hold true for children with developmental dysarthria in congenital disorders such as cerebral palsy. The majority of clients with dysarthria, acquired or developmental, will likely benefit more from the direct modification of speech sounds when they are responsive to intervention and the introduction of behavioral adaptations or compensatory strategies (e.g., rate control, volume control, postural adjustment) to improve overall speech intelligibility and communication effectiveness (Hustad, 2010). Based on the existing literature, it appears that the use of nonspeech oral–motor exercises is no longer recommended as standard practice in the treatment of dysarthria.

Text Box 8.2. How do I measure this?

Recently, a kindergarten student diagnosed with a functional phonological disorder came to my caseload with the following goals on his current Individualized Education Program:

1. Johnny will increase intelligibility to at least 70% without context cues by reducing instances of stopping to less than 20% of the time and instances of cluster reduction to less than 35% of the time. Baseline level of mastery: Intelligible 20–30% of the time.

2. Johnny will improve his tongue and lip strength, range of motion, and sequential movements while in therapy, as seen by increased intelligibility to 70%. Baseline level of mastery: Decreased strength, range of motion, and ability to perform sequential movements; intelligibility approximately 30%.

Goal number one, although problematic because it did not meet the minimal standards of a measurable and well-written objective, had just enough information to allow the first author to compare Johnny's baseline speech intelligibility with his current level of intelligibility as a gross measure of progress. However, goal number two put the first author in a precarious situation because she had no way of measuring progress. The baseline information indicating that Johnny had "decreased strength, range of motion, and ability to perform sequential movements" was not objective, specific, or measurable. It did not give her a true baseline measurement of the selected "target" skills. The goal that Johnny should "improve his tongue and lip strength, range of motion, and sequential movements while in therapy, as seen by increased intelligibility to 70%" was also not objective or measurable. How was she supposed to determine whether his tongue had become stronger or had a wider range of motion or his sequential movements had improved from his initial baseline? Did she need specialized equipment to measure strength and range (equipment she did not have)? And how would an increase in Johnny's intelligibility to 70% be an indicator of improved lip strength, range of motion, and sequential movements?

To further complicate things, in the first author's professional opinion, Johnny's oral–motor skills were sufficiently developed to support speech production. And what was she supposed to do about all the current evidence that has demonstrated over and over that nonspeech oral–motor exercises are not effective in the treatment of speech sound disorders? She quickly scheduled an IEP meeting with Johnny's parents and other team members to develop new goals. The existing goal number one was broken down into two goals, one targeting specific consonants affected by the stopping phonological error pattern and a second one targeting specific consonant clusters affected by consonant cluster reduction. Goal number two was eliminated.

In the treatment of cleft lip and palate it has been established that although the velopharyngeal (VP) mechanism can be strengthened, added strength will not improve speech production (Lof, 2009). Golding-Kushner (2001) stated that although blowing, yawning, whistling, sucking, cheek puffing, swallowing, gagging, and icing exercises have been suggested to improve or strengthen velopharyngeal closure and speech, multiview videofluoroscopy has shown that VP function for such nonspeech movements is different from VP movements for speech. Over time, speech–language pathologists have gained an understanding that the timing, the range, and even the neural control mechanisms for speech and nonspeech velopharyngeal closure are distinct (Clark, 2003; Dworkin, Marunick, & Krouse, 2004; Forrest, 2002; Glaze, 2009; Ruscello, 2008a). Glaze (2009) wrote that if the goal is to improve speech functioning, then the clinician must target speech itself.

Considering the lack of empirical evidence for the efficacy of nonspeech oral–motor exercises in the treatment of speech sound disorders, what then might be the motivating factors influencing their use by approximately 70–85% of speech–language pathologists? Kamhi (2008) conjectures that clinicians may be unclear about the distinction between oral–motor techniques that directly involve speech production and nonspeech oral–motor techniques that bear no relation to speech production. Clinicians also may think that nonspeech oral–motor exercises are a part of the shaping that is so frequently used in teaching correct speech sound production, that they are a way of breaking down complex speech sound production into its basic and discrete skills. Unfortunately, this is a misinterpretation of shaping. The basic, discrete, and simple skills used in the initial stage of shaping must be related to the final target. NSOME are not related to the final target; speech-related motor skills are.

As Kamhi (2008) further suggests, clinicians' desire to provide what may be considered the most current, state-of-the-art, popular, broad-based, eclectic, and "engaging" treatment, with the goal of appearing up to date and innovative, may also be a factor. This desire may be influenced by promotional materials, advertising, convention exhibits, Web sites, and other sources that advocate the use of nonspeech oral–motor activities and may sell related products (e.g., horns, straws, whistles, bite blocks, massagers).

Consistent with our previous stance on the treatment of speech sound discrimination, we recommend direct treatment of speech production, as the evidence favors it. The training of a presumed essential skill that is supposed to have an effect on speech sound production skills must be justified by controlled evidence that shows that such training is necessary to effect improvement under articulation treatment. There is no such evidence; in addition, there is plenty of evidence to show that children improve immensely with articulation and phonological treatment without NSOME. At this point, the burden lies on the proponents of NSOME, direct or indirect, to advance the empirical research needed to justify their use. Controlled experimental studies isolating the discrete use of NSOME and its effect on speech production must be conducted and replicated. In the absence of such research, clinicians may target only those oral–motor movements that are directly involved in the production of the speech sounds that need to be taught to children.

··

ACTIVITY

Give an example of a nonspeech oral–motor exercise and an example of an oral–motor phonetic placement cue that could be used to establish /θ/.

··

Chapter Summary

• Various approaches to speech sound production have evolved over the decades. Some programs are based on years of empirical research; others have evolved primarily from uncontrolled clinical data such as case studies; and still others are based on clinical experience or expert advocacy.

• When carefully examined, many of the approaches share several features, such as the selection of target behaviors and the use of antecedent stimuli, modeling, corrective feedback, and reinforcement. Most treatment programs differ in what they teach, not how they teach.

- Baker and McLeod (2011) identified 42 different speech sound disorder treatment approaches with varying quantities and levels of evidence; they recommend increased publication of rigorous and well-designed comparative studies.

- Specific treatment programs include the traditional, concurrent, cycles, contrast, complexity, stimulability, core vocabulary, and naturalistic speech intervention approaches.

- Currently, controversies surround language-based intervention treatment approaches and nonspeech oral–motor exercises.

- Specific program components sometimes contradict each other.

- The **traditional approach**, sometimes called the **motor-based approach**, has a long history in the field of speech–language pathology, since the early 1900s, and is most often associated with Charles Van Riper. Its hallmark is a hierarchical progression through five major phases: sensory–perceptual training or ear training, production training for sound establishment, production training for sound stabilization, transfer and carry-over training, and maintenance of the learned behaviors. Its basic framework of treatment has stood the test of time, although some components, specifically sensory–perceptual training, are now considered nonessential due to lack of empirical support.

- The **concurrent treatment approach** is a newer approach that challenges the traditional organization of treatment from simple to complex tasks. Instead, it uses a randomized, variable, and concurrent practice of target sound(s) at various response complexity levels. The effectiveness of this method has been studied under well-controlled experimental conditions that have resulted in positive treatment outcomes and have been replicated with various disorders, age groups, and treatment settings. Studies clearly describe the treatment methods.

- Hodson and Paden (1983, 1991) advanced a speech sound production program that combines linguistic and motor-oriented methods of remediation. Now known as the **cycles approach**, it uses sound awareness training, production training, and semantic awareness contrasts (minimal pairs) to establish target stimulable phonological skills. The remediation is planned around cycles as opposed to a specific mastery criterion. A **modified cycles approach** was developed by Tyler et al. (1987). Experimental studies evaluating the independent effectiveness of the many components included in the cycles approach have yet to be advanced and are a primary weakness of the approach.

- The varied **phonological contrast approaches** include the *minimal pair intervention method, maximal contrast method, multiple contrasts method,* and the *empty set.* These approaches have gained wide acceptance and clinical implementation. Contrast treatment approaches are some of the most systematically investigated methods of speech sound disorder treatment.

- The classic version of the **minimal pair intervention method** requires the use of word pairs that contrast the child's typical (error) production and the target production (single feature contrast). It may include perceptual plus production training or simply production training. To date, there is no compelling evidence to support perceptual training, so that step is often omitted.

- In the **maximal contrast method**, also known as **maximal opposition**, the minimal word pairs selected for phonological treatment have multiple feature contrasts. Contrasting word pairs may differ in manner, place, and voicing, in addition to other distinctive features. Rather than the child's errors, a sound the child produces correctly though it is maximally different from the error (target sound) is used for comparison with the target word.

- In the **multiple contrast method**, commonly known as the **multiple opposition method**, selection of a target sound for treatment is similar to that of the minimal pair approach but differs from it by creating minimal contrasting pairs for *all* or most of the errors and training them simultaneously.

- In the **empty set**, two error (target) sounds that are maximally opposed are selected for training in contrasting word pairs.

- The **complexity approach** focuses on *what* is targeted rather than *how* it is targeted. It is a speech production–oriented approach that has assembled strong empirical support and repeatedly demonstrated that more complex linguistic input (e.g., nonstimulable sounds, consistently erred sounds, later developing sounds) promotes greater generalization. Complex targets may be taught in a contrasting or noncontrasting format.

- Miccio and Elbert (1996) developed a speech sound disorder treatment program that focuses on enhancing the stimulability of nonstimulable sounds, aptly called the **stimulability approach**. The primary goal of this approach is to increase the child's phonetic inventory by establishing motor production of all nonstimulable error sounds. This approach lacks strong empirical support and is based mostly on case studies.

- The **core vocabulary approach** is an intervention method that seeks to establish consistent word production in children with moderate to severe speech sound disorders who display inconsistent production of words across three temporally separated attempts. Poor consistency in word production may affect the child's speech intelligibility. This approach lacks strong empirical support, and experimental studies evaluating its effectiveness are currently limited to one.

- Camarata (1993, 1995) recommends his **naturalistic speech intervention approach** to help improve a child's overall intelligibility and speech sound accuracy using a two-tier approach. This program uses **natural recasts** (corrective feedback given to the child in a naturalistic fashion without requiring the child to imitate the adult model). Experimental research evaluating the effectiveness of this approach is currently limited.

- **Language-based** speech sound production treatment approaches have produced inconsistent research data. It is unclear from evidence accrued so far that it is more efficacious to treat phonological skills indirectly than it is to treat them directly. In routine clinical practice of children who have language and phonological disorders, both kinds of skills may be simultaneously targeted (e.g., plurals and final /s/ or final clusters, regular past tense and final /t/ and /d/).

- According to current research, the use of **nonspeech oral–motor exercises** for the treatment of speech sound production skills across various disorders such as functional articulation disorder, phonological disorder, childhood apraxia of speech, dysarthria, and cleft palate is considered unnecessary and against best practice. The burden is on its proponents to offer strong experimental research to justify the use of such exercises.

PHONOLOGICAL AWARENESS
AND SPEECH SOUND DISORDERS

Write to be understood, speak to be heard, read to grow . . .
—*Lawrence Clark Powell*

A phonological phenomenon during the early elementary school years that has received much attention in recent years is *phonological* or *phonemic awareness* (J. L. Anthony & Francis, 2005; Gillon, 2004; Goswami & Bryant, 1990; Stackhouse, 1997). The concept was developed in the 1970s by L. Y. Liberman (1973) and quickly became one of the most researched constructs related to literacy skills; currently, more than a thousand studies are available on phonological awareness and related topics.

Phonological awareness (PA) refers to a child's knowledge that words are created from sounds and sound combinations; it is a knowledge of phonemes, phoneme onset and rime, syllables, and the occurrence of rhyme. It may also be thought of as a child's knowledge of *underlying sound representations* in the mind. In the vast literature on this topic, the reader may come across the term *phonemic awareness*, which can refer to a subskill of phonological awareness. Phonemic awareness is a child's recognition of individual phonemes and their role in forming different words. Another term in currency is *phonological processing*; this term means the same as phonological awareness, except that the orientation seems to be cognitive, with an emphasis on cognitive processes involved in understanding and analyzing sounds, syllables, rhymes, and word structures. Yet another term frequently used is *sensitivity to sounds and word structures*; this term means the same as *phonological awareness* (J. L. Anthony & Francis, 2005; Lonigan, Burgess, Anthony, & Barker, 1998). We use the expression phonological awareness in this chapter as the general term and the term *phonemic awareness* when referring specifically to that subskill.

A child with good PA, for example, could identify that the first sound in the word *bat* is /b/ and the last sound in the word *stop* is /p/. In essence, the child can break down the word and analyze its individual components. Robertson and Salter (1997) describe PA as "the knowledge of meaningful sounds, or phonemes, in our language and how those sounds blend together to form syllables, words, phrases, and sentences" (p. 5). In other words, PA is the awareness of the sound structures of spoken words (Gillon, 2004). At the skill level, PA refers to a speaker's recognition, discrimination, and manipulation of sounds (J. L. Anthony & Francis, 2005).

Although we have given some general definitions of PA in the previous paragraph, there is much controversy about its precise definition. There is plenty of disagreement as to what specific skills represent PA (J. L. Anthony & Lonigan, 2004). Some include all sub-syllabic skills (phonemic and onset–rime skills) in their definition, and some include only phoneme-level skills (Morais, 1991a). Still others include everything—subsyllabic-, syl-labic-, and word-related skills (Goswami & Bryant, 1990). Opinions differ on the relation-ship between different kinds of phonological awareness skills (PAS). Some believe that they are interrelated; others believe that at least some of the skills are independent (e.g., rhyme awareness and phonemic awareness) (Yopp, 1988). J. L. Anthony and Lonigan (2004), after a careful reanalysis of the results of four relatively large studies on the development of PA, concluded that PA is either a collection of related skills or the same skill measured differ-ently. They also concluded that it is a skill related to reading and spelling.

....

ACTIVITY

Briefly describe the different names given to phonological awareness; of those different names, which ones can be distinguished from each other?

....

Phonological awareness may be a part of the child's metalinguistic skills. *Metalinguistics* refers to an analysis of language, obviously through language itself. Metalinguistic skills would be an individual's ability to analyze, think about, talk about, and write about lan-guage. *Metaphonological* refers more specifically to the metalinguistics of phonology—that is, being able to talk about, describe, and analyze phonological aspects of one's language.

Our review of research suggests that the relevance of PA for speech sound disorders has been overstated. Therefore, we offer only a limited discussion of PA in this book, be-cause of the following arguments:

• PA is more relevant to language and literacy skills than to typical or impaired speech sound production skills (J. L. Anthony & Lonigan, 2004; Carroll, Snowling, Hulme, & Stevenson, 2003; Lonigan et al., 1998; Morais, 1991b). Phonological impair-ment alone is not predictive of literacy impairment (R. L. Peterson, Pennington, Shrib-erg, & Boada, 2009; Raitano, Pennington, Tunick, Boada, & Shriberg, 2004). That PA is more relevant to literacy skills means only, in our view, that the two form a single set of skills, not that PA is the cause of literacy skills. A child's "knowledge" of sounds in words (phonemic awareness) is part of, not a cause of or a precursor to, successful reading, for example. A child may be taught either to identify sounds in words or to read words. The latter strategy is more effective and economical. Incidentally, direct literacy training may also teach the child that words are made of sounds and sounds may be manipulated to change words.

• Not all children with pure speech sound disorders have a significant deficit in PA (Rvachew, Chiang, & Evans, 2007).

• Routine assessment and treatment of PA in children with speech sound disorders is not essential (Keilmann & Wintermeyer, 2008). It is not at all clear in what kinds of special cases it may be justified.

• PA treatment is offered to improve reading and other literacy skills, not to im-prove speech sound production skills or language skills. However, critical reviewers have concluded that there may be some positive findings, though little conclusive evidence, that

PA interventions "enable students to catch up in phonological or reading skills to typically developing peers" (Al Otaiba, Puranik, Zilkowski, & Curran, 2009, p. 107).

- Even though children with severe SSDs exhibit PA deficiencies, the treatment priority is intervention for speech sound production. PA treatment by itself does not correct speech sound errors. After PA treatment, the clinician may have the same job of treating the production of speech sounds. It is efficient and economical to move directly and quickly to teaching speech sound productions.

- In children who have a coexisting SSD and language disorder, PA intervention is a part of language–literacy intervention, not SSD intervention. As noted before, even in such cases, it may be more efficient to directly teach reading and writing skills rather than presumed "underlying skills" such as PA.

We will elaborate on some of these observations in the coming sections. Clinicians can gain additional information on PA in various language- and literacy-related writings, as well as sources dedicated to the topic (e.g., Gillon, 2004; Justice, 2006; Pence, 2007; Stahl & McKenna, 2006; Torgesen & Mathes, 2000).

Observable Skills of Phonological Awareness

Phonological awareness, phonemic awareness, phonological or phonemic sensitivity, and phonological processing are not operational (measurable) concepts; they cannot be directly observed or measured. Phonological representation, which is assumed to underlie these phenomena, also is not observable. These variously named phenomena refer to mental entities, and these mental entities are inferred from children's skills that may be observed and measured (Anthony, Lonigan, Burgess, Driscoll, & Phillips, 2002). The skills believed to indicate these inferred entities are grouped into three main classes:

1. *Rhyme awareness*—This is thought to be the awareness of words that do and do not rhyme. Specific skills that represent this awareness include correct identification of words that sound alike (rhyme; e.g., *hat*, *mat*, *cat*), producing words that rhyme with the stimulus word (e.g., the clinician says, "Tell me words that rhymes with *hat*"), and sorting out rhyming words from nonrhyming words (also described as *rhyme oddity*). When children begin to break the words into single or groups of sounds that rhyme or do not rhyme, they are believed to also recognize the syllable *onset* and *rime* distinction, described next.

2. *Syllable awareness*—This is thought to be the awareness that words are made up of syllables and that syllables in words may be divided or counted. A child may verbally count the syllables in stimulus words or may tap or clap once for each syllable in spoken words. Syllables also may be divided into onset and rime units. The *onset* portion of a syllable is the single consonant or consonant cluster that launches it; the onset typically precedes a vowel. The vowel plus the succeeding consonant that follows it make up the *rime* unit in a syllable. Not all English syllables have an onset; those that begin with a vowel (e.g., *in* or *at*) do not have an onset (which has to be the initial consonant or consonant cluster). All English syllables have a rime unit. The child who can isolate the initial

consonants and the following vowels and consonants is said to have onset–rime knowledge. Note the difference between *rhyme* (the same sound shared by two words—e.g., *cat* and *hat*) and *rime* (the vowel–consonant unit that follows the initial onset consonant or consonants in a syllable). Generally, rhyming words have a different onset (initial consonant or consonant cluster) but the same rime. The different initial sounds in *cat* and *hat* end in the same rime, *at* in both words. Thus, *at* in both words may be described as rime as well as rhyme; for that reason, the words *rime* and *rhyme* are sometimes used synonymously, or confused.

3. *Phoneme awareness*—Also called *phonemic awareness*, this is thought to be the awareness of individual phonemes in words. This awareness is indicated by such skills as pointing to or saying successive words that begin with the same sound (*alliteration*, as in *big brown bear*); naming the sound at the beginning, end, or middle of a word (*phoneme isolation*); blending two or more sounds that are temporally separated by a few seconds into a word (*phoneme blending)*; breaking down a word into its individual sound components (*phoneme segmentation*); changing a phoneme in a word to change the word itself (*phoneme manipulation*); and altering a word by omitting a sound in it (*phoneme elision or deletion*).

....

ACTIVITY

Compare and contrast the three major kinds of phonological awareness.

....

Print awareness is another skill often discussed in the context of phonological awareness and literacy. It refers to the early literacy skill of naming the letters of the alphabet. We have not included a discussion of this skill mainly because it is even more directly related to reading than the other skills described in this chapter.

PA is inferred from many other kinds of skills. We sample them in the section "Assessing Phonological Awareness" later in this chapter. Skills that index PA are interrelated. For instance, various skills listed under phoneme awareness (e.g., phoneme blending, manipulation, and segmentation) may be related. As noted, rhyme and syllable awareness are also interrelated. Nonetheless, their complexity varies, and the ages at which the two sets of skills are mastered vary; their acquisition rates may also differ. Some investigators believe that all individual skills described so far are so close to each other that PA is actually a single skill set, as described in a later section entitled "Phonological Awareness as a Unitary Skill."

Phonological Awareness Skill Learning

A general learning pattern is that children initially master larger phonological awareness skill components (such as word and syllable discrimination) and progressively become skillful in identifying and manipulating smaller units (such as onsets, rimes, and phonemes). Children become aware of words, syllables, and phonemes in that order (Lonigan et al., 1998; Lonigan, Anthony, Phillips, Purpura, & Wilson, 2009; Melby-Lervag, Lyster, &

Hulme, 2012; Robertson & Salter, 1995; Treiman & Zukowski, 1996). Another pattern is that children can discriminate between words that sound different or similar before they can manipulate individual sounds within words. In other words, rhyme recognition is learned before phoneme recognition or manipulation (Carroll et al., 2003; Gillon, 2004). Sound blending may be learned sooner than sound segmentation. Instead of moving through categorical stages of learning, children seem to acquire higher complexity skills while still getting better at lower complexity skills (J. L. Anthony & Francis, 2005).

Regardless of their oral language skills, children from middle- to upper-income families may have better PAS than those from lower-income families. Most studies have not reported a significant difference in PAS between boys and girls (Gillon, 2004). Variability in performance on phonological awareness tasks is generally very marked until age 4. Skills begin to stabilize after that age.

Cross-linguistic studies have identified some common general trends in the acquisition of PAS. For instance, Spanish-speaking children also learn such PAS as rhyme, alliteration, and syllable identification sooner than phoneme segmentation and manipulation; the latter skills are more likely to be learned only after explicit literacy instruction (Carillo, 1994; Gonzalez & Garcia, 1995).

Second-language learners of English (L2) with a primary home language (L1) may gain PAS proficiency that is comparable to that of primary English learners after only 1 year of schooling. For instance, studies on 6- and 7-year-old bilingual children speaking Punjabi (L1) and English (L2) or French (L1) and English (L2) have reported English PAS that are comparable to the skills of native English-speaking children (Chaippe & Siegel, 1999; Comeau, Cormier, Grandmaison, & Lacroix, 1999). In all children, better reading skills were correlated with better PAS.

Child's Language Characteristics Influence PAS Learning

Although general patterns of learning are evident, there are individual differences within and across languages. This suggests that each child's language and home environment have an effect on the acquisition of PAS. It is now clear from developmental research that the nature of the ambient language affects the rate at which a child acquires PAS. Syllable-related PAS are acquired sooner when syllables in the child's language are highly salient, compared to a language in which syllables are less salient. Compared to the English or French language, for example, Turkish, Greek, and Italian have better-defined syllable boundaries, simple syllable structures, and fewer vowels. Children speaking the latter languages are known to acquire syllable structure awareness skills sooner than those who speak English or French. Another language feature that might influence specific PAS is the number of onset consonant clusters in the child's language. For example, English has only 31 onset clusters, whereas Czech has 258. Consequently, English-speaking children identify single-consonant onsets at an earlier age than Czech children, who identify consonant cluster onsets at an earlier age. In essence, frequency of usage in the language helps develop PAS. Most every other phonological awareness skill studied cross-linguistically has shown this differential influence of the child's language skills, dispelling any notion of an innate phonological awareness. See J. L. Anthony and Francis (2005) for a review of studies related to these observations.

Another language-related variable is the **grapheme–phoneme consistency**, which varies across languages. An individual letter of a printed alphabet is called a **grapheme**. The alphabetic letters (graphemes) of some languages are more phonetic than others; more phonetic alphabets better represent speech sounds. In essence, the greater the grapheme–phoneme consistency, the lower the pronunciation confusion. The German alphabet, for example, is more phonetic, with greater grapheme–phoneme consistency, than the English alphabet, which does not well represent the English phonemes. Consequently, German-speaking children in their first year of schooling have better PAS than English-speaking children. If children speaking a language with poor letter–sound correspondence and low PAS begin to learn another language with a better correspondence, their PAS improves rapidly (DeJong & VanDerLeij, 2003; Durgunoglu & Oney, 1999). J. L. Anthony and Francis (2005) report that even literate adults may have difficulty with certain aspects of PAS, suggesting once again that PAS is not a prerequisite for literacy and oral language proficiency. Although preschoolers who can recognize phonemes and rhyming words have an advantage in learning to read and write, children and adults can be highly literate and verbally competent without being skillful in syllabification or onset–rime recognition.

Children generally are better able to identify or manipulate sounds in the initial and final positions in clusters than those in the medial position. PAS that help identify voice and voiceless features seem to be more difficult than identifying manner differences. PAS regarding more easily produced sounds (e.g., glides and nasals) may be more advanced at given ages than those related to obstruents (Treiman, Broderick, Tincoff, & Rodriguez, 1998).

Children whose language skills are advanced also have better PAS than those whose language skills are average or below average. For example, children who have a larger receptive or expressive vocabulary also exhibit better large-segment (syllable and word) PAS (Carroll et al., 2003).

Literacy Instruction Accelerates PAS

The claim that PAS is more closely related to reading and writing than to speech sound production is supported by the PAS learning literature. With exposure to spoken language, children learn only minimal and simpler PAS. Because of coarticulation effects, syllables and phonemes are not as explicit in running speech as they are in literacy instruction. Explicit reading and writing lessons, on the other hand, include information on syllables, words, and sounds and sound changes that create rhymes or change parts of words. Therefore, it is the written language instruction that accelerates the learning of PAS. When children learn to name the letters of the alphabet and the sounds they represent, their PAS improves significantly (Lonigan et al., 2009; Melby-Lervag et al., 2012).

The observation that exposure to oral language to some extent and explicit literacy instruction to a greater degree are related to PAS acquisition raises questions about the usual claim that PA is an underlying skill of literacy. PA is most likely a consequence of language experience—the initial implicit and subsequent formal instruction. It is unlikely that PA is a cause of anything; probably it is a consequence of having acquired language skills. Additional support for this interpretation comes from observations cited earlier: Children with higher language skills have higher PAS; presumably these children never had any direct PAS intervention. An important implication for SLPs is that it is better to teach speech sound production to children with SSD, language skills to children with language impairment, and direct literacy skills (reading and writing) to all children. If this is done well, PA might take care of itself. We will return to this issue in the section "Critical Evaluation of Phonological Awareness Intervention" later in the chapter.

Rhyme Recognition Skills Are Learned Relatively Early

Factor analysis has revealed that rhyme and syllable recognition skills are actually part of larger unit awareness compared to awareness of smaller units such as phonemes. Word and syllable recognition and rhyme awareness are related skills. Rhyme awareness scores are correlated with speech perception (receptive language skills) and short-term memory measures. Rhyme awareness is especially highly correlated with a child's vocabulary (Lonigan et al., 2009).

Generally, kindergarten children do well in rhyming words, identifying the number of syllables in words, blending syllables into words, and segmenting words into syllables (Robertson & Salter, 1995). Children in the age range of 2 to 3 years begin to understand words as discrete units of language. About 41% of children as young as 2 years may recognize two words that rhyme in a set of three (e.g., *fish*, *dish*, *book*) (Carroll et al., 2003; Lonigan et al., 1998). In one study, 61% of 3-year-olds correctly judged whether two words rhymed, and 35% of the same children suggested one rhyming word (Chaney, 1992). Similarly, most 3-year-olds begin to show a sense of alliteration (skill in telling which words share a phoneme in the initial, medial, or final word position), although they are more adept at identifying the initial phonemes in words.

A nonverbal response to rhyming stimuli can be observed in some 2-year-old children. For example, they may clap to rhythm. At the verbal level, *rhyme matching* may be observed in some 2-year-old children, as well. In this task, the child is asked which two of the three words presented rhyme (e.g., the clinician asks, "Which word rhymes with *cat—hat* or *ball*?"). Children in the age range of 2 to 3 years may match rhyming words with about 52% accuracy and increase to 70% accuracy between 4 and 5 years of age (Lonigan et al., 2009).

Detecting *rhyme oddity* seems to be a slightly more difficult task. The child has to specify which of the three presented words does not rhyme (e.g., "Which word does not rhyme—*cat, hat,* or *ball*?"). Accuracy for this rhyme oddity task is 38% for 2- to 3-year-olds and 48% for 4- to 5-year-olds. While 75% of 5-year-old children from middle-income families may be accurate in detecting rhyme oddity, less than 50% of children from low-income families may be accurate on this task. *Rhyme production*, saying words that rhyme with given target words (e.g., responding to such statements as "Tell me some words that rhyme with *cat*"), is an even more complex skill. Accuracy in producing at least one rhyming word for this task is only 35% at the age of 3 years (Carroll et al., 2003; Chaney, 1992; Lonigan et al., 1998).

Some investigators believe that rhyme recognition is not as strongly related to later reading and writing skills as phoneme recognition is. It is likely that rhyme recognition promotes phoneme recognition skills (Gillon, 2004). If so, rhyme recognition has an indirect contribution to later literacy skills. A different view that is gaining support is that all PAS are related to reading and writing because PAS is a unitary concept (J. L. Anthony et al., 2002; J. L. Anthony & Lonigan, 2004).

Syllable Recognition Skills Are Learned Relatively Late

Describing the number of syllables in a word and identifying the syllabic components of words are relatively easy for children. Although not as easy as clapping to rhythmic stimuli, these tasks are easier than phoneme segmentation. The simplest task in this category is to ask the child, "How many syllables are in the word *daddy*?" Fifty percent of 4-year-olds and 90% of 5-year-olds may correctly respond to such a question (J. L. Anthony & Francis, 2005). Four- to 5-year-olds may divide multisyllabic words into their components. For instance, they may separate *bat* and *man* in *batman*. At this level, children may not specify phonemes in syllables or manipulate them to change syllable structures.

Additional syllable recognition skills are intertwined with phoneme recognition skills. For example, syllable onset and rime recognition skills seem to interact with phoneme recognition skills. It is only when the phoneme recognition skill has improved that a child correctly segments syllables into their onset and rime components. Children are initially more successful at recognizing syllable onset and rime in singletons than in consonant clusters (Treiman & Zukowski, 1996).

There is limited research on the development of syllable recognition skills, as well as their relation to later literacy skills. Some investigators believe that syllable-level skills are not as good as phoneme-level skills in predicting later reading and writing skills (e.g., Muter, Hulme, Snowling, & Taylor, 1997). Others believe that PAS is a single factor and, therefore, all skill components are related to reading and writing (J. L. Anthony et al., 2002; J. L. Anthony & Lonigan, 2002). As described in a later section, "Phonological Awareness as a Unitary Skill," this latter view has been gaining strength through factor analysis of multiple study results.

Phoneme Recognition Skills Are Learned Last

Children do not demonstrate a clear awareness of phonemes until age 6 or 7 (E. W. Ball, 1993). Between 6 and 10 years of age, children learn to segment phonemes in a word (i.e., name individual phonemes in a word) and synthesize given phonemes into meaningful words. These two skills are called *phoneme segmentation* and *phonemic synthesis*, respectively. Most studies have concluded that this small-unit awareness follows the large-unit awareness of syllables and words (Carroll et al., 2003).

Children from upper-income levels may exhibit some level of phonemic awareness at a slightly earlier age than children from more disadvantaged backgrounds. Lonigan et al. (1998) reported that 5-year-old children from upper-income levels were able to correctly perform at least one phoneme deletion task. Data also suggest that children may learn phoneme blending earlier than phoneme elision (deletion) (Lonigan et al., 2009). Children learn to segment phonemes in words with no clusters earlier than words with clusters. Alliteration recognition is a skill that takes longer to learn. Some 2-year-olds may exhibit the skill, but even 5-year-olds perform it with only 50% accuracy (chance level).

Phoneme recognition skills improve significantly with literacy instruction. Generally, preschool children and nonreaders have difficulty with phoneme manipulation, segmentation, and deletion, although they may recognize some word-initial phonemes. Children with dyslexia score poorly on PAS. Similarly, illiterate adults also have difficulty with phoneme awareness tasks (Melby-Lervag et al., 2012). Learning to read, especially learning to spell, tends to improve phonemic awareness skills. This may be because in learning to spell words, children become more proficient in isolating sounds and letters in words, as well as in the alphabet.

Studies have consistently shown that phoneme-level skills are strong predictors of reading and writing. A child's skill in analyzing and breaking down words into their phonological components has been correlated with the acquisition of early reading skills (Catts, 1993; Robertson & Salter, 1997; Stackhouse, 1997; Swank, 1994; van Kleeck, 1995). In their meta-analysis of 235 studies, Melby-Lervag et al. (2012) showed that phoneme awareness scores are more highly correlated with later reading skills than rime awareness measures are. The authors caution that because the studies typically used the correlational research design, it is difficult to draw cause–effect relations. Reported data cannot rule out either one as the cause of the other: Preliteracy phonemic awareness skills, rudimentary in general, may be the cause or one of the causes of later reading skills. On the other hand, learning to read may be the cause of more sophisticated phonemic awareness skills. Another strong possibility is that there is no causal link between PAS and reading skills. Observed correlations between PAS and learning to read may be due to some other variable not measured. A sobering observation is that deaf children learn to read without phonemic awareness (Miller & Diane, 2011). Castles and Coltheart (2004), after a careful review of longitudinal and treatment studies on PAS and learning to read, concluded that "no study has provided unequivocal evidence that there is a causal link from competence in phonological awareness to success in reading and spelling acquisition" (p. 77). Yet another possibility also exists: Phonemic awareness (and other PAS) and reading skills may all be part of a single speech–language skill.

It should be evident that although some PAS are learned earlier than others, there are no discrete learning stages. The learning of different skills overlaps, and individual differences are significant. The clinician should consider individual differences in applying the general developmental trends just summarized. A preschool child whose home environment offered only a few literacy experiences, for example, cannot be expected to have the same phonological awareness skills as another child of the same age with extensive home literacy experiences.

....

ACTIVITY
Briefly describe the order in which major PA skills are learned.

....

Phonological Awareness as a Unitary Skill

Phonological awareness is typically operationalized as a set of distinct skills. Its division into three major sets of skills—rhyme, syllable, and phoneme awareness—with several subskills within each group, may give the impression that the skills are independent and that phonological awareness, sensitivity, knowledge, and processing are inferred from other skills. There is accumulating evidence that this may not be the case, that phonological awareness may constitute a single skill correlated with literacy skills (J. L. Anthony et al.,

2002). In other words, phonological awareness may be a unitary concept, as opposed to a collection of heterogeneous skills.

Factor analytic studies of PA skills in large numbers of children have demonstrated that multiple measures of phonological awareness are best explained as a single factor (see J. L. Anthony et al., 2002, and J. L. Anthony & Lonigan, 2002, for a comprehensive review of multiple studies). The reviewers of several comprehensive studies have concluded that although PA may be measured by tasks that involve detection, deletion, and blending at different levels of linguistic complexity (e.g., onset–rime, word, syllable, phoneme), these skills are not independent of each other. At different levels of linguistic development, children seem to present different skills; but it is likely the same skill, which increases in complexity. The apparent differences in the skills simply "reflect measurement artifacts" (J. L. Anthony et al., 2002, p. 87).

If PA is a single skill entity, correlated with reading and writing skills, it is plausible that it is part of literacy. All complex skills (such as reading and writing) are made up of simpler skills. Word-, syllable-, and phoneme-related skills might be simpler literacy skills learned earlier than reading and writing. Some of the PA skills (possibly rhyming and word recognition) can be implicitly learned with no specific instruction. Evidence suggests that complex PAS are related to advanced language skills, as well as formal literacy instruction (J. L. Anthony et al., 2002; J. L. Anthony & Lonigan, 2002). Therefore, it is likely that PA is simply a part of literacy, rather than something that is different from and thus related (correlated) to it.

Phonological Awareness and Speech Sound Production: Are They Related?

The relevance of PA to SSDs depends on a reliable and causal relationship between them. So far, the relationship found between PA and SSDs is correlational, not causative. All researchers recognize this, but many nonetheless imply a causal relation when they strongly recommend that clinicians and educators intervene to improve PA to improve speech sound production, language, and literacy skills. The assumption that an absence of PA is causally related to speech, language, and literacy skills forces the corollary that the same literacy skills in typical speakers are always caused by good PA. Do children with SSDs invariably have deficiencies in PA? Do typical speakers of all ages exhibit good PA?

Studies have reported positive correlations between severe phonological disorders in young children and poor phonological awareness (e.g., Bird & Bishop, 1992; Bird, Bishop, & Freeman, 1995; Carroll et al., 2003; Hodson, 1994, 1997; Dominick, Hodson, Coffman, & Wynne, 1993; Stackhouse, 1992; Webster & Plante, 1992). Children with language disorders who have concomitant phonological disorders also may exhibit poor phonological awareness skills (Bird & Bishop, 1992; Larrivee & Catts, 1999; Mann & Foy, 2003). Some studies have reported that poor phonological awareness skills in young children predict later problems in reading and spelling (e.g., E. W. Ball, 1993; Catts, 1991; Catts & Kamhi, 1986; Clarke-Klein & Hodson, 1995; Goldsworthy, 1996; Pratt & Brady, 1988; Stackhouse, 1997; Swank & Catts, 1994; J. Williams, 1984). In spite of such correlations, the relevance of PA to SSDs and typical speech sound production is unclear.

Phonological Awareness and Speech Sound Disorders

Evidence suggests that PA deficiencies and SSDs are not invariably associated. PA deficiencies in children who have a pure articulation disorder (no error patterns and reasonable intelligibility) may not be significant, and such children are not necessarily at risk for literacy problems (Catts, 1993). Two studies have found that phonological disorders do not predict later literacy skills in children (R. L. Peterson et al., 2009; Raitano et al., 2004), prompting the authors of this text to conclude that the presence of other deficits (e.g., language problems) is related to poor literacy. Any relation that exists between SSDs and PA is variable and inconsistent across children. For example, in their study on comparing phonological awareness therapy and speech production treatment for children, Hesketh, Adams, Nightingale, and Hall (2000) reported that some children with SSD had good PA; others had poor PA. They also reported that in their control group of typically developing children, some had good PA, and others had poor PA.

Additional support for the observation that a phonological disorder (PD) is not invariably associated with poor PA comes from a study by Rvachew (2007), in which 17 children with PD had low PA skills, but almost an equal number (16) had PD and good PA skills. These studies make it clear that PA skills may be good or deficient in children whose speech sound production skills are typical or atypical. Therefore, it is not possible to predict a child's PA from his or her speech sound production skills. This can only be interpreted to mean that PA skills and speech sound production skills are not systematically related in children.

There is accumulated evidence that SSDs may be treated effectively without teaching phonological awareness skills. Many single-subject experimental design studies have shown that such treatment procedures as instruction, modeling, demonstration of phonetic placement, and positive reinforcement and corrective feedback are effective in teaching correct production of speech sounds to children with SSDs. Treatment approaches that incorporate these behavioral methods (e.g., the contrast and complexity approaches; see Chapter 8) have been effective (Gierut, 1998). It is important to remember that many of these effective procedures do not include phonological awareness intervention (PAI).

Phonological Awareness in Typical Adult Speakers

Until recently, an ignored but important question was whether adults with typical or even superior speech–language skills have the level of PA proficiency that researchers have found in children with speech–language impairments. The outcome of nearly a dozen studies, reviewed by Brady et al. (2009), on phonological awareness and related skills of regular classroom teachers, as well as other people who specialize in literacy (reading and writing), has been disconcerting, though unsurprising upon some reflection. Results of those studies revealed that PA is generally low among classroom teachers, including experts in reading and writing. Concerned with this weak knowledge of PA among educators has led to the implementation of extensive professional development programs. An intensive program Brady et al. (2009) implemented to increase PA in teachers involved frequent classroom visits by PA experts over a period of an entire school year, plus a 2-day summer institute and monthly workshops. This program was successful in increasing teachers' PA. But the real intrigue is this: Why did the teachers need improved PA? Were they not able to teach reading and writing skills? If they had failed in teaching good reading and writing skills to their students, did the researchers first establish that it was due to a deficient PA? Perhaps even more important, had the teachers not acquired good reading and writing skills themselves, regardless of their low PA? One would assume that they had; if so, PA was unnecessary to learning good reading and writing skills. If PA was unnecessary to teachers, it should be so for their students. There should be a more direct path to first learning, and then teaching, reading and writing skills.

A study even more relevant to the present discussion was reported by Spencer, Schuele, Guillot, and Lee (2008). They assessed PA in SLPs and other educators with a paper-and-pencil measure on which the maximum score was 47. With a mean score of 37.34, SLPs outperformed other groups, but there still was room for improvement. The mean scores for the educators—kindergarten teachers, 29.47; first-grade teachers, 31.29; reading specialists, 30.62; and special education teachers, 29.05—suggested an even greater need for increasing PA. We raise the same questions about this study, however, as we have about the Brady et al. study, with two additional questions: Have SLPs not been effectively treating SSDs in children? Have they always taken the phonological awareness route to teach the correct production of speech sounds? Treatment efficacy research has clearly shown that speech sound disorders (including phonological error patterns) may be effectively remediated with no recourse to phonological awareness intervention (Gierut, 1998; see also Chapters 7 and 8).

ACTIVITY

Identify the implications, according to your thinking, of the finding that teachers and SLPs may need to improve their own phonological awareness.

Assessing Phonological Awareness

Phonological awareness may be assessed through standardized tests, criterion-referenced tools, such alternative procedures as dynamic assessment, and clinician-developed client-specific procedures. Several standardized tests that are dedicated to PA are now available. The major standardized tests are listed in Table 9.1.

Some language tests include subtests to assess PA. For instance, the *Clinical Evaluation of Language Fundamentals Preschool–Second Edition* (Wiig, Semel, & Secord, 2004) and the *Clinical Evaluation of Language Fundamentals–Fourth Edition* (Semel, Wiig, & Secord, 2003) include PA subtests. Such subtests are convenient to assess both language and PA in children.

Among the alternative assessment procedures, clinicians may consider **dynamic assessment** (Gutierrez-Clellen & Peña, 2001; Hegde & Pomaville, 2013) to find out how much assistance a child might need to demonstrate assessment targets. Dynamic assessment involves brief periods of intervention, if only in the form of graded prompts that might encourage correct responses from a child. One study (Spector, 1992) involved direct questions from the clinician to the child (e.g., "What is the first sound you hear in ____ [the target word]), then modeling (e.g., "Listen while I say the word slowly"), followed by

Table 9.1
PHONOLOGICAL AWARENESS ASSESSMENT INSTRUMENTS

Test	Skills Measured	Age or Grade Range
Comprehensive Test of Phonological Processing–Second Edition (Wagner, Torgesen, Rashotte, & Pearson, 2013)	Sound blending, matching, phoneme isolation, nonword segmenting, rapid naming	4 to 24 years, 11 months
Test of Phonological Awareness–Second Edition (Torgesen & Bryant, 2004)	Word-level phoneme identification in pictured stimuli	5 to 8 years
Pre-reading Inventory of Phonological Awareness (Dodd, Crosbie, McIntosh, Teitzel, & Ozanne, 2003)	Rhyme, sound and syllable segmentation, alliteration, sound isolation, letter–sound knowledge	4 to 6 years, 11 months
Phonological Awareness Test (Robertson & Salter, 2007)	Rhyming; invented spelling; phoneme deletion, blending, and manipulation	5 to 9 years
Test of Phonological Awareness Skills (Newcomer & Barenbaum, 2003)	Rhyming, incomplete words, sound sequencing, and sound deletion	5 to 10 years
Assessment of Sound Awareness and Production (Mattes, 1998)	Rhyming, isolating sounds in words, deleting sounds, replacing sounds in words, blending, identifying syllables	3 and up
Lindamood Auditory Conceptualization Test–Third Edition (Lindamood & Lindamood, 2004)	Phoneme discrimination and sound segmentation	5 to 18 years, 11 months
Test of Phonological Awareness in Spanish (Riccio et al., 2004)	Identifying initial and final sounds, rhyming, and deletion	4 years to 10 years, 11 months
Phonological Awareness Skills Program (Rosner, 1999)	Phoneme deletion from words and phoneme manipulation (substituting one phoneme for another)	4 to 10 years, 11 months

another question (e.g., "Can you tell me each sound in the word?"), and prompts ("There are two sounds in ____ [the target sound]), followed by a final question, "What are they?" The clinician also may ask the child to produce the sound sequence along with her. As can be seen from these examples, dynamic assessment goes beyond the typical assessment and offers modeling, prompts, and other forms of assistance to evoke the target responses. It may be noted that the authors of a recent study found that dynamic assessment offers no advantage when the child can perform tasks on more traditional assessment procedures (Kantor, Wagner, Torgesen, & Rashotte, 2011).

The clinician can also design **client-specific procedures** to evaluate individual children. In selecting stimulus materials and assessment procedures, the clinician should consult with the parents or caregivers and other professionals involved in the child's academic program such as reading specialists, resource specialists, and the regular education teacher. This approach will result in stimulus materials (e.g., words and pictures) that are especially relevant to the child, his or her family background, the home literacy environment, and academic demands placed on the child. While client-specific procedures are good for all children, they bear a special relevance to children of varied ethnocultural backgrounds for whom standardized tests of PA may be inappropriate. What follows is a brief outline of procedures the clinician may use in assessing the various elements of PA:

- *Rhyming*—the skill of identifying words that sound alike or rhyme
  - "Do the words *cat* and *hat* rhyme or sound alike?"
  - "Which word does not rhyme with the other words?"
  - "Tell me three words that rhyme with *hot*."
  - [The clinician selects pictures of words that rhyme and words that do not rhyme and places them in front of the child to sort.] "Put all the pictures whose names rhyme in one pile. Put the ones whose names don't rhyme in another pile."
- *Alliteration*—the skill of identifying words that begin or end with a certain sound
  - "Which words end with the /f/ sound?"
  - "Which words start with the /sh/ sound?"
  - "Does *bus* start with a /b/?"
  - "Tell me three words that start with /p/."
- *Phoneme isolation*—the skill of identifying whether a specific sound occurs in the beginning, end, or middle of a word
  - "Tell me if the /b/ is in the beginning, middle, or end of the word *bus*."
  - "What is the last sound in the word *pan*?"
- *Phoneme manipulation*—the skill of deleting, adding, or substituting a sound in a word to create other words
  - "What do you get if you take /h/ away from *hat*?"
  - "Say the word *man* without the /m/."
  - "Say *hit* without the last sound."
  - "Say *fat*. Now say *at*. What sound was left out on the second word?"
  - "Say *hat*. Now say it with a /b/ instead of an /h/ at the beginning."
- *Sound and syllable blending*—the skill of blending two or more sounds that are temporally separated by a few seconds into a word
  - "Listen carefully. What does *tea—cher* say?"
  - "Listen to me carefully. What does *h—a—t* say?"
- *Syllable and sound identification*—the skill of identifying the number of syllables or sounds in a word through clapping, finger tapping, or verbally stating it
  - "Tell me how many beats (syllables) there are in the word *hotdog*."
  - "Tell me how many sounds there are in the word *cat*."
- *Sound segmentation*—the skill of breaking down a word into its individual sound components

- ○ "What are the three sounds in the word *dog*?"
- ○ "What are the sounds in the word *house*?"

In analyzing and interpreting the assessment results, regardless of the procedure used, the clinician should take into consideration the speech sounds the child does not produce. For example, the child may not produce certain sounds in the word-initial and -final positions (initial or final consonant deletion). Obviously, when such missing sounds are the target sounds in PA assessment, the child may not give correct responses to such questions as "What is the first [or the last] sound in this word?" Similarly, a child might produce a single sound in place of many different sounds (e.g., /t/ for /g/ as in *tum* for *gum*, and /t/ for /k/ as in *tat* for *cat*). Unless error patterns are taken into consideration, responses may be misinterpreted. One way of minimizing misinterpretations is to evoke nonverbal tasks whenever possible from the child. For example, as described under "Rhyming" in the bulleted list above, the child can sort pictures of words that rhyme and separate them from pictures of those that do not rhyme.

....

ACTIVITY
Specify how a child's speech sound errors should be considered in assessing PA.

....

Teaching Phonological Awareness Skills

PA intervention (PAI) has been extensively researched in the context of literacy development and language impairments. The widely reported positive correlation between PA and later literacy skills (J. L. Anthony et al., 2002; J. L. Anthony & Lonigan, 2002) has generally been interpreted to mean that PA skills are prerequisites for literacy skills and, therefore, PAI is needed to promote literacy. An opposite interpretation is that PA, especially phoneme awareness skills, are a product of literacy instruction and, therefore, PAI is unnecessary; developmental data support this interpretation. As noted previously, children's PA accelerates when they begin to receive literacy instruction (see J. L. Anthony & Lonigan, 2002, and Melby-Lervag et al., 2012, for a review of studies).

Is PA causally linked to literacy skills? Castles and Coltheart (2004) critically reviewed studies on the hypothesized link between phonological awareness and success in learning to read. Based on an analysis of both longitudinal and experimental treatment studies, they concluded that "no study has provided unequivocal evidence that there is a causal link from competence in phonological awareness to success in reading and spelling acquisition" (p. 77). That there is a positive correlation between PA and literacy skills does not mean that the former is the cause of the latter. It does not mean that PA should be increased to promote literacy. Bus and van IJzendoorn (1999) made a meta-analysis of experimental training studies on the relation between early reading skills and phonological awareness skills and concluded that phonological awareness is not a sufficient condition for early reading.

As a consequence of the large amount of advocacy articles printed in speech–language pathology publications, SLPs seem to believe that (1) PAI is necessary to promote literacy skills; (2) it is effective in achieving that goal; and, therefore (3) it is an essential part of treatment for SSDs. Unfortunately, available evidence does not support any of these beliefs. There are many studies on PAI, possibly showing that PA can be improved when deficient (see Al Otaiba et al., 2009; Bus & van IJzendoorn, 1999; Melby-Lervag et al., 2012; Troia, 1999, for a comprehensive review of studies). A careful evaluation of the research, however, shows that the studies have significant methodological problems and have not demonstrated the superiority of PA over direct treatment of communication disorders or literacy skills.

The more straightforward view, based on research favorable to SLPs, is that it is better to teach speech sound productions, language skills, reading, and writing directly, instead of spending time on presumed underlying skills. Nonetheless, it may be minimally claimed by the investigators that it is *possible* to teach specific phonological awareness skills (Kirk & Gillon, 2007, among many others), although such a possibility is not a justification for teaching them, as we discuss in a later section, entitled "Critical Evaluation of Phonological Awareness Intervention."

Overview of Phonological Awareness Intervention

The detailed activities used to teach children PA are too numerous to summarize in this chapter. In general, clinicians design activities that help promote skills thought to be prerequisites for reading. These skills include rhyming, alliteration, sound and syllable blending, sound and syllable segmentation, phoneme isolation, phoneme identification, phoneme manipulation, and so forth. Parents can easily be trained to facilitate such basic skills as rhyming, syllable identification, and phoneme isolation in the home environment.

Those who advocate PAI suggest that the clinician follow a sequence of teaching such that children who enter the first grade will have attained most of the critical PA skills presumed to be needed to learn reading and writing skills. For instance, Schuele and Boudreau (2008) suggest the following graded sequence of targeting skills in PAI:

- **Preschool children** may be taught to match rhyming words, sort sounds in words, and segment words into syllables.
- **Early kindergarten children** may be taught to judge and match rhyming words, produce rhyming words upon request.
- **Middle kindergarten children** may be taught to match simple words that have the same initial and final sounds and segment sounds in similar word positions.
- **Late kindergarten children** may be taught to segment and blend more complex words (CV, VC, CVC words with two or three sounds).
- **Early first-grade children** may be taught to segment and blend words with sound clusters.

Once the target skills are selected for a child, clinicians can use the same procedure that they typically use to teach speech sound production. The clinician would develop stimulus materials to evoke the target skills, clearly identify the skills that the client is expected to learn, model the expected responses, provide reinforcing contingencies and corrective feedback, and arrange the sequence of training so that it progresses from simple to complex, as just summarized from Schuele and Boudreau (2008). Stimulus materials used in teaching PA skills include pictures that represent target words, printed words that rhyme, words that have the same and different sounds in initial and final positions, a range of words that vary in complexity (e.g., from simple single-syllable words to multisyllable words and words with sound clusters), appropriate reinforcers and forms of corrective feedback; see Chapter 7 for suggestions.

It is essential to establish a reliable baseline before starting intervention. The same stimulus items, words, and pictures may be used to establish baselines of rhyming skills, phoneme segmentation tasks, and any other targets selected for teaching. Teaching is initiated after base rates have been established.

Representative treatment methods are illustrated in several published studies and reviews (e.g., Denne, Langdown, Pring, & Roy, 2005; Gillon, 2000; Herbers, Paden, & Halle, 1999; Laing & Espeland, 2005; Schuele & Boudreau, 2008; Swanson, Hodson, & Schommer-Aikins, 2005). There is general agreement that active teaching with corrective feedback and positive reinforcement (sometimes described as *scaffolding*), are essential to teach the PA skills. The importance of initially modeling and gradually fading the modeled stimulus is highlighted by Wanzek, Dickson, Bursuck, and White (2000). We offer some suggestions for teaching selected PAS in the following lists.

Teaching **rhyming skills** may use the behavioral techniques known to be effective in teaching speech sound production skills (see Chapter 7 for details). Specific illustrations include the following (note that the clinician first describes each specific target skill):

- *Rhyme recognition*—Say, "Some words have the same sounds at the end. For example, the words *mom* and *Tom* end with the same sounds. We say that words that end with the same sounds rhyme. Now you tell me, do *Jen* and *Ben* rhyme?"

  - Praise the child for a correct response (e.g., say, "Very good—they do rhyme!"); give corrective feedback for an incorrect response (e.g., "They do rhyme; they both end with *en*, don't they?").

  - Present the next trial (with the same or different rhyming pairs).

  - Get at least three correct responses on each pair you present.

- *Rhyme and non-rhyme discrimination*—Say, "Some words rhyme, but others don't. For example, *cat* and *hat* rhyme, but *cat* and *dog* don't rhyme. Why don't they rhyme?" Praise or give corrective feedback. Then give a new exemplar (e.g., *bat* and *pillow*) and ask the child whether they rhyme. Praise or give corrective feedback. Present the next trial.

- *Rhyming word production*—Say, "When you know which words rhyme and which don't, you can think of many rhyming words. Tell me a word that rhymes with *ball*." Praise or give corrective feedback. The next possible steps are as follows:

  - Say, "Tell me which one does not rhyme: *tin, pin, ball*." Praise or give corrective feedback. Teach additional exemplars.

  - Say, "Tell me a word that does not rhyme with *ball*." Praise or give corrective feedback. Teach additional exemplars.

Teaching **phonemic awareness** follows similar steps of describing the specific skill, modeling it, asking the child to produce the skill, and providing a reinforcer or corrective feedback. Some examples follow:

- *Initial phoneme recognition*—Say, "Some words start with the same sounds; others start with different sounds. For example, *soup* and *soap* start with the same sound. Right?" Praise or give corrective feedback. Give repeated trials for similar and different initial sounds in words, as in the following examples:

  o Say, "Do *bud* and *bus* start with the same sound?" Praise or give corrective feedback. Repeat trials or give additional exemplars.

  o Say, "Do *Tom* and *Don* start with the same sound?" Praise or give corrective feedback. Repeat trials or give additional exemplars.

- *Final phoneme recognition*—Use the same procedure as in the previous target, with word-final phonemes as the target.

Teaching **phoneme manipulation skills** to children with SSDs may involve nonverbal responses to avoid errors in scoring their responses. The clinician may devise such nonverbal responses as manipulating alphabet blocks that would simulate phoneme manipulations. For example, the child may be asked to put together, in sequence, the alphabet blocks /m/, /o/, /m/ to create the word *mom*. Similarly, the child may be asked to add or remove letters (blocks) to teach various kinds of phoneme manipulation skills.

See Schuele and Boudreau (2008) for additional information on teaching a variety of phonological awareness skills. See also Torgesen and Mathes (2000) and Gillon (2004) for different treatment procedures.

ACTIVITY
Identify the general procedures you would use to teach PA.

Critical Evaluation of Phonological Awareness Intervention

Research supports the statement that it is possible to improve PAS in children who are deficient in them. Stronger claims must be evaluated carefully. There are a number of issues that SLPs treating SSDs need to consider. There is also a simple way of looking at this controversy; see Text Box 9.1.

SLPs treating SSDs first need to consider the nature of PAI. PAI is generally confounded with speech sound (or literacy) training. Some level of speech sound production training is inherent to it (Gillon, 2000; Herbers et al., 1999; Swanson et al., 2005). For instance, colored blocks that represent different phonemes can be used to teach *phoneme manipulation skills*. The child is asked to "show /p/ /p/"; the child is then asked to *say* /p/ /p/ and finally is asked to bring two blocks that represent the sound. To teach phoneme contrasts, the child may be asked to say and bring blocks that represent /p/ and /s/. In teaching correct identification of initial and final sounds in words, the clinician may ask, "Do *cat* and

---

Text Box 9.1. Flight from speech, language, and literacy teaching

What should we teach children with speech, language, and literacy problems? One would think that the answer is quite obvious: teach speech, language, and literacy skills. But many theoreticians suggest that that is not good enough. It is also necessary to teach some other skill, an underlying skill—generally a skill that hides behind the speech, language, and literacy skills. Many speech–language pathologists embrace this view. Instead of directly teaching the skills whose deficiency has triggered the diagnosis of a communication disorder, clinicians may target correlated, presumed to be underlying, theoretically suggested, behind-the-scene skills, hoping that somehow that will result in improved speech, language, and literacy skills. Phonological awareness intervention is one example of this trend. Nonspeech oral–motor exercises are another example.

Even before analyzing the research evidence, however, clinicians might ask themselves a simple question: Is it not more efficient to teach speech sound production than some other correlated skill to remediate speech sound disorders? Is it not more efficient to teach reading and writing than some other underlying skill? Many theoretically prompted target skills are a distraction from teaching speech, language, and literacy skills.

---

cow start with the same sound?" Before answering the question, the child is asked to *say* the two words first. Or the clinician might say, "The word *cat* starts with the /k/ sound. What is the sound that starts the word *cat*?" The child produces the /k/ sound (and may also say the word *cat*) and receives positive reinforcement (or corrective feedback if the response is incorrect) (Wanzek et al., 2000). Similarly, in sound segmentation treatment, the child is instructed to *say* the words slowly to separate the sounds (e.g., "b-a-r-n"). In linking speech sounds to print, the clinician may say, "Show me *at*," to which the child is asked first to respond by *saying* "at" and then putting the representative letter blocks in their correct order (Gillon, 2000). Any improvement in speech production skills, which have been reported in several studies on PAI, may actually be due to inherent speech training in those studies. The effect of speech sound production in PAI is less than remarkable because it is an indirect and inefficient method of teaching the correct production of speech sounds. Direct speech sound production training would be more effective and efficient in eliminating speech sound errors.

Second, SLPs need to consider that very few studies with experimental and control groups or single-subject experimental designs have established the actual effectiveness of PAI, rather than mere improvement under uncontrolled conditions. A few studies that did use a group experimental design have produced disappointing results. For example, Nancollis, Lawrie, and Dodd (2005) reported that preschool children who received training on phonological rhyme awareness and nonword spelling did not do as well as children in a control group who did not receive such training. When they assessed the treated children 2 years later, the awareness training had had little or no effect on later literacy development and may actually "have interfered with the acquisition of phoneme awareness" (p. 325). Hesketh et al. (2000) reported that children in the age range of 3-6 to 5-0 years who received either metaphonological treatment (mostly phonological awareness treatment) or regular articulation treatment did not differ in phonological awareness. Not surprisingly, the children who received articulation treatment had better articulation scores than those who received the awareness training. In their review of studies, Schuele and

Boudreau (2008) found that most studies report group findings, but that "some children have shown minimal growth after phonological awareness intervention" (p. 8). PA does not seem to respond to treatment as well as it is generally believed; again, as Schuele and Boudreau (2008) have pointed out, children with the lowest level of phonological awareness at base rate remain so after the treatment. Consequently, there is the typical call for either more or more intense PAI or a program of research to find out why PA does not improve with intervention as much as it should to facilitate literacy skills or speech sound production skills. There may be a simple explanation: PA is not useful in the everyday life of children or adults, and speech sound production and reading and writing are acquired without it; hence, PA is relatively insensitive to treatment.

Third, SLPs need to consider the conflicting evidence about the widely held belief that PAI and speech sound production (or literacy) have a reciprocal relationship—that is, that improvement in one will cause improvement in the other. Hesketh et al. (2000) found that children receiving exclusive "articulation therapy clearly received metaphonological [PA] benefit from it" and speech–language therapy improved PA; therefore, they wrote, "It does not appear that metaphonological therapy is necessary to achieve this improvement" (p. 347). On the contrary, a study by Herbers et al. (1999) has shown that speech production training may not always lead to phonological awareness, and one by Denne et al. (2005) has demonstrated that phonological awareness training does not necessarily improve speech production or literacy skills. Existing evidence suggests that PAI is an unnecessary exercise that takes valuable time away from direct speech–language treatment.

Fourth, studies on special populations cast serious doubts on the relation between PA and speech, language, and literacy skills. For instance, individual case studies have shown that precocious learners of reading may exhibit advanced literacy skills but little or no PA (e.g., Fletcher-Flinn & Thompson, 2000). Up to 3.5% of the population of young children learn to read or write precociously (Jackson, 1992); this means that many children do so without the benefit of PA. Another study has shown that children with Down syndrome who learn to read well may still score poorly on phonological awareness tests (Cossu, Rossini, & Marshall, 1993). Also, the reader may recall our earlier discussion of studies reporting deficient PA in teachers and special educators, including specialists in reading.

Fifth, the long-term effects of PAI are inadequately studied, and the available evidence is unimpressive. A study on oral language and PA intervention showed that the intervention was disappointing in producing long-term effects on language and literacy skills (Henning, McIntosh, Arnott, & Dodd, 2010). As noted previously, any positive effect reported, even on a short-term basis, may be confounded with speech sound or literacy instruction, because most treatment studies have simultaneously treated PA and literacy skills and then claimed that the offered treatment resulted in improved literacy skills (Gillon, 2000; Herbers et al., 1999; Swanson et al., 2005). Such results do not necessarily justify PAI. A treatment study by Keilmann and Wintermeyer (2008) in which 218 preschool children received specialized phonological awareness training reported that "a specialized training program to improve phonological awareness as a basis for reading and writing . . . seems to be unnecessary" (p. 73).

We do not believe that phonological awareness should be taught for its own sake. If taught, it should be as an aid for speech production or literacy skills. Negative evidence, as summarized, suggests that caution is needed in embracing phonological awareness training.

Several questions need to be answered before clinicians spend time on it: Is it possible to teach phonological awareness without involving speech production or literacy skills? If so, what is the effect of such training on speech production and literacy skills? Is it more or less effective to offer direct literacy skill training, without phonological awareness training, to improve literacy skills? Is it more or less effective to offer direct speech production training, without phonological awareness training, to improve speech production? If direct treatment can improve both speech production skills and literacy skills (especially reading), what is the need for phonological awareness training? Because available evidence does not clearly answer these questions, additional controlled and replicated research is needed to justify PAI.

Until better-controlled experimental studies produce contradictory evidence, we will continue to suggest that good speech production skills and literacy skills can exist with little or no PA. Intervention for PA may not lead to correct speech sound production or long-term literacy gains. Therefore, we conclude that children with SSDs should be taught speech production skills explicitly, and we agree with Cossu and colleagues' (1993) conclusion that "reading should be taught by teaching reading skills (including letter–sound correspondences), not phonological awareness skills" (p. 129).

....

ACTIVITY

Give two reasons you would teach phonological awareness skills. Give two reasons you would not teach phonological awareness skills.

....

Chapter Summary

- **Phonological awareness (PA)** is the knowledge that words are created from sounds and sound combinations; it refers to a set of skills in recognizing and manipulating the smaller units of words.

- PA is more relevant to language and literacy skills than to speech sound production and speech sound disorders (SSDs). Children with SSDs may have good or poor PA—so PA and SSDs are not systematically related.

- PA is inferred from a set of observable skills in recognizing, discriminating, and manipulating elements of words. These skills include *rhyme awareness*, *syllable awareness*, and *phoneme awareness.*

- **Rhyme awareness** refers to a child's skill in identifying words that do or do not rhyme. Rhyming words usually have different initial consonants (onset) but the same rime (vowels and consonants that follow).

- **Syllable awareness** is the skill of breaking words into syllables and counting the syllables in words. The skill of separating the onset from the rime is also a part of this awareness.

- **Phoneme awareness** refers to the skill of specifying individual sounds of words, deleting specific sounds in words, blending sounds temporally separated by the examiner, changing a phoneme to change the entire word, and so forth.

- Children recognize the larger units (words and syllables) before the smaller units (phonemes). Languages with prominent syllable boundaries and good grapheme–phoneme consistency, along with literacy instruction, have positive effects on PA learning.

- Rhyme recognition is learned before syllable recognition, and phoneme recognition is learned last. Evidence suggests that these are not independent skills but parts of a unitary skill.

- The relation between PA and SSDs is weak and perhaps not of much clinical significance. Children with SSDs may have high or low PA. Even teachers may have relatively low PA, suggesting PA is not necessary to acquire speech sound production or literacy skills.

- PAS may be assessed through standardized tests, dynamic assessment, and client-specific procedures.

- In analyzing the assessment data, the clinician should take into consideration the child's speech sound errors. If not, results may be misinterpreted.

- Intervention for PA is largely justified to promote better reading, writing, and spelling. No treatment evidence suggests that teaching PA is sufficient to eliminate SSDs; SSDs are eliminated only by teaching speech sound productions. Meta-analysis of many studies has concluded that PA intervention has not been shown to be effective in promoting literacy skills and that it is better to teach literacy skills directly.

GLOSSARY

abducted: Open, drawn apart; as in *abducted vocal folds*. See also *adducted*.

accessory nerve XI: Classified as a cranial nerve, it is both a cranial and a spinal nerve that supplies the muscles of the pharynx, soft palate, head, and shoulders.

acoustic: Pertaining to sound.

acoustics: A branch of phonetics that pertains to the study of the science of sound. It includes the study of the origin, transmission, modification, and effects of sound vibrations.

acoustic nerve VIII: See *vestibular acoustic nerve VIII*.

acoustic phonetics: A branch of phonetics dedicated to the study of the science of sound. See *acoustics*.

acoustic reflex: Reflexive contraction of the tensor tympani and the stapedius muscles triggered by loud sounds and noises.

ACT program: A program used in the treatment of childhood apraxia of speech that uses hand motions to prompt the articulatory movements and manner of production of the target productions.

Adam's apple: The lay term for the thyroid notch in the larynx.

adaptation: In articulation, the process by which sounds are affected by or take on the properties of other surrounding sounds. The perceptual property of the sound may be unaffected.

addition: A form of articulation error; a superfluous sound that does not belong in a word (e.g., in *biga* for *big*).

adducted: Closed or nearly closed, as in *adducted vocal folds*.

advanced word forms: Words used by a young child that have an advanced pronunciation in comparison to the rest of the child's phonological system. The use of such forms may disappear as the child's phonological system matures. Synonym: *progressive idioms*.

afferent: The flow of information toward the cell body.

affricates: A group of consonants with the characteristics of stops and fricatives.

age of customary production: The age at which approximately 50% of children produce a particular singleton sound.

age-equivalent: A type of standardized test score that is calculated based on the age that an average person earns a given score within the tested population.

age of mastery: The age at which approximately 90% of children produce a particular singleton sound.

air conduction: Sound traveling through the medium of the air; air-conducted sound reaches the cochlea through the outer and middle ear.

allographs: Different letters (alphabetic symbols) and letter combinations that can be used to represent the same sound (phoneme) in a specific language.

allophones: Variations of a phoneme.

allophonic variations: Articulatory or perceptual variations of the same phoneme, often caused by the sound's phonetic environment. Such variations do not change the meaning of a word.

alternating motion rates: Alternating repetitive movements of the tongue. Part of diadochokinetic testing by successive repetition of the same syllable sequence (e.g., /pʌ pʌ pʌ pʌ/, /tʌ tʌ tʌ tʌ/, and /kʌ kʌ kʌ kʌ/).

alveolar process: The outer edges of the maxillary bone (upper jaw) that house the molar, bicuspid, and cuspid teeth.

alveolar ridge: A ridge on the maxilla that overlies the roots of the teeth, most often located behind the upper anterior teeth. In most people it serves as the point of articulation for the English sounds /s/, /z/, /t/, /d/, /n/, /l/.

alveolar sounds: The consonant sounds /s/, /z/, /t/, /d/, /n/, /l/ made by placing the tongue against the alveolar ridge.

amplitude: Magnitude or range of movement of sound waves; the greater the amplitude, the louder the sound is perceived.

anatomy: Structure of an organism; the science pertaining to the structure of organisms.

aneurysm: Circumscribed dilation of an artery. Formed by a stretching of its walls; can be suggestive of a condition in which the weakened blood vessel may burst.

ankyloglossia: Limited movement of the tongue tip due to an abnormally short lingual frenulum; also known as a *tongue-tie*.

anoxia: Lack of or deficiency of oxygen, a potential cause of brain damage.

antecedent event: A stimulus presented before a target response is produced or attempted.

antecedent stimulus: A stimulus that precedes or accompanies a behavior and may exert discriminative control over that behavior.

anterior feature: Distinctive feature characteristic of sounds made in the front region of the mouth, generally at the alveolar ridge or forward. See also *distinctive features*.

anticipatory substitution: Sound substitution created by the coarticulatory effects of a sound that follows the target sound.

aperiodic: Sound vibrations (or other events) that do not repeat themselves at regular intervals; aperiodic sound is perceived noise.

aphasia: An acquired language disorder due to brain damage or disease; a variety of difficulties in formulating, expressing, and understanding language.

aphonia: Loss of voice.

applied phonetics: A branch of phonetics dedicated to the practical application of the knowledge gained from experimental, articulatory, acoustic, and perceptual phonetics.

apraxia: A disorder of sequenced movements of body parts in the absence of muscle weakness, incoordination, or paralysis; an acquired motor programming disorder. See also *oral apraxia*, *limb apraxia*, and *apraxia of speech*.

apraxia of speech: A sensorimotor disorder of speech, characterized by impaired ability to position the speech muscles and sequence the muscle movements (respiratory, laryngeal, and oral) necessary for volitional production of sounds and words.

approximants: Sounds produced by an "approximating" contact between the two articulators that form them; includes liquids and glides.

aprosody: Loss of the melody of speech (prosody). A less severe form is referred to as *dysprosody* (disordered prosody).

arresting sound: A consonant sound that closes a syllable.

articulation: In speech, movement of the speech mechanism to produce the sound of speech. One of the four basic processes involved in speech production.

articulation disorders: Problems in producing speech sounds.

articulator-bound features: Sound features produced by the action of a single articulator.

articulator-free features: Sound features produced by the actions of multiple articulators.

articulators: Organs of the speech production mechanism that help produce meaningful sound by interrupting the flow of exhaled air or by narrowing the space for its passage. The articulators include the lips, tongue, velum, jaw, hard palate, alveolar ridge, and teeth.

articulatory models: A model of speech production that seeks to explain only the articulatory speech movements.

articulatory phonetics: A branch of phonetics that focuses on how a speaker makes speech sounds; also termed *physiologic phonetics*.

arytenoid cartilages: Two small, pyramid-shaped cartilages capable of various kinds of movements; the vocal folds move accordingly because of their attachment to the arytenoids.

assessment: In articulation, the process followed and the procedures used to identify the presence or absence of an articulation or phonological disorder.

assimilation: The effect one speech sound has on another when produced in close sequence, such that the sounds become more like each other. The effect can be so extensive that it can be perceptually identified. See also *progressive assimilation* and *regressive assimilation*.

association fibers: Neural fibers that connect different parts of the brain within the two hemispheres.

ataxia: Disturbed balance and abnormal gait caused by damage to the cerebellum.

ataxic dysarthria: A motor speech disorder associated with ataxia. See also *dysarthria*.

athetosis: A neurological disorder characterized by slow, involuntary, writhing, and "wormlike" movements.

atrophy: Degeneration or wasting away of muscle, tissues, or organs. Muscular atrophy often occurs in paralysis.

audible nasal emission: Noise that can be heard of the air escaping through the nose.

audiogram: A graph that shows the results of various hearing tests.

audiologist: A specialist in the study of hearing and in the assessment and rehabilitation of hearing impairment.

audiology: The study and understanding of normal and disordered hearing and the rehabilitation of individuals with hearing loss.

audiological evaluation: Procedures used to measure hearing ability. Such procedures most often include but are not limited to pure-tone air- and bone-conduction thresholds; speech reception and discrimination scores; and discrimination of speech in the presence of noise.

audiological screening: A quick procedure performed to determine the need for further audiological evaluation. Testing is typically restricted to 500, 1,000, 2,000, and 4,000 Hz at 20–25 dB and performed in a quiet but not soundproof environment.

auditory bombardment: Procedure by which a child is provided with amplified auditory stimulation for a particular sound that is being taught.

auditory training: A rehabilitative process of training a person with hearing loss to listen to amplified sounds, recognize their meanings, and distinguish one sound from another.

aural rehabilitation: An educational process designed to improve the communicative abilities of a person with hearing loss; it includes auditory training, counseling, and speech–language therapy.

auricle: The most visible part of the outer ear, also known as the *pinna*.

automatic speech: Linguistic material often produced with minimal volitional control; may include such utterances as consecutive numbers, days of the week, expletives, verses, prayers, songs, and various kinds of common expressions.

autonomic nervous system: A system of nerves divided into sympathetic and parasympathetic branches that controls many involuntary functions of the body.

babbling: The playful vocal sounds that babies produce beginning at about 6 to 7 months of age.

back feature: A distinctive feature that characterizes sounds made in the back part of the oral cavity; the body of the tongue is retracted from the neutral position /ə/ during the production of sounds containing the back distinctive feature.

basal ganglia: Structures deep within the brain that help integrate motor impulses.

baselines: Measures of a child's target behaviors or treatment objectives before those behaviors are taught; they help the clinician establish client improvement, clinical effectiveness, and professional accountability.

base rating: The process followed by a clinician to obtain baseline measures of a child's target behaviors before those behaviors are taught. See also *baselines*.

basilar membrane: The floor of the cochlea, containing the organ of Corti and its several thousand hair cells that respond to sound.

behavioral approach: A treatment method that explicitly uses the principles and procedures of operant conditioning and learning.

behavioral principles: Concepts and procedures of operant conditioning and learning; frequently used in the treatment of communication disorders.

Bernoulli effect: Increased velocity and decreased pressure when gasses or liquids move through a constricted passage.

bifid uvula: A split uvula, suggesting that there may be a cleft underneath the tissue covering the palate.

bifurcation: Division or forking into two branches. The trachea bifurcates into two bronchi.

bilabial: Involving both lips; bilabial sounds are produced primarily by the two lips.

bilateral: On both sides, as in *bilateral cleft lip* or *bilateral hearing loss*.

bilingual: Of two languages; often refers to a person who speaks two languages.

binary classification system: A (+) and (–) value system that identifies whether a specific feature is present or absent in a sound. See also *distinctive features*.

blends: Two or more consonant sounds made next to each other with no vowel separation (e.g., /tr/, /pl/, /str/). See also *cluster*.

bone conduction: A process of conducting sound through bone vibrations.

booster treatment: A short period of intervention that may be necessary to reestablish previously trained skills that have diminished or regressed after initial dismissal from treatment.

bound morpheme: A morpheme that cannot convey meaning by itself; for example, the regular plural /s/ in the word cats. A bound morpheme is attached to a free morpheme for meaning.

brain stem: The collective term for the medulla, the pons, and the midbrain structures of the central nervous system.

breathiness: The voice quality that results when air escapes through partially open vocal folds.

broad phonetic transcription: The act of writing a phoneme into special phonetic symbols enclosed between virgules (slash marks); it can be interpreted only by someone familiar with the phonology of the language transcribed (e.g., /bot/ for *boat*; /ʃɪp/ for *ship*).

Broca's aphasia: Nonfluent, predominantly expressive aphasia. Associated with a lesion in the third frontal convolution of the dominant hemisphere. Characterized by problems with initiation of sound sequences in words and restricted grammar and vocabulary. Verbal output is often limited to expression of high-frequency content words. Auditory comprehension is relatively unaffected, allowing the individual to communicate information through yes–no or multiple-choice questions; writing is often affected.

Broca's area: A center for motor speech control within the frontal lobe of the language-dominant hemisphere in the brain.

bronchi: Primary divisions of the trachea that penetrate the lungs, one for the right lung and the other for the left lung; they serve to transport air to and from the lungs.

buccinator: A large, flat muscle that makes up most of the cheeks.

bulbar palsy: Paresis and atrophy of the muscles of the lips, tongue, mouth, and larynx as a result of lesions in the motor centers of the medulla oblongata.

canonical babbling: Infant vocalizations that include adult-like sounds and syllables; infraphonological stage 4.

carrier phrases: Short, repetitive phrases used as stimuli in speech sound production training as a transition level from words to sentences. Only a single word is changed as the target word exemplars are practiced in sequence. The child begins to predict the structure of the phrase and readily repeats it. Examples: "I see the [target exemplar]," "I want the [target exemplar]," "Can I have the [target exemplar]?"

carryover: The regular use of newly learned speech or language skills in everyday situations.

cartilage: Tough connective tissues, as in the thyroid cartilage, which is one of the cartilages of the larynx.

cavity: A hollow space within the body; a structure within the body containing other structures, as in the oral cavity, which contains the tongue, hard palate, soft palate, and so forth.

centering diphthongs: Diphthongs in which one of the stressed vowels combines with schwar /ɚ/. Synonym: *rhotic diphthongs.*

central nervous system: The brain and the spinal cord.

cerebellum: A structure below the brain and behind the brain stem that regulates equilibrium, body posture, and coordinated fine motor movements.

cerebral hemispheres: The two halves of the brain divided by the longitudinal or intrahemispheric fissure.

cerebral palsy: Brain damage suffered during infancy or the prenatal period and the resulting paralysis and problems of physical growth, locomotion, communication, and sensory issues.

cerebrospinal fluid: A clear fluid that surrounds and cushions the cerebrum.

cerebrum: The biggest of the central nervous system structures and the most important for speech, language, and hearing.

childhood apraxia of speech (CAS): A childhood motor speech disorder affecting the motor programming of the articulators; it primarily affects articulation and prosody. Also termed *developmental apraxia of speech* and *developmental verbal dyspraxia.*

chronic otitis media: The permanent rupture of the tympanic membrane with or without middle ear disease.

clarification request: A form of verbal corrective feedback that seeks to clarify the client's verbal output. At times, this type of feedback helps clients correct their own productions without additional feedback from the clinician.

Class I malocclusion: Misalignment of some individual teeth though the two arches are normally aligned.

Class II malocclusion: The upper jaw is protruded, and the lower jaw is retracted or receded.

Class III malocclusion: The upper jaw is receded, and the lower jaw is protruded.

cleft palate: Failure of the premaxilla to fuse with the maxillary bone and/or failure of the palatine process to fuse at the midline.

closed syllable: Vowel followed by a singleton consonant or consonant cluster.

closed-syllable word: A word that ends in a singleton consonant or consonant cluster (e.g., *pot, stop, must, last*).

closing interview: An interview conducted with the child's parents and relevant others involved in the child's life (e.g., teachers) in which the clinician presents the assessment findings and makes recommendations. Also known as *final interview.*

cluster: Two or more consonant sounds made next to each other with no vowel separation. See also *blends.*

cluster reduction: Omission of one or more consonants of a cluster (e.g., *top* for *stop*).

cluster simplification: Omission or substitution of one or more sound segments in a consonant cluster; can be considered a phonological process if it occurs frequently in a child's phonological system.

coarticulation: Articulatory movements for one phone that are carried over into the production of previous or subsequent phones; influence of one phone on another in perception or production.

cochlea: The main inner ear structure of hearing; it looks like the shell of a snail and is filled with a fluid called endolymph.

cochlear implant: An electronic device that is surgically placed in the cochlea and other parts of the ear of a deaf person and delivers the sound directly to the acoustic nerve endings in the cochlea.

coda: Consonant segment or consonant cluster that follows the nucleus (vowel or diphthong) of a syllable.

code switching: Changing from one language or dialect to another during a conversation.

cognates: Consonants produced in the same place and manner, except that one is voiceless and the other is voiced; in phonetic transcription they are typically written in pairs, with the voiceless sound given first (e.g., /p-b/, /wh-w/, /f-v/, /t-d/, /s-z/, /k-g/, /ʃ-ʒ/, /tʃ-dʒ/, /θ-ð/).

cognitive model of development: Theory proposing that children actively test hypotheses regarding phonological constraints and systems.

commissural fibers: The fibers that connect the two hemispheres of the brain.

communication: A form of social behavior; exchange of information.

communication board: An apparatus used by a person with limited verbal expression to communicate his or her needs, thoughts, and ideas. It may contain the letters of the alphabet, numbers, or commonly used words and phrases.

compensatory articulation: Correct or markedly improved production of sounds through unusual methods of articulation by a child with defective speech structures.

complementary distribution: Sounds that cannot be interchanged in a certain position; allophones that together cover all possible positional occurrences but do not appear in the same linguistic environment.

complete cleft of the palate: Total separation of the two palatal shelves of the hard palate.

complex tone: In acoustics, a sound wave characterized by combined pure tones; it has more than one pitch and contains components of different frequencies.

concurrent treatment: Simultaneous training of a target sound at different levels of response complexity.

conductive hearing loss: Diminished conductance of sound to the middle or inner ear due to the abnormalities of the external auditory canal, the eardrum, or the ossicular chain of the middle ear.

congenital: Present from birth but not necessarily genetic. See also *congenital disorder*.

congenital disorder: A disorder noticed at the time of birth or soon thereafter.

congenitally deaf: A condition of being born deaf.

connectionist model: A computer simulation model of speech production that emphasizes learning through environmental interactions and closely knit and interconnected neural networks.

consonant: A conventional speech sound made by certain movements of the articulatory muscles that alter, interrupt, or obstruct the expired airstream; defined according to manner of production, place of articulation, and voicing dimensions.

consonantal feature: A distinctive feature applied to sounds that have a marked constriction along the midline region of the vocal tract. Includes all consonant sounds except /h/, /w/, and /j/.

consonant deletion: A phonological process that describes the omission of initial or final consonants of words; a phonological problem. See also *final-consonant deletion* and *initial-consonant deletion*.

consonant harmony: An assimilation phonological process that affects manner of production or place of articulation; includes labial assimilation, velar assimilation, nasal assimilation, and alveolar assimilation.

consonant sequence reduction: The omission of one or more sound segments from two or more adjoining consonants.

constraints: Presumed limitations on sounds and sound patterns that are either allowed or prohibited in all and specific languages; a part of the nonlinear phonological theory, especially optimality theory.

contextual testing: A special assessment procedure that helps identify a facilitative phonetic context for correct production of a particular phoneme.

contextual training: A method of teaching speech sounds using contexts in which a target sound is correctly produced.

contiguous assimilation: A type of assimilation in which the affected sound and the sound that caused the change are adjacent to each other, with no interfering sound between them.

contingency priming: A procedure in which children in therapy are trained to prompt others to reinforce their own newly acquired behaviors.

continuant: Distinctive feature applied to sounds made with an incomplete point of constriction; flow of air is not entirely stopped. Continuant sounds are /w/, /f/, /v/, /θ/, /ð/, /s/, /z/, /l/, /ʃ/, /ʒ/, /j/, /r/.

contralateral: Refers to the opposite side, as in *contralateral motor control*. See also *ipsilateral*.

contrast therapy approach: A cognitive–linguistic approach to the treatment of articulation and phonological disorders; incorporates structured activities to increase awareness of the semantic distinction between the error production and the target.

conversational probe: A measure in which the clinician collects one or several conversational speech samples and then analyzes them for generalized responding of the trained target sounds or speech skills in untrained words, situations, response complexity levels, and so forth in the absence of any special prompting or reinforcement.

core vocabulary intervention (program): A speech sound intervention approach in which the child's inconsistent error productions are targeted for consistency training through a functional core vocabulary of approximately 70 words.

coronal feature: A distinctive feature used in reference to sounds made with the tongue blade raised above the neutral position required for the production of /ə/. Includes consonants /θ/, /ð/, /t/, /d/, /s/, /z/, /n/, /l/, /r/, /ʃ/, /ʒ/, /tʃ/, /dʒ/.

corrective feedback: A treatment procedure by which a client is provided with specific verbal, visual, or written feedback about the acceptability of a response immediately after the response is made.

corrective set: A technique used in the traditional intervention approach in which the clinician purposely misarticulates the target sound and asks the child to correct it.

cranial nerves: Nerves that emerge out of holes (foramina) in the base of the skull; they play a major role in speech production.

craniofacial anomalies: Birth defects of the skull and face.

Creutzfeldt-Jakob disease: Transmissible disease of the brain characterized by spongiform encephalopathy (spongelike appearance of the brain), progressive vacuolation (empty spaces) in the gray matter, and the death of nerve cells.

cricoarytenoid joint: A joint that connects the arytenoids to the cricoid cartilage and permits circular and sliding movements.

cricoid cartilage: A cartilage of the larynx and also the top ring of the trachea.

cricothyroid joint: A joint that connects the cricoid with the thyroid cartilage; permits back-and-forth movements.

cricothyroid muscle: A muscle that lengthens and tenses the vocal folds.

criterion of performance: The level of accuracy (e.g., 80% correct) in the production of a target behavior taught in treatment.

cross-sectional method: A research method in which many subjects, selected from different age levels, are studied simultaneously for a relatively brief duration. See also *longitudinal method*.

cued speech: Speech produced with manual cues that represent the sound of speech; it supplements and improves speech reading.

deaf: A person whose hearing loss typically exceeds 70 dB and who cannot hear or understand conversational speech under normal circumstances.

decibel (dB): A basic unit to measure the intensity of sound; it is ⅒ of a bel, the basic unit of measurement named after Alexander Graham Bell.

delayed imitation: In speech sound production therapy, the child's delayed imitation of the modeled target response. See also *imitation*.

dementia: General mental deterioration due to neurological or psychological factors. Among the symptoms associated with dementia are disorientation, impaired memory, impaired judgment, and deteriorating intellect.

denasalization: Substitution of an oral sound for a nasal sound (e.g., *tep* for *ten*); a problem of articulation.

dependent variable: Behaviors taught to clients by clinicians; effects of a behavior or event studied by scientists.

developmental apraxia of speech (DAS): See *childhood apraxia of speech*.

developmental dysarthria: A motor speech disorder associated with congenital and perinatal conditions that affect nervous system support for the speech musculature, or disorders acquired in childhood before speech is fully developed; commonly seen in cerebral palsy. See also *dysarthria* and *cerebral palsy*.

developmental verbal dyspraxia: See *childhood apraxia of speech*.

diacritical markers: Special symbols used in narrow phonetic transcription to depict the articulatory or perceptual features of a phone.

diadochokinetic syllable rates: The speed at which a speaker can repeat selected syllables (e.g., pʌ-tə-kə).

diadochokinetic testing: A special procedure used to evaluate the client's ability to rapidly alternate and sequence repetitive articulatory movements; helps assess the functional and structural integrity of the lips, jaw, and tongue through rapid repetitions of syllables.

diagnosis: A clinical judgment about the presence or absence of a disorder; also a description of the severity and nature of the disorder.

diagnostic audiological evaluation: See *audiological evaluation*.

dialect: Variation of speech within a specific language. Every dialect may has its own unique phonologic, semantic, morphologic, syntactic, and pragmatic characteristics.

diaphragm: A thick dome-shaped muscle that separates the stomach from the thorax, important for respiration.

diencephalon: A structure of the brain stem; it includes the thalamus and the hypothalamus.

differential diagnosis: In speech sound assessment, the clinician's attempt to differentiate various disorders such as articulation disorder, phonological disorder, childhood apraxia of speech, and developmental dysarthria.

diphthong: A combination of two pure vowels. See also *monophthong*.

diplegia: Paralysis of either the legs or the arms.

diplophonia: The production of two tones due to the simultaneous vibration of the ventricular vocal folds and the true vocal folds.

discontinuity theory: Theory indicating that speech sounds are not shaped out of the early vocalizations found in the babbling stage.

discrete trial: Structured opportunity to produce a selected target behavior.

discrete trial probe: A measure of response generalization in which a clinician selects stimulus items that have not received prior training and administers them similarly to baseline trials; however, in discrete probe trials, there is no modeling, positive reinforcement for correct responses, or corrective feedback for incorrect responses. See also *baselines*.

discriminative stimuli: Persons, objects, and physical settings that are associated with a reinforced response; the response is more likely to occur in the presence of such stimuli.

distinctive feature approach: An articulation–phonological treatment approach based on the distinctive features or phonemic contrasts of sounds; the goal of treatment is to establish missing distinctive features that create contrasts between words.

distinctive features: Unique characteristics that distinguish one phoneme from another.

distortions: Imprecise productions of speech sounds.

doubling: A phonological process characterized by reduplication or doubling of a syllable; often alters a single-syllable word form into a multisyllable production (e.g., [dada] for *dog* and [baba] for *ball*).

Down syndrome: A particular genetically inherited condition of mental retardation.

DTTC program: A comprehensive cuing program that shapes the movement gestures for speech production and the effective use of those gestures in the context of speech.

duration: A property of sound; a measure of time during which vibrations are sustained. Vowels have longer duration than consonants.

dynamic sphincteroplasty: A surgical procedure in which muscle flaps from the posterior tonsillar pillars are brought together with a short posterior pharyngeal wall flap to reduce the size of the central port during speech production.

dysarthria: A group of motor–speech disorders that are due to paralysis, weakness, or incoordination of speech muscles caused by central or peripheral nerve damage. There are at least six types of dysarthria: flaccid, ataxic, spastic, hypokinetic, hyperkinetic, and mixed.

dysphonia: A general term for a disordered voice.

dysprosody: Disordered prosody. See also *aprosody*.

echoic: An imitative verbal response; the stimulus and the response are the same.

echolalia: "Parrotlike" repetition of what is heard; an early sign of autism.

efferent nerves: Nerves that conduct impulses from the central nervous system to the peripheral organs.

electromyography: A technique of sensing, amplifying, and recording electrical activity of the muscles.

elicited responses: Reflexive responses triggered by stimuli; for example, the dilation of the pupil in response to light. See also *evoked responses*.

empty set: A contrast phonological treatment approach in which two error sounds with maximal feature distinction are paired for training.

endolymph: A kind of fluid that fills the cochlea.

endoscopes: Mechanical devices used to illuminate and examine internal organs by conducting light to and from an organ via thin fiberoptic tubes that are inserted either through the mouth (oral endoscopy) or through the nose (nasal endoscopy).

epilepsy: A seizure disorder caused by an excessive electrical discharge of damaged or abnormal brain cells, resulting in convulsion in the body.

esophagus: The flexible tube through which food reaches the stomach.

etiology: The study of causes of diseases and disorders.

eustachian tube: Also known as the *auditory tube*, it connects the middle ear with the nasopharynx and helps maintain a balanced air pressure within and outside the middle ear.

evoked responses: Responses that are not imitated, not reflexive, but learned; they are produced in relation to various discriminative stimuli.

evoked trial: A structured opportunity for the production of the target behavior; certain stimuli are arranged so that the target response is likely to occur.

exemplar: A response that illustrates the target behavior.

expansions: Vocal play and exploration during the infraphonological stage 3.

experimental phonetics: A branch of phonetics dedicated to the development of scientific methods for the study of speech sounds.

explicit learning: Learning speech and language skills (or any other skills) through explicit instruction, as in second-language learning with the help of a teacher. See also *implicit learning*.

external auditory meatus: Also known as the *ear canal*, it is a muscular tube that resonates the sound that enters it.

extrapyramidal system: A neural pathway that carries motor impulses from the brain to various muscles via several relay stations (hence also known as the *indirect system*). See also *pyramidal system*.

extrinsic muscles of the larynx: Laryngeal muscles with at least one attachment to structures other than the larynx. See also *intrinsic muscles of the larynx*.

facial nerve VII: A cranial nerve that controls a variety of facial expressions and movements.

facilitative phonetic context: A surrounding sound or group of sounds that has a positive influence on the production of a misarticulated sound.

faithfulness constraint: A restrictive rule of optimality theory that postulates that speech production should be faithful to the input.

feature geometry: A theory of phonology purporting that feature combinations of a sound segment are hierarchically organized.

final consonant deletion: A phonological process affecting the production of final consonants. Patterned deletion of consonant sounds in the final position of words.

finger spelling: A form of sign language in which the words are spelled in the air with the fingers.

fistula: A minute opening sometimes left after cleft palate surgery.

fissures: Relatively deep valleys of the brain that form boundaries of broad divisions of the cerebrum. See also gyrus.

flaccid dysarthria: A type of dysarthria associated with disorders of the lower motor neuron. Speech is characterized by marked hypernasality and nasal emission; breathiness may be present during phonation; audible inspiration may be perceived; consonant production is imprecise.

flaccid paralysis: Muscles that are too soft and flabby, caused by a lesion in the lower motor neurons.

follow-up assessment: A quick procedure after initial dismissal that helps the clinician determine whether the child requires additional treatment.

foot: In the metric theory of phonology, a timing unit that consists of a stressed syllable and one or more unstressed syllables.

foramina: An opening or hole.

fossilized word forms: See *frozen word forms*.

Fragile X syndrome: A genetic condition involving changes in part of the X chromosome that is the most common form of inherited intellectual disability (mental retardation) in boys.

free morpheme: A morpheme that can stand alone and mean something. See also *bound morpheme*.

frenulum: A small cord of tissue that extends from the floor of the mouth to the midline inferior surface of the tongue blade; if too short, it may restrict the elevation and extension of the tongue, which may or may not affect articulation.

frequency: In reference to sound, the number of times a cycle of vibration repeats itself within a second.

frequency of occurrence: In articulation and phonology, the number of times a particular phonological process occurs.

fricatives: A category of speech sounds produced by severely constricting the oral cavity and forcing the air through the point of constriction.

frontal lobe: The largest of the four lobes of the cerebrum, containing the primary motor cortex and Broca's area, which is especially important for speech production.

fronting: Substituting sounds produced in the front of the mouth for sounds produced in the back of the mouth; classified as a phonological process that occurs in both normally developing children and children with phonological disorders.

frozen word forms: Words that children continue to mispronounce despite the development of a more advanced phonological system; such words are likely related to names of familiar people or pets and are used often. Synonym: *regressive idioms.*

functional articulation disorders: Disorders that do not have a demonstrable organic or neurological cause.

functional speech sound disorders: See *functional articulation disorders.*

functional unit: A class or a group of verbal responses that have similar stimulus conditions and consequences.

fundamental frequency: The average rate at which given vocal folds vibrate, or the lowest frequency component of a complex tone.

generalization: The production of untrained (new) behaviors following training of similar behaviors, or the production of trained behaviors when shown new stimuli not used in training.

generalized production: Production of behaviors that have not been taught because of similar behaviors that have been taught; generalized productions are a treatment goal that may save much time and training effort.

glides: Speech sounds that are produced by gradually changing the shape of the articulators.

glossectomy: The surgical removal of the tongue and floor of the mouth.

glossopharyngeal nerve IX: A cranial nerve that supplies the tongue and pharynx.

glottal sounds: Sounds that are produced by keeping the vocal folds open and letting the air pass through; because this results in friction noise, glottals are also fricatives.

glottis: An opening that results when the vocal folds are abducted.

grapheme–phoneme consistency: Correspondence between the letters of the alphabet and the sounds they represent.

gyrus: A ridge on the cortex; the cortex has many *gyri* (plural).

hair cells: Hairlike structures (*cilia*) found on the organ of Corti that respond to sound vibrations.

hard of hearing: Term used to describe a person with a hearing loss within the range of 25 dB to 95 dB; a person who is hard of hearing has some useful hearing.

hard palate: The roof of the mouth and the floor of the nasal cavity; the point of constriction for several sounds, including /ʃ/, /ʒ/, /dʒ/, /tʃ/.

harshness: Roughness of the voice; undesirable vocal quality due mainly to irregular vibrations of the vocal folds.

hearing level: The lowest intensity of a sound necessary to stimulate the auditory system.

hearing screening: A brief testing procedure that separates those who have normal hearing from those who must be tested in detail (because they are suspected to have hearing loss).

hemiplegia: Paralysis of either the left or the right half of the body.

hertz (Hz): The name for cycles per second.

high-amplitude sucking method: An operant conditioning method of studying speech discrimination in infants by measuring their sucking rates when various sounds and syllables are presented and sucking responses positively reinforced.

high feature: Distinctive feature term referring to sounds made with the tongue elevated above the neutral position required for /ə/. The high-consonant sounds are /ʃ/, /ʒ/, /j/, /tʃ/, /dʒ/, /k/, /g/, /ŋ/.

historical phonetics: A branch of phonetics dedicated to studying how sounds change over time.

hoarse: A voice quality that includes both breathiness and harshness.

homonymy: The loss of linguistic contrast between two or more words due to the presence of phonological processes.

hyoid bone: A U-shaped bone that floats under the jaw; the muscles of the tongue and various muscles of the skull, larynx, and jaw are attached to this bone.

hyperkinesia: Increased (exaggerated or too much) body movement.

hypernasality: Excessive nasal resonance on non-nasal speech sounds.

hypoglossal nerve XII: A cranial nerve that innervates the tongue.

hypokinesia: Reduced (diminished or too little) range and force of muscle movements.

hyponasality: Too little nasal resonance on the nasal sounds of a language; may result from a cold or other condition obstructing the nasal passages.

hypothalamus: A structure within the diencephalon of the central nervous system; it helps integrate the actions of the autonomic nervous system and controls emotional experiences.

hypothesis of discontinuity: See *discontinuity theory*.

idiopathic: Of unknown cause or origin.

idiopathic speech sound disorders: Speech sound disorders of unknown origin (with no identified cause).

idiosyncratic: A structural or behavioral characteristic peculiar to an individual or group.

idiosyncratic error patterns (processes): Phonological error patterns or processes that are unique to an individual child and are not common in the typical course of development.

imitation: In speech sound production therapy, the child's response to the clinician's model of the target production.

immediate imitation: In speech sound production therapy, the child's immediate imitation of the modeled target response. See also *imitation*.

implicit learning: The view that caregivers and others teach speech and language skills to children implicitly, not by explicit instruction. See *explicit learning*.

inappropriate communicative behaviors: A client's typical behaviors in place of appropriate speech–language behaviors; in articulation therapy, a client's sound substitutions, omissions, or distortions; in phonological therapy, a child's absence of distinctive features or use of phonological processes.

incomplete cleft palate: The partial fusing of the two palatal shelves of the hard palate.

incus: The second and middle bone of the ossicular chain in the middle ear. See also *malleus* and *stapes*.

independent analysis: In articulation–phonological assessment, a description of the client's speech production errors without reference to the adult model; most clinically useful with very young children or children with significantly decreased speech intelligibility.

individualized education program: A federally and state-mandated program for children with disabilities and special needs who qualify for special education services in the public school system.

individualized family service plan: A federally and state-funded individualized education plan for a young child, with an emphasis on family needs, services, and family members' participation.

Individuals with Disabilities Education Act: Federal legislation that demands the provision of special education services to children with disabilities and special needs in the public schools; includes children with speech and language disorders.

information-getting interview: One of the first steps of a formal speech–language assessment, during which the clinician collects important background information from the client or the client's parents.

infraphonological stages: Stages of early infant vocalizations observed prior to canonical babbling.

initial consonant deletion: A phonological process affecting the production of initial consonants; patterned deletion of consonant sounds in the initial position of words.

instructions: In speech–language treatment, verbal stimuli that help facilitate a client's actions (i.e., production of a target sound).

integral stimulation: A treatment approach that uses a hierarchy of steps and gets more difficult as clinician modeling and cuing is faded. Originally applied to acquired apraxia of speech by Rosenbek et al. (1973), but now also used in childhood apraxia of speech.

intelligibility: How understandable a person's speech is to family members, strangers, and other listeners.

intensity: Magnitude of sound; sounds that are perceived as louder are greater in intensity.

interaction hypothesis: A view that emphasizes the role of social interaction between native and non-native speakers in bilingual language learning.

interdental sound: Sound made by lightly placing the tip of the tongue between the upper and lower central incisors; English interdental sounds include voiced /ð/ and voiceless /θ/.

interfering behaviors: Verbal and nonverbal behaviors that interrupt the treatment process, such as crying, off-seat behavior, excessive verbal interruptions, and inattention to task.

interlanguage: A second language whose mastery is still in progress.

internal auditory meatus: The opening through which the auditory nerve exits the inner ear.

International Phonetic Alphabet (IPA): A set of phonetic symbols, each of which stands for only one speech sound.

interrupted feature: Distinctive feature term applied to sounds produced by complete blockage of the airstream at their point of constriction; such sounds are the stops /t/, /d/, /k/, /g/, /p/, /b/ and the affricates /tʃ/, /dʒ/.

intervocalic: In articulation, singleton consonants or consonant blends that occur between vowels or diphthongs.

intonation: System within a language relating to pitch, stress, and juncture of the spoken language; pattern of pitch and stress in the flow of a person's speech.

intrinsic muscles of the larynx: Muscles that begin and end within the larynx and include the thyro-arytenoid, the cricothyroid, the posterior cricoarytenoid, the lateral cricoarytenoid, and the interarytenoid muscles. See also *extrinsic muscles of the larynx.*

ipsilateral: On the same side of the body. See also *contralateral.*

jargon: In speech and language development, verbal behavior by young children that begins about 10 months out of the variegated babbling stage; productions are characterized by strings of sounds and syllables with a variety of stress and intonational patterns. Often overlaps with the early period of meaningful speech. Also called conversational babble and modulated babble.

jaundice: A yellow discoloration of the skin, mucous membranes, and whites of the eyes caused by increased amounts of bilirubin in the blood.

juncture: A suprasegmental device that helps make semantic or grammatical distinctions in speech, including brief pauses to signal what might be represented by punctuation marks in written English.

kernicterus: A condition that is marked by the deposit of bile pigments in the nuclei of the brain and spinal cord and by degeneration of nerve cells, and usually occurs in infants.

kinesthetic cues: In articulation therapy, visual or verbal cues that focus on the position of the articulators or their correct pattern of movements to teach the correct production of a speech sound.

key words: A word or words in which a typically misarticulated sound is made correctly; can be used in therapy to stabilize the production of the sound across words.

labiodental sounds: Sounds that are produced by the lips and teeth.

labyrinth (of the temporal lobe): A fluid-filled system of interconnecting canals and passages that houses structures of the inner ear.

language: A system of symbols and codes in communication; a form of social behavior shaped and maintained by a verbal community.

language assessment: A process of observation and measurement of a client's language behaviors; typically, it precedes the development of a language treatment program.

language sampling: A procedure of recording a person's language behaviors under relatively normal conditions and, whenever possible, in conversational speech; part of a language assessment.

laryngologist: A medical specialist who treats throat problems.

laryngopharynx: The structure above the larynx and below the oropharynx.

larynx: A tubelike structure in the neck that includes various muscles, along with the vocal folds, cartilages, and membranes.

lateral cricoarytenoid muscle: A paired muscle that brings the vocal folds together (an adductor).

laterals: Sounds that are produced by letting air escape through the sides of the tongue; the English /l/ is a lateral.

lax vowels: Vowel sounds that are made without added muscle tension and have a short duration. The vowels typically described as lax include /ɪ/, /ɛ/, /æ/, /ʊ/, /ɑ/, /ɚ/, /ə/, /ʌ/.

levator veli palatini: A paired muscle that elevates the soft palate.

limb apraxia: The inability of some patients to move a limb voluntarily that cannot be accounted for by muscle weakness, incoordination, or paralysis.

linear phonological theories: Theories presuming that phonological properties are linear strings of segments and that sound segments are a bundle of independent features or characteristics.

lingua-alveolar sounds: Sounds produced by raising the tip of the tongue to make contact with the alveolar ridge immediately behind the front teeth.

linguadental sounds: Sounds produced by the tongue as it makes contact with the upper teeth.

lingua-palatal sounds: Sounds produced by the tongue as it comes in contact with the hard palate, located just behind the alveolar ridge.

linguavelar sounds: Sounds produced by the back of the tongue as it raises to make contact with the velum (soft palate).

linguistic-based approaches: In articulation–phonological therapy, treatment programs or approaches with the underlying philosophy that children's production errors result from phonological processes or rules of the adult system that have not yet been learned or fully acquired, or have been suppressed.

linguistics: The study of language, its structure, and the rules that govern that structure.

linguists: Professionals who specialize in linguistics.

liquids: Speech sounds produced with the least restriction of the oral cavity; also called *semivowels*. The English /r/ and /l/ are liquids.

longitudinal fissure: A fissure that divides the cerebrum into the left and right hemispheres.

longitudinal method: A procedure of studying one or a few subjects for an extended period of time to document changes in selected variables. Children's acquisition of language may be studied longitudinally. See also *cross-sectional method*.

long-term goals: Broadly defined speech and language behaviors that a client needs to learn in order to improve his or her overall communication competence.

loudness: A perceived characteristic of sound. Loudness is determined by the intensity of the sound signal; loudness of phonation or speech is determined by the degree of subglottal air pressure.

low feature: Distinctive feature term used to describe sounds made with the tongue lowered for the neutral position of /ə/. In American English, only the consonant /h/ has the low feature.

lower motor neuron damage: Neurological damage to the nerve fibers that descend from the central nervous system and exit the neuraxis (brain and spinal cord) to communicate with the cranial and spinal nerves.

maintenance procedures: Treatment procedures used to enhance the client's use of the target behaviors in extraclinical settings across time.

malleus: The first bone of the ossicular chain, located in the middle ear and attached to the tympanic membrane. See also *incus* and *stapes*.

malocclusions: Deviations in the shape and dimensions of the upper and lower jaw bones, the positioning of individual teeth, and the relation between the two jaws.

mandible: The lower jaw, which forms the floor of the mouth and houses the lower set of teeth.

mandibular processes: Two of a number of bulges that develop during the third week of embryonic growth; this process results in the mandible, lower lip, and the chin.

manner of production: The degree of and type of constriction of the vocal tract while producing certain speech sounds.

manual guidance: Any procedure in which the clinician uses his or her hands and fingers to physically guide and shape a correct response from a client.

marginal babbling: Infant vocal productions characterized by CV and VC syllable sequences that begin at about 4 months of age.

marked: Features of sound systems that are unique to a given language; presumably learned, not innate; contrasted with *unmarked*.

markedness constraint: A speech production requirement of optimality theory that restricts or generates productions that adhere to the principle of well formedness; contrasted with *faithfulness constraint*.

mastication: The act of chewing.

maxillae: A pair of large facial bones that form a major portion of the hard palate and the upper jaw.

maxillary processes: Two of a number of bulges that develop during the third week of embryonic growth; they give rise to the face, mouth, cheeks, and the sides of the upper lip.

maximal contrast method (maximal opposition): A method of selecting word pairs for phonological treatment that contain multiple feature contrasts or maximal opposition between contrasted phonemes.

McDonald's sensory–motor approach: A motor-based articulation therapy approach with the view that the syllable is the basic unit of training and that certain phonetic contexts can be used to facilitate correct production of the error sound.

mean length of utterance (MLU): The average length of a speaker's utterances as measured in terms of morphemes.

meatus: An anatomic channel or passageway between confining walls within the body.

medulla: The uppermost portion of the spinal cord, which enters the cranial cavity; it controls breathing and other vital functions of the body.

meningitis: An infectious disease that destroys the layers of the membrane (meninges) that surround and protect the brain.

metalinguistics: The study of the conscious awareness of language as a tool and the ability to reflect on language.

metaphonological: A subcomponent of metalinguistics; the ability to reflect on sounds and words.

metric theory: A nonlinear phonological theory that suggests a hierarchy based on feet, syllables, and segments; emphasizes the syllable structure and stress patterns of words in a language.

metathesis: A phonological process characterized by the reversal of two sounds in a word that may or may not be adjacent to each other (e.g., *pots* for *post*).

metathetic error: The reversal of two sounds within a word that may or may not be adjacent to each other.

midbrain: Also known as the *mesencephalon*, a narrow structure that lies above the pons and links the higher centers of the brain with the lower centers.

minimal contrast approach (method): See *minimal pair intervention method*.

minimal pairs: Morphemes that are similar except for one sound (e.g., *mit-sit, hot-pot, bake-bait*); a method of selecting word pairs for treatment.

minimal pair intervention method: A method of selecting word pairs for phonological treatment that contain one or two acoustic feature contrasts between the contrasted phonemes.

mixed nerves: Nerve fibers that carry sensory as well as motor impulses.

modeled trial: A prearranged opportunity for the production of a target behavior during which the clinician provides a model and the client is instructed to imitate the modeled production.

modeling: A treatment procedure used to facilitate a target production; the clinician models the target behavior, and the client is instructed to imitate the clinician.

modulated babble: See *jargon*.

monolingual: Refers to the use or knowledge of one language.

monophthong: Term used in reference to pure vowels.

monoplegia: Paralysis of only one limb.

morpheme: The smallest meaningful unit of a language.

morphology: The study of word structures.

morphophonemics: Sound alterations that result from joining one morpheme with another; morphophonemic rules specify how sounds are produced in combination in morphemes.

moto-kinesthetic cues: Cues provided by the clinician to teach the placement of sounds. The clinician touches and manipulates the client's articulators to facilitate correct production of the target sound. Moto-kinesthetic cues are often accompanied by auditory and visual cues.

moto-kinesthetic method: A procedure of teaching the correct production of speech sounds; the clinician manually moves the articulators to provide motor and kinesthetic feedback to the client.

motor-based approaches: In articulation therapy, treatment programs or approaches that focus on teaching the motor behaviors associated with the production of speech sounds; often considered "traditional" articulation treatment approaches.

motor control model: A theory of speech production based on the neural control of speech muscles.

motor nerves: Nerve fibers that carry impulses for movement from the brain to the muscles.

motor program: A hypothetical structural and functional unit that specifies a sequence of articulatory movements needed to produce specific speech targets.

motor speech disorders: Speech disorders that result from central or peripheral nervous system damage. Apraxia of speech and dysarthria are motor speech disorders. Also known as *neurogenic speech disorders*.

motor unit: Neurological term referring to the motor nuclei, cranial nerve, myoneural junction, and muscle, which together constitute the motor unit.

multidisciplinary evaluation team (MET): A group of persons, including teachers, parents, and qualified specialists, who evaluate the abilities and needs of a child to determine whether the child meets eligibility criteria for special education services under an Individualized Education Program in his or her public school.

multidisciplinary evaluation team meeting: A special meeting in which test results are shared by the multidisciplinary evaluation team and eligibility for special education services is determined. See also *multidisciplinary evaluation team (MET)*.

multilingual: Refers to the knowledge or use of more than two languages; a multilingual person is one who uses three or more languages.

multiple contrast method (the multiple oppositions approach): A method of selecting target sounds for treatment that is similar to the minimal pairs approach but differs by creating minimal pairs for all or most of the errors simultaneously.

multiple-phoneme approach: A highly structured motor-based articulation approach developed to meet the needs of children with multiple articulation errors; key features of the multiple-phoneme approach are the simultaneous teaching of multiple phonemes, a systematic application of behavioral principles, and an analysis of sound production in conversational speech.

multiple sclerosis: A neurological disorder characterized by a progressive and deteriorating muscular disability produced by an overgrowth of the myelin sheath surrounding the nerve tracts;

paralysis, muscular tremors, and dysarthria may be associated to varying degrees depending on the site of lesion.

myoelastic-aerodynamic theory of phonation: A theory that states that vocal fold vibrations are due to air pressure, the difference between positive and negative pressure, and the elasticity of the muscles.

myofunctional therapy: Treatment aimed at correcting a tongue thrust or myofunctional imbalance.

narrow phonetic transcription: A detailed form of recording a speech sound or utterance using the symbols of the International Phonetic Alphabet and special diacritic markers; transcription is enclosed in brackets to highlight the allophonic features or variations of a phoneme (e.g., [kʰout] for coat would indicate an aspirated production of the /k/ sound).

nasal emission: Excessive airflow through the nose that can often be measured and perceived; heard most frequently during the production of voiceless plosives and fricatives; typically indicative of an incomplete seal between the oral and the nasal cavities; often associated with cleft palate speech and some types of dysarthria.

nasal feature: A distinctive feature applied to sounds resonated in the nasal cavity. The nasal sounds include /m/, /n/, and /ŋ/.

nasals: Speech sounds with nasal resonance added to them; produced while keeping the velopharyngeal port open.

nasopharynx: The section of the pharynx that lies just behind the nasal cavities.

naturalistic speech intervention approach: A speech intervention approach in which the child's overall speech intelligibility is targeted first, followed by speech sound accuracy; new speech behaviors are established and strengthened through speech recasts. See also *natural recast*.

naturalness and markedness: A phonological theory that postulates that some phonological properties are common among languages, hence natural (unmarked), while other properties are unique to given languages (marked).

natural phonology: A theory of articulatory and phonological development; describes universal phonological processes as phonetically determined variables that lead to children's simplified speech sound production processes (patterns).

natural recast: A technique used in speech and language teaching to correct the child's errors in such a way that communication is not interrupted.

nerve cells: Specialized cells that make up the central nervous system; basic building blocks in the CNS responsible for receiving, transmitting, and synthesizing information; each nerve cell consists of a single axon, a cell body, dendrite(s), and many terminal knobs.

nervous system: An organization of nerves according to some structural, spatial, and functional principles.

neurologist: A medical specialist who diagnoses and treats disorders of the nervous system.

neuron: A single nerve cell. See also *nerve cells*.

neuropathology: The nature of a disease or damage and the structural and functional changes in the nervous system that result from disease processes.

neurotransmitter: A chemical substance that activates the receptive sites of nerve cells and helps generate the electrical nerve impulses necessary for stimulation of the nerve cell body.

noncontiguous assimilation: A type of assimilation in which the assimilated sound and the sound causing the assimilation are separated by an intervening sound.

nonlinear phonological theory: The theoretical assumption that segmental and suprasegmental phonological properties are organized hierarchically; includes metric theory, optimality theory, and feature geometry theory.

nonphonemic diphthong: Diphthongs that do not contrast meaning in words when they are interchanged with their pure-vowel counterpart; the only two American English nonphonemic diphthongs are /ei/ and /ou/.

nonreduplicated babbling: See *variegated babbling*.

nonreflexive vocalizations: Infant vocal productions that are nonreflexive in nature, including such productions as cooing, vocal play, marginal babbling, reduplicated babbling, variegated babbling, and jargon.

nonspeech oral–motor exercises (NSOME): Nonspeech activities (e.g., lip puckering and stretching and tongue retraction and elevation) that involve sensory stimulation to or movements of the lips, jaw, tongue, soft palate, larynx, and respiratory muscles with the intent of influencing the physiologic underpinnings of the speech mechanism and thus improving speech sound production.

nonverbal corrective feedback: A treatment procedure by which corrective feedback is provided through nonverbal means such as facial expressions, gestures, and other signals.

norms: Standards or patterns derived from a representative sampling of median achievement of a large group; a range of statistical information against which individual performance can be compared.

nucleus: 1. The controlling center of the neuron. 2. The vowel or diphthong that follows the initial consonant or blend in a syllable.

obstruents: Distinctive feature term used for consonants that are made with complete closure or narrow constriction of the oral cavity so that the airstream is stopped or friction noise is produced; obstruents include stops, fricatives, and affricates.

obturator: A prosthetic device used to cover the cleft of the hard palate and help achieve better velopharyngeal closure.

occipital lobe: One of the four lobes of the cerebral cortex; located at the lower back portion of the head just above the cerebellum; primarily concerned with vision.

occlusion: The manner in which the upper and lower dental arches meet each other.

omission: An absence of a required sound in a word position; a type of articulation error.

onset: One of the components of the syllable; the consonant or consonant cluster that initiates the syllable.

open-ended questions: Questions designed to encourage a full, meaningful answer.

open syllable: A syllable that ends in a vowel or a diphthong.

open-syllable word: A word that ends with an open syllable. See also *open syllable*.

operant: A class of behaviors that can be increased or decreased by arranging certain consequences.

operant conditioning: A procedure of creating, increasing, or decreasing behaviors by arranging certain stimulus conditions and immediate consequences.

optimality theory: A nonlinear phonological theory of language capacity; it suggests that grammars are a set of conflicting constraints. A generator and an evaluator help produce speech that results in a violation of the least number of grammatical constraints.

optimal output form: An assumption of the optimality theory that states that the most desirable speech output (optimal output) is the one that violates the least number of conflicting grammatical constraints.

oral apraxia: An inability to move the muscles of oral structures for nonspeech purposes in the absence of muscle weakness, incoordination, or paralysis. See also *apraxia of speech* and *limb apraxia*.

oral astereognosis: An inability to discriminate among and identify the types, locations, and sensations of various objects in the oral cavity.

oral form recognition: The ability to identify and discriminate among the locations and sensations of objects placed in the mouth with no visual information. Synonym: *oral stereognosis*.

orbicularis oris: The muscle that makes up the lips.

organic: Relating to an organ or structure of the body.

organic articulation disorder: An inability to produce correctly all or some of the standard sounds of a language as a result of anatomic, physiologic, or neurological causes.

organic speech sound disorder: See *organic articulation disorder.*

organ of Corti: The inner ear's structure of hearing; it contains the hair cells that respond to sound.

orofacial examination: A procedure conducted to rule out gross organic problems of the face and mouth that may be associated with disorders of communication.

orthodontics: The study and treatment of deviations of dental structures.

orthodontist: A dental specialist who moves the oral structures with the help of specially constructed devices.

ossicular chain: A set of three tiny bones (the malleus, incus, and stapes) found in the middle ear; the chain that conducts sound to the inner ear.

otitis media: An infection of the middle ear; a frequent cause of conductive hearing loss in children.

oval window: An opening to, and a part of, the inner ear.

overdifferentiation: Making an unnecessary distinction between allophonic variations of a phoneme. See *underdifferentiation.*

paired-stimuli approach: A motor-based articulation treatment approach that depends on the identification of a key word to teach correct production of a target sound in other contexts.

palatine bone: A part of the hard palate.

palatine process: The central, platelike portion of the maxillary bones; embryonically identified as the secondary palate, it forms the major portion of the roof of the mouth and the hard palate.

palatoglossus: A muscle that lowers the soft palate and elevates the dorsum of the tongue.

palatogram: An impression made by the tongue on an artificial palate.

palatopharyngeus: A muscle that lowers the soft palate and moves the pharyngeal walls inward.

palilalia: A speech disorder in which a word, phrase, or sentence is said repeatedly with increasing speed and declining distinctiveness; often associated with Parkinson's disease.

palsy: Paralysis.

parallel distribution processing: A computer term also used in explaining speech production; implies that speech processing and production are made possible by units that exist in parallel and process multiple bits of information simultaneously, making it possible to produce speech at the normally fast rate.

paraphasia: A word substitution problem found frequently in aphasic persons who can speak fluently and grammatically.

paraplegia: Paralysis of the legs only.

parietal lobe: One of the four lobes of the cerebral cortex; it lies behind the frontal lobe and integrates such body sensations as pain, touch, and temperature.

Parkinson's disease: A degenerative disease of the nervous system whose symptoms include rigidity of posture, hand tremors, and speech disorders (hypokinetic dysarthria).

partial assimilation: In articulation, a physiologic occurrence in which a sound takes on some of the characteristics of a neighboring sound.

pattern analysis: In articulation–phonological assessment, the clinician's attempt to identify any patterned or systematic modifications in the client's speech production errors.

percentage of occurrence: When conducting a phonological process analysis, the actual percentage with which the child uses a particular phonological process; calculated by determining the number of times the child uses a particular phonological process and dividing that number by the total number of opportunities for occurrence of the process.

percentile ranking: A statistical ranking on a standardized norm-referenced test that indicates the proportion of students in the norm group that scored the same or lower than the target student. For example, a test score that is greater than or equal to 75% of the scores of people taking the test is said to be at the 75th percentile rank. Not to be confused with percent correct, which relates to the proportion of correct answers.

perception: The process by which people select, organize, integrate, and interpret sensory information into a meaningful and coherent picture of the world around them.

perceptual phonetics: A branch of phonetics that studies the perception of sounds by the listener, including sound awareness and sound interpretation.

perilymph: The fluid that fills the canals that lie within the inner ear.

perinatal: Pertaining to the period immediately before and after birth.

periodic: The patterned repetition of the vibrations of a complex tone, which is a sound that consists of different frequencies. See also *complex tone*.

peripheral hearing problems: Reduced hearing ability due to pathologies in the outer, middle, or inner ear (excluding the auditory nerve).

peripheral nervous system: A collection of nerves that are outside the skull and the spinal column; includes the cranial nerves, the spinal nerves, and portions of the autonomic nerves.

pharyngeal flap surgery: A surgical procedure to reduce hypernasality due to a short velum. A muscular flap is raised from the back wall of the throat and attached to the soft palate.

pharyngeal fricatives: Consonant sounds produced by lingual–pharyngeal contact and an unusual tongue configuration; often an associated compensatory error in children with cleft palate.

pharyngoplasty: A set of surgical procedures used to improve the functioning of the velopharyngeal mechanism by implanting various substances (including Teflon) into the pharyngeal wall to make it bulge.

pharynx: The throat.

phonate: To produce sound.

phonation: One of the four basic speech processes; the production of voice through vocal fold vibration.

phone: In the study of speech production, a single speech sound represented by a single symbol in a phonetic system.

phoneme: A group or family of very closely related speech sounds that vary slightly in their production but are sufficiently similar acoustically that the listener perceives them as the same sound. For example, whether /t/ in *cat* is aspirated or unaspirated, the listener perceives the sound as /t/.

phoneme isolation: A phonological awareness skill of identifying whether a specific sound occurs in the beginning, end, or middle of a word.

phoneme manipulation: A phonological awareness skill of deleting, adding, or substituting a sound in a word to create other words.

phonemic awareness: A person's knowledge of phonemes and their role in forming syllables and words. See *phonological awareness*.

phonemic diphthong: A diphthong that cannot be reduced to its pure-vowel components without affecting the meaning of the words in which it occurs.

phonemic inventory: In a phonological analysis, an inventory of sounds that a child uses contrastively to signal a difference in the meanings of words.

phonemics: Study of the sound system and sound differences in a language.

phonemic transcription: Recording of a speech sound or speech unit into phonemic symbols, which are enclosed between virgules (slash marks); such recording indicates the phoneme to which the sound belongs. Synonym: *broad transcription*.

phonetic inventory: A person's repertoire of speech sounds; sounds that a person can produce with appropriate articulation although not always contrastively.

phonetic inventory analysis: An independent analysis that identifies the repertoire of sounds the child can produce with appropriate articulation without reference to the adult target. See also *phonetic inventory.*

phonetic placement method: A procedure of teaching a target sound by describing and demonstrating in front of a mirror how that sound is produced correctly.

phonetics: Study of speech sounds, their production and acoustic properties, and the written symbols used to represent their production.

phonetic transcription: See *narrow phonetic transcription.*

phonological awareness: Knowledge of sounds, syllables, sound combination rules, rhyme, and onset. See *phonemic awareness.*

phonological disorders: Errors of many phonemes that form patterns or clusters.

phonological mean length of utterance (PMLU): A measure of whole-word complexity in which the length of the child's words and the correct consonants in each production are divided by the total numbers of words in the sample.

phonological process analysis: In articulation–phonological assessment, the classification of sound errors according to operating phonological processes and their frequencies.

phonological processes: Many ways or patterns of simplifying difficult sound productions by omissions or substitutions.

phonology: The study of knowledge underlying speech sounds, sound patterns, and the rules used to create words with those sounds.

phonotactic constraints: Linguistic restriction in the way phonemes of a specific language can be arranged to form syllables.

phonotactics: Rules for how sounds can be combined to form syllables and how those sounds can be distributed; some rules vary across languages.

phrase: An utterance that is grammatically incomplete (e.g., "The boy").

physical prompts: In articulation therapy, visual signs or gestures that help a client visualize correct production of the target sound.

physical stimulus generalization: In articulation–phonological therapy, a client's production of the target sounds in untrained words.

physiological phonetics: See *articulatory phonetics.*

Picture Exchange Communication System (PECS) program: An augmentative and alternative picture exchange communication system used with children who have limited speaking ability.

pinna: See *auricle.*

pitch: A sensation determined by the frequency of sound vibration; the greater the frequency, the higher the perceived pitch.

place of articulation: One of three factors used to classify consonants; refers to the place of articulatory contact or constriction.

plosive sound: A stop consonant produced when the impounded air pressure behind the point of constriction is released through the oral cavity; not all stop consonants are plosive in nature.

pons: The structure that bridges the two halves of the cerebellum.

positive reinforcement: A method of increasing a response by presenting something desirable immediately after that response is made; a frequently used positive reinforcer is verbal praise.

posterior cricoarytenoid muscle: A muscle that pulls the vocal folds apart (an abductor).

postnatal: The period beginning immediately after the birth of a child and extending for about 6 weeks.

postvocalic: A consonant or consonant blend produced after a vowel or a diphthong; postvocalic sounds terminate the syllable.

poverty of stimulus: A nativist view that asserts that the environment does not provide enough stimuli or information to teach speech and language skills. See also *wealth of stimulus.*

pragmatics: The study of the rules that govern the use of language in social situations.

prefix: A morpheme added at the beginning of a base morpheme.

prelingual: The period before the acquisition of language, as in *prelingually deaf.*

prelinguistic: Refers to a period before the acquisition of language, as in *prelinguistic speech.*

premaxilla: The front portion of the maxillary bone.

prenatal: Preceding birth; occurring or existing before birth.

presbycusis: A common type of sensorineural hearing loss among the elderly.

pressure: Force, distributed over a certain area.

pressure consonants: Consonant sounds produced with a buildup of intraoral pressure, which include fricatives, stops, and affricates.

prevocalic: In speech production, a consonant or consonant blend occurring before a vowel or diphthong; prevocalic sounds initiate the syllable.

primary auditory cortex: An area within the temporal lobe concerned with hearing.

primary motor cortex: An area within the frontal lobe that controls voluntary movement.

primary palate: An embryonic structure from which the upper lip and the alveolar process evolve.

probe procedure: A clinical procedure used to assess the generalized production of the trained target behavior to untrained sounds, words, sentences, audiences, settings, and so forth.

prognosis: A statement about the future course of a disorder when certain therapeutic steps are taken or when nothing is done.

prognostic variables: Factors that can positively or negatively influence the improvement of a child's speech sound production skills. See *prognosis.*

programmed learning: A method of mastering various skills by the systematic use of operant conditioning principles.

progressive assimilation: A type of assimilation in which a sound takes on the articulatory or acoustic qualities of a preceding sound.

progressive idioms: See *advanced word forms.*

projection fibers: Neural pathways to and from the brain stem and spinal cord, as well as the sensory and motor areas of the cortex.

prompts: Hints or "cues" used in treatment to draw a target response from a client.

PROMPT program: A dynamic tactile treatment approach for motor speech disorders based on touch pressure and kinesthetic and proprioceptive cues; trained speech–language pathologists manually guide the articulators to help the child produce sounds or words.

proportion of whole-word correctness (PWC): A whole-word measure that examines the proportion in which sound segments are produced correctly within a word.

proportion of whole-word proximity (PWP): A whole-word measure that examines the proximity of a child's word to the adult target or determines how closely the child's attempt and the adult target match.

proportion of whole-word variability (PWV): The variability with which the whole word, not just a sound segment, is produced from one attempt to another.

proprioceptive cues: In speech sound training, images and other sensory cues that prompt correct movements of the articulator for speech sound production.

prosodic view of development: A theoretical view that states that children's acquisition of phonological skills begins with the mastery of certain initial words, which are schemata of adult forms.

prosody: Variations in rate, pitch, loudness, stress, intonation, and rhythm of continuous speech.

prosthesis: A device developed and fitted to compensate for missing or deformed structures.

protowords: Consistent sound patterns produced by young children that are semantically potent (carry meaning) but are not modeled after any adult words.

pseudobulbar palsy: Paralysis of the muscles of mastication, articulation, and swallowing as a result of neurological damage to both hemispheres of the brain.

punisher: In behavior modification terms, any stimulus that decreases a behavior when it is presented upon the behavior's occurrence.

punishment: A procedure designed to decrease the frequency of selected behaviors by arranging an immediate consequence for those behaviors.

pure tone: A tone of single frequency.

pure-tone audiometry: Audiometry in which tones of various frequencies and intensities are used as auditory stimuli in the measurement of a person's hearing ability.

pure vowels: Vowel sounds that maintain a relatively unchanged quality across the syllables in which they are produced.

pyramidal system: A bundle of nerve fibers that originate in the motor cortex and travel to the brain stem; it is the primary pathway of impulses for voluntary movement (also called the *direct system*). See also *extrapyramidal system*.

quadriplegia: Paralysis of all four limbs.

range of motion: The limitations within which a motion or movement may occur.

raspberries: In speech and language development, bilabial fricative sounds produced by young infants in the vocal play stage.

real words: See *true words*.

recast: A corrective reformulation of a child's utterance without requiring the child to imitate.

recurrent laryngeal nerve: A branch of the cranial nerve X (vagus); it moves down the chest cavity and then reverses its course back to the laryngeal and pharyngeal areas; it innervates many intrinsic laryngeal muscles and palatal muscles.

reduplicated babbling: Infant vocal productions in which a series of consonant–vowel syllables are repeated (e.g., *ma-ma*, *pa-pa*, *bo-bo*); such productions begin at about 7 months of age.

referent: An object, event, person, or abstraction represented by a symbol, verbal or otherwise.

reflexive vocalizations: Automatic responses produced by an infant that reflect his or her physical state, including crying, burping, coughing, and hiccuping.

register: A variation of language use depending on a particular speaking situation such as the audience (who), topic (what), purpose (why), and location (where).

regressive assimilation: A type of assimilation in which a sound takes on some or all of the articulatory or acoustic features of a following sound.

regressive idioms: See *frozen word forms*.

regressive substitution: Sound substitution in which a phoneme is affected by a sound that occurs earlier in the word; a speech characteristic of verbal apraxia.

reinforcer: An event that follows a response and thereby makes that response more likely in the future.

relational analysis: A comparison of a child's productions to the adult target forms within a specific linguistic community to identify errors of articulation and the operation of phonological processes.

releasing sound: A consonant sound that begins a syllable.

reliability: The consistency with which an event is repeatedly measured.

resonance: Forced vibration of a structure that is related to the source of sound; vibration of cavities below and above the larynx (source of sound).

respiration: One of the four basic speech processes. This system provides the air supply necessary for vocal fold vibration and speech production.

response cost: Taking a reinforcer away from a child every time a particular response is made in order to decrease that response.

response topography: In speech sound training, the specific linguistic level of training or generalized responding (e.g., syllables, words, sentences, conversational speech).

rhotic: Distinctive feature term used for the /r/ consonant and its various allophonic variations.

rhotic diphthongs: See *centering diphthongs*.

rhyming: A phonological awareness skill in identifying words that sound alike, or rhyme.

rib cage: Also known as the *thoracic cage*, a cylinder-like structure of 12 ribs that houses vital organs, including the heart and the lungs.

rime: A collective term for the nucleus and coda components of a syllable.

Rochester method: A means of communication that combines finger spelling and oral speech.

round feature: Distinctive feature term applied to sounds made with the lips rounded or protruded; includes the consonants /r/ and /w/ and the vowels /u/, /ʊ/, /o/, /ɔ/, and /ɝ/.

rule extraction: A scientific analysis of behaviors that detects patterns in them; in phonology, rules extracted from speech are questionably attributed to children who produce speech.

rule-following (rule-governed): Description of behavior that explicitly follows a rule that has been taught to the behaving organism; a questionable description when applied to speech and language production.

schwa: Name for the neutral vowel /ə/.

schwar: Name for the stressed vowel /ɝ/.

screening: A brief procedure that helps determine whether a person should be assessed at length.

secondary palate: Hard palate.

semantics: The study of the meaning of language.

semicircular canals: Structures of the inner ear responsible for maintaining balance (equilibrium).

semivowel: A consonant sound made by maintaining the vocal tract briefly in the vowel-like position needed for the following vowel in a syllable; term used for /w/, /j/, and sometimes /l/ and /r/.

sensorineural hearing loss: Diminished hearing due to damaged hair cells of the cochlea or the auditory portion of the cranial nerve VIII. See also *conductive hearing loss*.

sensory–motor approach: Motor-based articulation approach based on the assumption that the syllable is the basic unit of training and that phonetic contexts can be used to facilitate correct production of the target sound. Synonym: *McDonald's sensory–motor approach*.

sensory nerves: The cranial nerves that carry sensory information from a sense organ to the brain.

sensory perceptual training: A step typically included in the traditional articulation therapy approach; the goal is to increase the child's awareness of his own sound errors by incorporating ear-training activities such as sound identification and discrimination.

septum: The structure that divides the nasal cavities.

sequential bilingualism: The linguistic process of learning to speak a second language after one language has been mastered.

sequential motion rates: Rapid movements from one articulatory posture to another by repetition of different syllable chains. Part of diadochokinetic testing by repetitive movement of the syllable sequence /pʌtəkə/.

serous otitis media: A disease of the middle ear, in which it becomes inflamed and filled with thick or watery fluid.

servosystem model: A theory that explains speech production based on hypothesized feedback mechanisms in regulating articulatory movements.

shadowing: A technique used in the traditional intervention approach in which the clinician says the target sentence and then provides the child with a signal indicating that it is his or her turn. Also known as *echo speech*.

shaping: See *successive approximation*.

short-term objectives: In articulation–phonological therapy, the sounds, phonological rules, and other behaviors selected for training that support long-term goals or final target behaviors.

sibilants: Distinctive feature term applied to high-frequency consonant sounds that have a more strident quality and longer duration than most other consonants; most phoneticians classify /s/, /z/, /ʃ/, /ʒ/, /tʃ/, /dʒ/ in this category.

silent nasal emission: Inaudible leakage of air through the nose during the production of non-nasal speech sounds.

simultaneous bilingualism: The linguistic process of learning two languages at the same time.

slow-motion speech: A technique used in the traditional intervention approach in which the clinician and the child say the target sentence at the same time using a very slow rate of speech.

sociolinguistic or sociophonetic theories: A group of theories that emphasize learning of speech sounds (as against innate flourish) in social communicative interactions.

soft palate: A flexible muscular structure at the juncture of the oropharynx and the nasopharynx; also known as the velum, it may be lowered to open the velopharyngeal port or raised to close it.

soft neurological signs: Mild neurological abnormalities that are undetectable or difficult to identify during specialized testing (e.g., via CT scan). Neurological damage may be presumed based on some abnormal behaviors (e.g., fine motor problems).

sonorant: A consonant sound produced with a relatively unobstructed flow of air at the point of constriction, including the following: /m/, /n/, /ŋ/, /l/, /r/, /j/, /w/.

sound: Waves of disturbance in the molecules of a gas, a liquid, or a solid created by the vibrations of an object and the sensation felt by the hearing mechanism due to those vibrations.

sound approximation: Production of a misarticulated sound that approaches the target or standard production of that phoneme.

sound segmentation: A phonological awareness skill of breaking down a word into its individual sound components.

spastic dysphonia: A voice disorder caused by very tight closure (adduction) of the vocal folds and characterized by a strangled, squeezed, choppy, harsh, and breathy voice.

spastic paralysis: A form of paralysis due to lesions in the upper motor neurons characterized by too rigid muscles.

spasticity: Increased tone or rigidity of muscles.

spectogram: Photograph of the pressure waves of a particular sound.

spectrum: Pattern of physical energy across a frequency range for a particular sound.

speech: Production of phonemes; articulated sounds and syllables. See also *language*.

speech bulb: A prosthetic device that contains a palatal retainer and a pharyngeal extension and is placed behind the soft palate; it helps to eliminate or reduce hypernasality in children with velopharyngeal insufficiency.

speech–language pathologist: A specialist in the study, assessment, and treatment of speech–language (communication) disorders.

speech–language pathology: The study of human communication and its disorders and the assessment and treatment of those disorders.

speech perception: The identification of speech sounds from acoustic cues.

speech reading: A method of understanding speech by looking at the face of the speaker; a skill used by people with hearing loss to understand speech.

speech recast: A technique used in speech sound training to correct the child's sound errors in such a way that communication is not interrupted. See also *natural recast*.

spreading activation: A speech production model that proposes that when a phoneme is activated, all the features and syllables attached to it are also activated.

standard score: A statistical measure in standardized norm-referenced tests that indicates by how many standard deviation an individual's test score is above or below the mean.

stapedius muscle: A small muscle attached to the stapes in the middle ear; in response to loud sounds, it normally contracts to stiffen the ossicular chain.

stapes: One of the three bones of the ossicular chain in the middle ear. See also *incus* and *malleus*.

startle reflex: An infant's automatic response to loud sound, involving sudden movement that suggests a jumping response.

statistical learning theory: A theory based on the frequency with which a child hears specific speech and language elements and thus learns to produce them.

stimulability: The extent to which a misarticulated sound can be produced correctly by imitation or other cues.

stimulability intervention approach (program): A speech sound intervention program in which the stimulability of multiple target sounds is enhanced to a low production level so that the sounds then become part of the child's phonetic inventory.

stopping: Phonological process term used to describe patterned substitutions of stop consonants for fricatives and affricates.

stops: Speech sounds produced by completely stopping the airflow; also known as *stop-plosives*.

stress: A suprasegmental device that gives prominence to certain syllables within a sequence of syllables.

stress-timed languages: Languages across the world in which stressed syllables tend to be produced at regular intervals, including English, German, Russian, and Arabic.

stridents: Consonant sounds made by forcing the airstream through a small opening, which results in intense noise; the consonant sounds are /f/, /v/, /s/, /z/, /ʃ/, /ʒ/, /tʃ/, /dʒ/.

submucous cleft: An opening in the palate that is covered by a mucous membrane.

substitution: The production of a wrong sound in place of a right one.

successive approximation: A treatment technique for establishing a target behavior not in the client's repertoire; the client's target responses are progressively shaped to match the final target behavior. Synonym: *shaping*.

suffix: A morpheme added at the end of a word.

sulcus: A shallow valley on the surface of the brain; the brain has many *sulci* (plural). See also *fissures*.

supplementary motor cortex: An area of the frontal lobe that is thought to be involved in the motor planning of meaningful speech.

suprasegmentals: The prosodic features of a language, including stress, intonation, timing, duration, and juncture.

suspected developmental apraxia of speech: See *childhood apraxia of speech*.

syllabic speech sound: A vowel sound that creates the syllable; sometimes refers to consonants that take on a syllable-forming status (e.g., /l/ in the second syllable of the word *handle*).

syllable: The combination of a consonant and a vowel.

syllable-timed languages: Languages across the world in which syllables (stressed and unstressed) are produced at regular intervals; includes such languages as French, Italian, Greek, Spanish, Turkish, and Hindi.

syllable word shapes: Organization of consonants and vowels in a syllable (e.g., CVC = consonant, vowel, consonant; CCVC = consonant, consonant, vowel, consonant).

synapse: The juncture at which the neurons communicate with each other.

synaptic cleft: The tiny gap (space) between two neurons.

syntax: The arrangement of words to form meaningful sentences; a part of grammar.

target behavior: A behavior that a client is taught and expected to learn.

temporal lobe: One of the four lobes of the cerebral cortex; it contains the primary auditory cortex and Wernicke's area.

temporomandibular joint: The joint between the mandible and the temporal bone.

tense feature: Distinctive feature term applied to sounds that are made with a relatively greater degree of tension or contraction at the root of the tongue, including the consonants /p/, /t/, /k/, /tʃ/, /dʒ/, /ʃ/, /f/, /s/, /l/, /θ/ and the vowels /i/, /e/, /o/, /u/, /ʌ/, /ɝ/.

tensor tympani: A muscle in the middle ear that tenses the eardrum.

tensor veli palatini: A pair of muscles that stretch the soft palate.

thalamus: A part of the diencephalon that lies above the brain stem; the thalamus integrates sensory information and relays it to various parts of the cerebral cortex.

threshold of hearing: An intensity level at which a tone is faintly heard at least 50% of the time it is presented.

time-out: A procedure used to decrease the frequency of an error response; every time an error response is made, a brief period of no reinforcement or silence is imposed.

tongue thrust: A pattern of deviant or reverse swallow in which the tongue pushes against the teeth.

total assimilation: In articulation, a physiologic occurrence in which a sound takes on all of the characteristics of a neighboring sound, thus becoming identical to a neighboring sound (e.g., the /k/ of *cat* totally assimilating to the /t/ that follows to produce *tat*).

total communication: A method of communication that simultaneously uses speech, manual signs, and finger spelling.

trachea: A tube formed by a ring of cartilages leading to the lungs.

traditional treatment approach: A highly structured classic approach to the treatment of articulation disorders that progresses from sensory perceptual training to production training and then from the sound in isolation to the maintenance of learned behaviors in nonclinical settings across time.

training broad approach: An articulation–phonological treatment approach in which several target sounds are taught at the same time.

transfer: The extension of newly learned behaviors from one setting (usually the clinical setting) to various other settings.

treatment: The techniques, strategies, and approaches used to create positive change in a child's skills.

treatment objectives: The skills selected for training.

treatment procedures: Special techniques a clinician uses to effect changes in child behaviors.

treatment program: A comprehensive plan of treatment.

treatment variables: The presumed causes for positive changes in target behavior(s) under treatment conditions.

trigeminal nerve V: A cranial nerve that supplies many structures of the face; controls jaw and tongue movements.

true words: Words used by young children that have semantic consistency and closely match adult production in their phonological and articulatory features. Synonym: *real words*.

tympanic membrane: The thin, semitransparent, cone-shaped eardrum, which is highly sensitive to sound.

underdifferentiation: Failure to distinguish two phonemes in a second language because they are not differentiated in the first. See *overdifferentiation*.

underlying processes: The deep phonological patterns in children's production errors.

unilateral: One sided.

unilateral cleft: A cleft on one side of the alveolar ridge and the lip.

unison speech: A technique used in the traditional intervention approach in which the clinician uses hand tapping or other signals of rhythm for sentence production; the child follows the clinician's physical movements and prosody to repeat the sentence in unison with the clinician.

unmarked: Features of sound systems that are shared by many languages of the world (also called *natural*); thought to be innate; contrasted with *marked*.

unrounded vowels: Vowels made without lip rounding: /i/, /ɪ/, /ɛ/, /e/, /ɑ/, /æ/, /ɚ/, /ə/, /ʌ/.

usage-based theory of phonology: Theory in which children learn to produce speech and language features they hear more frequently than others; similar to the statistical learning theory.

utterance: An isolated unit of verbal expression preceded and followed by silence. An utterance may be made up of a single word, phrase, clause, or sentence.

vagus nerve X: A cranial nerve that supplies many organs, including the larynx, the pharynx, the base of the tongue, and the external ear.

validity: The degree to which a test or other measuring instrument measures what it claims to measure.

variegated babbling: Infant vocalizing that typically begins at about 9 months of age; characterized by the production of vowel, consonant–vowel, and some consonant–vowel–consonant syllable combinations, with varying consonants and vowels from one syllable to another.

velar fronting: Phonological process characterized by the substitution of alveolar consonants for velar sounds; typical substitutions include d/g, t/k, and n/ŋ; however, others may be observed.

velocity: Quickness or speed of motion.

velopharyngeal closure: The physiologic act of closing the nasal cavity from the oral cavity so that air is directed through the mouth rather than the nose; closure is achieved by intricate upward, backward, and lateral movements of the velum and various pharyngeal muscles.

velopharyngeal incompetence: Poor movement of the velopharyngeal structures, usually due to a neurological disorder or injury (as in cerebral palsy, stroke, or traumatic brain injury).

velopharyngeal insufficiency: An anatomical deficiency in the soft palate (velum) or superior constrictor muscle, resulting in the inability to achieve velopharyngeal closure and often resulting in hypernasal speech; often associated with a cleft palate.

velopharyngeal port: The structure that connects the oral and nasal passages; it may be closed or opened by various muscle actions.

velum: The soft palate; formed by muscles that help raise and lower it.

ventricles: The small spaces in the skull that are filled with cerebrovascular spinal fluid.

verbal antecedent: A verbal stimulus that precedes or accompanies a behavior and may exert discriminative control over that behavior. See also *antecedent stimulus*.

verbal apraxia: Difficulty in initiating and executing the movement patterns necessary to produce speech when there is no paralyis, weakness, or incoordination of speech muscles; thought to be due to the brain's disturbed motor planning.

verbal corrective feedback: Verbal information provided to a client when a target or other behavior is inadequate, inappropriate, or unacceptable.

verbal prompt: A verbal hint or "cue" used to draw a target response from a client; it may include the use of vocal emphasis and the provision of verbal information (e.g., "When you make your /s/, remember that your tongue stays inside your mouth").

vestibular acoustic nerve VIII: The vestibular branch of this cranial nerve, which is concerned with balance, body position, and movement.

vestibular system: An inner ear structure containing three semicircular canals; the system is concerned with balance, body position, and movement.

virgules: Slash marks used to enclose phonemic symbols.

visually reinforced head turn method: An operant conditioning method of studying infant speech perception by reinforcing a head turn response to new or changed sound or syllable presentation.

vocal emphasis: A treatment technique by which a clinician increases his or her vocal intensity to highlight a target behavior; in articulation therapy, a clinician would say the target sound more loudly or prolong production of the target sound.

vocal folds: A pair of thin muscles in the larynx whose vibrations are the source of voice. Also termed *vocal cords*.

vocalic: Distinctive feature term used for sounds made without marked constriction of the vocal tract; includes all vowels and the consonants /l/ and /r/.

vocalis muscles: The vibrating parts of the vocal folds; also known as the *thyroarytenoid muscles*.

vocal tract model: A theory of voice and speech that is mainly concerned with the shaping of the pharyngeal, oral, and nasal cavities in voice and speech production.

voiced sounds: Sounds made with vocal fold vibration.

voiceless sounds: Sounds made without vocal fold vibration.

voicing: The presence of vocal fold vibrations in the production of speech sounds. Also termed voice.

volitional speech: Speech productions made under voluntary control.

vowel: A speech sound produced with an unrestricted passage of the airstream through the oral cavity; a syllable-forming sound.

vowel diagram: A schematic arrangement of the vowels of a given language; also known as a *vowel chart*.

vowel quadrant: A schematic representation of the tongue positions for the four extreme points of vowel production /i/, /u/, /æ/, and /ɑ/.

wealth of stimulus: The view that the environment provides plenty of stimuli and information from which children learn their speech and language skills. See also *poverty of stimulus*.

Wernicke's area: A center in the temporal lobe thought to be responsible for both understanding and formulating speech.

whole-word accuracy (WWA): Pertaining to accurate production of all the sounds within a word.

whole-word transcription: A method of phonetic transcription in which the entire word, as opposed to a specific unit, is recorded for a detailed phonological analysis.

word-based phonological theory: A theory that states that words, not segments, are the initial phonological learning units.

Abbs, J. H. (1996). Mechanisms of speech motor execution and control. In N. J. Lass (Ed.), *Principles of experimental phonetics*. St. Louis, MO: Mosby.

Acevedo, M. (1991, November). *Spanish consonants among groups of Head Start children*. Paper presented at the annual convention of the American Speech-Language-Hearing Association, Atlanta.

Air, H., Wood, A. S., & Neils, J. R. (1989). Considerations for organic disorders. In N. A. Creaghead, P. W. Newman, & W. A. Secord (Eds.), *Assessment and remediation of articulatory and phonological disorders* (2nd ed.). Columbus, OH: Merrill.

Allen, G. (1984). Some tips on tape recording speech–language samples. *Journal of the National Student Speech-Language-Hearing Association, 12*, 10–17.

Allen, M. (2012). Intervention efficacy and intensity for children with speech sound disorders. *Journal of Speech, Language, and Hearing Research.* doi:10.1044/1092-4388(2012/11-0076)

Almost, D., & Rosenbaum, P. (1998). Effectiveness of speech intervention for phonological disorders: A randomized controlled trial. *Developmental Medicine and Child Neurology, 40*, 319–325.

Al Otaiba, S., Puranik, C., Zilkowski, R., & Curran, T. (2009). Effectiveness of early phonological interventions for students with speech and language impairments. *Journal of Special Education, 43*(2), 107–128.

Amayreh, M. M. (2003). Completion of the consonant inventory of Arabic. *Journal of Speech, Language, and Hearing Research, 46*, 517–529.

Amayreh, M. M., & Dyson, A. T. (1998). The acquisition of Arabic consonants. *Journal of Speech, Language, and Hearing Research, 41*, 642–653.

American Speech-Language-Hearing Association. (1983). *Social dialects: A position paper*. Rockville, MD: Author.

American Speech-Language-Hearing Association. (1989). Report of ad hoc committee on labial-lingual posturing function. *ASHA, 31*, 92–94.

American Speech-Language-Hearing Association. (2004). Preferred practice patterns for the profession of speech-language pathology [Preferred Practice Patterns]. Available from www.asha.org/policy

American Speech-Language-Hearing Association. (2006). 2006 Schools survey report: Caseload characteristics. Rockville, MD: Author.

American Speech-Language-Hearing Association. (2007). Childhood apraxia of speech: Position statement. Available from www.asha.org/policy

Andrews, N., & Fey, M. (1986). Analysis of the speech of phonologically impaired children in two sampling conditions. *Language, Speech, and Hearing Services in Schools, 17*, 187–198.

Anthony, A. D., Boggle, T., Ingram, T. S., & McIsac, M. W. (1971). The Edinburgh Articulation Test. Edinburgh, UK: E. and S. Livingstone.

Anthony, J. L., & Francis, D. J. (2005). Development of phonological awareness. *Current Directions in Psychological Sciences, 14*, 255–259.

Anthony, J. L., & Lonigan, C. J. (2004). The nature of phonological awareness: Converging evidence from four studies of preschool and early grade school children. *Journal of Educational Psychology, 96*, 43–55.

Anthony, J. L., Lonigan, C. J., Burgess, S. R., Driscoll, K., Phillips, B. M., & Cantor, B. J. (2002). Structure of preschool phonological sensitivity: Overlapping sensitivity to rhyme, words, syllables, and phonemes. *Journal of Experimental Child Psychology, 82,* 65–92.

Archangeli, D. (1988). Aspects of underspecification theory. *Phonology Yearbook, 5,* 183–207.

Archangeli, D., & Pulleyblank, D. (1994). *Grounded phonology.* Boston: MIT Press.

Arlt, P. B., & Goodban, M. T. (1976). A comparative study of articulation acquisition as based on a study of 240 normals, aged three to six. *Language, Speech, and Hearing Services in Schools, 7,* 173–180.

Arndt, W. B., Elbert, M., & Shelton, R. L. (1970). Standardization of a test of oral stereognosis. In J. Bosman (Ed.), *Second symposium on oral sensation and perception.* Springfield, IL: Charles C. Thomas.

Arndt, W. B., Elbert, M., & Shelton, R. L. (1971). Prediction of articulation improvement with therapy from early lesson sound production task scores. *Journal of Speech and Hearing Research, 14,* 149–153.

Bailey, J. S., Timbers, G. D., Phillips, E. L., & Wolf, M. M. (1971). Modification of articulation errors of predelinquents by their peers. *Journal of Applied Behavioral Analysis, 4,* 266–281.

Baker, E. (2010). Minimal pair intervention. In S. F. Warren & M. E. Fey (Series Eds.) & A. L. Williams, S. McLeod, & R. J. McCauley (Vol. Eds.), *Intervention for speech sound disorders in children* (pp. 41–72). Baltimore: Brookes.

Baker, E., & McLeod, S. (2011). Evidence-based practice for children with speech sound disorders: Part 1 narrative review. *Language, Speech, and Hearing Services in Schools, 42,* 102–139.

Baker, E., & Williams, A. L. (2010). Complexity approaches to intervention. In S. F. Warren & M. E. Fey (Series Eds.) & A. L. Williams, S. McLeod, & R. J. McCauley (Vol. Eds.), *Intervention for speech sound disorders in children* (pp. 95–115). Baltimore: Brookes.

Baker, R. D., & Ryan, B. P. (1971). *Programmed conditioning for articulation.* Monterey, CA: Monterey Learning Systems.

Baldwin, J. D., & Baldwin, J. I. (2000). *Behavior principles in everyday life* (4th ed.). Boston: Pearson.

Ball, E. W. (1993). Assessing phoneme awareness. *Language, Speech, and Hearing Services in Schools, 24,* 130–139.

Ball, M. J., & Kent, R. D. (1997). *The new phonologies.* San Diego, CA: Singular.

Ball, M. J., Muller, N., & Rutter, B. (2010). *Phonology for communication disorders.* New York: Psychology Press.

Ball, M. J., & Rahilly, J. (1999). *Phonetics: The science of speech.* London: Arnold.

Bankson, N. W., & Bernthal, J. E. (1990a). *Bankson-Bernthal test of phonology.* Chicago: Riverside Press.

Bankson, N. W., & Bernthal, J. E. (1990b). *Quick screen of phonology.* Chicago: Riverside Press.

Bankson, N. W., & Bernthal, J. E. (2004). Treatment approaches. In N. W. Bernthal & J. E. Bankson (Eds.), *Articulation and phonological disorders* (5th ed.). Boston: Allyn & Bacon.

Bankson, N., & Byrne, M. (1972). The effect of a timed correct sound production task on carryover. *Journal of Speech and Hearing Research, 15,* 160–168.

Barlow, J. A. (2001). Case study: Optimality theory and the assessment and treatment of phonological disorders. *Language, Speech, and Hearing Services in Schools, 32,* 242–256.

Barlow, J. A., & Gierut, J. A. (1999). Optimality theory in phonological acquisition. *Journal of Speech, Language, and Hearing Research, 42,* 1482–1498.

Barlow, J. A., & Gierut, J. A. (2002). Minimal pair approaches to phonological remediation. *Seminars in Speech and Language, 23*(1), 57–67.

Bartoshuk, A. (1964). Human neonatal cardiac responses to sound: A power function. *Psychonomic Science, 1,* 151–152.

Baru, A. V. (1975). Discrimination of synthesized vowels [a] and [I] with varying parameters in dog. In G. Fant & M. A. Tatham (Eds.), *Auditory analysis and the perception of speech*. London: Academic.

Bashir, A. S., Grahamjones, F., & Bostwick, R. Y. (1984). A touch-cue method of therapy for developmental verbal apraxia. In W. H. Perkins & J. H. Northern (Eds.), *Seminars in speech and language* (pp. 127–137). New York: Thieme-Stratton.

Bassi, C. (1983). Development at 4 years. In J. V. Irwin & S. P. Wong (Eds.), *Phonological development in children 18 to 72 months*. Carbondale: Southern Illinois University Press.

Bates, E. (1997). On language savants and the structure of the mind. *International Journal of Bilingualism, 1*(2), 163–179.

Battle, D. E. (2002). *Communication disorders in multicultural populations* (3rd ed.). Boston: Butterworth-Heinemann.

Bauman-Waengler, J. (1994). Normal phonological development. In R. J. Lowe (Ed.), *Phonology: Assessment and intervention applications in speech pathology*. Baltimore: Williams & Wilkins.

Bauman-Waengler, J. (2011, November). *Articulation disorders in school-age children: Disregarded language problems*. Paper presented at the Annual Convention of the American Speech-Language-Hearing Association, San Diego, CA.

Bayles, K., & Harris, G. (1982). Evaluating speech and language skills in Papago Indian children. *Journal of American Indian Education, 21*(2), 11–20.

Behrman, A. (2012). *Speech and voice science* (2nd ed.). San Diego, CA: Plural.

Bench, J. (1969). Audio-frequency and audio-intensity discrimination in the human neonate. *International Audiology, 8*, 615–625.

Bennett, C. W. (1974). Articulation training in two hearing impaired girls. *Journal of Applied Behavioral Analysis, 7*, 439–445.

Bernhardt, B. (1992). The application of nonlinear phonological theory to intervention with one phonologically disordered child. *Clinical Linguistics & Phonetics, 6*, 283–316.

Bernhardt, B. (1994). The prosodic tier and phonological disorders. In M. Yavas (Ed.), *First and second language phonology* (pp. 149–172). San Diego, CA: Singular.

Bernhardt, B., & Stemberger, J. P. (1998). *Handbook of phonological development: From the perspective of constraint-based nonlinear phonology*. San Diego, CA: Academic Press.

Bernhardt, B., & Stemberger, J. P. (2000). *Workbook in nonlinear phonology for clinical application*. Austin, TX: PRO-ED.

Bernhardt, B., & Stemberger, J. P. (2011). Constraint-based nonlinear phonological theories: Applications and implications. In M. J. Ball, M. R. Perkins, & S. Howard (Eds.), *The handbook of clinical linguistics* (pp. 423–438). Malden, MA: Wiley-Blackwell.

Bernhardt, B., & Stoel-Gammon, C. (1994). Nonlinear phonology: Introduction and clinical application. *Journal of Speech and Hearing Research, 37*, 123–143.

Best, C. T., McRoberts, G. W., Lafleur, R., & Silver-Isenstadt, J. (1995). Divergent developmental patterns for infants' speech perception of two nonnative consonant contrasts. *Infant Behavior and Development, 18*, 339–350.

Bhatnagar, S. C. (2012). *Neuroscience for the study of communicative disorders* (4th ed.). Baltimore: Lippincott Williams & Wilkins.

Bird, J., & Bishop, D. V. M. (1992). Perception and awareness of phonemes in phonologically impaired children. *European Journal of Disorders of Communication, 27*, 289–311.

Bird, J., Bishop, D. V. M., & Freeman, N. H. (1995). Phonological awareness and literacy development in children with expressive phonological impairments. *Journal of Speech and Hearing Research, 38*, 446–462.

Birnholz, J. C., & Benacerraf, B. B. (1983). The development of human fetal learning. *Science, 222*, 516–518.

Blache, S. E., Parsons, C. L., & Humphreys, J. M. (1981). A minimal-word-pair model for teaching the linguistic significance of distinctive feature properties. *Journal of Speech and Hearing Disorders, 46*, 291–296.

Blakeley, R. W. (2001). *Screening test for developmental apraxia of speech* (2nd ed.). Austin, TX: PRO-ED.

Bleile, K. M. (1996). *Articulation and phonological disorders: A book of exercises* (2nd ed.). Clifton Park, NY: Thomson Delmar Learning.

Bleile, K. M. (2006). *The late 8*. San Diego, CA: Plural.

Blevins, J. (2004). *Evolutionary phonology: The emergence of sound patterns*. Cambridge, UK: Cambridge University Press.

Blevins, J. (2006). An overview of evolutionary phonology. *Theoretical Linguistics, 32*, 117–166.

Bloch, R., & Goodstein, L. (1971). Functional speech disorders and personality: A decade of research. *Journal of Speech and Hearing Disorders, 36*, 295–314.

Bloom, K. (1988). Duration of early vocal sounds. *Infant Behavior and Development, 12*, 245–250.

Bloom, K., Russell, A., & Wassenberg, K. (1987). Turn taking affects the quality of infant vocalizations. *Journal of Child Language, 14*, 211–227.

Bondarenko, K. (2011). *Speech sound acquisition of two year olds*. Unpublished master's thesis, William Paterson University of New Jersey, Wayne.

Boone, D. R., & McFarlane, S. C. (2000). *The voice and voice therapy* (6th ed.). Englewood Cliffs, NJ: Prentice Hall.

Bradley, D. P. (1989). A systematic multiple-phoneme approach. In N. A. Creaghead, P. W. Newman, & W. A. Secord (Eds.), *Assessment and remediation of articulatory and phonological disorders* (2nd ed.). Columbus, OH: Merrill.

Brady, S., Gillis, M., Smith, T., Lavalette, M. E., Liss-Bronstein, L., Lowe, E., et al. (2009). First grade teachers' knowledge of phonological awareness and code concepts: Examining gains from an intensive form of professional development and corresponding teacher attitudes. *Reading and Writing, 22*, 425–455.

Brice, A. E. (2002). *The Hispanic child: Speech, language, culture, and education*. Boston: Allyn & Bacon.

Brice, A. E., & Brice, R. G. (2009). *Language development: Monolingual and bilingual acquisition*. Boston: Allyn & Bacon.

Bricker, W. A. (1967). Errors in the echoic behavior of preschool children. *Journal of Speech and Hearing Research, 10*, 67–76.

Bridger, W. (1961). Sensory habituation and discrimination in the human neonate. *American Journal of Psychiatry, 117*, 991–996.

Broomfield, J., & Dodd, B. (2004). The nature of referred subtypes of primary speech disability. *Child Language Teaching and Therapy, 20*, 135–151.

Broomfield, J., & Dodd, B. (2005). Clinical effectiveness. In B. Dodd (Ed.), *Differential diagnosis and treatment of children with speech disorder* (pp. 211–230). London: Whurr.

Browman, C. P., & Goldstein, L. (1986). Toward an articulatory phonology. *Phonology Yearbook, 3*, 219–252.

Browman, C. P., & Goldstein, L. (1992). Articulatory phonology: An overview. *Phonetica, 49*, 155–190.

Buckley, M., & Landis, G. H. (2009). Surgical repair of the cleft lip and palate: Procedures and issues. In K. T. Moller & L. E. Glaze (Eds.), *Cleft lip and palate: Interdisciplinary issues and treatment* (2nd ed., pp. 483–512). Austin, TX: PRO-ED.

Bunta, F., Fabiano-Smith, L., Goldstein, B., & Ingram, D. (2009). Phonological whole-word measures in 3-year-old bilingual children and their age-matched monolingual peers. *Clinical Linguistics and Phonetics, 23*, 156–175.

Burdick, C. K., & Miller, J. D. (1973). New procedures for training chinchillas for psychoacoustic experiments. *Journal of the Acoustical Society of America, 54,* 789–792.

Burdick, C. K., & Miller, J. D. (1975). Speech perception in the chinchilla: Discrimination of sustained /a/ and /i/. *Journal of the Acoustical Society of America, 58,* 415–427.

Bus, A. G., & van IJzendoorn, M. H. (1999). Phonological awareness and early reading: A meta-analysis of experimental training studies. *Journal of Educational Psychology, 91,* 403–414.

Butterworth, B., & Harris, M. (1994). *Principles of developmental psychology.* Hove, East Sussex, UK: Erlbaum.

Bybee, J. (2001). *Phonology and language use.* Cambridge, UK: Cambridge University Press.

Bybee, J. (2006). *Frequency of use and the organization of language.* Oxford, UK: Oxford University Press.

Bzoch, K. R. (Ed.). (2004). *Communicative disorders related to cleft lip and palate* (5th ed.). Austin, TX: PRO-ED.

Calvert, D. (1982). Articulation and hearing impairments. In L. Lass, J. Northern, D. Yoder, & L. McReynolds (Eds.), *Speech, language and hearing* (Vol. 2). Philadelphia: Saunders.

Camarata, S. (1993). The application of naturalistic conversation training to speech production in children with speech disabilities. *Journal of Applied Behavior Analysis, 26,* 173–182.

Camarata, S. (1995). A rationale for naturalistic speech intelligibility intervention. In S. F. Warren & J. Reichle (Series Eds.) & M. E. Fey, J. Windsor, & S. F. Warren (Vol. Eds.), *Communication and language intervention series: Vol. 5. Language Intervention: Preschool through the elementary years* (pp. 63–84). Baltimore: Brookes.

Camarata, S. (1996). On the importance of integrating naturalistic language, social intervention, and speech intelligibility training. In L. Koegel, R. Koegel, & G. Dunlap (Eds.), *Positive behavior support: Including people with difficult behavior in the community* (pp. 333–351). Baltimore: Brookes.

Camarata, S. (2002). *Treating speech disorders in preschool children.* Paper presented at the Disabilities Conference, Johns Hopkins University, Baltimore.

Camarata, S. (2010). Naturalistic intervention for speech intelligibility and speech accuracy. In S. F. Warren & M. E. Fey (Series Eds.) & A. L. Williams, S. McLeod, & R. J. McCauley (Vol. Eds.), *Intervention for speech sound disorders in children* (pp. 381–405). Baltimore: Brookes.

Camarata, S., Nelson, K. E., & Camarata, M. (1994). Comparison of conversational-recasting and imitative procedures for training grammatical structures in children with specific language impairment. *Journal of Speech and Hearing Research, 37,* 1414–1423.

Campbell, T. F., Dollaghan, C. A., Rockette, H. E., Paradise, J. L., Feldman, H. M., Shriberg, L. D., et al. (2003). Risk factors for speech delay of unknown origin in 3-year-old children. *Child Development, 74,* 346–357.

Capelli, R. (1985). *Experimental analysis of morphological acquisition.* Unpublished master's thesis, California State University, Fresno.

Cardona, G. (1998). *Panini: A survey of research.* New Delhi: Motilal Banarsidas.

Carillo, M. (1994). Development of phonological awareness and reading acquisition: A study in Spanish language. *Reading and Writing: An Interdisciplinary Journal, 6,* 279–298.

Carr, E. G., Levin, L., McConnachie, G., Carlson, J. I., Kemp, D. C., & Smith, C. E. (1994). *Communication-based intervention for problem behavior.* Baltimore: Brookes.

Carrier, J. K. (1970). A program of articulation therapy administered by mothers. *Journal of Speech and Hearing Disorders, 35,* 344–353.

Carroll, J. M., Snowling, M. J., Hulme, C., & Stevenson, J. (2003). The development of phonological awareness in preschool children. *Developmental Psychology, 39,* 913–923.

Carter, A. (1974). *The development of communication in the sensorimotor period: A case study.* Unpublished doctoral dissertation, University of California, Berkeley.

Carter, A. (1979). Prespeech meaning relations: An outline of one infant's sensorimotor morpheme development. In P. Fletcher & M. Garman (Eds.), *Language acquisition*. Cambridge, UK: Cambridge University Press.

Carter, E. T., & Buck, M. W. (1958). Prognostic testing for functional articulation disorders among children in the first grade. *Journal of Speech and Hearing Disorders, 23*, 124–133.

Caruso, A. J., & Strand, E. A. (Eds.). (1999). *Clinical management of motor speech disorders in children.* New York: Thieme.

Castles, A., & Coltheart, M. (2004). Is there a causal link from phonological awareness to success in learning to read? *Cognition, 91*, 77–111.

Catts, H. (1991). Facilitating phonological awareness: Role of speech–language pathologists. *Language, Speech, and Hearing Services in Schools, 22*, 196–203.

Catts, H. (1993). The relationship between speech–language impairments and reading disabilities. *Journal of Speech and Hearing Research, 36*, 948–958.

Catts, H., & Kamhi, A. (1988). The linguistic basis of reading disorders: Implications for the school speech–language pathologist. *Language, Speech, and Hearing Services in Schools, 17*, 329–341.

Chaippe, P., & Siegel, L. S. (1999). Phonological awareness and reading acquisition in English- and Punjabi-speaking Canadian children. *Journal of Educational Psychology, 91*, 20–28.

Chan, A., & Li, D. (2000). English and Cantonese phonology in contrast: Explaining Cantonese ESL learners' English pronunciation problems. *Language, Culture, and Curriculum, 13*(1), 67–85.

Chaney, C. (1992). Language development, metalinguistic skills, and print awareness in 3-year-old children. *Applied Psycholinguistics, 13*, 485–514.

Cheng, L. L. (1991). *Assessing Asian language performance: Guidelines for evaluating limited-English-proficient students.* Oceanside, CA: Academic Communication Associates.

Cheng, L. L. (Ed.). (1995). *Integrating language and learning for inclusion: An Asian-Pacific focus.* San Diego, CA: Singular.

Cheng, L. L. (2002). Asian and Pacific American cultures. In D. E. Battle (Ed.), *Communication disorders in multicultural populations* (3rd ed.). Boston: Butterworth-Heinemann.

Chomsky, N. (1957). *Syntactic structures.* The Hague, Netherlands: Mouton.

Chomsky, N. (1965). *Aspects of the theory of syntax.* Cambridge, MA: MIT Press.

Chomsky, N. (1981). *Lectures on government and binding.* Dordrecht, Netherlands: Foris.

Chomsky, N., & Halle, M. (1968). *The sound pattern of English.* New York: Harper & Row.

Christiansen, M. H., & Chater, N. (2008). Language as shaped by the brain. *Behavioral and Brain Sciences, 31*, 489–558.

Chumpelik, D. (1984). The PROMPT system of therapy: Theoretical framework and applications for developmental apraxia of speech. *Seminars in Speech and Language, 5*, 139–153.

Ciolli, L., & Seymour, H. (2004). Dialect identification versus evaluation of risk in language screening. *Seminars in Speech and Language, 25*(1), 33–40.

Clark, H. M. (2003). Neuromuscular treatments for speech and swallowing: A tutorial. *American Journal of Speech–Language Pathology, 12*, 400–415.

Clark, H. M. (2010). Nonspeech oral motor intervention. In S. F. Warren & M. E. Fey (Series Eds.) & A. L. Williams, S. McLeod, & R. J. McCauley (Vol. Eds.), *Intervention for speech sound disorders in children* (pp. 579–599). Baltimore: Brookes.

Clarke-Klein, S., & Hodson, B. (1995). A phonologically based analysis of misspellings by third graders with disordered-phonology histories. *Journal of Speech and Hearing Research, 38*, 839–849.

Clements, G. N. (1985). The geometry of phonological features. *Phonology Yearbook, 2*, 305–328.

Clements, G. N. (1995). Constraint-based approaches to phonology. *Proceedings of the XIIIth International Congress of Phonetic Sciences, 3*, 66–73.

Clements, G. N., & Keyser, S. (1983). *CV phonology: A generative theory of the syllable.* Cambridge, MA: MIT Press.

Cole, P., & Taylor, O. (1990). Performance of working class African American children on three tests of articulation. *Language, Speech, and Hearing Services in Schools, 21,* 171–176.

Comeau, L., Cormier, P., Grandmaison, E., & Lacroix, D. (1999). A longitudinal study of phonological processing skills in children learning to read in a second language. *Journal of Educational Psychology, 91,* 29–43.

Comrie, B. (Ed.). (1990). *The world's major languages.* New York: Oxford University Press.

Conley, D. (1966). *The effects of using standardized instructions to evaluate speech correction procedures.* Unpublished master's thesis, Arizona State University, Tempe.

Coplan, J., & Gleason, J. R. (1988). Unclear speech: Recognition and significance of unintelligible speech in preschool children. *Pediatrics, 82,* 447–452.

Cossu, G., Rossini, F., & Marshall, J. C. (1993). When reading is acquired but phonemic awareness is not: A study of literacy in Down's syndrome. *Cognition, 46*(2), 129–138.

Costello, J., & Bosler, C. (1976). Generalization and articulation instruction. *Journal of Speech and Hearing Disorders, 41,* 359–373.

Costello, J., & Ferrer, J. (1976). Punishment contingencies for the reduction of incorrect responses during articulation instruction. *Journal of Communication Disorders, 9,* 43–61.

Costello, J., & Hairston, J. (1976). Concurrent modification of incorrect responses and off-task behaviors occurring during articulation instruction. *Journal of Communication Disorders, 9,* 175–190.

Costello, J., & Onstine, J. (1976). The modification of multiple articulation errors based on distinctive feature theory. *Journal of Speech and Hearing Disorders, 41,* 199–215.

Craig, H. K., Thompson, C. A., Washington, J. A., & Potter, S. L. (2003). Phonological features of child African American English. *Journal of Speech, Language, and Hearing Research, 66,* 623–635.

Craig, H. K., & Washington, J. A. (2002). Oral language expectations for African American preschoolers and kindergartners. *American Journal of Speech–Language Pathology, 11,* 59–70.

Craig, H. K., & Washington, J. A. (2004). Grade-related changes in the production of African American English. *Journal of Speech, Language, and Hearing Research, 47,* 450–463.

Craig, H. K., Washington, J. A., & Thompson, C. A. (2002). Oral language expectations for African American children in grades 1 through 5. *American Journal of Speech–Language Pathology, 14,* 119–130.

Crawford, J. (1995). Endangered Native American languages: What is to be done and why? *Bilingual Research Journal, 19,* 17–38.

Creaghead, N. A., Newman, P. W., & Secord, W. A. (1989). *Assessment and remediation of articulatory and phonological disorders* (2nd ed.). Columbus, OH: Merrill.

Crosbie, S., Holm, A., & Dodd, B. (2005). Intervention for children with severe speech disorder: A comparison of two approaches. *International Journal of Language and Communication Disorders, 40,* 467–491.

Crowe Hall, B. J. (1991). Attitudes of fourth and sixth graders toward peers with mild articulation disorders. *Language, Speech, and Hearing Services in Schools, 22,* 334–340.

Crystal, D. (1987). *The Cambridge encyclopedia of language.* Cambridge, UK: Cambridge University Press.

Culatta, B., Setzer, L., & Horn, D. (2005). Meaning-based intervention for a child with speech and language disorders. *Topics in Language Disorders, 25*(4), 388–401.

Curtis, J. F., & Hardy, J. C. (1959). A phonetic study of misarticulation of /r/. *Journal of Speech and Hearing Research, 2,* 244–257.

Dagenais, P. (1995). Electropalatography in the treatment of articulation/phonological disorders. *Journal of Communication Disorders, 28,* 303–329.

Dalbor, J. (1980). *Spanish pronunciation: Theory and practice* (2nd ed.). New York: Holt, Rinehart, and Winston.

Darley, F., Aronson, A., & Brown, J. (1969a). Clusters of deviant speech dimensions in the dysarthrias. *Journal of Speech and Hearing Research, 12*, 462.

Darley, F., Aronson, A., & Brown, J. (1969b). Differential diagnostic patterns of dysarthria. *Journal of Speech and Hearing Research, 12*, 246.

Darley, F., Aronson, A., & Brown, J. (1975). *Motor speech disorders*. Philadelphia: Saunders.

Davis, B. L., Jakielski, K., & Marquardt, T. P. (1998). Developmental apraxia of speech: Determiners of differential diagnosis. *Clinical Linguistics and Phonetics, 12*, 25–45.

Davis, B. L., & MacNeilage, P. F. (1995). The articulatory basis of babbling. *Journal of Speech and Hearing Research, 38*, 1199–1211.

Davis, B. L, MacNeilage, P. F., Matyear, C. L., & Powell, J. K. (2000). Prosodic correlates of stress in babbling: An acoustical study. *Child Development, 71*(5), 1258–1270.

Dean, E., Howell, J., Hill, A., & Waters, D. (1990). *Metaphon resource pack*. Windsor, UK: NFER-Nelson.

DeCasper, A., & Fifer, W. (1980). Of human bonding: Newborns prefer their mothers' voices. *Science, 208*, 1174–1176.

DeCasper, A., & Spence, M. (1986). Prenatal maternal speech influences newborns' perception of speech sounds. *Infant Behavior and Development, 9*, 133–150.

DeCesari, R. (1985). *Experimental training of grammatical morphemes: Effects on the order of acquisition*. Unpublished master's thesis, California State University, Fresno.

DeFina, A. A. (1992). *Portfolio assessment: Getting started*. New York: Scholastic Professional Books.

Dehaene-Lambertz, G., Hertz-Pannier, L., & Dubois, J. (2006). Nature and nurture in language acquisition: Anatomical and functional brain-imaging studies in infants. *Trends in Neurosciences, 29*(7), 367–373.

Dehaene-Lambertz, G., Hertz-Pannier, L., Dubois, J., & Dehaene, S. (2008). How does early brain organization promote language acquisition in humans? *European Review, 16*(4a), 399–411.

DeJong, P. F., & VanDerLeij, A. (2003). Developmental changes in the manifestation of a phonological deficit in dyslexic children learning to read a regular orthography. *Journal of Educational Psychology, 95*, 22–40.

Dekkers, J., van der Leeuw, F., & van der Weijer, J. (2000). *Optimality theory: Phonology, syntax, and acquisition*. Oxford, UK: Oxford University Press.

de Lacy, P. (2006). *Markedness: Reduction and preservation in phonology*. Cambridge, UK: Cambridge University Press.

De la Fuente, M. T. (1985). *The order of acquisition of Spanish consonant phonemes by monolingual Spanish speaking children between the ages of 2.0 and 6.5*. Unpublished doctoral dissertation, Georgetown University, Washington, DC.

Dell, G. S. (1986). A spreading activation theory of retrieval in sentence production. *Psychological Review, 93*, 283–321.

Denne, M., Langdown, N., Pring, T., & Roy, P. (2005). Treating children with expressive phonological disorders: Does phonological awareness therapy work in the clinic? *International Journal of Communication Disorders, 40*(4), 493–504.

Dillard, J. L. (1972). *Black English: Its history and usage in the United States*. New York: Random House.

Dinnsen, D. A. (2008). Fundamentals of optimality theory. In D. A. Dinnsen & J. A. Gierut (Eds.), *Optimality theory, phonological acquisition and disorders* (pp. 3–36). London: Equinox.

Dinnsen, D. A., Chin, S. B., & Elbert, M. (1992). On the lawfulness of change in phonetic inventories. *Lingua, 86*, 207–222.

Dinnsen, D. A., & Gierut, J. A. (Eds.). (2008). *Optimality theory, phonological acquisition and disorders.* London: Equinox.

Dinnsen, D. A., & Gierut, J. A. (2011). Optimality theory: A clinical perspective. In M. J. Ball, M. R. Perkins, N. Muller, & S. Howard (Eds.), *The handbook of clinical linguistics* (pp. 439–451). Malden, MA: Wiley-Blackwell.

Dodd, B. (Ed.). (2005). *Differential diagnosis and treatment of children with speech disorders* (2nd ed.). London: Whurr.

Dodd, B. (2011). Differentiating speech delay from disorder: Does it matter? *Topics in Language Disorders, 31*(2), 96–111.

Dodd, B., & Bradford, A. (2000). A comparison of three therapy methods for children with different types of developmental phonological disorders. *International Journal of Language and Communication Disorders, 35,* 189–209.

Dodd, B., Crosbie, S., McIntosh, B., Teitzel, T., & Ozanne, A. (2003). *Pre-reading inventory of phonological awareness.* San Antonio, TX: Pearson Assessment.

Dodd, B., Holm, A., Crosbie, S., & McIntosh, B. (2010). A core vocabulary approach for management of inconsistent speech disorder. *Advances in Speech–Language Pathology, 8,* 220–230. In S. F. Warren & M. E. Fey (Series Eds.) & A. L. Williams, S. McLeod, & R. J. McCauley (Vol. Eds.), *Intervention for speech sound disorders in children* (pp. 117–136). Baltimore: Brookes.

Dodd, B., Huo, Z., Crosbie, S., Holm, A., & Ozanne, A. (2006). *Diagnostic evaluation of articulation and phonology.* San Antonio, TX: Pearson Assessment.

Dodd, B., & Iacono, T. (1989). Phonological disorders in children: Changes in phonological process use during treatment. *British Journal of Communication Disorders, 24,* 333–351.

Dodd, B., McCormack, P., & Woodyatt, G. (1994). An evaluation of an intervention program: The relationship between children's phonology and parents' communicative behavior. *American Journal of Mental Retardation, 98,* 632–645.

Dominick, M., Hodson, B., Coffman, G., & Wynne, M. (1993, November). *Metaphonological awareness performance and training: Highly unintelligible prereaders.* Poster presented at the annual meeting of the American Speech-Language-Hearing Association, Anaheim, CA.

Donegan, P. J., & Stampe, D. (1979). The study of natural phonology. In D. A. Dinnsen (Ed.), *Current approaches to phonological theory.* Bloomington: Indiana University Press.

Dore, J., Franklin, M. B., Miller, R. T., & Ramer, A. L. (1976). Transitional phenomena in early language acquisition. *Journal of Child Language, 3,* 13–28.

Dubois, E. M., & Bernthal, J. E. (1978). A comparison of three methods of obtaining articulatory responses. *Journal of Speech and Hearing Disorders, 43,* 295–305.

Duffy, J. R. (2005). *Motor speech disorders: Substrates, differential diagnosis, and management* (2nd ed.). St. Louis, MO: Mosby.

Durgunoglu, A., & Oney, B. (1999). Cross-linguistic comparison of phonological awareness and word recognition. *Reading and Writing, 11,* 281–299.

Dworkin, J. P., Marunick, M. T., & Krouse, J. H. (2004). Velopharyngeal dysfunction: Speech characteristics, variable etiologies, evaluation techniques, and differential treatments. *Language, Speech, and Hearing Services in Schools, 35,* 333–352.

Dyson, A. T. (1986). Development of velar consonants among normal two-year-olds. *Journal of Speech and Hearing Research, 29,* 493–498.

Dyson, A. T., & Paden, E. P. (1983). Some phonological acquisition strategies used by two-year-olds. *Journal of Childhood Communication Disorders, 7,* 6–18.

Earnest, M. M. (2001). *Preschool motor speech evaluation and intervention.* Austin, TX: PRO-ED.

Edeal, D. M., & Gildersleeve-Neumann, C. E. (2011). The importance of production frequency in speech therapy for childhood apraxia of speech. *American Journal of Speech–Language Pathology, 20,* 95–110.

Edwards, H. T. (2003). *Applied phonetics: The sounds of American English* (3rd ed.). Albany, NY: Thomson Delmar Learning.

Edwards, J., & Beckman, M. E. (2008). Methodological questions in studying consonant acquisition. *Clinical Linguistics & Phonetics, 22*, 937–956.

Edwards, M. L. (1983). Selection criteria for developing therapy goals. *Journal of Childhood Communication Disorders, 7*, 36–45.

Edwards, M. L., & Bernhardt, B. (1973). *Phonological analyses of the speech of four children with language disorders.* Unpublished paper, Stanford University, Palo Alto, CA.

Eilers, R. E. (1980). Infant speech perception: History and mystery. In G. Yeni-Komshian, J. Kavanagh, and C. A. Ferguson (Eds.), *Child phonology: Vol. 2. Perception.* New York: Academic Press.

Eilers, R. E., & Minifie, F. (1975). Fricative discrimination in early infancy. *Journal of Speech and Hearing Research, 18*, 158–167.

Eilers, R. E., & Oller, D. K. (1976). The role of speech discrimination in developmental sound substitutions. *Journal of Child Language, 3*, 319–329.

Eilers, R. E., Wilson, W., & Moore, J. (1977). Developmental changes in speech discrimination in infants. *Journal of Speech and Hearing Research, 20*, 766–780.

Eimas, P. (1974). Auditory and linguistic processing of cues for places of articulation by infants. *Perception Psychophysiology, 16*, 513–521.

Eimas, P., Siqueland, E., Jusczyk, P., & Vigorito, J. (1971). Speech perception in infants. *Science, 146*, 668–670.

Eisenberg, R. (1976). *Auditory competence in early life: The roots of communicative behavior.* Baltimore: University Park Press.

Elbert, M., Dinnsen, D. A., Swartzlander, P., & Chin, S. B. (1990). Generalization to conversational speech. *Journal of Speech and Hearing Disorders, 55*, 694–699.

Elbert, M., & Gierut, J. (1986). *Handbook of clinical phonology: Approaches to assessment and treatment.* Austin, TX: PRO-ED.

Elbert, M., & McReynolds, L. V. (1975). Transfer of /r/ across contexts. *Journal of Speech and Hearing Disorders, 40*, 380–387.

Elbert, M., & McReynolds, L. V. (1978). An experimental analysis of misarticulating children's generalization. *Journal of Speech and Hearing Disorders, 44*, 459–471.

Elbert, M., Powell, T. W., & Swartzlander, P. (1991). Toward a technology of generalization: How many exemplars are sufficient? *Journal of Speech and Hearing Research, 34*, 81–87.

Elfenbein, J. L. (1994). Monitoring preschoolers' hearing aids: Issues in program design and implementation. *American Journal of Audiology, 3*(2), 65–70.

Elliot, G. B., & Elliot, K. A. (1964). Some pathological, radiological and clinical implications of the precocious development of the human ear. *Laryngoscope, 74*, 1160–1171.

Ellis, N. C. (2011). Implicit and explicit SLA and their interface. In C. Sanz & R. P. Leow (Eds.), *Implicit and explicit language learning: Conditions, processes, and knowledge in SLA and bilingualism* (pp. 35–47). Washington, DC: Georgetown University Press.

Ellison, T. M. (2000). The universal constraint set: Convention, not fact. In J. Dekkers, F. van der Leeuw, & J. van de Weijer (Eds.), *Optimality theory: Phonology, syntax, and acquisition.* Oxford, UK: Oxford University Press.

Elowson, A. M., Snowdon, C. T., & Lazaro-Perea, C. (1998). 'Babbling' and social context in infant monkeys: Parallels to human infants. *Trends in Cognitive Sciences, 2*(1), 31–37.

Engel, D. C., Brandriet, S. E., Erickson, K. M., Gronhoud, K. D., & Gunderson, G. D. (1966). Carryover. *Journal of Speech and Hearing Disorders, 31*, 227–233.

Evans, N., & Levinson, S. C. (2009). The myth of language universals: Language diversity and its importance for cognitive science. *Behavioral and Brain Sciences, 32*, 429–492.

Fabiano-Smith, L., & Goldstein, B. A. (2010a). Early-, middle-, and late-developing sounds in monolingual and bilingual children: An exploratory investigation. *American Journal of Speech–Language Pathology, 19*, 66–77.

Fabiano-Smith, L., & Goldstein, B. A. (2010b). Phonological acquisition in bilingual Spanish–English speaking children. *Journal of Speech–Language and Hearing Research, 53*, 160–178.

Fairbanks, G. (1954). Systematic research in experimental phonetics: 1. A theory of the speech mechanism as a servosystem. *Journal of Speech and Hearing Disorders, 19*, 133–139.

Fairbanks, G., & Green, E. (1950). A study of minor organic deviations in 'functional' disorders of articulation: 2. Dimension and relationship of the lips. *Journal of Speech and Hearing Disorders, 15*, 165–168.

Fairbanks, G., & Lintner, M. (1951). A study of minor organic deviations in functional disorders of articulation. *Journal of Speech and Hearing Disorders, 16*, 273–279.

Faircloth, M. A., & Faircloth, S. R. (1970). An analysis of the articulatory behavior of a speech-defective child in connected speech. *Journal of Speech and Hearing Disorders, 35*, 51–61.

Fant, G. (1960). *Acoustic theory of speech production*. The Hague: Mouton.

Fant, G. (1989). Speech research in perspective. *STL-QPSR, 4*, 1–7.

Felsenfeld, S., McGue, M., & Broen, P. A. (1995). Familial aggregation of phonological disorders: Results from a 28-year follow-up. *Journal of Speech and Hearing Research, 38*, 1091–1107.

Ferguson, C. A. (1978). Learning to pronounce: The earliest stages of phonological development in the child. In F. D. Minifie & L. L. Lloyd (Eds.), *Communicative and cognitive abilities: Early behavioral assessment*. Baltimore: University Park Press.

Ferguson, C. A. (1986). Discovering sound units and constructing sound systems: It's child's play. In J. S. Perkell & D. H. Klatt (Eds.), *Invariance and variability of speech processes*. Hillsdale, NJ: Erlbaum.

Ferguson, C. A., & Farwell, C. B. (1975). Words and sounds in early language acquisition. *Language, 51*, 419–439.

Ferrier, E., & Davis, M. (1973). A lexical approach to remediation of final sound omissions. *Journal of Speech and Hearing Disorders, 38*, 126–130.

Fey, M. E. (1986). *Language intervention with young children*. Boston: Allyn & Bacon.

Fey, M. E., Cleave, P. L., Ravida, A. I., Long, H. S., Dejmal, A. E., & Easton, E. L. (1994). Effects of grammar facilitation on the phonological performance of children with speech and language impairments. *Journal of Speech and Hearing Research, 37*, 594–607.

Fisher, H., & Logemann, J. (1971). *The Fisher-Logemann test of articulation competence*. Austin, TX: PRO-ED.

Fisichelli, R. M. (1950). *An experimental study of the prelinguistic speech development of institutionalized infants*. Unpublished doctoral dissertation, Fordham University, New York.

Fitch, J. L. (1973). *Voice and articulation*. In B. B. Lahey (Ed.), *The modification of language behavior*. Springfield, IL: Charles C. Thomas.

Fletcher, S. G. (1972). Time-by-count measurement of diadochokinetic syllable rate. *Journal of Speech and Hearing Research, 15*, 763–770.

Fletcher, S. G. (1978). *Time-by-count measurement of diadochokinetic syllable rate*. Austin, TX: PRO-ED.

Fletcher-Flinn, C. M., & Thompson, G. B. (2000). Learning to read with underdeveloped phonemic awareness but lexicalized phonological decoding: A case study of a 3-year-old. *Cognition, 74*, 177–208.

Flexer, C., Gillette, Y., & Wray, D. (1997). Communicative management of persons with multiple disabilities. In C. T. Ferrand & R. L. Bloom (Eds.), *Introduction to organic and neurogenic disorders of communication: Current scope and practice*. Needham Heights, MA: Allyn & Bacon.

Flipsen, P., Jr. (2006). Measuring the intelligibility of conversational speech in children. *Clinical Linguistics and Phonetics, 20*, 303–312.

Flipsen, P., & Gildersleeve-Neumann, C. (2009). *Childhood apraxia of speech: Some basics of assessment and treatment.* Paper presented at the American Speech-Language-Hearing Association Convention, New Orleans, LA.

Fluharty, N. (2000). *Fluharty preschool speech and language screening test* (2nd ed.). Austin, TX: PRO-ED.

Forrest, K. (2002). Are oral–motor exercises useful in the treatment of phonological/articulatory disorders? *Seminars in Speech and Language, 23*(1), 15–25.

Forrest, K. (2003). Diagnostic criteria of developmental apraxia of speech used by clinical speech–language pathologists. *American Journal of Speech–Language Pathology, 12*, 376–380.

Forrest, K., Dinnsen, A., & Elbert, M. (1997). Impact of substitution patterns on phonological learning by misarticulating children. *Clinical Linguistics and Phonetics, 11*, 63–76.

Freed, D. (2012). *Motor speech disorders* (2nd ed.). Clifton Park, NY: Delmar Cengage Learning.

Fry, D. B. (1965). The dependence of stress judgments on vowel formant structures. In E. Zwirner & W. Bethge (Eds.), *Proceedings of the Sixth International Congress of Phonetic Sciences.* Basel, Switzerland: Karger.

Fudala, J. B. (2000). *Arizona articulation proficiency scale* (3rd ed.). Torrance, CA: Western Psychological Services.

Fuller, D. R., Pimentel, J. T., & Peregoy, B. M. (2011). *Applied anatomy and physiology for speech–language pathology and audiology.* Baltimore: Lippincott Williams and Wilkins.

Gallagher, T. M., & Shriner, T. H. (1975a). Articulatory inconsistencies in the speech of normal children. *Journal of Speech and Hearing Research, 18*, 168–175.

Gallagher, T. M., & Shriner, T. H. (1975b). Contextual variables related to inconsistent /s/ and /z/ production in the spontaneous speech of children. *Journal of Speech and Hearing Research, 18*, 623–633.

Gammon, S., Smith, P., Daniloff, R., & Kim, C. (1971). Articulation and stress juncture production under oral anesthetization and masking. *Journal of Speech and Hearing Research, 14*, 271–282.

Garn-Nunn, P. G., & Lynn, J. M. (2004). *Calvert's descriptive phonetics* (3rd ed.). New York: Thieme.

Gerken, L., & Aslin, R. N. (2005). Thirty years of research on infant speech perception: The legacy of Peter W. Jusczyk. *Language Learning and Development, 1*, 5–21.

Gibbon, F. (1999). Undifferentiated lingual gestures in children with articulation/phonological disorders. *Journal of Speech, Language, and Hearing Research, 42*, 382–397.

Gibbon, F. E. (2002). Features of impaired tongue control in children with phonological disorders. In F. Windsor, L. Kelly, & N. Hewlett (Eds.), *Investigations in clinical linguistics and phonetics* (pp. 299–309). Mahwah, NJ: Erlbaum.

Gibbon, F. E. (2007). Research and practice in developmental phonological disorders. In M. C. Pennington (Ed.), *Phonology in context* (pp. 245–278). New York: Palgrave Macmillan.

Gierut, J. A. (1985). *On the relationship between phonological knowledge and generalization learning in misarticulating children.* Doctoral dissertation, Indiana University, Bloomington.

Gierut, J. A. (1989). Maximal opposition approach to phonological treatment. *Journal of Speech and Hearing Disorders, 54*, 9–19.

Gierut, J. A. (1990). Differential learning of phonological oppositions. *Journal of Speech and Hearing Research, 33*, 540–549.

Gierut, J. A. (1991). Homonymy in phonological change. *Clinical Linguistics and Phonetics, 5*, 119–137.

Gierut, J. A. (1992). The conditions and course of clinically induced phonological change. *Journal of Speech and Hearing Research, 35*, 1049–1063.

Gierut, J. A. (1998). Treatment efficacy: Functional phonological disorders in children. *Journal of Speech, Language, and Hearing Research, 41,* S85–S100.

Gierut, J. A. (1999). Syllable onsets: Clusters and adjuncts in acquisition. *Journal of Speech, Language, and Hearing Research, 42,* 708–726.

Gierut, J. A. (2001). Complexity in phonological treatment: Clinical factors. *Language, Speech, and Hearing Services in Schools, 32,* 229–241.

Gierut, J. A. (2004, Summer). Clinical application of phonological complexity. *CSHA Magazine, 16,* 6–7.

Gierut, J. A. (2005). Phonological intervention: The how or the what? In S. F. Warren & M. E. Fey (Series Eds.) & A. G. Kamhi & K. E. Pollock (Vol. Eds.), *Communication and language intervention series: Phonological disorders in children—Clinical decision making in assessment and intervention* (pp. 201–210). Baltimore: Brookes.

Gierut, J. A. (2007). Phonological complexity and language learnability. *American Journal of Speech–Language Pathology, 16*(1), 6–17.

Gierut, J. A. (2008). Phonological disorders and the developmental archive. In D. A. Dinnsen & J. A. Gierut (Eds.), *Optimality theory, phonological acquisition, and disorders* (pp. 37–92). London: Equinox.

Gierut, J. A., & Champion, A. H. (2001). Syllable onset II: Three element clusters in phonological treatment. *Journal of Speech, Language, and Hearing Research, 44,* 886–904.

Gierut, J. A., Elbert, M., & Dinnsen, D. (1987). A functional analysis of phonological knowledge and generalization learning in misarticulating children. *Journal of Speech and Hearing Research, 30,* 462–479.

Gierut, J. A., & Morrisette, M. L. (2005). The clinical significance of optimality theory for phonological disorders. *Topics in Language Disorders, 25*(3), 266–280.

Gierut, J. A., Morrisette, M. L., & Champion, A. H. (1999). Lexical constraints in phonological acquisition. *Journal of Child Language, 26,* 261–294.

Gierut, J. A., Morrisette, M. L., Hughes, M. T., & Rowland, S. (1996). Phonological treatment efficacy and developmental norms. *Language, Speech, and Hearing Services in Schools, 27,* 215–230.

Gierut, J. A., Morrisette, M. L., & Ziemer, S. M. (2010). Nonwords and generalization in children with phonological disorders. *American Journal of Speech–Language Pathology, 19,* 167–177.

Gierut, J. A., & Neumann, H. J. (1991). Teaching and learning /θ/: A nonconfound. *Clinical Linguistics and Phonetics, 6,* 191–200.

Gildersleeve, C., Davis, B., & Stubble, E. (1996, November). *When monolingual rules do not apply: Speech development in a bilingual environment.* Paper presented at the annual convention of the American Speech-Language-Hearing Association, Seattle, WA.

Gildersleeve-Neumann, C., & Davis, B. (1998, November). *Learning English in a bilingual preschool environment: Change over time.* Paper presented at the annual convention of the American Speech-Language-Hearing Association, San Antonio, TX.

Gillon, G. T. (2000). The efficacy of phonological awareness intervention for children with spoken language impairment. *Language, Speech, and Hearing Services in Schools, 31,* 126–141.

Gillon, G. T. (2004). *Phonological awareness: From research to practice.* New York: Guilford Press.

Glaze, L. E. (2009). Behavioral approaches to treating velopharyngeal dysfunction and nasality. In K. T. Moller & L. E. Glaze (Eds.), *Cleft lip and palate: Interdisciplinary issues and treatment* (2nd ed., pp. 415–452). Austin, TX: PRO-ED.

Golding-Kushner, K. J. (1997). Cleft lip and palate, craniofacial anomalies, and velopharyngeal insufficiency. In C. T. Ferrand & R . L. Bloom (Eds.), *Introduction to organic and neurogenic disorders of communication: Current scope and practice.* Boston: Allyn & Bacon.

Golding-Kushner, K. J. (2001). *Therapy techniques for cleft palate and related disorders.* San Diego, CA: Singular.

Goldman, R., & Fristoe, M. (2000). *The Goldman-Fristoe test of articulation* (2nd ed.). Circle Pines, MN: American Guidance Service.

Goldsmith, J. A. (1979). *Autosegmental phonology.* New York: Garland Press.

Goldsmith, J. A. (1990). *Autosegmental and metrical phonology.* Oxford, UK: Blackwell.

Goldsmith, J. A. (1999). *Phonological theory: The essential readings.* Oxford, UK: Blackwell.

Goldstein, B. A. (1988). *The evidence of phonological processes of 3- and 4-year-old Spanish speakers.* Unpublished master's thesis, Temple University, Philadelphia.

Goldstein, B. A. (1993). *Phonological patterns in speech-disordered Puerto Rican Spanish-speaking children.* Unpublished doctoral dissertation, Temple University, Philadelphia.

Goldstein, B. A. (1995). Spanish phonological development. In H. Kayser (Ed.), *Bilingual speech–language pathology: An Hispanic focus.* San Diego, CA: Singular.

Goldstein, B. A. (2000). *Cultural and linguistic diversity resource guide for speech–language pathology.* San Diego, CA: Singular.

Goldstein, B. A. (2004). *Bilingual language development and disorders in Spanish–English speakers.* Baltimore: Brookes.

Goldstein, B. A., Fabiano, L., & Washington, P. S. (2005). Phonological skills in predominantly English-speaking, predominantly Spanish-speaking, and Spanish–English bilingual children. *Language, Speech, and Hearing Services in Schools, 36,* 201–218.

Goldstein, B. A., & Iglesias, A. (1996). Phonological patterns in normally developing 4-year-old Spanish-speaking preschoolers of Puerto Rican descent. *Language, Speech, and Hearing Services in the Schools, 27*(1), 82–90.

Goldstein, B. A., & Iglesias, A. (2006). *Contextual probes of articulation competence–Spanish.* Greenville, SC: Super Duper Publications.

Goldstein, B. A., & Pollock, K. (2000). Vowel errors in Spanish-speaking children with phonological disorders: A retrospective, comparative study. *Clinical Linguistics and Phonetics, 14*(3), 217–234.

Goldstein, H., & Gierut, J. (1998). Outcomes measurement in child language and phonological disorders. In C. M. Frattali (Ed.), *Measuring outcomes in speech–language pathology.* New York: Thieme.

Goldstein, M. H., King, A. P., & West, M. J. (2003). Social interaction shapes babbling: Testing parallels between birdsong and babbling. *Proceedings of the National Academy of Sciences, 100*(13), 8030–8035.

Goldston, C. (1996). Direct optimality theory: Representation as pure markedness. *Language, 72,* 713–748.

Gonzalez, A. (1981). *A descriptive study of phonological development in normal speaking Puerto Rican preschoolers.* Unpublished doctoral dissertation, Pennsylvania State University, State College.

Gonzalez, J. E. J., & Garcia, C. R. H. (1995). *Effects of word linguistic properties on phonological awareness in Spanish children. Journal of Educational Psychology, 87,* 193–201.

Gordon-Brannan, M. (1994). Assessing intelligibility: Children's expressive phonologies. *Topics in Language Disorders, 14,* 17–25.

Gorlin, R. J., & Baylis, A. L. (2009). Embryologic and genetic aspects of clefting and selected craniofacial anomalies. In K. T. Moller & L. E. Glaze (Eds.), *Cleft lip and palate: Interdisciplinary issues and treatment* (2nd ed., pp. 103–169). Austin, TX: PRO-ED.

Goswami, U., & Bryant, P. E. (1990). *Phonological skills and learning to read.* Hillsdale, NJ: Erlbaum.

Gottesman, I., & Gould, T. D. (2003). The endophenotype concept in psychiatry: Etymology and strategic intentions. *American Journal of Psychiatry, 160,* 636–645.

Gracco, V. L. (1990). Characteristics of speech as a motor control system. In G. E. Hammond (Ed.), *Cerebral control of speech and limb movements.* Amsterdam: Elsevier Science Publishers.

Greenberg, J. H. (1987). *Language in the Americas.* Palo Alto, CA: Stanford University Press.

Greenlee, M. (1973). Some observations on initial English consonant clusters in a child two to three years old. *Papers and Reports on Child Language Development, 6,* 85–100.

Greenlee, M. (1974). Interacting processes in the child's acquisition of stop-liquid clusters. *Papers and Reports on Child Language Development, 7,* 85–100.

Grunwell, P. (1982). *Clinical phonology.* London: Croom Helm.

Grunwell, P. (1985). *Phonological assessment of child speech (PACS).* Windsor, UK: NFER-Nelson.

Grunwell, P. (1987). *Clinical phonology* (2nd ed.). London: Croom Helm.

Grunwell, P. (1990). *Developmental speech disorders.* Edinburgh: Churchill Livingstone.

Grunwell, P. (1997a). Developmental phonological disability: Order or disorder. In B. W. Hodson & M. L. Edwards (Eds.), *Perspectives in applied phonology.* Gaithersburg, MD: Aspen.

Grunwell, P. (1997b). Natural phonology. In M. J. Ball & R. D. Kent (Eds.), *The new phonologies: Developments in clinical linguistics.* San Diego, CA: Singular.

Gussmann, E. (2002). *Phonology: Analysis and theory.* Cambridge, UK: Oxford University Press.

Gutierrez-Clellen, V., & Peña, E. (2001). Dynamic assessment of diverse children: A tutorial. *Language, Speech, and Hearing Services in Schools, 32,* 212–224.

Haelsig, P. C., & Madison, C. L. (1986). A study of phonological processes exhibited by 3-, 4-, and 5-year-old children. *Language, Speech, and Hearing Services in the Schools, 17,* 107–114.

Hall, P. K. (2000). A letter to the parent(s) of a child with developmental apraxia of speech: Part I. Speech characteristics of the disorder. *Language, Speech, and Hearing Services in the Schools, 31,* 169–172.

Hall, P. K., Jordan, L. S., & Robin, D. A. (2007). *Developmental apraxia of speech: Theory and clinical practice* (2nd ed.). Austin, TX: PRO-ED.

Halle, M. (1992). Phonological features. In *International encyclopedia of linguistics* (Vol. 3). Oxford, UK: Oxford University Press.

Halliday, M. A. K. (1975). *Learning how to mean: Explorations in the development of language.* London: Edwards Arnold.

Hansen Edwards, J. G. (2006). *Acquiring a non-native phonology: Linguistic constraints and social barriers.* New York: Continuum.

Hanson, M. L. (1994). Oral myofunctional disorders and articulatory patterns. In J. Bernthal & N. Bankson (Eds.), *Child phonology: Characteristics, assessment, and intervention with special populations* (pp. 29–53). New York: Thieme.

Hare, G. (1983). Development at 2 years. In J. V. Irwin & S. P. Wong (Eds.), *Phonological development in children 18 to 72 months.* Carbondale: Southern Illinois University Press.

Harley, T. A. (2008). *The psychology of language: From data to theory* (3rd ed.). London: Taylor and Francis.

Harris, G. A. (1998). American Indian cultures: A lesson in diversity. In D. E. Battle (Ed.), *Communication disorders in multicultural populations* (2nd ed.). Boston: Butterworth-Heinemann.

Haspelmath, M. (2006). Against markedness (and what to replace it with). *Journal of Linguistics, 42,* 25–70.

Hauner, K. K. Y., Shriberg, L. D., Kwiatkowski, J., & Allen, C. T. (2005). A subtype of speech delay associated with developmental psychosocial involvement. *Journal of Speech, Language, and Hearing Research, 48,* 635–650.

Hayden, D., & Square, P. (1994). Motor speech treatment hierarchy: A systems approach. *Clinics in Communication Disorders, 4,* 175–182.

Hayden, D., & Square, P. (1999). *Verbal motor production assessment for children.* San Antonio, TX: Psychological Corporation.

Hayes, B. (1988). Metrics and phonological theory. In F. Newmeyer (Ed.), *Linguistics: The Cambridge survey: Vol. 2. Linguistic theory: Extensions and implications*. Cambridge, UK: Cambridge University Press.

Haynes, S. (1985). Developmental apraxia of speech: Symptoms and treatment. In D. F. Johns (Ed.), *Clinical management of neurogenic communicative disorders* (2nd ed.). Boston: College-Hill Press.

Haynes, W., & Moran, M. (1989). A cross-sectional developmental study of final consonant production in southern black children from preschool through third grade. *Language, Speech, and Hearing Services in Schools, 20*(4), 400–406.

Healy, T., & Madison, C. (1987). Articulation error migration: A comparison of single word and connected speech samples. *Journal of Communication Disorders, 20*, 129–136.

Hecht, M., Collier, M., & Ribeau, S. (1993). *African American communication*. Newbury Park, CA: Sage.

Hegde, M. N. (1998). *Treatment procedures in communicative disorders*. Austin, TX: PRO-ED.

Hegde, M. N. (2003). *Clinical research in communicative disorders: Principles and strategies* (3rd ed.). Austin, TX: PRO-ED.

Hegde, M. N. (2008). *Hegde's pocketguide to assessment in speech–language pathology*. Albany, NY: Thomson Delmar.

Hegde, M. N. (2010a). *A coursebook on scientific and professional writing for speech–language pathology* (3rd ed.). Albany, NY: Thomson Delmar.

Hegde, M. N. (2010b). *Introduction to communicative disorders* (4th ed.). Austin, TX: PRO-ED.

Hegde, M. N. (2010c). Language and grammar: A behavioral analysis. *Journal of Speech–Language Pathology and Applied Behavior Analysis, 5*, 90–113.

Hegde, M. N., & Davis, D. (2010). *Clinical methods and practicum in speech–language pathology* (5th ed.). Clifton Park, NY: Delmar Cengage Learning.

Hegde, M. N., & Maul, C. A. (2006). *Language disorders in children: An evidence-based approach to assessment and treatment*. Boston: Allyn & Bacon.

Hegde, M. N., & Pomaville, F. (2013). *Assessment of communication disorders in children: Resources and protocols* (2nd ed.). San Diego, CA: Plural.

Helfrich-Miller, K. R. (1994). Melodic intonation therapy for developmental apraxia. *Clinics in Communication Disorders, 4*, 175–182.

Henning, C., McIntosh, B., Arnott, W., & Dodd, B. (2010). Long-term outcome of oral language and phonological awareness intervention with socially disadvantaged preschoolers: The impact on language and literacy. *Journal of Research in Reading, 33*, 231–246.

Herbers, H. M., Paden, E. P., & Halle, J. W. (1999). Phonological awareness and production: Change during intervention. *Language, Speech, and Hearing Services in Schools, 30*, 50–60.

Hesketh, A., Adams, C., Nightingale, C., & Hall, R. (2000). Phonological awareness therapy and articulation training approaches for children with phonological disorders: A comparative outcome study. *International Journal of Language and Communication Disorders, 35*(3), 337–354.

Hetzron, R. (1990). Semitic languages. In B. Comrie (Ed.), *The world's major languages*. New York: Oxford University Press.

Hewlett, N. (1988). Acoustic properties of /k/ and /t/ in normal and phonologically disordered speech. *Clinical Linguistics and Phonetics, 2*, 29–45.

Hickman, L. (1997). *Apraxia profile*. San Antonio, TX: Psychological Corporation.

Highwater, J. (1975). *Indian America*. New York: David McKay.

Hixon, T. J., Weismer, G., & Hoit, J. D. (2013). *Preclinical speech science* (2nd ed.). San Diego, CA: Plural.

Hodge, M., Salonka, R., & Kollias, S. (2005, November). *Use of nonspeech oral–motor exercises in children's speech therapy*. Poster presented at the annual meeting of the American Speech-Language-Hearing Association, San Diego, CA.

Hodge, M. M., & Wellman, L. (1999). Management of children with dysarthria. In A. J. Caru..
& E. A. Strand (Eds.), *Clinical management of motor speech disorders in children*. New York:
Thieme.

Hodson, B. W. (1986). *Assessment of phonological processes–Spanish*. San Diego, CA: Los Amigos Association.

Hodson, B. W. (1989). Phonological remediation: A cycles approach. In N. A. Creaghead, P. W.
Newman, & W. A. Secord (Eds.), *Assessment and remediation of articulatory and phonological
disorders* (2nd ed.). Columbus, OH: Merrill.

Hodson, B. W. (1994). Helping children become intelligible and literate: The role of phonology.
Topics in Language Disorders, 14, 1–6.

Hodson, B. W. (1997). Disordered phonologies: What we have learned about assessment and treatment. In B. W. Hodson & M. L. Edwards (Eds.), *Perspectives in applied phonology*
(pp. 197–224). Gaithersburg, MD: Aspen.

Hodson, B. W. (2004). *Hodson assessment of phonological patterns* (3rd ed.). Austin, TX: PRO-ED.

Hodson, B. W., & Paden, E. P. (1981). Phonological processes which characterize unintelligible and
intelligible speech in early childhood. *Journal of Speech and Hearing Disorders, 46*, 369–373.

Hodson, B. W., & Paden, E. P. (1983). *Targeting intelligible speech: A phonological approach to remediation*. San Diego, CA: College-Hill Press.

Hodson, B. W., & Paden, E. P. (1991). *Targeting intelligible speech: A phonological approach to remediation* (2nd ed.). Austin, TX: PRO-ED.

Hoffman, P. R. (1983). Interallophonic generalization of /r/ training. *Journal of Speech and Hearing
Disorders, 48*, 215–221.

Hoffman, P. R., Norris, J. A., & Monjure, J. (1990). Comparison of process targeting and whole
language treatment for phonologically delayed preschool children. *Language, Speech, and
Hearing Services in Schools, 21*, 102–109.

Hoffman, P. R., Schuckers, G. H., & Ratusnik, D. L. (1977). Contextual-coarticulatory inconsistency of /r/ misarticulation. *Journal of Speech and Hearing Research, 20*, 631–643.

Holm, A., Crosbie, S., & Dodd, B. (2005). Treating inconsistent speech disorders. In B. Dodd
(Ed.), *Differential diagnosis and treatment of children with speech disorder* (pp. 182–201). London:
Whurr.

Holm, A., Crosbie, S. & Dodd, B. (2007). Differentiating normal variability from inconsistency
in children's speech: Normative data. *International Journal of Language and Communication
Disorders, 42*, 467–486.

Holm, A., & Dodd, B. (1999). An intervention case study of a bilingual child with phonological
disorder. *Child Language Teaching and Therapy, 15*, 139–158.

Houston, D. (2005). Speech perception in infants. In D. B. Pisoni & R. E. Remez (Eds.), *Handbook
of speech perception* (pp. 417–448). Oxford, UK: Blackwell.

Houston, D. (2011). Infant speech perception. In R. Seewald & A. M. Tharpe (Eds.), *Comprehensive
handbook of audiology* (pp. 47–62). San Diego, CA: Plural.

Howard, I. S., & Messum, P. (2011). Modeling the development of pronunciation in infant speech
acquisition. *Motor Control, 15*, 85–117.

Hudak, T. J. (1990). Thai. In B. Comrie (Ed.), *The world's major languages* (pp. 757–777). New York:
Oxford University Press.

Hume, E. (2004). Deconstructing markedness. *Berkeley Linguistics Society, 30*.

Hume, E. (2011). Markedness. In M. Van Oostendorp, C. Ewen, E. Hume, & K. Rice (Eds.), *The
Blackwell companion to phonology* (Vol. 1, pp. 79–106). New York: Wiley.

Hustad, K. (2010). Childhood dysarthria. In K. M. Yorkson, D. R. Beukelman, E. A. Strand, & M.
Hakel (Eds.), *Management of motor speech sound disorders in children and adults* (3rd ed.). Austin,
TX: PRO-ED.

Hustad, K., & Weismer, G. (2007). A continuum of interventions for individuals with dysarthria: Compensatory and rehabilitative approaches. In G. Weismer (Ed.), *Motor speech disorders* (pp. 261–303). San Diego, CA: Plural.

Hwa-Froelich, F., Hodson, B. W., & Edwards, H. T. (2002). Characteristics of Vietnamese phonology. *American Journal of Speech–Language Pathology, 11,* 264–273.

Iglesias, A. (2002). Latino culture. In D. E. Battle (Ed.), *Communication disorders in multicultural populations* (3rd ed.). Boston: Butterworth-Heinemann.

Ingram, D. (1976). *Phonological disability in children.* New York: American Elsevier.

Ingram, D. (1981). *Procedures for the phonological analysis of children's language.* Baltimore: University Park Press.

Ingram, D. (2000, June). *The measurement of whole word productions.* Paper presented to the Child Phonology Conference, University of Northern Iowa, Cedar Falls.

Ingram, D. (2002). The measurement of whole-word productions. *Journal of Child Language, 29,* 713–733.

Ingram, D., & Ingram, K. D. (2001). A whole-word approach to phonological analysis and intervention. *Language, Speech, and Hearing Services in Schools, 32,* 271–283.

Irwin, J. V., & Weston, A. J. (1975). *Paired stimuli kit.* Milwaukee, WI: Fox Point.

Irwin, J. W., & Wong, S. P. (Eds.). (1983). *Phonological development in children 18 to 72 months.* Carbondale: Southern Illinois University Press.

Irwin, O. C. (1947a). Infant speech: Consonant sounds according to manner of articulation. *Journal of Speech and Hearing Disorders, 12,* 402–404.

Irwin, O. C. (1947b). Infant speech: Consonantal sounds according to place of articulation. *Journal of Speech and Hearing Disorders, 12,* 397–401.

Irwin, O. C. (1948). Infant speech: Development of vowel sounds. *Journal of Speech and Hearing Disorders, 13,* 31–34.

Irwin, O. C. (1952). Speech development in the young child: Some factors related to the speech development of the infant and young child. *Journal of Speech and Hearing Disorders, 17,* 269–279.

Irwin, O. C., & Chen, H. P. (1946). Infant speech: Vowel and consonant frequency. *Journal of Speech and Hearing Disorders, 11,* 123–125.

Iuzzini, J., & Forrest, K. (2010). Evaluation of a combined treatment approach for childhood apraxia of speech. *Clinical Linguistics and Phonetics, 24*(4–5), 335–345.

Jackson, N. E. (1992). Precocious reading of English: Origins, structure, and predictive significance. In P. S. Klein & A. J. Tannenbaum (Eds.), *To be young and gifted* (pp. 171–203). Norwood, NJ: Ablex.

Jakobson, R. (1968). *Child language, aphasia and phonological universals* (A. R. Keiler, Trans.). The Hague, Netherlands: Mouton. (Original work published 1941)

Jakobson, R., Fant, G., & Halle, M. (1952). *Preliminaries to speech analysis: The distinctive features and their correlates.* Cambridge, MA: MIT Press.

Jakobson, R., & Halle, M. (1956). *Fundamentals of language.* The Hague, Netherlands: Mouton.

James, D., van Doorn, J., & McLeod, S. (2002). Segment production in mono-, di- and polysyllabic words in children aged 3–7 years. In F. Windsor, L. Kelly, & N. Hewlett (Eds.), *Themes in clinical phonetics and linguistics* (pp. 287–298). Hillsdale, NJ: Erlbaum.

Jelm, J. M. (2001). *Verbal dyspraxia profile.* DeKalb, IL: Janelle.

Jensen, P., Williams, W., & Bzoch, K. (1975, November). *Preference of young infants for speech vs. nonspeech stimuli.* Paper presented at the annual American Speech and Hearing Association Convention, Washington, DC.

Jimenez, B. C. (1987). Acquisition of Spanish consonants in children aged 3–5 years, 7 months. *Language, Speech, and Hearing Services in the Schools, 18*(4), 357–363.

Joffe, B., & Pring, T. (2008). Children with phonological problems: A survey of clinical practice. *International Journal of Language and Communication Disorders, 43,* 154–164.

Johansson, W., Wendenburg, E., & Westin, B. (1964). Measurement of tone response by the human fetus. *Acta Otolaryngology of Stockholm, 57*, 188–192.

Johnson, J., Winney, B., & Pederson, O. (1980). Single word versus connected speech articulation testing. *Language, Speech, and Hearing Services in Schools, 11*, 175–179.

Johnston, J. (1983). What is language intervention? The role of theory. In J. Miller, D. Yoder, & R. Scheifelbusch (Eds.), *Contemporary issues in language intervention, ASHA Reports 12*, 52–57.

Jordan, G. (2004). *Theory construction in second language acquisition.* Philadelphia: John Benjamins.

Julien, H. M., & Munson, B. (2012). Modifying speech to children based on their perceived phonetic accuracy. *Journal of Speech, Language, and Hearing Research, 55*, 1836–1849.

Jusczyk, P. W., & Luce, P. A. (2002). Speech perception and spoken word recognition: Past and present. *Ear & Hearing, 23*(1), 2–40.

Jusczyk, P., Rosner, B., Cutting, J., Foard, C., & Smith, L. (1977). Categorical perception of nonspeech sounds by 2-month-old infants. *Perceptual Psychophysics, 21*, 50–54.

Justice, L. M. (2006). *Clinical approaches to emergent literacy intervention.* San Diego, CA: Plural.

Kager, R. (1999). *Optimality theory.* Cambridge, UK: Cambridge University Press.

Kaiser, A. P., & Gray, D. B. (1993). *Enhancing children's communication: Research foundation for intervention.* Baltimore: Brookes.

Kamhi, A. (2006). Treatment decisions for children with speech-sound disorders. *Language, Speech, and Hearing Services in Schools, 37*, 271–279.

Kamhi, A. (2008). A meme's-eye view of nonspeech oral motor exercises. *Seminars in Speech and Language, 29*(4), 331–339.

Kamhi, A. G., Pollock, K. E., & Harris, J. L. (1996). *Communication development and disorders in African American children.* Baltimore: Brookes.

Kan, P. F., & Kohnert, K. (2005). Preschoolers learning Hmong and English: Lexical-semantic skills in L1 and L2. *Journal of Speech, Language, and Hearing Research, 48*, 372–383.

Kantor, P. T., Wagner, R. K., Torgesen, J. K., & Rashotte, C. A. (2011). Comparing two forms of dynamic assessment of preschool phonological awareness. *Journal of Learning Disabilities, 44*, 313–321.

Kaufman, N. (1995). *Kaufman speech praxis test for children.* Detroit, MI: Wayne State University Press.

Kaye, A. (1990). Arabic. In B. Comrie (Ed.), *The world's major languages.* New York: Oxford University Press.

Kayser, H. (1995). *Bilingual speech–language pathology: An Hispanic focus.* San Diego, CA: Singular.

Kayser, H. (1998). Hispanic cultures and language. In D. E. Battle (Ed.), *Communication disorders in multicultural populations.* Boston: Butterworth-Heinemann.

Keilmann, A., & Wintermeyer, M. (2008). Is a specialized training of phonological awareness indicated in every preschool child? *Folia Phoniatrica, 60*, 73–79.

Kenney, K. W., & Prather, E. M. (1986). Articulation development in preschool children: Consistency of productions. *Journal of Speech and Hearing Research, 29*, 29–36.

Kent, R. D. (1997). *The speech sciences.* Albany, NY: Thomson Delmar.

Kent, R. D., Adams, S. G., & Turner, G. S. (1996). Models of speech production. In N. J. Lass (Ed.), *Principles of experimental phonetics* (pp. 3–45). St. Louis, MO: Mosby.

Kent, R. D., & Bauer, H. R. (1985). Vocalizations of one-year-olds. *Journal of Child Language, 13*, 491–526.

Kent, R. D., Martin, R. E., & Sufit, R. L. (1990). Oral sensation: A review and clinical prospective. In H. Winitz (Ed.), *Human communication disorders* (Vol. 3). Norwood, NJ: Ablex.

Khan, L., & Lewis, N. (1986). *Phonological analysis*. Circle Pines, MN: American Guidance Service.

Khan, L., & Lewis, N. (2002). *The Khan–Lewis phonological analysis* (2nd ed.). Circle Pines, MN: American Guidance Service.

Kim, N. (1990). Korean. In B. Comrie (Ed.), *The world's major languages* (pp. 881–898). New York: Oxford University Press.

Kiparsky, P. (1982). Lexical morphology and phonology. In I. S. Yang (Ed.), *Linguistics in the morning calm* (pp. 3–91). Seoul, South Korea: Hanshin.

Kirk, C., & Gillon, G. T. (2007). Longitudinal effects of phonological awareness intervention on morphological awareness in children with speech impairment. *Language, Speech, and Hearing Services in Schools, 38*, 342–352.

Klein, H. B., Lederer, S. H., & Cortese, E. E. (1991). Children's knowledge of auditory/articulatory correspondence: Phonologic and metaphonologic. *Journal of Speech and Hearing Research, 34*, 559–564.

Klick, S. L. (1985). Adapted cuing technique for use in treatment of dyspraxia. *Language, Speech, and Hearing Services in School, 16*(4), 256–259.

Knock, T. R., Ballard, K. J., Robin, D. A., & Schmidt, R. A. (2000). Influence on order of stimulus presentation of speech motor learning: A principled approach to treatment of apraxia of speech. *Aphasiology, 14*, 653–668.

Koch, H. (1956). Sibling influence on children's speech. *Journal of Speech and Hearing Disorders, 21*, 322–329.

Koegel, R. L., Koegel, L. K., & Ingham, J. C. (1986). Programming rapid generalization of correct articulation through self-monitoring procedures. *Journal of Speech and Hearing Disorders, 51*, 24–32.

Koegel, R. L., Koegel, L. K., Voy, K. V., & Ingham, J. C. (1988). Within-clinic versus outside-of-clinic self-monitoring of articulation to promote generalization. *Journal of Speech and Hearing Disorders, 53*, 392–399.

Kohnert, K. (2007). *Language disorders in bilingual children and adults*. San Diego, CA: Plural.

Kornfeld, J. R. (1971). Theoretical issues in child phonology. *Papers of the 7th Regional Meeting, Chicago Linguistic Society*, 454–468.

Krashen, S. (1985). *The input hypothesis: Issues and implications*. New York: Longman.

Krauss, M. (n.d.). *Status of Native American language endangerment*. Retrieved from jan.ucc.nau .edu/~jar/SIL/Krauss.pdf

Kresheck, J. D., & Socolofsky, G. (1972). Imitative and spontaneous articulatory assessment of four-year-old children. *Journal of Speech and Hearing Research, 15*, 729–733.

Kuczwara, L. A., Brinholz, J. C., & Klodd, D. A. (1984). Auditory responsiveness in the fetus. *National Student Speech-Language-Hearing Association Journal, 14*, 12–20.

Kuehn, D. P., Lemme, M. L., & Baumgartner, J. M. (Eds.). (1989). *Neural bases of speech, hearing, and language*. Boston: College-Hill Press.

Kuhl, P. K. (1987). Perception of speech sounds in early infancy. In C. Salapatek & L. Cohen (Eds.), *Handbook of infant perception: Vol. 2. From perception to cognition*. New York: Academic Press.

Kuhl, P. K., & Miller, J. D. (1975). Speech perception by the chinchilla: Voiced–voiceless distinction in alveolar plosive consonants. *Science, 190*, 69–72.

Kuhl, P. K., & Miller, J. D. (1978). Speech perception by the chinchilla: Identification functions for synthetic VOT stimuli. *Journal of the Acoustical Society of America, 63*, 905–917.

Kuhl, P., & Padden, D. M. (1983). Enhanced discriminability at the phonetic boundaries for the place feature in macaques. *Journal of the Acoustical Society of America, 73*, 1003–1010.

Kummer, A. W. (2014). *Cleft palate and craniofacial anomalies: Effects on speech and resonance* (3rd ed.). Clifton Park, NY: Delmar Cengage Learning.

Ladefoged, P., & Maddieson, I. (1996). *The sounds of the world's languages.* Oxford, UK: Blackwell.

Laing, S. (2003). Assessment of phonology in preschool African American vernacular English speakers using an alternate response mode. *American Journal of Speech–Language Pathology, 12,* 273–281.

Laing, S., & Espeland, W. (2005). Low intensity phonological awareness training in a preschool classroom for children with communication impairments. *Journal of Communication Disorders, 38*(1), 65–82.

Langdon, H. W., & Cheng, L. L. (Eds.). (1992). *Hispanic children and adults with communication disorders.* Gaithersburg, MD: Aspen.

Larrivee, L., & Catts, H. (1999). Early reading achievement in children with expressive phonological disorders. *American Journal of Speech–Language Pathology, 8,* 118–128.

Lass, N., & Pannbacker, M. (2008). The application of evidence-based practice to nonspeech oral-motor treatments. *Language, Speech, and Hearing Services in Schools, 39,* 408–421.

Leap, W. L. (1993). *American Indian English.* Salt Lake City: University of Utah Press.

Lee, H. B. (1999). Korean. In *Handbook of the International Phonetic Association* (pp. 120–122). Cambridge, UK: Cambridge University Press.

Leman, W. (1980). *A reference grammar of the Cheyenne language.* Retrieved from http://www.language-archives.org/item/oai:sil.org:2188

Lenneberg, E. H. (1967). *Biological foundations of language.* New York: Wiley.

Leonard, L. B. (1985). Unusual and subtle phonological behavior in the speech of phonologically disordered children. *Journal of Speech and Hearing Disorders, 50,* 4–13.

Leonard, R. J. (1994). Characteristics of speech in speakers with oral/oralpharyngeal ablation. In J. Bernthal & N. Bankson (Eds.), *Child phonology: Characteristics, assessment, and intervention with special populations.* New York: Thieme.

Leopold, W. F. (1947). *Speech development of a bilingual child: A linguist's record: Vol. 2. Sound-learning in the first two years.* Evanston, IL: Northwestern University Press.

Levitt, H., & Stromberg, H. (1983). Segmental characteristics of speech of hearing-impaired children: Factors affecting intelligibility. In I. Hochberg, H. Levitt, & M. Osberger (Eds.), *Speech of the hearing impaired.* Baltimore: University Park Press.

Lewis, B. A. (1992). Pedigree analysis of children with phonology disorders. *Journal of Learning Disabilities, 25,* 586–597.

Lewis, B. A. (2010). Genetic influences on speech sound disorders. In R. Paul & P. Flipsen, Jr. (Eds.), *Speech sound disorders in children* (pp. 51–69). San Diego, CA: Plural.

Lewis, B. A., Avrich, A. A., Freebairn, L. A., Taylor, H. G., Iyengar, S. K., & Stein, C. M. (2011). Subtyping children with speech sound disorders by endophenotypes. *Topics in Language Disorders, 31*(2), 112–127.

Lewis, B., Ekelman, B., & Aram, D. (1989). A familial study of severe phonological disorders. *Journal of Speech and Hearing Research, 32,* 713–724.

Lewis, B. A., Freebairn, L., Hansen, A., Iyengar, S., & Taylor, G. (2004). School-age follow-up of children with childhood apraxia of speech. *Language, Speech, and Hearing Services in Schools, 35,* 122–140.

Lewis, B. A., Freebairn, L., Hansen, A., Miscimarra, L., Iyengar, S., & Taylor, G. (2007). Speech and language skills of parents of children with speech sound disorders. *American Journal of Speech–Language Pathology, 16,* 108–118.

Lewis, B., & Freebairn-Farr, L. (1991). *Preschool phonology disorders at school age, adolescence, and adulthood.* Paper presented at the convention of the American Speech-Language-Hearing Association, Atlanta, GA.

Lewis, B. A., Shriberg, L., Freebairn, L., Hansen, A., Stein, C., Taylor, G., et al. (2006). The genetic basis of speech sound disorders: Evidence from spoken and written language. *Journal of Speech, Language, and Hearing Research, 49,* 1294–1312.

Lewkowicz, D. J., & Hansen-Tift, A. M. (2012). Infants deploy selective attention to the mouth of a talking face when learning speech. *Proceedings of the National Academy of Science, 109,* 1431–1436.

Li, C., & Thompson, S. (1987). Chinese. In B. Comrie (Ed.), *The world's major languages* (pp. 811–833). New York: Oxford University Press.

Liberman, I. Y. (1973). Segmentation of the spoken word and reading acquisition. *Bulletin of the Orton Society, 23,* 65–77.

Liberman, M. (1970). The grammar of speech and language. *Cognitive Psychology, 1,* 301–323.

Liberman, M. (1975). *The intonational system of English.* New York: Garland.

Liberman, M., & Prince, A. (1977). On stress and linguistic rhythm. *Linguistic Inquiry, 8,* 249–336.

Linares, T. A. (1981). Articulation skills in Spanish-speaking children. In R. V. Padilla (Ed.), *Ethnoperspectives in bilingual education research: Vol. 3. Ethnoperspectives in bilingual education research: Bilingual education technology.* Ypsilanti: Michigan State University.

Lindamood, P. C., & Lindamood, P. (2004). *Lindamood auditory conceptualization test* (3rd ed.). Austin, TX: PRO-ED.

Ling, D., & Ling, A. (1978). *Aural habilitation: The foundations of verbal learning in hearing-impaired children.* Washington, DC: A.G. Bell Association for the Deaf.

Lippke, B. A., Dickey, S. E., Selmar, J. W., & Soder, A. L. (1997). *Photo articulation test* (3rd ed.). Austin, TX: PRO-ED.

Locke, J. L. (1980a). The inference of speech perception in the phonologically disordered child: I. A rationale, some criteria, the conventional tests. *Journal of Speech and Hearing Disorders, 45,* 431–444.

Locke, J. L. (1980b). The inference of speech perception in the phonologically disordered child: II. Some clinically novel procedures, their use, some findings. *Journal of Speech and Hearing Disorders, 45,* 445–468.

Locke, J. L. (1983). *Phonological acquisition and change.* New York: Academic Press.

Lof, G. L. (2009, November). *Nonspeech oral motor exercises: An update on the controversy.* Paper presented at the American Speech-Language-Hearing Association Convention, New Orleans, LA.

Lof, G. L. (2012, April). *An evidence-based speech sound disorders update.* Workshop presented at the Manitoba Speech and Hearing Association, Winnipeg, Canada.

Lof, G. L., & Watson, M. (2008). A nationwide survey of nonspeech oral motor exercise use: Implications for evidence-based practice. *Language, Speech, and Hearing Services in Schools, 39,* 392–407.

Long, M. H. (1983). Native speaker/nonnative speaker conversation and the negotiation of comprehensible input. *Applied Linguistics, 4,* 126–141.

Long, M. H. (2000). Second language acquisition theories. In M. Byram (Ed.), *Encyclopedia of language teaching* (pp. 527–534). London: Routledge.

Long, S. H. (1994). Language and other special populations of children. In V. Reed (Ed.), *An introduction to children with language disorders* (2nd ed.). New York: Merrill.

Lonigan, C. J., Anthony, J. L., Phillips, B. M., Purpura, D. J., Wilson, S. B., & McQueen, J. D. (2009). The nature of preschool phonological processing abilities and their relation to vocabulary, general cognitive abilities, and print knowledge. *Journal of Educational Psychology, 101,* 345–358.

Lonigan, C. J., Burgess, S. R., Anthony, J. L., & Barker, T. A. (1998). Development of phonological sensitivity in 2- to 5-year-old children. *Journal of Educational Psychology, 90,* 294–311.

Lowe, R. J. (1994). *Phonology: Assessment and intervention applications in speech pathology.* Baltimore: Williams & Wilkins.

Lowe, R. J. (1995). *Assessment link between phonology and articulation* (Rev. ed.). Moline, IL: LinguiSystems.

Lowe, R. J. (2012). *Workbook for the identification of phonological processes and distinctive features* (4th ed.). Austin, TX: PRO-ED.

Lowe, R. J., Knutson, P. J., & Monson, M. A. (1985). Incidence of fronting in preschool children. *Language, Speech, and Hearing Services in Schools, 16*, 119–123.

Lundeen, C. (1991). Prevalence of hearing impairment among school children. *Language, Speech, and Hearing Services in Schools, 32*, 87–96.

Maag, J. W. (1999). *Behavior management.* San Diego, CA: Singular.

Maas, E., & Farinella, K. A. (2012). Random versus blocked practice in treatment of childhood apraxia of speech. *Journal of Speech, Language, and Hearing Research, 55*, 561–578.

Maas, E., Robin, D., Austermann Hula, S., Freedman, S., Wulf, G., Ballard, K., et al. (2008). Principles of motor learning in treatment of motor speech disorders. *American Journal of Speech–Language Pathology, 17*, 277–298.

MacKay, I. (1987). *Phonetics: The science of speech production* (2nd ed.). Boston: Pearson.

Macken, M. A., & Barton, D. P. (1980). A longitudinal study of the acquisition of the voicing contrasts in American-English word-initial stops, as measured by voice onset time. *Journal of Child Language, 7*, 41–74.

Macken, M. A., & Ferguson, C. A. (1983). Cognitive aspects of phonological development: Model, evidence, and issues. In K. E. Nelson (Ed.), *Children's language* (Vol. 4). Hillsdale, NJ: Erlbaum.

Majorano, M., & D'Odorico, L. (2011). The transition into ambient language: A longitudinal study of babbling and first word production of Italian children. *First Language, 31*(1), 47–66.

Mann, V. A., & Foy, J. G. (2003). Phonological awareness, speech development, and letter knowledge in preschool children. *Annals of Dyslexia, 53*, 149–173.

Marquardt, T. P., Sussman, H. M., & Davis, B. L. (2001). Developmental apraxia of speech: Advances in theory and practice. In D. Vogel & M. P. Cannito (Eds.), *Treating disordered speech motor control* (2nd ed.). Austin, TX: PRO-ED.

Marshalla, P. (1996). *Oral–motor techniques in articulation therapy.* Temecula, CA: Speech Dynamics.

Mason, M., Smith, M., & Hinshaw, M. (1976). *Medida Española de Articulacion [Spanish Articulation Measure].* San Ysidro, CA: San Ysidro School District.

Mason, R. M. (1988). Orthodontic perspectives on orofacial myofunctional therapy. *International Journal of Orofacial Myology, 14*, 49–55.

Mason, R., & Proffit, W. (1974). The tongue-thrust controversy: Background and recommendations. *Journal of Speech and Hearing Disorders, 39*, 115–132.

Matheney, A., & Panagos, J. (1978). Comparing the effects of articulation and syntax programs on syntax and articulation improvement. *Language, Speech, and Hearing Services in Schools, 9*, 57–61.

Mattes, L. (1994). *Spanish articulation measures* (Rev. ed.). Oceanside, CA: Academic Communication Associates.

Mattes, L. J. (1995). *Spanish language assessment procedure* (3rd ed.). Oceanside, CA: Academic Communication Associates.

Mattes, L. J. (1998). *Assessment of sound awareness and production.* Oceanside, CA: Academic Communication Associates.

McAuliffe, M. J., & Ward, E. C. (2006). The use of electropalatography in the assessment and treatment of acquired motor speech disorders in adults: Current knowledge and future directions. *NeuroRehabilitation, 21*, 189–203.

McCabe, R. B., & Bradley, D. P. (1973). *The systematic multiphonemic approach to articulation therapy.* Short course presented at American Speech-Language-Hearing Association Southeastern Regional Conference, Atlanta.

McCabe, R. B., & Bradley, D. P. (1975). Systematic multiple phonemic approach to articulation therapy. *Acta Symbolica, 6*, 2–18.

McCarthy, J. (1988). Feature geometry and dependency: A review. *Phonetics, 43,* 84–108.

McCarthy, J., & Prince, A. (1993). *Prosodic morphology I: Constraint interaction and satisfaction* (Tech. Rep. No. 3). Piscataway, NJ: Rutgers Center for Cognitive Science.

McCarthy, J., & Prince, A. (1994). The emergence of the unmarked: Optimality in prosodic morphology. *Northeastern Linguistic Society, 24,* 333–379.

McCauley, R. J., & Strand, E. A. (2008). A review of standardized tests of nonverbal oral and speech motor performance in children. *American Journal of Speech–Language Pathology, 17,* 81–91.

McCauley, R. J., Strand, E., Lof, G. L., Schooling, T., & Frymark, T. (2009). Evidence-based systematic review: Effects of non-speech oral motor exercises on speech. *American Journal of Speech–Language Pathology.* doi:10.1044/1058-0360(2009/09-0006)

McCormack, P., & Dodd, B. (1998, September). *Is inconsistency in word production an artifact of severity in developmental speech disorders?* Poster presented at Child Language Seminar, Sheffield, England.

McCune, L., & Vihman, M. M. (2001). Early phonetic and lexical development: A productivity approach. *Journal of Speech, Language, and Hearing Research, 44,* 670–684.

McDonald, E. (1964). *Deep test of articulation.* Pittsburgh, PA: Stanwix House.

McDonald, E. T., & Aungst, L. (1970). Apparent independence of oral sensory functions and articulatory proficiency. In J. Bosma (Ed.), *Second symposium on oral sensation and perception.* Springfield, IL: Charles C. Thomas.

McEwen, F., Happe, F., Bolton, P., Bolton, P., Rijsdijk, F., Ronald, A., et al. (2007). Origins of individual differences in imitation: Links with language, pretend play, and socially insightful behavior in two-year-old twins. *Child Development, 78,* 479–492.

McIntosh, B., & Dodd, B. (2008). Evaluation of core vocabulary intervention for treatment of inconsistent phonological disorder: Three case studies. *Child Language Teaching and Therapy, 24,* 305–327.

McLaughlin, B., & Heredia, R. (1996). Information processing approaches to research on second language acquisition and use. In W. Ritchie & T. Bhatia (Eds.), *Handbook of second language acquisition.* San Diego, CA: Academic Press.

McLaughlin, S. (2006). *Introduction to language development* (2nd ed.). Albany, NY: Thomson Delmar.

McLaughlin, S. (2010). *Verbal Behavior* by B. F. Skinner: Contributions to analyzing early language learning. *Journal of Speech–Language Pathology and Applied Behavior Analysis, 5,* 114–149.

McLeod, S. (Ed.). (2007). *The international guide to speech acquisition.* Clifton Park, NY: Thomson Delmar Learning.

McLeod, S., van Doorn, J., & Reed, V. A. (2001). Consonant cluster development in two-year-olds: General trends and individual differences. *Journal of Speech, Language, and Hearing Research, 44,* 1144–1171.

McNutt, J. (1994). Generalization of /s/ from English to French as a result of phonological remediation. *Journal of Speech–Language Pathology and Audiology / Revue d'orthophonic et d'audiologie, 18,* 109–114.

McReynolds, L. (1972). Articulation generalization during articulation training. *Language and Speech, 15,* 149–155.

McReynolds, L., & Bennett, S. (1972). Distinctive feature generalization in articulation training. *Journal of Speech and Hearing Disorders, 37,* 462–470.

McReynolds, L., & Elbert, M. (1981a). Criteria for phonological process analysis. *Journal of Speech and Hearing Disorders, 46,* 197–204.

McReynolds, L., & Elbert, M. (1981b). Generalization of correct articulation in clusters. *Applied Psycholinguistics, 2,* 119–132.

McReynolds, L., & Engmann, D. (1975). *Distinctive feature analysis of misarticulations*. Baltimore: University Park Press.

McWhorter, J. (2000). *Spreading the word: Language and dialect in America*. Portsmouth, NH: Heinemann.

McWilliams, B. J., Morris, H. L., & Shelton, R. L. (1990). *Cleft palate speech* (2nd ed.). Philadelphia: B.C. Decker.

Mecham, M. (1996). *Cerebral palsy* (2nd ed.). Austin, TX: PRO-ED.

Mehler, J., Jusczyk, P., Lambertz, G., Halsted, N., Bertoncini, J., & Amiel-Tison, C. (1988). A precursor of language acquisition in young infants. *Cognition, 29,* 143–178.

Melby-Lervag, M., Lyster, S-A. H., & Hulme, C. (2012). Phonological skills and their role in learning to read: A meta-analytic review. *Psychological Bulletin, 138,* 322–352.

Menn, L. (1976). Evidence for an interactionist-discovery theory of child phonology. *Stanford Papers and Reports on Child Language Development, 12,* 169–177.

Menn, L. (1983). Development of articulatory, phonetic, and phonological capabilities. In B. Butterworth (Ed.), *Language production* (Vol. 2). London: Academic Press.

Menn, L. (2004). Saving the baby: Making sure that old data survive new theories. In R. Kager, J. Pater, & W. Zonneveld (Eds.), *Constraints in phonological acquisition* (pp. 54–77). New York: Cambridge University Press.

Menyuk, P. (1968). The role of distinctive features in children's acquisition of phonology. *Journal of Speech and Hearing Research, 11,* 138–146.

Meyer, P. G. (2000). Tongue, lip, and jaw differentiation and its relationship to orofacial myofunctional treatment. *International Journal of Orofacial Myology, 26,* 44–52.

Meyer, P. J. (2006). *Attitude is everything: If you want to succeed above and beyond* (Vol. 2). Merced, CA: Leading Edge.

Meza, P. (1983). *Phonological analysis of Spanish utterances of highly unintelligible Mexican-American children*. Unpublished master's thesis, San Diego State University, San Diego, CA.

Miccio, A. W. (2005). Components of phonological assessment. In S. F. Warren & M. E. Fey (Series Eds.) & A. G. Kamhi & K. E. Pollock (Vol. Eds.), *Communication and language intervention series: Phonological disorders in children—Clinical decision making in assessment and intervention* (pp. 163–173). Baltimore: Brookes.

Miccio, A. W. (2009). First things first: Stimulability therapy for children with small phonetic repertoires. In C. Bowen (Ed.), *Children's speech sound disorders* (pp. 96–101). Malden, MA: Wiley-Blackwell.

Miccio, A. W., & Elbert, M. (1996). Enhancing stimulability: A treatment program. *Journal of Communication Disorders, 29,* 335–351.

Miccio, A. W., & Scarpino, S. E. (2011). Phonological analysis, phonological processes. In M. J. Ball, M. R. Perkins, & S. Howard (Eds.), *The handbook of clinical linguistics* (pp. 412–422). Malden, MA: Wiley-Blackwell.

Miccio, A. W., & Williams, A. L. (2010). Stimulability intervention. In S. F. Warren & M. E. Fey (Series Eds.) & A. L. Williams, S. McLeod, & R. J. McCauley (Vol. Eds.), *Intervention for speech sound disorders in children* (pp. 179–202). Baltimore: Brookes.

Miller, J. D., & Kuhl, P. K. (1976). Speech perception by the chinchilla: A progress report on syllable-initial voiced-plosive consonants. *Journal of the Acoustical Society of America, 59,* S54(A).

Miller, J. L., Kent, R. D., & Atal, B. S. (Eds.). (1991). *Papers in speech communication: Speech perception*. Woodbury, NY: Acoustical Society of America.

Miller, P. C., & Diane, M. (2011). Phonemic awareness is not necessary to become skilled deaf reader. *Journal of Developmental and Physical Disabilities, 23,* 459, 476.

Mitchell, R., & Myles, F. (2004). *Second language learning theories* (2nd ed.). London: Arnold.

Moerk, E. L. (1983). *The mother of Eve—as a first language teacher*. Norwood, NJ: Ablex.

Moerk, E. L. (1989). The LAD was a lady and the tasks were ill-defined. *Developmental Review, 9,* 21–57.

Moerk, E. L. (1990). Three-term contingency patterns in mother–child verbal interactions during first language acquisition. *Journal of the Experimental Analysis of Behavior, 54,* 293–305.

Moerk, E. L. (1992). *A first language taught and learned.* Baltimore: Brookes.

Moerk, E. L. (1996). Input and learning processes in first language acquisition. In H. W. Rees (Ed.), *Advances in child development and behavior* (Vol. 26). New York: Academic Press.

Moerk, E. L. (2000). *The guided acquisition of first language skills.* Stamford, CT: Ablex.

Moller, K. T., & Glaze, L. E. (2009). *Cleft lip and palate: Interdisciplinary issues and treatment* (2nd ed.). Austin, TX: PRO-ED.

Moon, C., Cooper, R. P., & Fifer, W. P. (1993). 2-day-olds prefer their native language. *Infant Behavior and Development, 16*(4), 495–500.

Moon, C., & Fifer, W. P. (1990). Syllables as signals for 2-day-old infants. *Infant Behavior and Development, 13,* 377–390.

Morais, J. (1991a). Constraints on the development of phonological awareness. In S. A. Brady & D. P. Shankweiler (Eds.), *Phonological processes in literacy* (pp. 5–27). Hillsdale, NJ: Erlbaum.

Morais, J. (1991b). Phonological awareness: A bridge between language and literacy. In D. Sawyer & B. Fox (Eds.), *Phonological awareness in reading: The evolution of current perspectives* (pp. 31–72). New York: Springer-Verlag.

Morley, M. (1957). *The development and disorders of speech in childhood.* Edinburgh, UK: Churchill Livingstone.

Morrisette, M. L., & Gierut, J. A. (2002). Lexical organization and phonological change in treatment. *Journal of Speech, Language, and Hearing Research, 45,* 143–159.

Morrison, J., & Shriberg, L. (1992). Articulation testing versus conversational speech sampling. *Journal of Speech and Hearing Research, 35,* 259–273.

Morse, P. A. (1972). The discrimination of speech and non-speech stimuli in early infancy. *Journal of Exceptional Child Psychology, 14,* 477–492.

Moskowitz, A. (1973). Acquisition of phonology and syntax: A preliminary study. In G. Hinitikka, J. Moravcsik, & P. Suppes (Eds.), *Approaches to natural language.* Dordrecht, Holland: Reidel.

Mowrer, D. E. (1971). Transfer of training in articulation therapy. *Journal of Speech and Hearing Disorders, 36,* 427–445.

Mowrer, O. (1960). *Learning theory and symbolic processes.* New York: Wiley.

Muir, D., & Field, J. (1979). Newborn infants orient to sounds. *Child Development, 50,* 431–436.

Mullen, R., & Schooling, T. (2010). The national outcome measurement system for pediatric speech–language pathology. *Language, Speech, and Hearing Services in Schools, 41,* 44–60.

Munhall, K. G., & Johnson, E. K. (2012). Speech perception: When to put your money where the mouth is. *Current Biology, 22*(6), R190–R192.

Munson, B., Edwards, J., Schellinger, S., Beckman, M. E., & Meyer, M. K. (2010). Deconstructing phonetic transcription: Covert contrast, perceptual bias, and an extraterrestrial view of Vox Humana. *Clinical Linguistics and Phonetics, 24,* 245–260.

Murdoch, B. E., Porter, S., Younger, R., & Ozanne, A. (1984). Behaviors identified by South Australian clinicians as differentially diagnostic of developmental articulatory dyspraxia. *Australian Journal of Human Communication Disorders, 12*(2), 55–70.

Murdock, J. Y., Garcia, E. E., & Hardman, M. L. (1977). Generalizing articulation training with trainable mentally retarded subjects. *Journal of Applied Behavior Analysis, 10,* 717–733.

Muter, V., Hulme, C., Snowling, M., & Taylor, S. (1997). Segmentation, not rhyming, predicts early progress in learning to read. *Journal of Experimental Child Psychology, 65,* 370–398.

Nancollis, A., Lawrie, B, & Dodd, B. (2005). Phonological awareness intervention and the acquisition of literacy skills in children from deprived social backgrounds. *Language, Speech, and Hearing Services in Schools, 36,* 325–335.

Nathani, S., Ertmer, D., & Stark, R. (2006). Assessing vocal development in infants and toddlers. *Clinical Linguistics and Phonetics, 20,* 351–369.

Neel, A. T., & Palmer, P. M. (2012). Is tongue strength an important influence on rate of articulation in diadochokinetic and reading tasks? *Journal of Speech, Language, and Hearing Research, 55,* 235–246.

Nemoy, E., & Davis, S. (1937). *The correction of defective consonant sounds.* Boston: Expression.

Nemoy, E., & Davis, S. (1954). *The correction of defective consonant sounds* (Rev. ed.). Boston: Expression.

Netsell, R. (1986). *Neurobiologic view of speech production and the dysarthrias.* Boston: College-Hill Press.

Newbury, D. F., & Monaco, A. P. (2010). Genetic advances in the study of speech and language disorders. *Neuron, 68,* 309–320.

Newcomer, P., & Barenbaum, E. (2003). *Test of phonological awareness skills.* Austin, TX: PRO-ED.

Newman, P. W., & Creaghead, N. A. (1989). Assessment of articulatory and phonological disorders. In N. A. Creaghead, P. W. Newman, & W. A. Secord (Eds.), *Assessment and remediation of articulatory and phonological disorders* (2nd ed.). Columbus, OH: Merrill.

Newport, E., Gleitman, A., & Gleitman, L. (1977). Mother, I'd rather do it myself: Some effects and non-effects of maternal speech style. In C. Snow & C. Ferguson (Eds.), *Talking to children: Language input and acquisition.* New York: Cambridge University Press.

Nittrouer, S. (2001). Challenging the notion of innate phonetic boundaries. *Journal of the Acoustical Society of America, 110,* 1598–1605.

Nittrouer, S. (2002). From ear to cortex: A perspective on what clinicians need to understand about speech perception and language processing. *Language, Speech, and Hearing Services in Schools, 33,* 237–252.

Norris, J. A., & Hoffman, P. R. (1990). Language intervention within naturalistic environments. *Language, Speech, and Hearing Services in Schools, 21,* 72–84.

Ohala, J. J. (1980). Application of phonological universals in speech pathology. In N. J. Lass (Ed.), *Speech and language: Advances in basic research and practice* (Vol. 3, pp. 75–97). New York: Academic Press.

Ohala, J. J. (1986). Consumer's guide to evidence in phonology. *Phonology Year Book, 3,* 3–26.

Ohala, J. J. (1995). Phonetics of phonology. In G. Bloothooft, V. Hazan, D. Huber, & J. Listerri (Eds.), *European studies in phonetics and speech communication.* Utrecht, Netherlands: OTS Publications.

Ohala, J. J. (1996). Phonetics of sound change. In C. Jones (Ed.), *Historical linguistics: Problems and prospects* (pp. 237–278). London: Longman.

Ohala, J. J. (1997, August). Phonetics in phonology. In *Proceedings of the 4th Seoul International Conference on Linguistics* (pp. 45–50). Retrieved from http://www.linguistics.berkeley.edu/~ohala/papers/SEOUL1-phonet-phonol.pdf

Ohala, J. J. (2004). Phonetics and phonology then, and then, and now. In H. Quené & V. van Heuven (Eds.), *On speech and language: Studies for Sieb G. Nooteboom.* LOT Occasional Series 2. Utrecht, Netherlands: Netherlands Graduate School of Linguistics.

Ohala, J. J. (2005). Phonetic explanations for sound patterns: Implications for grammars of competence. In W. J. Hardcastle & J. M. Beck (Eds.), *A figure of speech. A festschrift for John Laver* (pp. 23–38). Mahwah, NJ: Erlbaum.

Ohde, R. N., & Sharf, D. J. (1992). *Phonetic analysis of normal and abnormal speech.* New York: Merrill.

Oller, D. K. (1980). The emergence of the sounds of speech in infancy. In G. Yeni-Komshian, J. Kavanagh, & C. A. Ferguson (Eds.), *Child phonology: Vol. 1. Production*. New York: Academic Press.

Oller, D. K. (2000). *The emergence of the speech capacity*. Mahwah, NJ: Erlbaum.

Oller, D. K., Eilers, R., Basinger, D., Steffens, M. L., & Urbano, R. (1995). Extreme poverty and the development of precursors to the speech capacity. *First Language, 15*(Part 2), 167–187.

Oller, D. K., Eilers, R., Steffens, M. L., Lynch, M. P., & Urbano, R. (1994). Speech-like vocalizations in infancy: An evaluation of potential risk factors. *First Language, 21*(Part 1), 33–58.

Oller, D. K., & Griebel, U. (2008). Contextual flexibility in infant vocal development and the earliest steps in the evolution of language. In D. K. Oller & U. Griebel (Eds.), *Evolution of communicative flexibility: Complexity, creativity, and adaptability in human and animal communication* (pp. 141–168). Cambridge, MA: MIT Press.

Oller, D. K., Wieman, L. A., Doyle, W. J., & Ross, C. (1976). Infant babbling and speech. *Journal of Child Language, 3*, 1–11.

Olmsted, D. (1971). *Out of the mouth of babes*. The Hague, Netherlands: Mouton.

Olswang, L. B., & Bain, B. A. (1985). The natural occurrence of generalization during articulation treatment. *Journal of Communication Disorders, 18*, 109–129.

O'Neill, J., & Conzemius, A. (2006). *The power of SMART goals: Using goals to improve student learning*. Bloomington, IN: Solution Tree.

Owens, R. (2005). *Language development: An introduction* (6th ed.). Boston: Allyn & Bacon.

Pagliarian, K. C. (2009). *Analysis of therapeutic efficacy in three phonological models of contrastive approach*. Unpublished dissertation, Federal University of Santa Maria, Santa Maria, Brazil.

Panagos, J., Quine, M., & Klich, R. (1979). Syntactic and phonological influences on children's articulation. *Journal of Speech and Hearing Research, 22*, 841–848.

Paradis, J. L., Dollaghan, C. A., Campbell, T. E., Feldman, H. M., Bernard, B. S., Colburn, D. K., et al. (2000). Language, speech sound production, and cognition in three-year-old children in relation to otitis media in their first three years of life. *Pediatrics, 105*, 1119–1130.

Paradis, J. L., & Genesee, F. (1996). Syntactic acquisition in bilingual children: Autonomous or interdependent? Studies in *Second Language Acquisition, 18*, 1–25.

Paterson, M. M. (1994). Articulation and phonological disorders in hearing-impaired school-aged children with severe and profound sensorineural losses. In J. E. Bernthal & W. Bankson (Eds.), *Child phonology: Characteristics, assessment, and intervention with special populations*. New York: Thieme.

Patkowski, M. S. (1994). The critical age hypothesis and interlanguage phonology. In M. Yavas (Ed.), *First and second language phonology*. San Diego, CA: Singular.

Patterson, J. L. (1999). What bilingual toddlers hear and say: Language input and word combinations. *Communication Disorders Quarterly, 2*(1), 32–38.

Paynter, E. T., & Bumpas, T. C. (1977). Imitative and spontaneous articulatory assessment of three-year-old children. *Journal of Speech and Hearing Disorders, 42*, 119–125.

Paynter, E. T., & Petty, N. A. (1974). Articulatory sound acquisition of two-year-old children. *Perceptual and Motor Skills, 39*, 1079–1085.

Pearson, B. Z. (2004). Theoretical and empirical bases for dialect-neutral language assessment: Contributions from theoretical and applied linguistics to communication disorders. *Seminars in Speech and Language, 25*(1), 13–25.

Pearson, B. Z., Velleman, S. L., Bryant, T. J., & Charko, T. (2009). Phonological milestones for African American English-speaking children learning Mainstream American English as a second dialect. *Language, Speech, and Hearing Services in Schools, 40*, 229–244.

Pence, K. (2007). *Assessment in early literacy*. San Diego, CA: Plural.

Pennington, L., Goldbart, J., & Marshall, J. (2004). Speech and language therapy to improve the communication skills of children with cerebral palsy. *Cochrane Database of Systematic Review*, 2, 1–51.

Pennington, L., Goldbart, J., & Marshall, J. (2005). Direct speech and language therapy for children with cerebral palsy: Findings from a systematic review. *Developmental Medicine and Child Neurology*, 47, 57–63.

Pennington, L., Smallman, C., & Farrier, F. (2006). Intensive dysarthria therapy for older children with cerebral palsy: Findings from six case studies. *Child Language Teaching Therapy*, 22, 255–273.

Pennington, M. C. (2007). The context of phonology. In M. C. Pennington (Ed.), *Phonology in context* (pp. 1–24). New York: Palgrave Macmillan.

Perez, E. (1994). Phonological differences among speakers of Spanish-influenced English. In J. E. Bernthal & N. W. Bankson (Eds.), *Child phonology: Characteristics, assessment, and intervention with special populations*. New York: Thieme.

Peterson, R. L., Pennington, B. F., Shriberg, L. D., & Boada, R. (2009). What influences literary outcome in children with speech sound disorders? *Journal of Speech, Language, and Hearing Research*, 52, 1175–1188.

Peterson-Falzone, S., Hardin-Jones, M. A., & Karnell, M. P. (2001). *Cleft palate speech* (3rd ed.). St. Louis, MO: Mosby.

Phillips, S. U. (1983). *The invisible culture: Communication in classroom and community on the Warm Springs Indian Reservation*. New York: Longman.

Pierce, J. R., & Hanna, I. V. (1974). *The development of a phonological system in English-speaking American children*. Portland, OR: HaPi Press.

Pigott, T., Barry, J., Hughes, B., Eastin, D., Titus, P., Stensil, H., et al. (1985). *Speech-ease screening inventory: K-1*. Austin, TX: PRO-ED.

Pollock, K. (2002). Identification of vowel errors: Methodological issues and preliminary data from the Memphis vowel project. In M. J. Ball & F. E. Gibbon (Eds.), *Vowel disorders* (pp. 83–113). Boston: Butterworth-Heinemann.

Pollock, K., & Berni, M. C. (2003). Incidence of non-rhotic vowel errors in children: Data from the Memphis vowel project. *Clinical Linguistics and Phonetics*, 17, 393–401.

Pollock, K., Meeks, M., Stepherson, E., & Berni, M. C. (2004, May). *Types of vowel errors in children: More data from the Memphis Vowel Project*. Paper presented at the annual Child Phonology Conference, Tempe, AZ.

Poole, E. (1934). Genetic development of articulation of consonant sounds in speech. *Elementary English Review*, 11, 159–161.

Powell, T. W. (1991). Planning for phonological generalization: An approach to treatment target selection. *American Journal of Speech–Language Pathology*, 1, 21–27.

Powell, T. W. (1996). Stimulability considerations in the phonological treatment of a child with a persistent disorder of speech-sound production. *Journal of Communication Disorders*, 29, 315–333.

Powell, T. W. (2003). Stimulability and treatment outcomes. *Perspectives on Language Learning and Education*, 10(1), 3–6.

Powell, T. W., & Elbert, M. (1984). Generalization following the remediation of early- and late-developing consonant clusters. *Journal of Speech and Hearing Disorders*, 49, 211–218.

Powell, T. W., Elbert, M., & Dinnsen, D. (1991). Stimulability as a factor in the phonologic generalization of misarticulating preschool children. *Journal of Speech and Hearing Research*, 34, 1318–1328.

Powell, T. W., & McReynolds, L. V. (1969). A procedure for testing position generalization from articulation training. *Journal of Speech and Hearing Disorders*, 12, 629–645.

Prather, E., Hedrick, D., & Kern, C. (1975). Articulation development in children aged two to four years. *Journal of Speech and Hearing Research, 40*, 55–63.

Pratt, A., & Brady, S. (1988). Relation of phonological awareness to reading disability in children and adults. *Journal of Educational Psychology, 80*, 319–323.

Preisser, D. A., Hodson, B. W., & Paden, E. P. (1988). Developmental phonology. *Journal of Speech and Hearing Disorders, 53*, 125–130.

Preston, J., & Edwards, M. L. (2010). Phonological awareness and types of sound errors in preschoolers with speech sound disorders. *Journal of Speech and Hearing Research, 53*, 44–60.

Preston, J. L., & Koenig, L. L. (2011). Phonetic variability in residual speech sound disorders: Exploration of subtypes. *Topics in Language Disorders, 31*(2), 168–184

Prezas, R. F., & Hodson, B. W. (2010). The cycles phonological remediation approach. In S. F. Warren & M. E. Fey (Series Eds.) & A. L. Williams, S. McLeod, & R. J. McCauley (Vol. Eds.), *Intervention for speech sound disorders in children* (pp. 137–157). Baltimore: Brookes.

Prince, A., & Smolensky, P. (1993). *Optimality theory: Constraint interaction in generative grammar* (Tech. Rep. No. 2). Piscataway, NJ: Rutgers Center for Cognitive Science.

Prosek, R., & House, A. (1975). Intraoral air pressure as a feedback cue in consonant production. *Journal of Speech and Hearing Research, 18*, 133–147.

Pruitt, S., & Oetting, J. (2009). Past tense marking by African American English-speaking children reared in poverty. *Journal of Speech, Language, and Hearing Research, 52*, 2–15.

Pullum, G. K., & Scholz, B. C. (2002). Empirical assessment of stimulus poverty arguments. *Linguistic Review, 19*, 9–50.

Raitano, N. A., Pennington, B. F., Tunick, R. A., Boada, R., & Shriberg, L. D. (2004). Pre-literacy skills of subgroups of children with speech sound disorders. *Journal of Child Psychology and Psychiatry, 45*, 821–835.

Raphael, L. J., Borden, G. J., & Harris, K. S. (2011). *A speech science primer.* Baltimore: Lippincott Williams & Wilkins.

Ray, E., & Heyes, C. (2011). Imitation in infancy: The wealth of the stimulus. *Developmental Science, 14*, 92–105.

Ray, J. (2002). Treating phonological disorders in a multilingual child: A case study. *American Journal of Speech–Language Pathology, 11*, 305–315.

Reber, A. S. (1993). *Implicit learning and tacit knowledge: An essay on the cognitive unconscious.* New York: Oxford University Press.

Reber, A. S. (2011). An epitaph for grammar: An abridged history. In C. Sanz & L. P. Leow (Eds.), *Implicit and explicit language learning: Conditions, processes, and knowledge in SLA and bilingualism* (pp. 23–34). Washington, DC: Georgetown University Press.

Reichle, J., & Wacker, D. P. (1993). *Communicative alternatives to challenging behavior.* Baltimore: Brookes.

Rescorla, L., & Lee, F. (2001). Language impairment in young children. In T. Layton, E. Crais, & L. Watson (Eds.), *Handbook of early language impairment in children: Nature.* Albany, NY: Delmar.

Reynolds, J. (1990). Abnormal vowel patterns in phonologically disordered children: Some data and a hypothesis. *British Journal of Disorders of Communication, 25*, 115–148.

Riccio, C. A., Imhoff, B., Hasbrouck, J. E., & Davis, G. N. (2004). *Test of phonological awareness in Spanish.* Austin, TX: PRO-ED.

Richards, J. (Ed.). (1974). *Error analysis: Perspectives on second language learning.* London: Longman.

Ringel, R., House, A., Burk, K., Dolinsky, J., & Scott, C. (1970). Some relation between orosensory discrimination and articulatory aspects of speech production. *Journal of Speech and Hearing Disorders, 35*, 3–11.

Roberts, J., Burchinal, M., & Foote, M. (1990). Phonological process decline from 2½ to 8 years. *Journal of Communication Disorders, 23*, 205–217.

Roberts, J., Long, S. H., Malkin, C., Barnes, E., Skinner, M., Hennon, E. A., & Anderson, K. (2005). A comparison of phonological skills of boys with Fragile X syndrome and Down syndrome. *Journal of Speech, Language, and Hearing Research, 48*, 980–995.

Roberts, J. E., Rosenfeld, R. M., & Zeisel, S. A. (2004). Otitis media and speech and language: A meta-analysis of prospective studies. *Pediatrics, 113*, 237–247.

Robertson, D., & Salter, W. (1995). *The phonological awareness kit.* East Moline, IL: LinguiSystems.

Robertson, D., & Salter, W. (1997). *The phonological awareness test.* East Moline, IL: LinguiSystems.

Robinson-Zanartu, C. (1996). Serving Native American children and families: Considering cultural variables. *Language, Speech, and Hearing Services in Schools, 27*, 373–384.

Romaine, S. (2003). Variation. In C. J. Doughty & M. H. Long (Eds.), *The handbook of second language acquisition* (pp. 409–435). Oxford, UK: Blackwell.

Roseberry-McKibbin, C. (1995). *Multicultural students with special language needs* (2nd ed.). Oceanside, CA: Academic Communication Associates.

Rosenbaum, P. L., Paneth, N., Leviton, A., Goldstein, M., & Bax, M. (2007). A report: The definition and classification of cerebral palsy. *Developmental medicine and child neurology, 49*(Suppl. 109), 8–14.

Rosenbek, J. C. (1985). Treating apraxia of speech. In D. F. Johns (Ed.), *Clinical management of neurogenic communicative disorders* (2nd ed.). Boston: College-Hill Press.

Rosenbek, J. C., Lemme, M. L., Ahern, M. B., Harris, E. H., & Wertz, R. T. (1973). A treatment for apraxia of speech in adults. *Journal of Speech and Hearing Research, 38*(4), 462–472.

Rosner, J. (1999). *Phonological Awareness Skills Program.* Austin, TX: PRO-ED.

Roth, F. P., & Worthington, C. K. (2011). *Treatment resource manual for speech–language pathology* (4th ed.). Clifton Park, NY: Delmar Cengage Learning.

Roulstone, S. S., Loader, S., Northstone, K., Beveridge, M., & the ALSPAC Team. (2002). The speech and language of children aged 25 months: Descriptive data from the Avon Longitudinal Study of Parents and Children. *Early Child Development and Care, 172*, 259–268.

Ruscello, D. M. (2008a). An examination of nonspeech oral motor exercise for children with velopharyngeal inadequacy. *Seminar in Speech and Language, 29*(4), 294–303.

Ruscello, D. M., (2008b). Oral–motor treatment issues related to children with developmental speech sound disorders. *Language, Speech, and Hearing Services in School, 39*, 380–391.

Ruscello, D. M., St. Louis, K. O., & Mason, N. (1991). School-age children with phonological disorders: Coexistence with other speech/language disorders. *Journal of Speech and Hearing Research, 34*, 236-242.

Rvachew, S. (1994). Speech perception training can facilitate sound production learning. *Journal of Speech and Hearing Research, 37*, 347–357.

Rvachew, S. (2007). Perceptual foundations of speech acquisition. In S. McLeod (Ed.), *The international guide to speech acquisition* (pp. 26-30). Clifton Park, NY: Thomson Delmar Learning.

Rvachew, S., & Brosseau-Lapré, F. (2010). Speech perception intervention. In A. L. Williams, S. McLeod, & R. J. McCauley (Eds.), *Intervention for speech sound disorders* (pp. 295–314). Baltimore, MD: Brookes.

Rvachew, S., & Brosseau-Lapré, F. (2012). *Developmental phonological disorders.* San Diego, CA: Plural.

Rvachew, S., Chiang, P., & Evans, N. (2007). Characteristics of speech errors produced by children with and without delayed phonological awareness skills. *Language, Speech, and Hearing Services in Schools, 38*, 60–71.

Rvachew, S., & Nowak, M. (2001). The effect of target behavior selection on phonological learning. *Language, Speech, and Hearing Services in Schools, 12*, 463–471.

Rvachew, S., Nowak, M., & Cloutier, G. (2004). Effects of phonemic perception training on speech production and phonological awareness skills of children with expressive phonological delay. *American Journal of Speech–Language Pathology, 13*, 250–263.

Rvachew, S., Rafaat, S., & Martin, M. (1999). Stimulability, speech perception skills, and treatment of phonological disorders. *American Journal of Speech–Language Pathology, 8*, 33–43.

Saaristo-Helin, K. (2009). Measuring phonological development: A follow-up study of five children acquiring Finnish. *Language and Speech, 52*, 55–77.

Saaristo-Helin, K., Savinainen-Makkonen, T., & Kunnari, S. (2006). The phonological mean length of utterance: Methodological challenges from a crosslinguistic perspective. *Journal of Child Language, 33*, 179–190.

Saben, C. B., & Ingham, J. C. (1991). The effects of minimal pairs treatment on the speech-sound production of two children with phonologic disorders. *Journal of Speech and Hearing Research, 34*, 1023–1040.

Saffran, J. R. (2003). Statistical language learning: Mechanisms and constraints. *Current Directions in Psychological Science, 12*, 110–114.

Saffran, J. R., Newport, E. L., Aslin, R. N., Tunick, R. A., & Barrueco, S. (1997). Incidental language learning: Listening (and learning) out of the corner of your ear. *Psychological Science, 8*, 101–105.

Sampson, G. (1997). *Educating Eve*. London: Cassell.

Sander, E. (1972). When are speech sounds learned? *Journal of Speech and Hearing Disorders, 37*, 55–63.

Sanz, C., & Leow, R. P. (Eds.). (2011). *Implicit and explicit language learning: Conditions, processes, and knowledge in SLA and bilingualism*. Washington, DC: Georgetown University Press.

Scherer, N. J. (1999). The speech and language status of toddlers with cleft lip and and/or palate following early vocabulary intervention. *American Journal of Speech–Language Pathology, 8*, 81–93.

Scheuermann, B. K., & Hall, J. K. (2008). *Positive behavioral supports for the classroom*. Columbus, OH: Pearson.

Schlinger, H. D. (2010). Behavioral vs. cognitive views of speech perception and production. *Journal of Speech–Language Pathology and Applied Behavior Analysis, 5*, 150–165.

Schmidt, L. S., Howard, B. H., & Schmidt, J. F. (1983). Conversational speech sampling in the assessment of articulation proficiency. *Language, Speech, and Hearing Services in Schools, 14*, 210–214.

Schuele, C. M., & Boudreau, D. (2008). Phonological awareness intervention: Beyond the basics. *Language, Speech, and Hearing Services in Schools, 39*, 3–20.

Schumann, J. (1978). *The pidginisation process: A model for second language acquisition*. Rowley, MA: Newbury House.

Schwartz, R. G. (1992). Clinical application of recent advances in phonological theory. *Language, Speech, and Hearing Services in Schools, 23*, 269–276.

Scripture, M., & Jackson, E. (1927). *A manual of exercises for the correction of speech disorders*. Philadelphia: F. A. Davis.

Secord, W. A. (1981). *Test of minimal articulation competence*. San Antonio, TX: Psychological Corporation.

Secord, W. A. (1989). The traditional approach to therapy. In N. A. Creaghead, P. W. Newman, & W. A. Secord (Eds.), *Assessment and remediation of articulatory and phonological disorders* (2nd ed.). Columbus, OH: Merrill.

Secord, W. A., Boyce, S. E., Donohue, J. S., Fox, R. A., & Shine, R. E. (2007). *Eliciting sound: Techniques and strategies for clinicians* (2nd ed.). Clifton Park, NY: Delmar Cengage Learning.

Secord, W., & Donohue, J. (2002). *Clinical assessment of articulation and phonology.* Austin, TX: PRO-ED.

Secord, W. A., & Shine, R. E. (1997). *Secord articulation contextual test.* Greenville, SC: Super Duper Publications.

Seikel, J. A., Drumright, D. G., & Seikel, P. (2014). *Essentials of anatomy and physiology for communicative disorders* (2nd ed.). Albany, NY: Thomson Delmar Learning.

Seikel, J. A., King, D. W., & Drumright, D. G. (2010). *Anatomy and physiology for speech, language, and hearing* (4th ed.). Albany, NY: Thomson Delmar Learning.

Selby, J. C., Robb, M. P., & Gilbert, H. R. (2000). Normal vowel articulations between 16 and 36 months of age. *Clinical Linguistics and Phonetics, 14,* 255–256.

Semel, E., Wiig, E., & Secord, W. (2003). *Clinical evaluation of language fundamentals* (4th ed.). San Antonio, TX: Psychological Corporation.

Seymour, H. N. (2004). A noncontrastive model for assessment of phonology. *Seminars in Speech and Language, 25*(1), 91–99.

Seymour, H. N., & Pearson, B. Z. (2004). Steps in designing and implementing an innovative assessment instrument. *Seminars in Speech and Language, 25*(1), 27–31.

Seymour, H. N., Roeper, T., & de Villiers, J. (2000). *Dialect sensitive language test.* Unpublished manuscript.

Seymour, H. N., Roeper, T., de Villiers, J., & de Villiers, P. (2003). *Diagnostic evaluation of language variation–Screening test.* San Antonio, TX: Pearson.

Seymour, H. N., Roeper, T., de Villiers, J., & de Villiers, P. (2005). *Diagnostic evaluation of language variance–Norm referenced.* San Antonio, TX: Pearson.

Seymour, H. N., & Seymour, C. M. (1981). Black English and Standard American English contrasts in consonantal development for four- and five-year-old children. *Journal of Speech and Hearing Disorders, 46,* 276–280.

Shekar, C., & Hegde, M. N. (1995). India: Its people, culture, and languages. In L. L. Cheng (Ed.), *Integrating language and learning for inclusion.* San Diego, CA: Singular.

Shekar, C., & Hegde, M. N. (1996). Cultural and linguistic diversity among Asian Indians: A case of Indian English. *Topics in Language Disorders, 16*(4), 54–64.

Shelton, R., Elbert, M., & Arndt, W. B. (1967). A task for evaluation of articulation change: II. Comparison of task scores during baseline and lesson series testing. *Journal of Speech and Hearing Research, 10,* 578–585.

Shelton, R., Johnson, A., & Arndt, W. B. (1977). Delayed judgment speech-sound discrimination and /r/ or /s/ articulation status and improvement. *Journal of Speech and Hearing Research, 20,* 704–717.

Shibatani, M. (1990). Japanese. In B. Comrie (Ed.), *The world's major languages.* New York: Oxford University Press.

Shriberg, L. D. (1975). A response evocation program for /ɚ/. *Journal of Speech and Hearing Disorders, 40,* 92–105.

Shriberg, L. D. (1993). Four new prosody-voice measures for genetics research and other studies in developmental phonological disorders. *Journal of Speech and Hearing Research, 36,* 105–140.

Shriberg, L. D. (1994). Five subtypes of developmental phonological disorders. *Clinics and Communication Disorders, 4*(1), 38–53.

Shriberg, L. D. (2010). Childhood speech sound disorders: From postbehaviorism to the postgenomic era. In R. Paul & P. Flipsen, Jr. (Eds.), *Speech sound disorders in children* (pp. 1–34). San Diego, CA: Plural.

Shriberg, L. D., Aram, D. M., & Kwiatkowski, J. (1997a). Developmental apraxia of speech: I. Descriptive and theoretical perspectives. *Journal of Speech and Hearing Research, 40,* 273–286.

Shriberg, L. D., Aram, D. M., & Kwiatkowski, J. (1997b). Developmental apraxia of speech: II. Toward a diagnostic marker. *Journal of Speech and Hearing Research, 40,* 286–312.

Shriberg, L. D., Aram, D. M., & Kwiatkowski, J. (1997c). Developmental apraxia of speech: III. A subtype marked by inappropriate stress. *Journal of Speech and Hearing Research, 40,* 313–337.

Shriberg, L. D., & Austin, D. (1998). Comorbidity of speech and language disorders: Implications for a phenotype marker for speech delay. In R. Paul (Ed.), *Exploring the speech–language connection* (pp. 73–117). Baltimore: Brookes.

Shriberg, L. D., Fourakis, M., Hall, S., Karlsson, H. B., Lohmeier, L., Mcsweeny, J., et al. (2010). Extensions to the speech disorders classification system. *Clinical Linguistics & Phonetics, 24*(10), 795–824.

Shriberg, L. D., Friel-Patti, S., Flipsen, P., Jr., & Brown, R. L. (2000). Otitis media, fluctuant hearing loss, and speech–language outcomes: A preliminary structural equation model. *Journal of Speech, Language, and Hearing Research, 43,* 100–120.

Shriberg, L. D., Gruber, F. A., & Kwiatkowski, J. (1994). Developmental phonological disorders III: Long-term speech sound normalization. *Journal of Speech and Hearing Research, 37,* 1151–1177.

Shriberg, L. D., & Kent, R. D. (2013). *Clinical phonetics* (4th ed.). Boston: Allyn & Bacon.

Shriberg, L. D., & Kwiatkowski, J. (1980). *Natural process analysis.* New York: Wiley.

Shriberg, L. D., & Kwiatkowski, J. (1982). Phonological disorders III: A procedure for assessing severity of involvement. *Journal of Speech and Hearing Disorders, 47,* 256–270.

Shriberg, L. D., & Kwiatkowski, J. (1990). Self-monitoring and generalization in preschool speech-delayed children. *Language, Speech, and Hearing Services in Schools, 21,* 157–170.

Shriberg, L. D., & Kwiatkowski, J. (1994). Developmental phonological disorders I: A clinical profile. *Journal of Speech and Hearing Research, 37,* 1100–1126.

Shriberg, L. D., Kwiatkowski, J., & Gruber, F. A. (1994). Developmental phonological disorders II: Short-term speech sound normalization. *Journal of Speech and Hearing Research, 37,* 1127–1150.

Shriberg, L. D., Lewis, B. A., Tomblin, J. B., McSweeny, J. L., Karlsson, H. K., & Scheer, A. R. (2005). Toward diagnostic and phenotypic markers for genetically transmitted speech delay. *Journal of Speech, Language, and Hearing Research, 48,* 834–852.

Shriberg, L. D., Thielke, H., Kwiatkowski, J., Kertoy, M. K., Katcher, M. L., et al. (2000). Risk for speech disorder associated with early recurrent otitis media with effusion: Two retrospective studies. *Journal of Speech, Language, and Hearing Research, 43,* 79–99.

Shriberg, L. D., Tomblin, J. B., & McSweeny, J. L. (1999). Prevalence of speech delay in 6-year-old children and comorbidity with language impairment. *Journal of Speech, Language, and Hearing Research, 42,* 1461–1481.

Shriberg, L. D., & Widder, C. (1990). Speech and prosody characteristics of adults with mental retardation. *Journal of Speech and Hearing Research, 33,* 627–653.

Shukla, S. (2006). Panini. In K. Brown (Ed.), *Encyclopedia of language and linguistics* (2nd ed., pp. 153–155). New York: Elsevier.

Shultz, S., & Vouloumanos, A. (2010). Three-month-olds prefer speech to other naturally occurring signals. *Language Learning and Development, 6*(4), 141-257.

Siegel, G. M., Winitz, H., & Conkey, H. (1963). The influence of testing instruments on articulatory responses of children. *Journal of Speech and Hearing Disorders, 28,* 67–76.

Silverman, D. (2011). Usage-based phonology. In N. C. Kula, B. Bortma, & K. Nasukawa (Eds.), *Continuum companion to phonology* (pp. 369–455). London: Continuum International.

Silverman, F. H., & Paulus, P. G. (1989). Peer reactions to teenagers who substitute /w/ for /r/. *Language, Speech, and Hearing Services in Schools, 20,* 219–221.

Singh, S. (1976). *Distinctive features: Theory and validation.* Baltimore: University Park Press.

Singh, S., & Frank, D. C. (1972). A distinctive feature analysis of the consonantal substitutions pattern. *Language and Speech, 15*, 209–218.

Sinnott, J. M., & Mosteller, K. W. (2007). A vowel identification procedure for gerbils. *Journal of the Acoustical Society of America, 122*, 2947.

Skahan, S. M., Watson, M., & Lof, G. L. (2007). Speech–language pathologists' assessment practices for children with suspected speech sound disorders: Results of a national survey. *American Journal of Speech–Language Pathology, 16*, 246–259.

Skelly, M., Spector, D., Donaldson, R., Brodeur, A., & Paletta, F. (1971). Compensatory physiologic phonetics for the glossectomee. *Journal of Speech and Hearing Research, 36*, 101–114.

Skelton, S. L. (2004). Concurrent task sequencing in single-phoneme phonologic treatment and generalization. *Journal of Communication Disorders, 37,* 131–155.

Skelton, S. L., & Funk, T. (2004). Teaching speech sounds to young children: A pilot study of concurrent treatment using randomly ordered, variable-complexity task sequences. *Perceptual & Motor Skills, 99*(2), 602–604.

Skelton, S. L., & Hagopian, A. L. (2013). *Using randomized variable practice in the treatment of childhood apraxia of speech.* Unpublished manuscript, California State University, Fresno.

Skelton, S. L., & Kerber, J. R. (2005, November). *Using concurrent treatment to teach multiple phonemes to phonologically-disordered children.* Poster presented at the American Speech-Language-Hearing Association Convention, San Diego, CA.

Skelton, S. L., & Price, J. R. (2006, November). *A preliminary comparison of concurrent and traditional speech sound treatment.* Poster presented at the American Speech-Language-Hearing Association Convention, Miami, FL.

Skelton, S. L., & Resciniti, D. N. (2009, November). *Using a motor learning treatment with phonologically disordered children.* Poster presented at the American Speech-Language-Hearing Association Convention, New Orleans, LA.

Skelton, S. L., & Richard, J. T. (2013). *The speech improvement class: Use of a motor learning treatment for speech sound disorders in small groups.* Unpublished manuscript, California State University, Fresno.

Skinner, B. F. (1957). *Verbal behavior.* New York: Appleton Century.

Small, L. H. (2012). *Fundamentals of phonetics* (3rd ed.). Boston: Allyn & Bacon.

Smit, A. B. (1986). Ages of speech sound acquisition: Comparisons and critiques of several normative studies. *Language, Speech, and Hearing Services in Schools, 17*, 175–186.

Smit, A. B. (1993a). Phonologic error distributions in the Iowa–Nebraska articulation norms project: Consonant singletons. *Journal of Speech and Hearing Research, 36*, 533–547.

Smit, A. B. (1993b). Phonologic error distributions in the Iowa–Nebraska articulation norms project: Word-initial consonant clusters. *Journal of Speech and Hearing Research, 36*, 931–947.

Smit, A. B. (2004). *Articulation and phonology resource guide for school-age children and adults.* Albany, NY: Thomson Delmar.

Smit, A. B., Hand, L., Freilinger, J. J., Bernthal, J. E., & Bird, A. (1990). The Iowa articulation norms project and its Nebraska replication. *Journal of Speech and Hearing Disorders, 55*, 779–798.

Smith, M. W., & Ainsworth, S. (1967). The effects of three types of stimulation on articulatory responses of speech defective children. *Journal of Speech and Hearing Research, 10*, 333–338.

Snow, C. (1977). The development of conversation between mothers and babies. *Journal of Child Language, 4*, 1–22.

Snow, K. (1963). A detailed analysis of articulation responses of normal first grade children. *Journal of Speech and Hearing Research, 6*, 277–290.

Snow, K., & Milisen, R. (1954). The influence of oral versus pictorial representation upon articulation testing results [Monograph]. *Journal of Speech and Hearing Disorders, 4*, 29–36.

So, L., & Dodd, B. (1994). Phonologically disordered Cantonese-speaking children. *Clinical Linguistics and Phonetics, 8,* 235–255.

Spector, J. (1992). Predicting progress in beginning reading: Dynamic assessment of phonemic awareness. *Journal of Educational Psychology, 84,* 353–363.

Spence, M. J., & Freeman, M. S. (1996). Newborn infants prefer the maternal low-pass filtered voice, but not the maternal whispered voice. *Infant Behavior & Development, 19,* 199–212.

Spencer, E. J., Schuele, C. M., Guillot, K. M., & Lee, M. W. (2008). Phonemic awareness skills of speech–language pathologists and other educators. *Language, Speech, and Hearing Services in Schools, 39,* 512–520.

Spriestersbach, D. C., & Curtis, J. F. (1951). Misarticulation and discrimination of speech sounds. *Quarterly Journal of Speech, 37,* 483–491.

Spring, D. R., & Dale, P. S. (1975). Discrimination of stress early infancy. *Journal of Speech and Hearing Research, 20,* 224–231.

Square, P. A. (1999). Treatment of developmental apraxia of speech: Tactile-kinesthetic, rhythmic, and gestural approaches. In A. J. Caruso & E. A. Strand (Eds.), *Clinical management of motor speech disorders in children.* New York: Thieme.

Square, P., Chumpelik, D., & Adams, S. (1985). Efficacy of the PROMPT system of therapy for the treatment of acquired apraxia of speech. In R. Brookshire (Ed.), *Clinical aphasiology conference proceedings.* Minneapolis, MN: BRK.

Stackhouse, J. (1992). Developmental verbal dyspraxia: A longitudinal case study. In R. Campbell (Ed.), *Mental lives: Case studies in cognition.* Oxford, UK: Blackwell.

Stackhouse, J. (1997). Phonological awareness: Connecting speech and literacy problems. In B. Hodson & M. Edwards (Eds.), *Perspectives in applied phonology.* Gaithersburg, MD: Aspen.

Stackhouse, J., & Wells, B. (1997). *Children's speech and literacy difficulties: Vol. 1. A psycholinguistic framework.* London: Whurr.

Stahl, K., & McKenna, M. (2006). *Reading research at work: Foundations of effective practice.* New York: Guilford Press.

Stampe, D. (1969). The acquisition of phonetic representation. *Papers from the fifth regional meeting of the Chicago Linguistic Society* (pp. 433–444). Chicago: Chicago Linguistic Society.

Stampe, D. (1979). *A dissertation on natural phonology.* New York: Garland.

Stark, R. (1978). Features of infant sounds: The emergence of cooing. *Journal of Child Language, 5,* 379–390.

Stark, R. (1979). Prespeech segmental feature development. In P. Fletcher & M. Garman (Eds.), *Language Acquisition.* Cambridge, UK: Cambridge University Press.

Stark, R. (1980). Stages of speech development in the first year of life. In G. Yeni-Komshian, J. Kavanagh, & C. A. Ferguson (Eds.), *Child phonology: Vol. 1. Production.* New York: Academic Press.

Stein, C. M., Schick, J. H., Taylor, H. G., Shriberg, L. D., Millard, C., Kundtz-Kluge, A., et al. (2004). Pleiotropic effects of a chromosome 3 locus on speech-sound disorder and reading. *American Journal of Human Genetics, 74,* 283–297.

Steriade, D. (1987). Redundant values. In A. Bosch, B. Need, & E. Schiller (Eds.), *Papers from the parasession on autosegmental and metrical phonology* (pp. 339–362). Chicago: Chicago Linguistic Society.

Steriade, D. (1990). *Greek prosodies and the nature of syllabification* (Doctoral dissertation, Massachusetts Institute of Technology, 1982). New York: Garland Press.

Stern, D. (1977). *The first relationship.* Cambridge, MA: Harvard University Press.

Stevens, K., & Keyser, S. (1989). Primary features and their enhancement in consonants. *Language, 65,* 81–106.

Stinchfield, S., & Young, E. (1938). *Children with delayed or defective speech: Motor-kinesthetic factors in training.* Stanford, CA: Stanford University Press.

St. Louis, K. O., & Ruscello, D. (2000). *Oral speech mechanism screening examination* (3rd ed.). Austin, TX: PRO-ED.

Stockman, I. J. (1996). Phonological development and disorders in African American children. In A. G. Kamhi, K. E. Pollock, & J. L. Harris (Eds.), *Communication development and disorders in African American children.* Baltimore: Brookes.

Stockman, I. J. (2006). Evidence for a minimal competence core of consonant sounds in the speech of African American children: A preliminary study. *Clinical Linguistics & Phonetics, 20*(10), 723–749.

Stockman, I. J. (2008). Toward validation of a minimal competence phonetic core for African American children. *Journal of Speech, Language, and Hearing Research, 51,* 1244–1262.

Stockman, I. J. (2010). A review of developmental and applied language research on African American children: From a deficit to difference perspective on dialectal differences. *Language, Speech and Hearing Services in the Schools, 41,* 23–38.

Stockman, I. J., Karasinski, L., & Guillory, B. (2008). The use of conversational repairs by African American preschoolers. *Language, Speech and Hearing Services in the Schools, 39,* 461–474.

Stockwell, R. P., & Bowen, J. D. (1983). *The sounds of English and Spanish.* The Hague, Netherlands: Mouton.

Stoel-Gammon, C. (1984, July 8–13). *Phonetic inventories, 15–24 months: A longitudinal study.* Paper presented at the Third International Congress for the Study of Child Language, Austin, TX.

Stoel-Gammon, C. (1985). Phonetic inventories, 15–24 months: A longitudinal study. *Journal of Speech and Hearing Research, 28,* 505–512.

Stoel-Gammon, C. (1987). Phonological skills of two-year-olds. *Language, Speech, and Hearing Services in Schools, 18,* 323–329.

Stoel-Gammon, C. (2001). Transcribing the speech of young children. *Topics in Language Disorders, 21,* 12–21.

Stoel-Gammon, C., & Cooper, J. A. (1981, August 9–14). *Individual differences in early phonological and lexical development.* Paper presented at the Second International Congress for the Study of Child Language, Vancouver, BC.

Stoel-Gammon, C., & Cooper, J. A. (1984). Patterns of early lexical and phonological development. *Journal of Child Language, 11,* 247–271.

Stoel-Gammon, C., & Dunn, C. (1985). *Normal and disordered phonology in children.* Austin, TX: PRO-ED.

Stoel-Gammon, C., & Pollock, K. (2011). Vowel development and disorders. In M. J. Ball, M. R. Perkins, N. Muller, & S. Howard (Eds.), *The handbook of clinical linguistics* (pp. 525–548). Malden, MA: Wiley-Blackwell.

Stoel-Gammon, C., Stone-Goldman, J., & Glaspey, A. (2002). Pattern-based approaches to phonological therapy. *Seminars in Speech and Language, 23,* 3–13.

Stokes, S. F., Klee, T., Carson, C. P., & Carson, D. (2005). A phonemic implicational hierarchy of phonological contrasts for English-speaking children. *Journal of Speech, Language, and Hearing Research, 48*(4), 817–833.

Strand, E. A., & Debertine, P. (2000). The efficacy of integral stimulation intervention with developmental apraxia of speech. *Journal of Medical Speech–Language Pathology, 8*(4), 295–300.

Strand, E. A., & McCauley, R. J. (2008, August 12). Differential diagnosis of severe speech impairment in young children. *The ASHA Leader.*

Strand, E. A., McCauley, R. J., Weigand, S. D., Stoeckel, R. B., & Bass, B. S. (2012). A motor speech assessment for children with severe speech disorders: Reliability and validity of evidence. *Journal of Speech, Language, and Hearing Research.* doi:10.1044/1092-4388(2012/12-0094)

Strand, E. A., & Skinder, A. (1999). Treatment of developmental apraxia of speech: Integral stimulation methods. In A. J. Caruso & E. A. Strand (Eds.), *Clinical management of motor speech disorders in children* (pp. 109–148). New York: Thieme.

Strand, E. A., & Stoeckel, R. (2006). Treatment of severe childhood apraxia of speech: A treatment efficacy study. *Journal of Medical Speech–Language Pathology, 14*(4), 297–308.

Strecker, D. (1990). Tai languages. In B. Comrie (Ed.), *The world's major languages.* New York: Oxford University Press.

Swank, L. (1994). Phonological coding abilities: Identification of impairments related to phonologically based reading problems. *Topics in Language Disorders, 14,* 56–71.

Swank, L., & Catts, H. (1994). Phonological awareness and written word decoding. *Language, Speech, and Hearing Services in Schools, 25,* 9–14.

Swanson, T. J., Hodson, B. W., & Schommer-Aikins, M. (2005). An examination of phonological awareness treatment outcomes for seventh-grade poor readers from a bilingual community. *Language, Speech, and Hearing Services in Schools, 36,* 336–345.

Taelman, H., Durieux, G., & Gillis, S. (2005). Notes on Ingram's whole-word measures for phonological development. *Journal of Child Language, 32,* 391–405.

Teaser, B. (2000). On the role of optimality and strict domination in language learning. In J. Dekkers, F. van der Leeuw, & J. van de Weijer (Eds.), *Optimality theory: Phonology, syntax, and acquisition.* Oxford, UK: Oxford University Press.

Templin, M. C. (1947). Spontaneous versus imitated verbalization in testing articulation in preschool children. *Journal of Speech and Hearing Disorders, 12,* 293–300.

Templin, M. C. (1957). *Certain language skills in children: Their development and interrelationships.* Institute of Child Welfare Monograph Series No. 26. Minneapolis, MN: University of Minnesota Press.

Terrel, S., Arensberg, K., & Rosa, M. (1992). Parent–child comparative analysis: A criterion referenced method for the nondiscriminatory assessment of a child who spoke a relatively uncommon dialect of English. *Language, Speech, and Hearing Services in Schools, 23,* 34–42.

Thompson, C. A., Craig, H. K., & Washington, J. A. (2004). Variable production of African American English across oracy and literacy contexts. *Language, Speech, and Hearing Services in Schools, 35,* 269–283.

Thompson, L. C. (1965). *A Vietnamese grammar.* Seattle: University of Washington Press.

Tomasello, M. (2005). *Constructing a language: A usage-based theory of language acquisition.* Cambridge, MA: Harvard University Press.

Toombs, M., Singh, S., & Hayden, M. (1981). Markedness of features in the articulatory substitutions of children. *Journal of Speech and Hearing Disorders, 46,* 184–191.

Torgesen, J. K., & Bryant, B. R. (2004). *Test of phonological awareness* (2nd ed.). Austin, TX: PRO-ED.

Torgesen, J. K., & Mathes, P. G. (2000). *A basic guide to understanding, assessing, and teaching phonological awareness.* Austin, TX: PRO-ED.

Trehub, S. (1976). The discrimination of foreign speech contrasts by infants and children. *Child Development, 47,* 466–472.

Treiman, R., Broderick, V., Tincoff, R., & Rodriguez, L. (1998). Children's phonological awareness: Confusion between phonemes that differ only in voicing. *Journal of Experimental Child Psychology, 68,* 3–21.

Treiman, R., & Zukowski, A. (1996). Children's sensitivity to syllables, onset, rimes, and phonemes. *Experimental Child Psychology, 61,* 193–215.

Troia, G. A. (1999). Phonological awareness intervention research: A critical review of the experimental methodology. *Reading Research Quarterly, 34,* 28–52.

Trubetzkoy, N. S. (1969). *Principles of phonology* (C. A. M. Baltaxe, Trans.). Berkeley: University of California Press. (Original work published 1939)

Tsao, F-M., Liu, H-M., & Kuhl, P. K. (2004). Speech perception in infancy predicts language development in the second year of life: A longitudinal study. *Child Development, 75*(4), 1067–1084.

Tsugawa, L. (2002). *Spanish preschool articulation test.* Billings, MT: Lexicon Press.

Twain, M. (1985). *The adventures of Huckleberry Finn.* New York: Penguin. (Original work published 1884)

Tyler, A. A. (2002). Language-based intervention for phonological disorders. *Seminars in Speech and Language, 23,* 69–81.

Tyler, A. A. (2005). Promoting generalization: Selecting, scheduling, and integrating goals. In A. Kamhi & K. Pollock (Eds.), *Phonological disorders in children: Clinical decision making in assessment and intervention.* Baltimore: Brookes.

Tyler, A. A., Edwards, M. L., & Saxman, J. H. (1987). Clinical application of two phonologically based treatment procedures. *Journal of Speech and Hearing Disorders, 52,* 393–409.

Tyler, A. A., & Figurski, G. R. (1994). Phonetic inventory changes after treating distinctions along an implicational hierarchy. *Clinical Linguistics and Phonetics, 8*(2), 91–107.

Tyler, A. A., Lewis, K. E., Haskill, A. M., & Tolbert, L. C. (2002). Efficacy of cross-domain effects of a morphosyntax and a phonology intervention. *Language, Speech, and Hearing Services in Schools, 33,* 52–66.

Tyler, A. A., Lewis, K., & Welch, C. (2003). Predictors of phonological change following intervention. *American Journal of Speech–Language Pathology, 12,* 289–298.

Tyler, A. A., & Sandoval, K. T. (1994). Preschoolers with phonological and language disorders: Treating different linguistic domains. *Language, Speech, and Hearing Services in Schools, 25,* 215–234.

Tyler, A., & Watterson, K. (1991). Effects of phonological versus language intervention in preschoolers with both phonological and language impairment. *Child Language and Teaching Therapy, 7,* 141–160.

Tyler, A., Williams, M., & Lewis, K. (2006). Error consistency and the evaluation of treatment outcomes. *Clinical Linguistics & Phonetics, 20*(6), 411–422.

Udvari, A., & Thousand, J. (1995). Promising practices that foster inclusive education. In R. Villa & J. Thousand (Eds.), *Creating an inclusive school.* Alexandria, VA: Association for Supervision and Curriculum Development.

U.S. Bureau of the Census. (2010). *Statistical abstract of the United States.* Washington, DC: U.S. Government Printing Office.

van Keulen, J. E., Weddington, G. T., & Dubois, C. E. (1998). *Speech, language, learning and the African American child.* Needham Heights, MA: Allyn & Bacon.

van Kleeck, A. (1995). Emphasizing form and meaning repeatedly in prereading and early reading instruction. *Topics in Language Disorders, 16,* 27–49.

Van Riper, C. (1939). *Speech correction: Principles and methods.* Englewood Cliffs, NJ: Prentice Hall.

Van Riper, C., & Emerick, L. (1984). *Speech correction: An introduction to speech pathology and audiology.* Englewood Cliffs, NJ: Prentice Hall.

Van Riper, C., & Erickson, R. (1996). *Speech correction: An introduction to speech pathology and audiology* (9th ed.). Englewood Cliffs, NJ: Prentice Hall.

Van Riper, C., & Irwin, J. (1958). *Voice and articulation.* Englewood Cliffs, NJ: Prentice Hall.

Velleman, S. L., & Strand, K. (1994). Developmental verbal dyspraxia. In J. E. Bernthal & W. Bankson (Eds.), *Child phonology: Characteristics, assessment, and intervention with special populations* (pp. 110–139). New York: Thieme.

Velleman, S. L., & Vihman, M. L. (2007). Phonology in infancy and early childhood: Implications for theories of language learning. In M. C. Pennington (Ed.), *Phonology in context* (pp. 25–50). New York: Palgrave Macmillan.

Vihman, M. M. (1998). Early phonological development. In J. E. Bernthal & N. W. Bankson (Eds.), *Articulation and phonological disorders*. Boston: Allyn & Bacon.

Vihman, M. M., Ferguson, C. A., & Elbert, M. (1986). Phonological development from babbling to speech: Common tendencies and individual differences. *Applied Psycholinguistics, 7,* 3–40.

Vihman, M. M., & Greenlee, M. (1987). Individual differences in phonological development: Ages one to three years. *Journal of Speech and Hearing Research, 30,* 503–521.

Vihman, M. M., Macken, M. A., Miller, R., Simmons, H., & Miller, J. (1985). From babbling to speech: A reassessment of the continuity issue. *Language, 61,* 395–443.

Vogel, D., & Cannito, M. P. (2001). *Treating disordered speech motor control* (2nd ed.). Austin, TX: PRO-ED.

Wagner, R., Torgesen, J., Rashotte, C., & Pearson, N. (2013). *Comprehensive test of phonological processing* (2nd ed.). Torrance, CA: Western Psychological Services.

Wanzek, J., Dickson, S., Bursuck, W., & White, J. (2000). Teaching phonological awareness to students at risk for reading failure: An analysis of four instructional programs. *Learning Disabilities Research & Practice, 15,* 153–173.

Waring, R., Fisher, J., & Atkin, N. (2001). The articulation survey: Putting numbers to it. In L. Wilson & S. Hewat (Eds.), *Proceedings of the 2001 Speech Pathology Australian National Conference: Evidence and innovation* (pp. 145–151). Melbourne, Australia.

Warlaumont, A. S., Westermann, G., Buder, E. H., & Oller, D. K. (2013). Prespeech motor learning in a neural network using reinforcement. *Neural Networks, 38,* 64–75.

Washington, J., & Craig, H. (1992). Articulation test performance of low-income, African American preschoolers with communication impairments. *Language, Speech, and Hearing Services in the Schools, 23,* 203–207.

Washington, J. A., & Craig, H. K. (2002). Morphosyntactic forms of African American English used by young children and their caregivers. *Applied Psycholinguistics, 23,* 209–231.

Waterson, N. (1971). Child phonology: A prosodic view. *Journal of Linguistics, 7,* 179–211.

Watson, M., & Terrell, P. (2012). Longitudinal changes in phonological whole-word measures in 2-year-olds. *International Journal of Speech–Language Pathology, 14*(4), 351–362.

Webb, W. G., & Adler, R. (2007). *Neurology for the speech–language pathologist* (5th ed.). Boston: Butterworth-Heinemann.

Webster, P. E., & Plante, A. S. (1992). Effects of phonological impairment on word, syllable, and phoneme segmentation and reading. *Language, Speech, and Hearing Services in Schools, 23,* 176–182.

Weiner, F. (1979). *Phonological process analysis.* Baltimore: University Park Press.

Weiner, F. (1981). Treatment of phonological disability using the method of meaningful minimal contrast: Two case studies. *Journal of Speech and Hearing Disorders, 46,* 97–103.

Weiner, F., & Bankson, N. (1978). Teaching features. *Language, Speech, and Hearing Services in Schools, 9,* 29–34.

Weinreich, U. (1953). *Languages in contact.* The Hague, Netherlands: Mouton.

Weismer, G. (2006). Philosophy of research in motor speech disorders. *Clinical Linguistics and Phonetics, 20*(5), 315–349.

Weiss, C. E., Gordon, M. E., & Lillywhite, H. S. (1987). *Clinical management of articulatory and phonologic disorders* (2nd ed.). Baltimore: Williams & Wilkins.

Welker, G. (1996). *Native American languages.* Retrieved from FTP:indians.org/welker.americans.htm

Wellman, B., Case, I., Mengert, I., & Bradbury, D. (1931). Speech sounds of young children. *University of Iowa Studies in Child Welfare, 5*(2).

Wepman, J. M., & Reynolds, W. M. (1986). *Wepman's auditory discrimination test* (2nd ed.). Torrance, CA: Western Psychological Services.

Werker, J., & Tees, R. (1984). Cross-language speech perception: Evidence for perceptual reorganization during the first year of life. *Infant Behavior and Development, 7*, 49–64.

Westby, C., & Vining, C. B. (2002). Living in harmony: Providing services to Native American children and families. In D. E. Battle (Ed.), *Communication disorders in multicultural populations* (3rd ed., pp. 138–178). Boston: Butterworth-Heinemann.

Westermann, G., Ruh, N., & Plunkett, K. (2009). Connectionist approaches to language learning. *Linguistics, 47*, 413–452.

Weston, A. J., & Irwin, J. V. (1971). Use of paired stimuli in modification of articulation. *Perceptual Motor Skills, 32*, 947–957.

Wiig, E., Semel, E., & Secord, W. (2004). *Clinical evaluation of language fundamentals preschool* (2nd ed.). San Antonio, TX: Psychological Corporation.

Wilcox, K. A., & Morris, S. E. (1995). Speech outcomes of the language-focused curriculum. In M. Rice & K. Wilcox (Eds.), *Building a language-focused curriculum for the preschool classroom: A foundation for lifelong communication.* Baltimore: Brookes.

Williams, A. L. (1991). Generalization patterns associated with training least phonological knowledge. *Journal of Speech and Hearing Research, 34*, 722–733.

Williams, A. L. (2000). Multiple oppositions: Theoretical foundations for an alternative contrastive intervention approach. *American Journal of Speech–Language Pathology, 9*, 282–288.

Williams, A. L. (2003). *Speech disorders resource guide for preschool children.* Albany, NY: Thomson Delmar.

Williams, A. L. (2006a). *SCIP: Sound Contrasts in Phonology* [version 1]. Greenville, SC: Thinking Publications.

Williams, A. L. (2006b). A systematic perspective for assessment and intervention: A case study. *Advances in Speech–Language Pathology, 8*(3), 245–256.

Williams, A. L. (2010). Multiple oppositions intervention. In S. F. Warren & M. E. Fey (Series Eds.) & A. L. Williams, S. McLeod, & R. J. McCauley (Vol. Eds.), *Intervention for speech sound disorders in children* (pp. 73–94). Baltimore: Brookes.

Williams, G., & McReynolds, L. (1975). The relationship between discrimination and articulation training in children with misarticulations. *Journal of Speech and Hearing Research, 18*, 401–412.

Williams, J. (1984). Phonemic analysis and how it relates to reading. *Journal of Learning Disabilities, 17*, 240–245.

Willis, W. (1992). Families with African American roots. In E. W. Lynch & M. A. Hanson (Eds.), *Developing cross-cultural competence: A guide for working with young children and their families.* Baltimore: Brookes.

Wilson, M. E. (1996). Arabic speakers: Language and culture, here and abroad. *Topics in Language Disorders, 16*(4), 65–80.

Wilson, W. F. (1998). Delivering speech–language and hearing services in the Arab world: Some cultural considerations. In D. E. Battle (Ed.), *Communication disorders in multicultural populations* (2nd ed.). Boston: Butterworth-Heinemann.

Winitz, H. (1969). *Articulatory acquisition and behavior.* Englewood Cliffs, NJ: Prentice Hall.

Winitz, H. (1984). Auditory considerations in articulation and training. In H. Winitz (Ed.), *Treating articulation disorders: For clinicians by clinicians.* Baltimore: University Park Press.

Winitz, H. (1989). Auditory considerations in treatment. In N. A. Creaghead, P. W. Newman, & W. A. Secord (Eds.), *Assessment and remediation of articulatory and phonological disorders* (2nd ed.). Columbus, OH: Merrill.

Winitz, H., & Irwin, O. C. (1958). Syllabic and phonetic structure of infants' early words. *Journal of Speech and Hearing Research, 1*, 250–256.

Wolfram, W. (1986). Language variation in the United States. In O. Taylor (Ed.), *Treatment of communication disorders in culturally and linguistically diverse populations*. San Diego, CA: College-Hill Press.

Wolfram, W. (1994). The phonology of a sociocultural society: The case of African American vernacular English. In J. E. Bernthal & N. W. Bankson (Eds.), *Child phonology: Characteristics, assessment, intervention with special populations*. New York: Thieme.

Yates, A. (1987). Current status and future directions of research on the American Indian child. *American Journal of Psychiatry, 144*, 1135–1142.

Yavas, M. (Ed.). (1994). *First and second language phonology*. San Diego, CA: Singular.

Yavas, M. (1998). *Phonology: Development and disorders*. San Diego, CA: Singular.

Yavas, M., & Goldstein, B. (1998). Phonological assessment and treatment of bilingual speakers. *American Journal of Speech–Language Pathology, 7*, 49–60.

Yoder, P., Camarata, S., & Gardner, E. (2005). Treatment effects on speech intelligibility and length of utterance in children with specific language and intelligibility impairments. *Journal of Early Intervention, 28*, 34–49.

Yopp, H. K. (1988). The validity and reliability of phonemic awareness tests. *Reading Research Quarterly, 23*, 159–177.

Yorkston, K. M., Beukelman, D., Strand, E. A., & Hakel, M. (2010). *Management of motor speech disorders in children and adults* (4th ed.). Austin, TX: PRO-ED.

Yoshikawa, Y., Asada, M., Hosada, K., & Koga, J. (2003). A constructivist approach to infants' vowel acquisition through mother–infant interaction. *Connection Science, 15*, 245–258.

Zehel, Z., Shelton, R. L., Arndt, W. B., Wright, V., & Elbert, M. (1972). Item context and /s/ phone articulation test results. *Journal of Speech and Hearing Research, 15*, 852–860.

Zimmerman, I., Steiner, V., & Evatt-Pond, R. (2012a). *Preschool language scale–Spanish* (5th ed.). San Antonio, TX: Psychological Corporation.

Zimmerman, I., Steiner, V., & Evatt-Pond, R. (2012b). *Preschool language scale–Spanish screening test* (5th ed.). San Antonio, TX: Psychological Corporation.

Zuniga, M. E. (1992). Families with Latino roots. In E. W. Lynch & M. J. Hanson (Eds.), *Developing cross-cultural competence*. Baltimore: Brookes.

In this index, the following abbreviations are used: *b* for text box, *f* for figure, and *t* for table.

Laryngeal nodes, 102, 123
Laryngeal structures, 23–24, 24f
Laryngeal vibration, 358
Larynx, 28f, 37, 37f
Lateral sulcus, 37, 37f, 38f
Latino children. *See also* Spanish language and dialects; Spanish-speaking children, 231–237
Learned versus innate behavior. *See also* hypothesis of discontinuity; universal grammar (UG), 105, 109–110, 129–130, 193–197, 198–206
Learning. *See* speech sound learning (SSL)
Learning disorders, 318
Let's Give It a Smile, 371
Let's Paste Spots on the Dalmatian, 371
LG. *See* liquid gliding (LG)
LI. *See* language disorders and language impairments (LI)
Ligature, 86
Linear phonological error pattern analysis, 282–284
Linear phonological theories (LPTs). *See also* distinctive features theory; natural phonological theory, 4, 8, 9, 108–113, 419
Ling system, 394
Lingua-alveolars. *See also* coronal place nodes
    acoustical qualities of, 68
    depalatalization and, 96
    overview of, 78
    in SSL, 149, 159, 166–167, 176
    stops and, 74
    substitution patterns and, 94
Linguadentals, 78
Linguapalatals, 78
Linguavelars. *See also* dorsal place nodes; velar assimilation; velar fronting (VF), 68, 78, 103, 120, 149, 159, 168
Linguistic decoder, 195–196
Linguistic rules, 132
Linguistic theories of SSL, 197–201
Linking, 103
Lip rounding, 85
Lips. *See also* cleft lip and palate, 28f, 29, 37, 37f, 176

Liquid deviations, 171, 172
Liquid gliding (LG). *See also* error patterns; phonological patterns (PP), 97, 117, 170, 172
Liquid nasalizations, 235
*LIQUIDS, 117, 121
Liquids. *See also* liquid gliding (LG)
    acoustical qualities of, 68
    age of mastery of, 168
    anatomy and physiology for, 68
    in cluster deletions and substitutions, 93, 94
    distinctive features of, 83
    markedness constraints and, 116, 117
    overview of, 77
    place of articulation in, 78
    in SSL, 142, 166, 168, 191
    vocalization and, 97–98
    vulnerability to, 297
Liquid simplifications, 232, 235
Lisps, 188, 297
Literacy-based approach. *See* phonological awareness intervention (PAI)
Literacy instruction, 458–459, 460–461
Literacy skills
    articulation disorders and, 185
    in developmental dysarthria, 389
    hearing impairments and, 328
    phonological awareness and, 454, 455, 457, 459, 462, 463, 464, 467
    print awareness, 456
Longitudinal methods of research, 157–159
Lower motor neurons, 48
LPTs. *See* linear phonological theories (LPTs)
Lungs, 20, 20f, 23

M

MAE. *See* Mainstream American English (MAE)
Magnetic resonance imaging, 271
Mainstream American English (MAE)
    AAE versus, 213, 214t, 216t, 218, 219, 221–222
    Native American languages versus, 228
    overview of, 208, 210

ABOUT THE AUTHORS

Adriana Peña-Brooks holds a master's degree in speech–language pathology from California State University–Fresno. She also holds a Certificate of Clinical Competence from the American Speech-Language-Hearing Association, licenses in speech–language pathology from the states of California and Arizona, and the Clinical Rehabilitation Services Credential from the state of California. She has previously worked as an instructor and clinical supervisor in the Department of Communicative Sciences and Disorders at California State University–Fresno. Subsequently, she has worked as a speech–language pathologist in a variety of clinical settings, with the majority of her experience in the public schools. Over the years, she has gained clinical expertise in assessing and treating a variety of communication disorders in children of varying ethnocultural backgrounds, and, throughout her career, she has assessed and treated hundreds of children with speech sound disorders. She has also worked extensively with adults who have neurogenic communication disorders. She has made various scholarly presentations at the local, state, and national levels. She is co-author of *Treatment Protocols for Articulation and Phonological Disorders* and *Articulation and Phonological Disorders: Assessment and Treatment Resource Manual*. She is a bilingual and bicultural speech–language pathologist who speaks, reads, and writes fluently in Spanish. Currently, she lives in Sahuarita, Arizona, balancing her time between raising her triplets, practicing in the public schools, and devoting her time to scholarly writing in speech–language pathology.

M. N. (Giri) Hegde, PhD, is professor emeritus of communication sciences and disorders at California State University–Fresno. He holds a master's degree in experimental psychology from the University of Mysore, India, a post-master's diploma in medical (clinical) psychology from Bangalore University, India, and a doctoral degree in speech–language pathology from Southern Illinois University at Carbondale. He is a specialist in fluency disorders, language disorders, research methods, and treatment procedures in communicative disorders. He has published many research articles on language and fluency disorders and has made numerous presentations to national and international audiences on various basic and applied topics in communicative disorders and experimental and applied behavior analysis. With his deep and wide scholarship, he has authored several highly regarded and widely used scientific and professional books, including *Treatment Procedures in Communicative Disorders, Clinical Research in Communicative Disorders, Introduction to Communicative Disorders, A Coursebook on Aphasia and Other Neurogenic Language Disorders, Assessment and Treatment of Language Disorders in Children, Clinical Methods and Practicum in Speech–Language Pathology, Treatment Protocols for Language Disorders in Children, A Coursebook on*

Scientific and Professional Writing in Speech–Language Pathology, A Coursebook on Language Disorders in Children, Hegde's PocketGuide to Treatment in Speech–Language Pathology, and *Hegde's PocketGuide to Assessment in Speech–Language Pathology.* He also has served on the editorial boards of scientific and professional journals and continues to serve as an editorial consultant to the *Journal of Fluency Disorders.*

Dr. Hegde is a recipient of various honors, including the Outstanding Professor Award from California State University–Fresno, CSU–Fresno Provost's Recognition for Outstanding Scholarship and Publication, a Distinguished Alumnus Award from the Southern Illinois University Department of Communication Sciences and Disorders, and an Outstanding Professional Achievement Award from District 5 of the California Speech-Language-Hearing Association. He is also a Fellow of the American Speech-Language-Hearing Association.